T0294831

SOFT TISSUE AUGMENTATION

PROCEDURES IN COSMETIC DERMATOLOGY

Procedures in Cosmetic Dermatology
Series Editors: Jeffrey S. Dover MD, FRCPC and Murad Alam MD, MSCI, MBA

Recently published volumes:

2023
Hair Restoration
First edition
Jeffrey S. Dover, MD, FRCPC and Murad Alam, MD, MSCI, MBA
ISBN 978-0-323-82921-2

2023
Botulinum Toxin
Fifth Edition
Alastair Carruthers, MA, BM, BCh, FRCPC, FRCP(Lon),
Jean Carruthers, MD, FRCS(C), FRC(Ophth),
Jeffrey S. Dover, MD, FRCPC,
Murad Alam, MD, MSCI, MBA, and Omer Ibrahim, MD
ISBN 978-0-323-83116-1

2023
Lasers, Lights, and Energy Devices
Fifth edition
Elizabeth L. Tanzi, MD, FAAD, Jeffrey S. Dover, MD, FRCPC, and Leah K. Spring, DO, FAAD
ISBN 978-0-323-82905-2

2020
Chemical Peels
Third edition
Suzan Obagi, MD
ISBN 978-0-323-65389-3

2017
Botulinum Toxin
Fourth edition
Alastair Carruthers, MA, BM, BCh, FRCPC, FRCP(Lon) and
Jean Carruthers MD, FRCS(C), FRC(Ophth)
ISBN 978-0-323-47659-1

2017
Soft Tissue Augmentation
Fourth edition
Jean Carruthers MD, FRCS(C), FRC(Ophth),
Alastair Carruthers, MA, BM, BCh, FRCPC, FRCP(Lon),
Jeffrey S. Dover, MD, FRCPC and Murad Alam, MD, MSCI, MBA
ISBN 978-0-323-47658-4

Forthcoming volumes:

2023
Advanced Lifting
First edition
Hooman Khorasani, MD and Eyal Levit, MD
ISBN 978-0-323-67326-6

2023
Cosmetic Procedures in Skin of Color
First edition
Andrew F. Alexis, MD, MPH
ISBN 978-0-323-83144-4

2024
Photodynamic Therapy
Third edition
Macrene Alexiades, MD, PhD
ISBN 978-0-443-10689-7

2024
Cosmeceuticals
Fourth edition
Zoe Diana Draelos, MD
ISBN 978-0-443-11808-1

PROCEDURES IN COSMETIC DERMATOLOGY

SOFT TISSUE AUGMENTATION

FIFTH EDITION

Edited by

Jean Carruthers, MD, FRCS(C), FRC(Ophth)
Clinical Professor
Ophthalmology
University of British Columbia
Vancouver, British Columbia
Canada

Alastair Carruthers, MA, BM, BCh, FRCPC, FRCP(Lon)
Emerite Professor of Dermatology and Skin Science
University of British Columbia
Vancouver, British Columbia
Canada

Jeffrey S. Dover, MD, FRCPC
Director
SkinCare Physicians
Chestnut Hill, Massachusetts
United States
Associate Clinical Professor of Dermatology
Department of Dermatology
Yale University School of Medicine
New Haven, Connecticut
United States
Adjunct Associate Professor of Dermatology
Department of Dermatology
Brown Medical School
Providence, Rhode Island
United States

Murad Alam, MD, MSCI, MBA
Professor and Vice-Chair
Department of Dermatology
Feinberg School of Medicine, Northwestern University
Chicago, Illinois
United States
Professor
Departments of Surgery, Otolaryngology, and Medical Social Sciences
Feinberg School of Medicine, Northwestern University
Chicago, Illinois
United States

Video Editor

Omer Ibrahim, MD
Associate
Dermatology
Chicago Cosmetic Surgery and Dermatology
Chicago, Illinois
United States

Series Editors

Jeffrey S. Dover, MD, FRCPC and Murad Alam, MD, MSCI, MBA

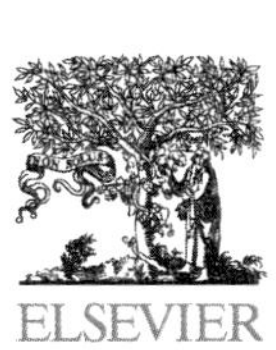

ELSEVIER

Elsevier
1600 John F. Kennedy Blvd.
Ste 1800
Philadelphia, PA 19103-2899

PROCEDURES IN COSMETIC DERMATOLOGY: SOFT TISSUE AUGMENTATION,
FIFTH EDITION ISBN: 978-0-323-83075-1

Notice

Practitioners and researchers must always rely on their own experience and knowledge in evaluating and using any information, methods, compounds or experiments described herein. Because of rapid advances in the medical sciences, in particular, independent verification of diagnoses and drug dosages should be made. To the fullest extent of the law, no responsibility is assumed by Elsevier, authors, editors or contributors for any injury and/or damage to persons or property as a matter of products liability, negligence or otherwise, or from any use or operation of any methods, products, instructions, or ideas contained in the material herein.

Previous editions copyrighted 2018, 2013, 2008 and 2005.

Content Strategist: Jessica L. McCool
Content Development Manager: Ranjana Sharma
Publishing Services Manager: Shereen Jameel
Project Manager: Gayathri S
Design Direction: Patrick C. Ferguson

Printed in India

Last digit is the print number: 9 8 7 6 5 4 3 2

CONTENTS

VIDEO CONTENTS

SERIES PREFACE

This new fifth edition of Procedures editions presents the increasing sophistication and scientific understanding of the effectiveness of all the new treatments developed by cosmetic dermatologic surgeons and their colleagues. Expert opinion has now been joined by data, mathematical significance, and fact. Scientific papers are judged on their level of evidence as well as how helpful they are in expanding our body of knowledge.

While many areas of the world are now dealing with aging populations, in North America the Millennials (B 1980–1995) have now overtaken the Boomers (B 1946–1964) as a proportion of the workforce and are increasingly interested in cosmetic treatments to delay and prevent the signs of aging. This new construct has been termed "Prejuvenation" (K. Arndt MD).

Never before has the cosmetic world been such a topic of fascination because of the attitudes of the Millennials in openly sharing their experiences over internet social platforms. If the Boomer generation felt that cosmetic treatments were an indulgence, Millennials feel that they are a normal part of personal wellness and healthcare.

The fifth edition of the Procedures in Cosmetic Dermatology series keeps you at the front edge of clinical knowledge and for those starting out in the field these texts quickly introduce you and bring you to the state of the art.

Our authors are leading dermatologists and cosmetic specialists in the field.

The general public view dermatologists as the experts in less invasive cosmetic procedures. A nationwide advanced fellowship program in cosmetic dermatologic surgery has been initiated to train the next generation of dermatologists to the highest standards.

Physicians need to be proficient in the latest methods for enhancing appearance and concealing the visible signs of aging.

To that end, we hope that you, our reader, find the books enjoyable and educational.

We thank our many contributors and wish you well on your journey of discovery.

Jeffrey S. Dover, MD, FRCPC and
Murad Alam, MD, MSCI, MBA

SERIES PREFACE FIRST EDITION

Although dermatologists have been procedurally inclined since the beginning of the specialty, particularly rapid change has occurred in the past quarter century. The advent of frozen section technique and the golden age of Mohs skin cancer surgery has led to the formal incorporation of surgery within the dermatology curriculum. More recently, technological breakthroughs in minimally invasive procedural dermatology have offered an aging population new options for improving the appearance of damaged skin.

Procedures for rejuvenating the skin and adjacent regions are actively sought by our patients. Significantly, dermatologists have pioneered devices, technologies, and medications, which have continued to evolve at a startling pace. Numerous major advances including virtually all cutaneous lasers and light-source-based procedures, botulinum exotoxin, soft tissue augmentation, dilute anesthesia liposuction, leg vein treatments, chemical peels, and hair transplants have been invented or developed and enhanced by dermatologists. Dermatologists understand procedures, and we have special insight into the structure, function, and working of skin. Cosmetic dermatologists have made rejuvenation accessible to risk-averse patients by emphasizing safety and reducing operative trauma. No specialty is better positioned than dermatology to lead the field of cutaneous surgery while meeting patient needs.

As dermatology grows as a specialty, an ever-increasing proportion of dermatologists will become proficient in the delivery of different procedures. Not all dermatologists will perform all procedures, and some will perform very few, but even the less procedurally directed among us must be well versed in the details to be able to guide and educate our patients. Whether you are a skilled dermatologic surgeon interested in further expanding your surgical repertoire, a complete surgical novice wishing to learn a few simple procedures, or somewhere in between, this book and this series are for you.

The volume you are holding is one of a series entitled "Procedures in Cosmetic Dermatology." The purpose of each book is to serve as a practical primer on a major topic area in procedural dermatology.

If you want to make sure you find the right book for your needs, you may wish to know what this book is and what it is not. It is not a comprehensive text grounded in theoretical underpinnings. It is not exhaustively referenced. It is not designed to be a completely unbiased review of the world's literature on the subject. At the same time, it is not an overview of cosmetic procedures that describes these in generalities without providing enough specific information to actually permit someone to perform the procedures. And importantly, it is not so heavy that it can serve as a doorstop or a shelf filler.

What this book and this series offer is a step-by-step, practical guide to performing cutaneous surgical procedures. Each volume in the series has been edited by a known authority in that subfield. Each editor has recruited other equally practical-minded, technically skilled, hands-on clinicians to write the constituent chapters. Most chapters have two authors to ensure that different approaches and a broad range of opinions are incorporated. On the other hand, the two authors and the editors also collectively provide a consistency of tone. A uniform template has been used within each chapter so that the reader will be easily able to navigate all the books in the series. Within every chapter, the authors succinctly tell it like they do it. The emphasis is on therapeutic technique; treatment methods are discussed with an eye to appropriate indications, adverse events, and unusual cases. Finally, this book is short and can be read in its entirety on a long plane ride. We believe that brevity paradoxically results in greater information transfer because cover-to-cover mastery is practicable.

We hope you enjoy this book and the rest of the books in the series and that you benefit from the many hours of clinical wisdom that have been distilled to produce it. Please keep it nearby, where you can reach for it when you need it.

Jeffrey S. Dover, MD, FRCPC and
Murad Alam, MD, MSCI
Year: 2005

PREFACE

"To improve is to change; to be perfect is to change often."

Winston Churchill

In this fifth edition of *Procedures in Cosmetic Dermatology*, everything indeed changed! This includes the development of new fillers, new understanding of safety and technique in the use of different cannulas and needles, new appreciation of the details of our evolving facial three-dimensional subcutaneous anatomy.

Diagnostic imaging with computed tomography (CT) scanning has shown bone remodeling of the facial skeleton starting about age 25 in women and 45 in men. Magnetic resonance imaging (MRI) scans have outlined the detailed anatomy of the facial fat pockets, which permit reflation techniques to be both exact and repeatable. Diagnostic Duplex ultrasonography has permitted visualization of the subcutaneous anatomy, including the all-important vasculature in its relationship to fat, bone, and the filler that has been injected.

Studies of patient-reported outcomes show that combination treatments (fillers plus neuromodulators and energy-based devices) not only give improved results but also improved patient satisfaction and retention.

An appreciation of the similarities and differences in treating facial skin in all Fitzpatrick and Glogau skin types allows culturally appropriate rejuvenation.

The concept of filler erasability has further elevated the popularity of hyaluronic acid (HA) fillers, and hyaluronidase is now in every office.

Longer-lasting semipermanent and permanent fillers also have their place in our therapeutic armamentarium. The calcium hydroxylapatite fillers, poly-L-lactic acid, liquid injectable silicone, and polymethylmethacrylate (PMMA) in bovine collagen suspension are all approved for facial augmentation, and we expect more classes of fillers to become available.

Finally, we turn to the most important concept of all: the feelings of our patients! The admixture of local anesthetic with fillers has indeed allowed many more patients to avail themselves of this successful cosmetic treatment.

The modern filler world has continued to advance rapidly. We hope that you enjoy this changed world as much as we do.

Jean Carruthers, MD, FRCS(C), FRC(Ophth)
Alastair Carruthers, MA, BM, BCh, FRCPC, FRCP(Lon)
Jeffrey S. Dover, MD, FRCPC
Murad Alam, MD, MSCI, MBA

CONTRIBUTORS

Murad Alam, MD, MSCI, MBA
Professor and Vice-Chair
Department of Dermatology
Feinberg School of Medicine
Northwestern University;
Professor
Departments of Surgery, Otolaryngology, and Medical Social Sciences
Feinberg School of Medicine, Northwestern University
Chicago, Illinois
United States

Andrew F. Alexis, MD, MPH
Vice-Chair
Dermatology
Weill Cornell Medicine;
Professor
Clinical Dermatology
Weill Cornell Medical College
New York, New York
United States

Raúl Alberto Banegas, MD
Director
Plastic Surgery
Centro Arenales, Buenos Aires
Argentina

Paola Barriera, MD
Dermatologist
Department of Dermatology
Cleveland Clinic Foundation
Cleveland, Ohio
United States

Katie Beleznay, MD, FRCPC
Dermatologist
Humphrey and Beleznay Cosmetic Dermatology;
Clinical Instructor
Department of Dermatology and Skin Science
University of British Columbia
Vancouver, British Columbia
Canada

Vince Bertucci, MD, FRCPC, FAAD
Founder & Medical Director
Bertucci Dermatology
Woodbridge, Ontario;
Instructor
Division of Dermatology
University of Toronto
Toronto, Ontario
Canada

Lauren Meshkov Bonati, MD
Dermatologic Surgeon
Cosmetic, Laser, and Mohs Surgery
Mountain Dermatology Specialists
Edwards, Colorado
United States

André Vieira Braz, MD
Clínica Dr Andre Braz
Rio de Janeiro, Brazil

Harold Brody, MD
Clinical Professor
Dermatology
Emory University School of Medicine
Atlanta, Georgia
United States

Adam K. Brys, MD
Dermatology Associates of Concord
Concord, Massachusetts
United States

Kimberly Butterwick, MD
Cosmetic Laser Dermatology
San Diego, California
United States

Alastair Carruthers, MA, BM, BCh, FRCPC, FRCP(Lon)
Emeritus Professor of Dermatology and Skin Science
University of British Columbia
Vancouver, British Columbia
Canada

Jean Carruthers, MD, FRCS(C), FRC(Ophth)
Clinical Professor
Ophthalmology
University of British Columbia
Vancouver, British Columbia
Canada

Annie Chiu, MD, FAAD
Director
Dermatology
The Derm Institute
Redondo Beach, California
United States

Sue Ellen Cox, MD
Founder and Medical Director
Dermatology
Aesthetic Solutions;
Affiliate Clinical Faculty
Department of Dermatology
Duke University;
Affiliate Clinical Faculty
Department of Dermatology
University of North Carolina
Chapel Hill, North Carolina
United States

Lauren Duffey Crow, MD, MPH
Resident in Dermatology
University of Pittsburgh Medical Center
Pittsburgh, Pennsylvania
United States

Luciana de Abreu, MD, MSc
Dermatologist
Private Practice
Rio de Janeiro, Brazil

Inayaguassu Moura de Lavôr, MD
Dermatologist
Dermatology
Private Practice
São Paulo, Brazil

Shraddha Desai, MD, FAAD
Clinical Instructor
Dermatology
Rush University
Chicago, Illinois;
Adjunct Clinical Professor
Dermatology
Loyola University
Maywood, Illinois;
Director
Dermatologic Cosmetic & Laser Surgery
Duly Health and Care
Naperville, Illinois
United States

Jeffrey S. Dover, MD, FRCPC
Director
SkinCare Physicians, Chestnut Hill, Massachusetts;
Associate Clinical Professor of Dermatology
Department of Dermatology
Yale University School of Medicine
New Haven, Connecticut;
Adjunct Associate Professor of Dermatology
Department of Dermatology
Brown Medical School
Providence, Rhode Island
United States

Karen Dover, MD
Physician, CEO & President
Dr Karen J Dover Laser and Cosmetic Medicine and Surgery
Ottawa, Ontario
Canada

Sabrina Fabi, MD
Volunteer Assistant Clinical Professor
Dermatology
University of California San Diego;
Associate
Dermatology
Cosmetic Laser Dermatology
San Diego, California
United States

Rebecca Fitzgerald, MD
Dermatology/Private Practice
Los Angeles, California
United States

Conor J. Gallagher, PhD
Vice President
Medical Affairs and Scientific Innovation
Revance Therapeutics Inc.,
Nashville, Tennessee
United States

Marguerite Germain, MD
Founder
Germain Dermatology
Mt Pleasant, South Carolina
United States

Katherine Given, MD, PhD, MBA, FAAD
Dermatologic Surgeon
Palo Alto Foundation Medical Group
Mountain View, California;
Clinical Instructor
University of California, San Francisco
Department of Dermatology
San Francisco, California
United States

David J. Goldberg, MD, JD
Cosmetic Dermatology and Clinical Research
Schweiger Dermatology Group;
Clinical Professor of Dermatology
Former Director of Mohs Surgery and Laser Research
Icahn School of Medicine;
Adjunct Professor of Law
Fordham Law School
New York, New York
United States

Courtney Gwinn, MD
Dermatologist
Chestnut Hill, Massachusetts
United States

Adele Haimovic, MD
Dermatologist
The Ronald O. Perelman Department of Dermatology
NYU Langone Health
New York, New York
United States

Kerry Heitmiller, MD, FAAD
Dermatology
Private Practice
Allura Skin & Laser Center
San Mateo, California
United States

Sara Hogan, MD
Assistant Health Sciences Clinical Professor
Dermatology
UCLA David Geffen School of Medicine
Los Angeles, California
United States

Shannon Humphrey, MD, FRPC
Clinical Associate Professor
Department of Dermatology and Skin Science
University of British Columbia;
Humphrey & Beleznay Cosmetic Dermatology
Vancouver, British Columbia
Canada

Omer Ibrahim, MD
Associate
Dermatology
Chicago Cosmetic Surgery and Dermatology
Chicago, Illinois
United States

Derek Jones, MD
Founder and Medical Director
Skin Care and Laser Physicians of Beverly Hills
Los Angeles, California
United States

Rohit Kakar, MD
Dermatologist
Bloomfield Hills, Michigan
United States

Joely Kaufman, MD
Director
Dermatology
Skin Associates of South Florida
Coral Gables, Florida
United States

Nisrine Kawa, MD, MPH
Resident physician
Yale New Haven Health
Waterbury Hospital
Waterbury, Connecticut
United States

Emily Keller, MD
IndyDerm
Greenwood, Indiana
United States

Femida Kherani, MD, FRCSC DiplABO
Clinical Associate Professor
Department of Ophthalmology & Visual Sciences
University of British Columbia
Vancouver, British Columbia
Canada

Shilpi Khetarpal, MD
Assistant Professor of Dermatology
Dermatology
Cleveland Clinic Foundation
Cleveland, Ohio
United States

David Kim, MD, MS
Dermatologist
Idriss Dermatology
New York, New York
United States

Karen Kim, MD
SkinCare Physicians
Chestnut Hill, Massachusetts
United States

Elizabeth Kream, MD
Dermatology
Cosmetic and Laser Surgery Fellow
New York, New York
United States

Steven Krueger, MD
Micrographic Surgery & Dermatologic Oncology Fellow
University of Massachusetts Medical School
Worcester, Massachusetts
United States

Val Lambros, MD
Private Practice Plastic Surgery
Newport Beach, California
United States

Margo Lederhandler, BA, MD
Dermatologist and Dermatologic Surgeon
Private Practice;
Assistant Professor of Clinical Dermatology
Department of Dermatology
Weill Cornell Medicine
New York, New York
United States

Kachiu C. Lee, MD, MPH
Dermatologist
Main Line Center for Laser Surgery
Ardmore, Pennsylvania
United States

Ming Lee, MD, FAAD
Dermatologist and Dermatologic Surgeon
The Gainesville Skin Cancer Center
Gainesville, Florida;
Dermatology Fellow
Department of Dermatology
Feinberg School of Medicine, Northwestern University
Chicago, Illinois
United States

Nicole Y. Lee, MD, MPH, FAAD
Dermatology
Wesson Dermatology
Great Neck, New York
United States

Steven Liew, MBBS, FRACS
Plasticsurgery
Shape Clinic
Sydney, New South Wales
Australia

Bassel H. Mahmoud, MD, PhD, FAAD
Associate Professor
Dermatology
University of Massachusetts
Worcester, Massachusetts
United States

Kavita Mariwalla, MD, FAAD
Director
Mariwalla Dermatology
West Islip, New York
United States

Rachel Miest, MD
Pariser Dermatology Specialists
Chesapeake, Virginia
United States

Ardalan Minokadeh, MD, PhD
Dermatologist
Skin Care and Laser Physicians of Beverly Hills
Los Angeles, California
United States

Gary D. Monheit, MD
Private Practice
Total Skin and Beauty Dermatology;
Clinical Professor
Department of Dermatology and Ophthalmology
University of Alabama at Birmingham
Birmingham, Alabama
United States

Laurel M. Morton, MD
Physician
Dermatology
SkinCare Physicians
Chestnut Hill, Massachusetts
United States

Farah Moustafa, MD, FAAD
Assistant Professor,
Director of Laser & Cosmetics
Dermatology
Tufts University School of Medicine
Boston, Massachusetts
United States

Diane K. Murphy, MBA
Consultant
Santa Barbara, California
United States

Rhoda S. Narins, MD, FAAD
Private Practice;
Director of Cosmetic Dermatology, PC
Clinical Professor of Dermatology
Ronald O. Perelman Department of Dermatology
New York University
New York, United States

David M. Ozog, MD
Chair
Department of Dermatology
Henry Ford Health
Detroit, Michigan
United States

Heidi B. Prather, MD, FAAD, FASDS
Cosmetic and Procedural Dermatologist
Westlake Dermatology
Austin, Texas
United States

Rachel Pritzker, MD, FAAD
Dermatologist
Chicago Cosmetic Surgery and Dermatology
Chicago, Illinois
United States

Saleh Rachidi, MD, PhD
Skin Laser and Surgery Specialists
New York, New York
United States

Kent Remington, MD
Remington Laser Dermatology Centre
Calgary, Alberta
Canada

Berthold Rzany, MD, ScM
Medizin am Hauptbahnhof
Wahlarztzentrum für Dermatologie & Venerologie
Wien, Austria

Mona Sadeghpour, MD
Dermatologist
SkinMed Institute
Lone Tree, Colorado
United States

Neil S. Sadick, MD, FACP, FAACS, FACPh, FAAD
Clinical Professor
Department of Dermatology
Cornell University Medical College
University of Minnesota
Minneapolis, Minnesota
United States

Nazanin Saedi, MD
Dermatologist
Dermatology Associates of Plymouth Meeting
Clinical Associate Professor of Dermatology
Thomas Jefferson University
Plymouth Meeting, Pennsylvania
United States

Matthew Sandre, HBMSc, BScN, MD
Dermatologist
Sunnybrook Health Sciences Centre;
Division of Dermatology
University of Toronto
Toronto, Ontario
Canada

Nowell Solish, MD FRCP
Associate Professor
Dermatology
University of Toronto
Toronto, Ontario
Canada

Nada Soueidan, MD
Dermatologist and Medical Director
Nu Yu Medical Center
Beirut, Lebanon;
Doha, Qatar;
Oujda, Morocco

Kathleen Suozzi, MD
Associate Professor
Department of Dermatology
Yale School of Medicine;
Director, Aesthetic Dermatology
Dermatology
Yale School of Medicine
New Haven, Connecticut
United States

Allison Sutton, MD, FRCPC
Founder and Medical Director
West Dermatology;
Clinical Instructor
Department of Dermatology and Skin Science
University of British Columbia
Vancouver, British Columbia
Canada

Ada Regina Trindade de Almeida, MD
Hospital do Servidor Publico Municipal de São Paulo
São Paulo- SP
Brazil

Neelam Vashi, MD
Boston University Cosmetic and Laser Center
Boston, Massachusetts
United States

Michelle Vy, MD
Department of Dermatology
University of California
Davis Medical Center
Sacramento, California
United States

Heidi A. Waldorf, MD
President
Waldorf Dermatology Aesthetics
Nanuet, New York
United States

Susan Weinkle, MD
Affiliate Clinical Professor
Department of Dermatology
University of South Florida
Tampa, Florida
United States

Britney N. Wilson, MD, MSc
Massachusetts General Hospital
Boston, Massachusetts
United States

Woffles T.L. Wu, MBBS, FRCSE, FAMS
Medical Director
Woffles Wu Aesthetic Surgery and Laser Centre
Singapore, Singapore

Daniel Yanes, MD
Dermatologist
MI Skin Dermatology
Washington, District of Columbia
United States

First, and most importantly, we dedicate this volume to our sons and their families. Our sons were young when the botulinum toxin story began and they have regarded the efforts of their parents to cope with this accidental discovery with tolerance and increasing pride over the years. We appreciate the support and encouragement they have given us. The love they have given us means we are indeed fortunate.

We have been fortunate to have an amazing series of mentors during our careers, Alan Scott and Barrie Jay for Jean and Ted Tromovitch, Sam Stegman, Rick Glogau, and Stuart Maddin for us both. The interest and imagination stirred by these individuals have been crucial.

Finally, we have been fortunate to work with outstanding people over the years in our various offices, as well as at the American Society for Dermatologic Surgery. They have all been a part of our story and have helped to create our careers and, hence, the volume that you are holding. Thanks to all of them!

Jean Carruthers MD, FRCS(C), FRC(Ophth) and
Alastair Carruthers, MA, BM, BCh, FRCPC, FRCP(Lon)

To my mentor Kenneth A. Arndt, a true scholar whose inquisitiveness, curiosity and enthusiasm, support, and friendship have guided me through my career.

To my father, Mark—a great teacher, listener, and role model.

And especially to my wife, Tania, for her never-ending encouragement, patience, support, love, and friendship and for being my moral compass.

Jeffrey S. Dover, MD, FRCPC

1

Introduction

Jean Carruthers and Alastair Carruthers

SUMMARY AND KEY FEATURES

- Knowledge of the subcutaneous neurovascular, bony, and muscular anatomy of each region of the face, along with an understanding of the exterior landmarks, is increasingly becoming important. An understanding of the aesthetic desires of each subject and careful targeted volumization is the key to aesthetic success with facial fillers.
- Understanding the different regional concepts of beauty and the use of validated assessment scales have aided in achieving optimal outcomes.
- Reversers and better pain management have enhanced augmentation procedures. Better understanding of anatomy and improved injection techniques may reduce, but have so far not eliminated, vascular occlusion complications.
- Three-dimensional fillers are now seen as stimulators of cutaneous neocollagenesis, thus improving the texture of facial skin from the "inside."

In 1885, two extremely powerful European figures, Kaiser Wilhelm and Chancellor Bismarck, decided to announce the new age of retirement, age 65 years. At that time, the median age in the population was 16 years. Nowadays, it is 29.6.

In addition, adults are currently working longer and living better and are much more educated about the ways to live a healthy lifestyle.

The new world of noninvasive rejuvenation is perfectly timed to assist all age groups to recover and maintain their youthful and empowered appearance.

In the American Society for Dermatologic Surgery (ASDS) Consumer Survey on Cosmetic Dermatologic Procedures, of 7315 individuals surveyed, 5 of 10 were considering a cosmetic procedure for aesthetic indications not only in the face but also over the entire body. They wished to look as young as they felt, to appear more attractive, and to feel more confident.

In 2014, nearly half of all cosmetic patients in the United States requesting noninvasive or minimally invasive interventions received multiple cosmetic procedures at the same time. They are also most interested in procedures that give little or no downtime.

Synthetic fillers, such as hyaluronans, calcium hydroxylapatite, poly-L-lactic acid, and silicone, allow three-dimensional volumization without a prior harvesting procedure. Local tumescent anesthesia liposuction allows autologous fat to be used for volumization.

The anatomic structures of facial aging of bone, fat, and skin have been further studied by computed tomography (CT), magnetic resonance imaging (MRI) scans, duplex ultrasound, and detailed anatomic cadaver dissection, which have allowed us to visualize accurately the underlying age-related changes. A new descriptive language of age-related facial changes using facial scales has been published, demonstrating their value in improving communication not only with our patients in our clinics but also with each other as we work together toward better treatments.

Patient-reported outcomes (PROs) have become the standard for assessing treatment outcomes from the patient's point of view. Published validated questionnaires, such as the Facial Line Outcomes (FLO) and Self-Perception of Age (SPA), can be used as easily in the clinic as in the research setting. Several validated PROs are used both by patients and by the treating and evaluating physician—such as the Lip Fullness Scale (LFS) and Look and Feel of the Lips (LAF) scale, as well as the severity scales for Perioral Lines at Rest (POL), Perioral Lines at Maximum Contraction (POLM), and Oral Commissure Severity (OCS) and the Face-Q scales. The recognition that the patient's opinion is all important and must thus be recorded, studied, and understood is a gift of the field of aesthetic medicine.

Patients prefer their treatments to be as pain-free as possible. In the past decade, we have learned that educating our subjects dramatically reduces their anxiety, as does topical chilling with ice and topical anesthesia and "talkesthesia." Pain control for facial injections has largely evolved away from trigeminal nerve blocks, with the common addition of lidocaine to injected fillers. The addition of saline or lidocaine with epinephrine to dilute the filler decreases cohesiveness, allowing for smooth delivery, the ability to distribute the product evenly by gentle massage, and vasoconstriction for safety.

Whereas it is necessary to use needles for intradermal injection of filler, larger-diameter (25 G) blunt tipped cannulas have been shown to be safer than 27 G cannulas or needles. In addition, excellent work using duplex ultrasonography can show the blood vessels in the facial region to be injected and thus help prevent embolic vascular occlusion. The inherent variability of vascular patterns between individuals and between the two sides of the same individual makes this modern ultrasound "the eye under the skin." Duplex ultrasound can also be used to locate filler that requires removal by hyaluronidase injection and one can within minutes see the restoration of the normal vascular pattern.

Reversibility has also become a cornerstone of facial filler injections. Hyaluronidase is an enzyme that will catabolize any hyaluronic acid (HA) filler, usually within 24 hours. New classes of fillers may be produced with custom-made "erasers" in the future. Posttreatment bruising can now be treated immediately using intense pulsed light at moderate settings, which allows the bruise to be absorbed within 24 to 48 hours instead of 7 to 10 days. New topical formulations activate macrophages to phagocytose red blood cells and also reduce time to bruise recovery.

All subjects are aware that they will see an immediate filler effect with the desired new contour. They may not be aware of the neocollagenesis that occurs with the filler apparently stimulating the development of new collagen in the dermis, which will subsequently give a more reflectant glowing facial skin.

The past century has seen an explosion of development of new fillers and their global acceptance by a patient population that would rather look restored and younger without the trauma and downtime of surgery. Indeed, the introduction of noninvasive or minimally invasive injectable procedures represents a significant shift in the approach to facial rejuvenation. According to the website of the ASDS, filler injections in 2019 have increased by 78% since 2012. The recent addition of sophisticated ultrasound imaging has made it possible to inspect subcutaneous anatomy both during and after filler injections so that subcutaneous vascular anatomy is understood with respect to aesthetic filler boluses.

This trend is bound to continue, as with the "ZoomDysmorphia" in our current pandemic, 87% of patients are coming in because they are spending 5 to 10 hours a day on videoconferencing where they are looking constantly at their and their colleagues' faces. Safe volume restoration in the face and other body areas will continue to be very popular, particularly as part of a comprehensive multifaceted aesthetic treatment plan.

FURTHER READING

ASDS Consumer Survery (2021). Sourced 13 Sep 2022 (www.asds.net). 70 percent of 3527 consumers surveyed were considering a cosmetic procedure on face and or body.

ASDS survey on dermatologic procedures. http://mobile.twitter.com. Accessed 13 September 2022.

Carruthers, J., Burgess, C., Day, D., et al. (2016). Consensus recommendations for combined aesthetic interventions in the face using botulinum toxin, fillers, and energy-based devices. *Dermatol Surg*, *0*, 1–12.

Carruthers, A., Carruthers, J., Hardas, B., et al. (2008). A validated lip fullness rating scale. *Dermatol Surg*, *34*(suppl 2), S161–S166.

Carruthers, A., Carruthers, J., Hardas, B., et al. (2008). A validated marionette lines rating scale. *Dermatol Surg*, *34*(suppl 2), S167–S172.

Carruthers, A., Carruthers, J., Hardas, B., et al. (2008). A validated crow's feet rating scale. *Dermatol Surg*, *34*(suppl 2), S173–S178.

Carruthers, A., Carruthers, J., Hardas, B., et al. (2008). A validated hand grading rating scale. *Dermatol Surg*, *34*(suppl 2), S179–S183.

Carruthers, J., Carruthers, A., Monheit, G. D., Davis, P. G., & Tardie, G. (2011). Multicenter, randomized, parallel-group study of onabotulinumtoxin A and hyaluronic acid dermal fillers (24-mg/mL smooth, cohesive gel) alone and in combination for lower facial rejuvenation: satisfaction and patient-reported outcomes. *Dermatol Surg*, *36*(suppl 4), 2135–2145.

Carruthers, J., Flynn, T. C., Geister, T. L., et al. (2012). Validated assessment scales for the mid face. *Dermatol Surg*, *38*, 320–332.

Carruthers, J. D. A., Glogau, R., & Blizter, A. (2008). Facial Consensus Group Faculty. Advances in facial rejuvenation: botulinum toxin type A, hyaluronic acid dermal fillers, and combination therapies: consensus recommendations. *Plast Reconstr Surg*, *121*(suppl 5), S5–S30.

Fagien, S., & Carruthers, J. (2008). A comprehensive review of patient reported satisfaction with botulinum toxin type A for aesthetic procedures. *Plast Reconstr Surg*, *122*, 1915–1925.

Pavicic, T., Webb, K. L., Frank, K., Gotkin, R. H., Tamura, B., & Cotofana, S. (2019). Arterial wall penetration forces in needles versus cannulas. *Plast Reconstr Surg*, *143*, 504e.

Schelke, L. W., Decates, T. S., & Velthuis, P. J. (2018). Ultrasound to improve the safety of hyaluronic acid filler treatments. *J Cosmet Dermatol*, 1–6.

Wikipedia. Median age of the world's population. https://en.m.wikipedia.org. Accessed March 29, 2021.

2

Fillers: Paradigm Shifts Produce New Challenges

Omer Ibrahim

SUMMARY AND KEY FEATURES

- A shift in treatment concept to include "recreate" in addition to "rejuvenate."
- The increased demand for minimally invasive aesthetic procedures in lieu of surgery has inspired the injector to adapt, evolve, and flourish as an artist.
- Newer products are niche variations of existing hyaluronic acid technology, and their varieties continue to expand on the market.
- Volume replacement gives satisfying aesthetic improvement unachievable by other means.
- More robust fillers require deeper application.
- Deeper placement involves exposure to vascular communications with retinal artery and branches of carotid artery.
- Newer treatment areas (e.g., temples, jawline, and nose) predispose to inherently different risks and potential side effects.
- Intravascular injection or vascular compression from robust agents can cause catastrophic consequences.
- Risk factors include filler particle size, pressure generated, and speed of injection.
- Clinicians must be aware of psychosocial impact of filler injections, and not pander to unrealistic societal perceptions of beauty.

"Let me be very clear. I am extremely happy with who I am and how I look, but sometimes you need a change. There's nothing wrong with wanting a different look from time to time."

Female patient, age 36 years, seen in consultation for jawline enhancement

According to the American Society for Dermatologic Surgery (ASDS) annual survey, 1.6 million soft-tissue filler procedures were performed in 2019, an increase of 78% since 2012 (Fig. 2.1). This boom in filler injections is likely due to a combination of increased demand, a heightened sense of self-awareness and beauty perception, and an ever-growing armamentarium of a variety of fillers at the injector's disposal. The clinician can now rejuvenate signs of aging ranging from the finest of lines to deep hollows. In addition to reversing signs of aging, the injector is now entrusted with the task of reshaping features of the face and recreating structures not originally present, a demand becoming increasingly popular among the social media-savvy and recently financially independent younger patient demographic. In this chapter, we will discuss a brief history of the evolution of fillers, the shift in beauty trends, and the physical risks and social implications of newer, "in-demand" procedures.

By 2010 and onward, fillers were moving from treatment of static wrinkles in the two-dimensional plane to correcting the three-dimensional volume changes in the aging face. What started out as very small and arbitrary amounts of material (0.5- and 1.0-mL syringes of bovine collagen or occasional microdroplets of silicone) in

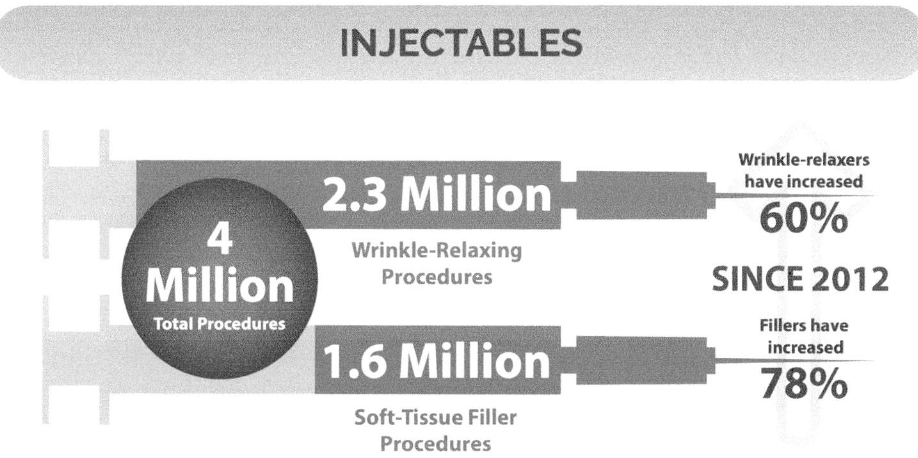

Fig. 2.1 Trends in injectable treatments between 2012 and 2019. (Courtesy of 2019 American Society for Dermatologic Surgery (ASDS) Survey on Dermatologic Procedures. http://asds.net/Procedures-Survey.)

the 1970s and an unblinking focus on the single line or small dermal acne scar suddenly blossomed into greater volumes of filler, especially with the introduction of hyaluronic acid (HA) gels. With the blockbuster aesthetic impact of botulinum toxin on the muscles of facial expression, the tools were at hand to address a second significant component of facial aging: the dramatic loss of subcutaneous and deep tissue volume associated with the aging face.

The single syringe of collagen commercially available for 25 years was completely inadequate to address the tasks at hand. The markets began to respond with a virtual flood of new filler products—HA gels, poly-L-lactic acid (PLLA), calcium hydroxylapatite (CaHA), and polymethylmethacrylate (PMMA). After 20 years of three fillers—collagen, silicone, and fat—the aesthetic market expanded in 5 years to more than 300 commercially available forms of injectable filler worldwide, with more coming every year.

The HA gels are now available in a variety of densities, with added lidocaine, and they constitute the lion's share of the filler market in North America at the present time. Although Restylane was the first HA filler product US Food and Drug Administration (FDA) approved to enter the US market, it was quickly followed by the Juvéderm family of fillers and has been joined by other injectable products of different compositions: Sculptra—a PLLA filler; Radiesse—a CaHA filler; Bellafill—a PMMA filler; and handful of other brands of HA gels of differing attributes.

As a result of the influx of new fillers, together with a heightened appreciation of the three-dimensional nature of volume loss in the aging face, there was a rapid increase in volume of material being injected into the deeper compartments of the face, frequently giving more significant and natural improvements to the aging face. Convex contours of the cheek in particular but also the temples, lips, tear troughs, were subtly restored to younger volumes in ways that traditional incisional surgery could not address. Whole new areas of application were suddenly available to the injector.

Homologous fat, which was a readily available by-product of liposuction techniques introduced in the early 1980s, was the only true volume injectable. Many liposuction surgeons tried various harvesting and processing techniques as they recycled the unwanted fat from abdomens and hips to various places on the face and body. However, for the most part, the results were inconsistently dependable and not long-lasting for the majority of patients and occasionally produced unwanted asymmetric outcomes. But the use of fat did increase further understanding of the nature and distribution of the subcutaneous fat compartments in the aging face. For example, noninvasive magnetic resonance imaging (MRI) and imaging techniques estimate the volume of the midface subcutaneous fat at somewhere between 13 and 17 mL per side—not a deficit likely to be repaired with a single syringe of any material!

HA fillers have become the dominant filler in the United States and global markets. They are stable at room temperature and available "off the shelf" and were manufactured in single preloaded syringes. They provide good reversibility with hyaluronidase, an important safety consideration. They provide more immediate "lift" than the collagen fillers that preceded them, have longer duration of action, and require no allergy skin testing prior to treatment. They are easily injected through small-gauge needles, 27 gauge and smaller. Because they are derived from bacteria, they do not share the problems of animal-derived proteins like collagen products.

The evolution of HA gel products has made some technologic improvements in the products. One approach has been to vary the concentration of the HA gel. Another is to vary the degree of cross-linking between the polymer chains, and another significant improvement was the addition of lidocaine for increased comfort of injection. Changes in density and cross-linking variously affect the rheology of the materials and can improve duration, lift, and ease of injection through small-gauge needles.

The challenge for the treating physician is to select the suitable agent and place it appropriately in the given anatomic location to produce the desired aesthetic result. In the 1970s and early 1980s when bovine collagen injections were in use, wrinkles were the aesthetic target, the placement was in the dermis, and the postinjection side effects were predictably local bruising at the site of injection. As the aesthetic range gradually included defects with some depth, like expression lines, vascular occlusions began to appear, particularly ischemic accidents in the supratrochlear vessels (from treatment of the glabellar lines), the angular branch of the facial artery (treatment of nasolabial folds), or the occlusion of the labial artery (lip augmentation).

These vascular accidents appeared to increase in number when the shift occurred from the original Zyderm collagen to Zyplast, a collagen product in which the collagen polymers were cross-linked to produce longer duration of effect. Zyplast was much more slippery than Zyderm, and injectors could inadvertently inject the entire syringe with one push on the plunger, potentially contributing to vascular accidents. Although debate swirled about the underlying cause of these occlusions (intravascular vs. extravascular compression, hemostatic effect of the collagen vs. mass effect of the bolus in the vessel), the nature of the phenomenon was that it was irreversible—nothing existed to dissolve the collagen, and it required the injection to occur below the dermis in the subcutaneous space, where the smaller arteries came close to the surface anatomy.

The evolution of use of the HA gel fillers followed the same process, although the dermal placement of these materials was certainly less common. Restylane, because of the particulate nature of the HA, produced a color shift known as the Tyndall effect when it was injected too superficially. However, it certainly did not take much time for the occlusive accidents to be seen with HA treatment of the glabellar creases, nasolabial folds at the base of the nose, and labial arteries, among others. The next evolutionary step was to use the HA fillers to go even deeper in the soft tissue to address true volume deficits: loss of premalar and malar fat, perioral volume loss, atrophy along the mandibular ridge, and loss of fat in the temples, forehead, and nose. As a result, the fillers on the market became more robust and versatile in nature, and the demand for not only rejuvenation but also recreation and reshaping exploded.

The advent of social media and the subsequent creation of photo editing and sharing platforms have undoubtedly shifted the public's perception of beauty. While some physical characteristics of beauty may remain constant across time and cultures, the emphasis on certain body parts or facial attributes has shifted. Nonsurgical rhinoplasties, chin augmentation, jawline refinement, and buttock augmentation are a few of the procedures that have been broadcasted on TV and social media platforms. Akin to adopting a new hairstyle at a salon, young patients are now pursuing tweaks in their features in order to achieve a "new look" (Figs. 2.2 and 2.3) In the seemingly blink of an eye, a celebrity can disappear and reemerge just a few days later with a sharper chin, a slimmer jawline, fuller lips, or an enhanced hourglass figure—gone are the days of paparazzi-sourced photos of celebrities wrapped in postsurgical bandages attempting to discreetly flee a medical facility. The exposure of minimally invasive enhancements on social media and the transparency by some celebrities have showcased to the public the versatility of fillers and demonstrated the range of possibilities of what can be done with the syringe in lieu of the scalpel. In turn, the filler industry responded: at least

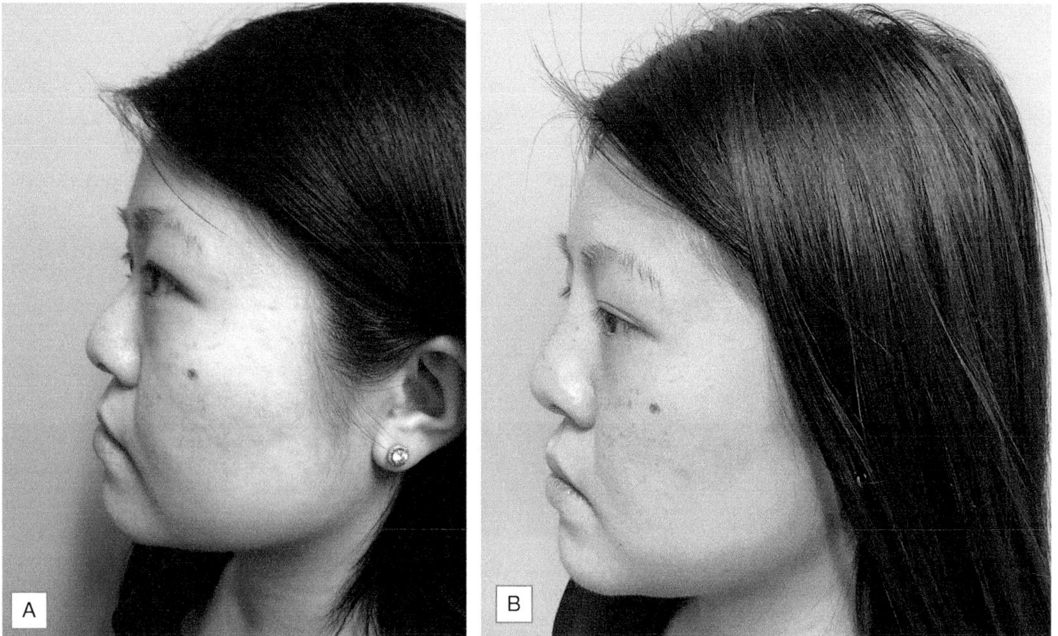

Fig. 2.2 Nasal reshaping using hyaluronic acid filler to increase bridge height and definition. (A) Prior to treatment. (B) Immediately after treatment. (Copyrights reserved by Omer Ibrahim, MD.)

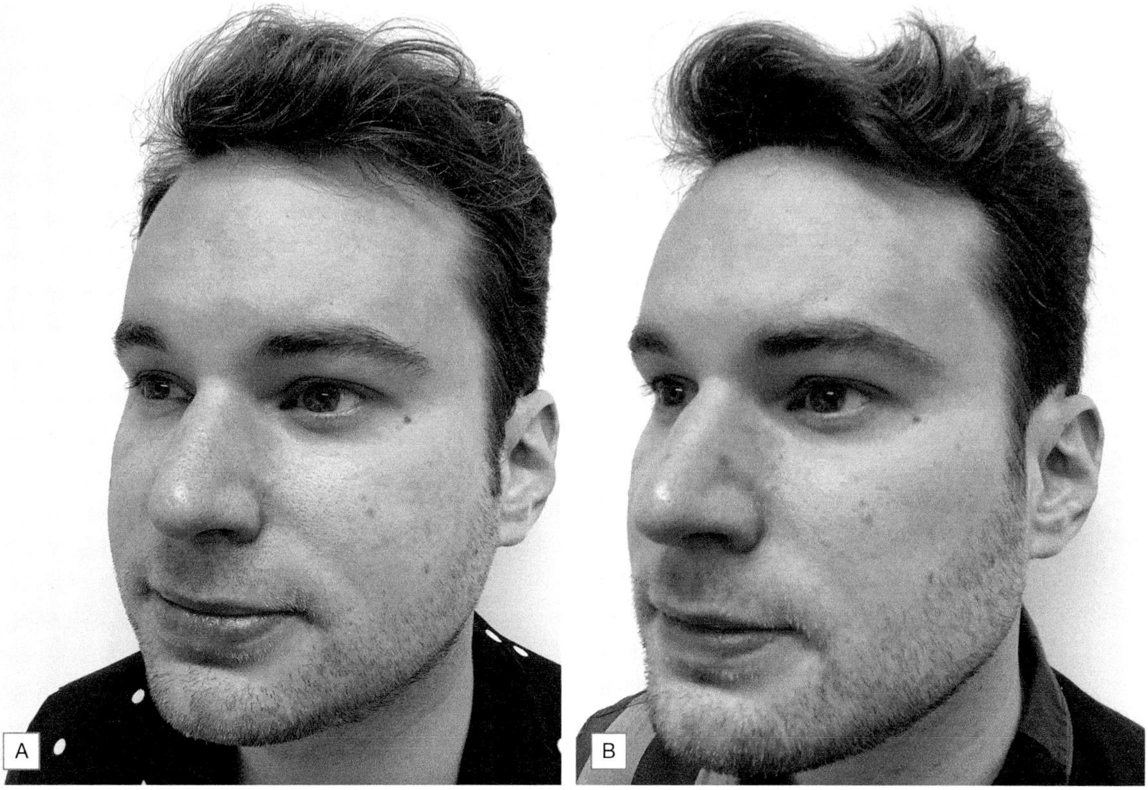

Fig. 2.3 Cheekbone and jawline treatment with hyaluronic acid filler in a young patient seeking a sharper, more "masculine" appearance. (A) Prior to treatment. (B) Two weeks after treatment. (Copyrights reserved by Omer Ibrahim, MD.)

two HA fillers (Voluma and Restylane Defyne) are now FDA approved for nonsurgical augmentation of the chin, and more are on the way. The role of contouring the lower face to achieve a freshly balanced profile has been solidified in the field. Now, the young millennial with newly acquired financial independence actively seeks rejuvenative as well as reimaginative procedures.

In order to address the demand for newer, en vogue procedures, the clinician must be aware of the physical risks and psychosocial implications of these treatments. Deeper placement of filler, especially in high-risk zones such as the nose, predisposes the injector to the risk of intravascular occlusion. Several superficial arteries of the facial vasculature are distal branches of the ophthalmic artery (supraorbital, supratrochlear, dorsal nasal, and angular artery of the nose) (Fig. 2.4). Intraarterial injection can lead to skin necrosis and even devastating ocular complications, including irreversible blindness. The danger is not limited to the arterial side of the circulation. In the temple area, a frequent site of unwanted atrophy and an aesthetic target for deep filler injections, the middle temporal vein (MTV) communicates with the cavernous sinus through the periorbital veins and the pulmonary artery via the internal jugular vein, requiring judicious placement of filler in the immediate periosteal space to avoid intravascular injection of the MTV and potential vision loss or pulmonary and cerebral embolism.

Unfortunately, only small amounts of filler are required to produce retrograde injection from the distal branches to the retinal artery, reportedly as little as 0.5 mL of material. Although, fortunately, these deep vascular complications with retrograde embolism are quite rare, they warrant a careful understanding of both the potentially problematic vasculature and available techniques to lessen the risk of the injections. The inextricable link between speed of injection and risk of side effect has been demonstrated in clinical trials. In addition,

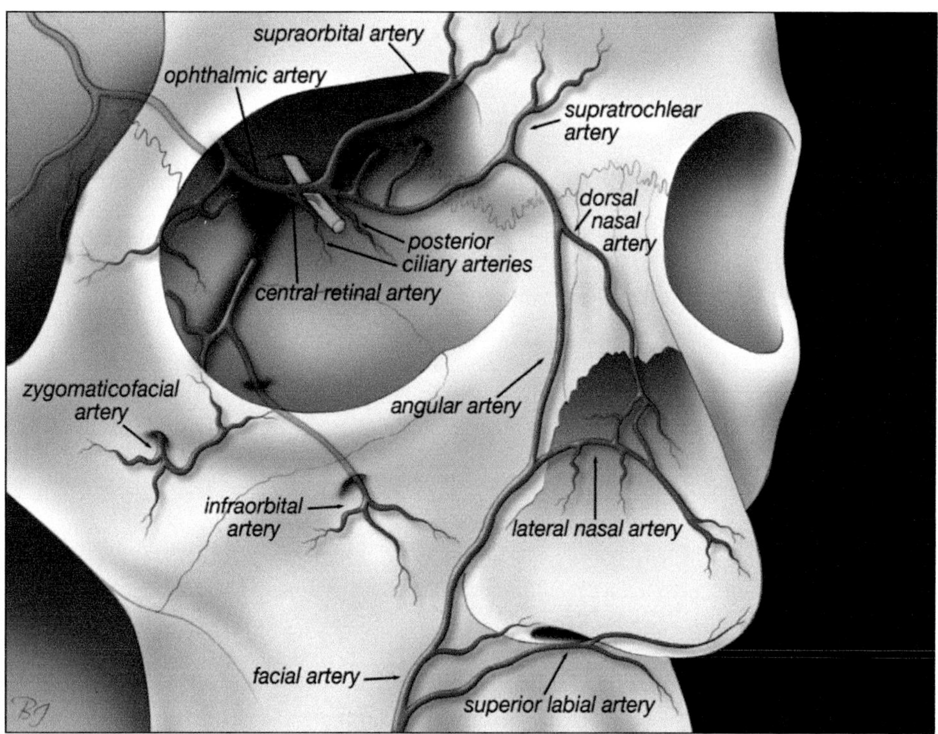

Fig. 2.4 The potential for retrograde communication and embolism to the central retinal artery can be traced to the facial artery, lateral nasal artery, dorsal nasal artery, infraorbital artery, zygomaticofacial artery, supratrochlear artery, supraorbital artery, and even the superior labial artery. (Reprinted from Lazzeri D, Agostini T, Figus M, Nardi M, Pantaloni M, Lazzeri S. Blindness following cosmetic injections of the face. *Plast Reconstr Surg*. 2012;129(4):995–1012. p 1006.)

suggestions have been made to use smaller syringes (reducing pressure), blunt cannulas (less chance of direct vessel cannulation), multiple small aliquots rather than large single amounts, aspiration before injection to confirm location of the needle tip, and moving the needle or cannula slightly while injecting to avoid intravascular puncture. When possible, consider injecting across the vessel's path rather than parallel to it to minimize intravascular injection.

Although vascular accidents have been reported with all manner of filler, fat clearly seems to run a higher risk, probably secondary to the higher pressures and larger particle sizes injected. Along with other permanent or semipermanent fillers, such as CaHA, PMMA, polylactic acid (PLA), and silicone, there is no chance of removing or dissolving the offending filler in case of vascular accident. HA gel fillers offer a chance to ameliorate some cases of vascular occlusion if the occlusion is in the superficial vasculature (e.g., glabellar ischemia, angular artery ischemia, or labial artery occlusion). In these cases, flooding the area with hyaluronidase and supportive care with aspirin and appropriate wound care may help minimize the damage.

However, if deeper vascular occlusion has occurred (vision changes, symptoms of stroke, etc.), time pressure is acute. Retinal ganglion cell death can occur in as early as 12 to 15 minutes. Emergency consultation with ophthalmology and neurology is required. Recovery of function is usually marginal at best. Use of hyaluronidase in the retro-orbital space may have theoretical benefit, but the use is not established.

In addition to the crucial need to be aware of the physical risks of filler injections, the unprecedented ubiquity of minimally invasive procedures on TVs, tablets, and phones has made the psychological and social impact of the injector even more powerful. Selfies and social media have been shown to increase patients' anxiety and dysmorphia and decrease their sense of self-worth, self-esteem, and confidence. These psychological factors can have devastating consequences such as self-harm and suicide. In this age of filters, photo editing, and unrealistic expectations set by some celebrities and influencers stands the clinician at a vital cusp: constantly teetering between elevating their practice and risking falling into pandering to impractical beauty ideals. The clinician must continuously evaluate and reevaluate the concerns of the patient and the source of those concerns, and ask: can I deliver an aesthetically pleasing, genuine result without feeding into unrealistic societal expectations and catering to an underlying dysmorphia? The line is blurry, but the responsibility to uphold ethical standards while providing patient education and delivering evidence-based treatment ultimately falls upon the clinician.

Despite the potential risks and psychosocial impacts of minimally invasive filler injections, the ever-growing breadth of fillers on the market, the changing patient demographic, and the evolving beauty trends have invigorated the aesthetic field. The injector can marry medicine, psychology, and art to rejuvenate, recreate, and reshape in unprecedented ways, and can do so safely and effectively with appropriate knowledge of risk, technique, and anatomy.

FURTHER READING

American Society for Dermatologic Surgery. (2021). *ASDS Survey on Dermatologic Procedures.* https://www.asds.net/medical-professionals/practice-resources/asds-survey-on-dermatologic-procedures.

Barrera, J. E., & Most, S. P. (2008). Volumetric imaging of the malar fat pad and implications for facial plastic surgery. *Arch Facial Plast Surg, 10*(2), 140–142.

Beleznay, K., Carruthers, J. D., Humphrey, S., & Jones, D. (2015). Avoiding and treating blindness from fillers: a review of the world literature. *Dermatol Surg, 41*(10), 1097–1117.

Chang, S. H., Yousefi, S., Qin, J., et al. (2016). External compression versus intravascular injection: a mechanistic animal model of filler-induced tissue ischemia. *Ophthal Plast Reconstr Surg, 32*, 261–266.

DeLorenzi, C. (2014). Complications of injectable fillers, part 2: vascular complications. *Aesthet Surg J, 34*(4), 584–600.

Fagien, S. (2016). Commentary on a rethink on hyaluronidase injection, intra-arterial injection and blindness. *Dermatol Surg, 42*(4), 549–552.

Glogau, R. G., & Kane, M. A. (2008). Effect of injection techniques on the rate of local adverse events in patients implanted with nonanimal hyaluronic acid gel dermal fillers. *Dermatol Surg, 34*(suppl 1), S105–S109.

Goodman, G. J., & Clague, M. D. (2016). A rethink on hyaluronidase injection, intraarterial injection, and blindness: is there another option for treatment of retinal artery embolism caused by intraarterial injection of hyaluronic acid? *Dermatol Surg, 42*(4), 547–549.

Harb, A., & Brewster, C. T. (2020). The nonsurgical rhinoplasty: a retrospective review of 5000 treatments. *Plast Reconstr Surg, 145*, 661–667.

Maymone, M. B. C., Laughter, M., Dover, J., & Vashi, N. A. (2019 Sep–Oct). The malleability of beauty: perceptual adaptation. *Clin Dermatol*, *37*(5), 592–596.

Perrett, D. I., May, K. A., & Yoshikawa, S. (1994). Facial shape and judgements of female attractiveness. *Nature*, *368*, 239–242.

Shome, D., Vadera, S., Male, S. R., & Kapoor, R. (2020). Does taking selfies lead to increased desire to undergo cosmetic surgery. *J Cosmet Dermatol*, *19*(8), 2025–2032.

Steinsapir, K. D. (2016). Treating filler related visual loss. *Dermatol Surg*, *42*(4), 552–554.

Tansatit, T., Apinuntrum, P., & Phetudom, T. (2015). An anatomical study of the middle temporal vein and the drainage vascular networks to assess the potential complications and the preventive maneuver during temporal augmentation using both anterograde and retrograde injections. *Aesthetic Plast Surg*, *39*(5), 791–799.

Tobalem, S., Schutz, J. S., & Chronopoulos, A. (2018). Central retinal artery occlusion—rethinking retinal survival time. *BMC Ophthalmol*, *18*(1), 101.

Wang, J. V., Rieder, E. A., Schoenberg, E., Zachary, C. B., & Saedi, N. (2020). Patient perception of beauty on social media: Professional and bioethical obligations in esthetics. *J Cosmet Dermatol*, *19*(5), 1129–1130.

3

Facial Beauty and the Central Role of Volume

Omer Ibrahim, Karen Kim, Neelam Vashi, and Karen Dover

SUMMARY AND KEY FEATURES

- Attractiveness appreciation is an innate human skill involving all the senses.
- Volume is important in many of the indicators of youth, maturity, attractiveness, symmetry, and gender differentiation.
- Bone and dentition resorb with age.
- Most major retaining ligaments induce deep facial grooves, as the face cascades forward and rotates inward with age.
- Facial fat compartments have deep and superficial elements, with the deeper ones particularly prone to atrophy and migration with aging.
- The use of soft tissue fillers can aid in combating these changes and facilitate a more graceful aging process.

INTRODUCTION

The quest for beauty is eternal, a phenomenon as old as time itself. It is universal, it knows no limits, it transcends all boundaries and borders, and it is essential to our existence, both as individuals and as a species. Since time immemorial, humans have relentlessly cultivated beauty in their physical surroundings, coveted it in their partners, sought it in their peers, and strived for it within themselves. Although certain beauty ideals have gone in and out of style over time, and some may have shown variations across cultures, the fundamentals have remained constant. Facial beauty is defined by certain tenets: symmetry, balance, harmony, synchrony of elements, homogeneity of color and texture, and smooth contours. An extremely important feature of restoration, enhancement or maintenance of facial beauty is judicious and strategic placement of volume, as it is responsible for achieving many of the desirable attributes. With a multitude of soft-tissue fillers, the clinician has an extensive armamentarium to address age-related changes in facial volume and hence modify patients' self-perception, self-esteem, and overall interaction with their external world. Central to this role is a deep understanding of beauty, as there is little doubt that it is beauty that we are ultimately seeking. To successfully manage patients and their aesthetic concerns, we must start by establishing why beauty exists, why its attainment is so important to our patients, how it evolves over time, and how best to address those predictable changes.

THE VERY EXISTENCE OF BEAUTY

The pursuit of beauty is an innate drive linked to survival itself. Connection is one of the most primal of human needs. We are programmed to communicate with one another and to bond from birth, and these tendencies are honed as life proceeds. We learn to modify our appearance and behavior very early in life to enhance positive human engagements, thus maximizing our survival tendencies. A child, at its youngest, understands that charm and attractiveness will beget nurturing connections, ones that are rewarded with love, food, protection, safety, and security. By recognizing what is good and bad around us in terms of beauty or ugliness, we are likely to choose good (or beautiful) and avoid bad or harmful (ugly). Many different professions have studied attractiveness and beauty—psychologists, neuroscientists, biologists, human behaviorists, anthropologists, dentists and orthodontists, dermatologists and surgeons, as well as other specialties—all approaching this topic from their unique perspectives. With the prospect for a more fulfilling life, enhanced purely by its presence or absence, beauty clearly has an important function.

PEARL 1 Attractiveness appreciation is an innate human skill involving all the senses, with predominance of the visual sense.

Given that our visual sense is such a dominant force, it is no surprise that our appreciation of facial appearance is rapid and efficient. Humans have profound needs to connect with one another and to belong and conform within a larger group. These needs manifest throughout all of life's stages, from early infancy to the playground days of childhood, from our romantic choices in adolescence and beyond, to the quest for social and professional circles in adulthood. The most direct and effective way to achieve this coveted interpersonal connection is through our faces and our facial expressions; therefore, maximizing facial attractiveness is of utmost importance to humans. Although facial movement and surface-related issues are undoubtedly important aspects to a beautiful face, volume and the resultant shape remain key components to the perception of a beautiful face (Fig. 3.1).Volume is central to rejuvenation of the aging face, or facial improvement at any age, and plays a pivotal role in our visual clues when assessing facial beauty.

PEARL 2 The appraisal of beauty and the recognition of another's face take only a fraction of a second. Brain responses to facial beauty have been widely studied. Magnetic resonance imaging (MRI) has shown that beauty results in widespread brainwave activity that directly correlates to the degree of facial attractiveness. In another study, performing a task was found to take longer if one was distracted by an attractive facial image, even if it was outside direct vision. In other words, facial beauty automatically overrides any other task performance.

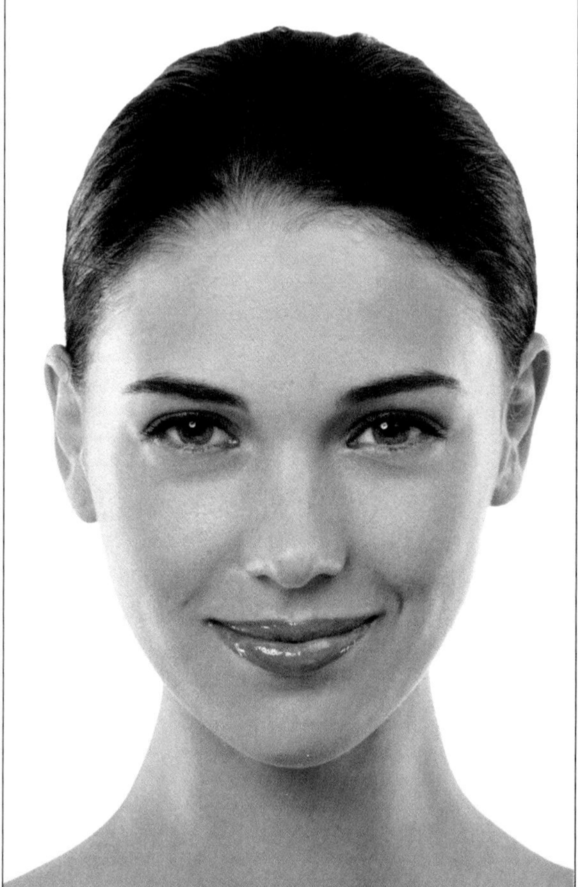

Fig. 3.1 Representation of a beautiful face.

PEARL 3 Although we very quickly assess beauty, the exact mechanism remains elusive.

What are the principles that underpin our understanding of beauty?

The total attractiveness of an individual is not quite the same as facial beauty. Attractiveness is multifactorial, more of the total package; it may relate to how a person moves, one's appearance of fitness, the manner of expression, or how one sounds or even thinks. It may relate to one's power or success, to reputation, how a person relates to others, and many other facets that go into the making of an individual. Mere physical beauty, combined with attractiveness, can lead to success and wealth in life. As it becomes clear, success begets beauty, which in turn begets more success. As such, reasonable dedication to one's physical appearance is a sound investment in one's future stability and financial security.

The introduction of photography and its rapid evolution and integration into our quotidian lives through smartphones and "selfies" have undoubtedly shaped our modern perception and understanding of beauty. Until almost 100 years ago, humans were not accustomed to seeing themselves represented in images. Self-portraits hung on the walls of mansions, palaces, and castles of the upper-class for centuries, but the average humans depended on their social interactions with their peers for self-validation and self-definition. After the invention of photography, the idea of seeing one's image in print became possible. Later, with the advent and worldwide distribution of smartphones, photography became ubiquitous, with most individuals capable of access within seconds to a device to photograph themselves, to check on their appearance, comparing themselves to the beauty ideals blasted on social platforms online, and to filter, modify, and modulate their appearance at will. The tsunami of selfies, filters-effects, editing options, and virtual, video-based meetings has led to a unique storm for distortion in self-perception, as these images alter one's external sense of self. The synchrony between inner and outer beauty is essential for a harmonious sense of self, and the omnipresence of self-imagery has created an imbalance in this relationship. This has resulted in an increase in displeasure with one's appearance, greater anxiety, and a surge in the desire to undergo cosmetic procedures in an attempt to rectify this perceived disparity. It should also be noted that the camera and lens with which one photographs significantly affect the resultant image, thus impacting one's self-perception. The choice of photographic hardware, further magnified by the software options, in conjunction with varying lighting conditions, can render a huge range in resultant images, altering facial angles and curves, shifting balance and shape, often creating fictitious issues, and false impressions for the viewer. These factors play significantly and regularly into the information received by the human psyche, as the barrage of sensory input rarely lets up.

These are important, game-changing considerations in the modern aesthetic arena, and patient expectations must be filtered through this new lens.

Attractiveness in humans is certainly not limited to the face. A determinant of female attractiveness and beauty is termed the "ogee curve." This curve is simply a convexity, followed by a concavity, which is best appreciated by the example of the classic 1950s pin-up, in which there is a convexity on either side of a concavity at the waistline. The waist–hip ratio (WHR) is one of the most alluring aspects of body attractiveness. The thrust, however, of this chapter is more specifically facial beauty and the role of volume in that beauty, and here, we witness volume-expanded ogee curves (Fig. 3.2) as clues to sexual maturity in the curve of the high cheekbones, eyelid–cheek junction, lips, and eyebrow.

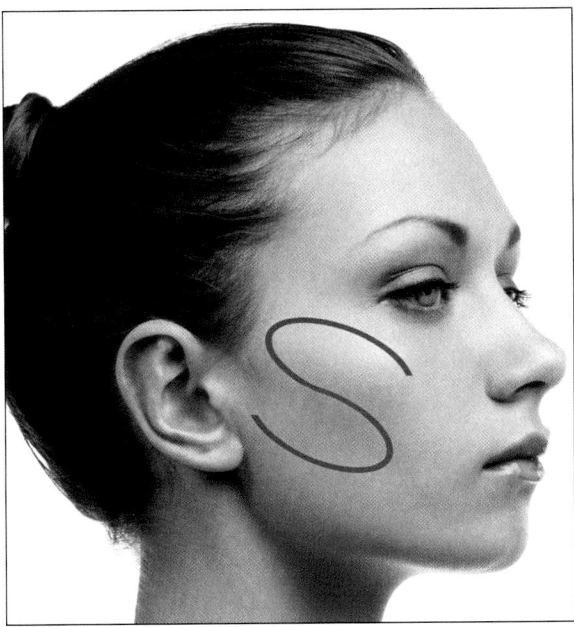

Fig. 3.2 Diagram of the ogee curve taking in the eyelid–cheek junction, high cheek bone, and the concavity inferior to this.

THE ROLE OF VOLUME IN THE APPRECIATION OF FACIAL BEAUTY

Volume provides the face its characteristic shape and is a prominent aspect of beauty. It is that concept that underpins much of what we perceive as the symmetry and geometry of facial attractiveness. This shape fluctuates with weight gain and loss, and with age, as tissues decrease in volume in some areas and appear to increase in others, thus contributing to the round shape of a more youthful face (Fig. 3.3) and the squaring off of an aging face.

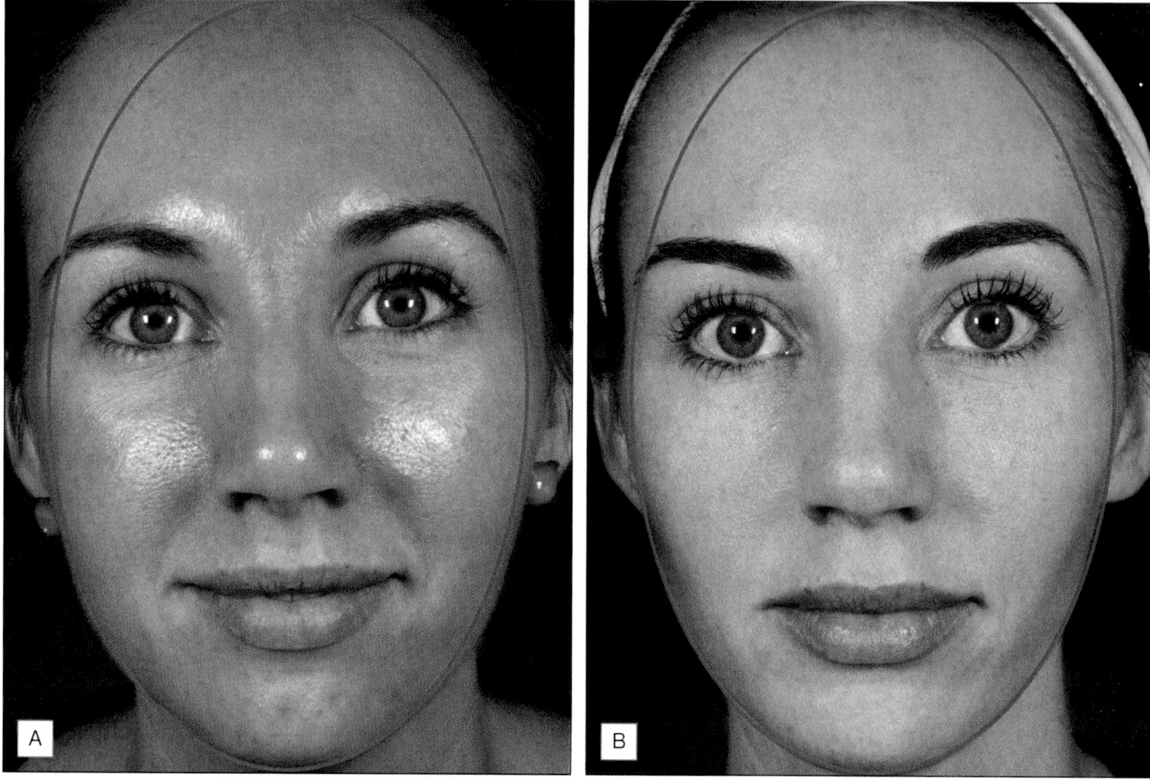

Fig. 3.3 Facial shape before (A) and after (B) weight loss, showing a change from round to oval.

PEARL 4 Volume is important in many of the indicators of youth, maturity, attractiveness, symmetry, and gender differentiation.

Volume is important in all the facial layers, from the underlying architectural structure of the bones and teeth to the muscle, fat, and the superficial layers of the skin. Most volume loss occurs deeply, with bony resorption around and within major facial orifices. The orbits expand and rotate, and the piriform aperture (Fig. 3.4) widens, allowing posterior displacement of the nasal base, with drooping of the nose and deepening of the nasolabial fold.

PEARL 5 Bone and dentition support the facial form and structure of overlying muscles and resorb with age, both periorificially and in the bones supporting mastication.

Dentition volume decreases and the mandibular and maxillary volumes diminish. Anterior projection of the periorbital zone occurs, with the midface, nose, perioral area, and the chin all suffering as a result. The decrease in volume of the large muscles of mastication, especially the masseter muscles, combined with the changes in the mandible, particularly the shortening in the posterior ramus height and body length, contribute to an increasingly obtuse mandibular angle. This has significant ramifications for the fading of beauty in older age, with the facial shape changing and the support for the lower face waning.

PEARL 6 The muscles of mastication, particularly the masseter and temporalis muscles, lose volume in the aging process.

Separate, facial fat compartments (Fig. 3.5) have been described in both the superficial and deep layers of the face, each with its defined pockets of fat, separated by retaining ligaments. These fat pads descend over time, with concurrent depletion of the contents, leading to a paucity of fat and cheek flattening. With this structural

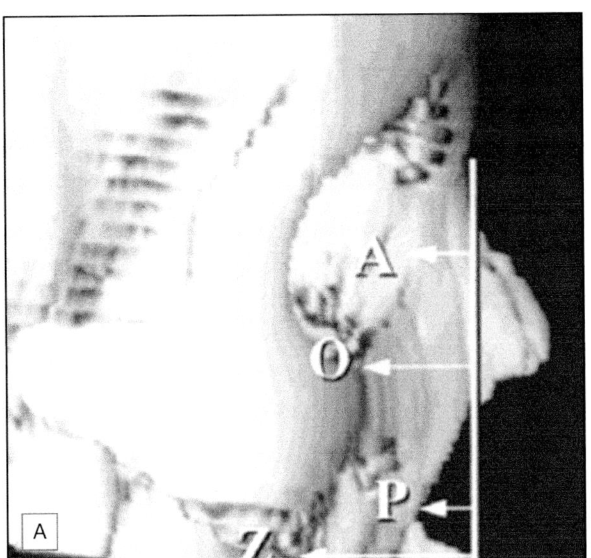

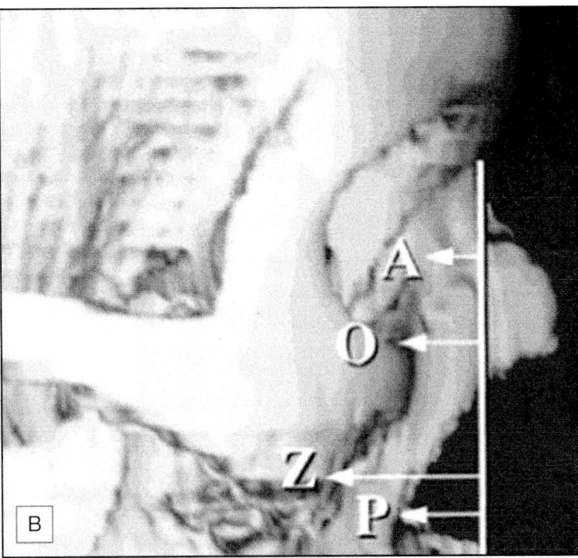

Fig. 3.4 The areas of the facial skeleton that selectively resorb with aging, with the size of the *arrows* indicating relative tendency for bone loss. A, nasal base; O, Orbit; P, piriform aperture; Z, zygoma. (From Mendelson B, Wong C. Changes in the facial skeleton with aging: implications and clinical applications in facial rejuvenation. *Aesth Plast Surg*. 2012;36:4:753–760.)

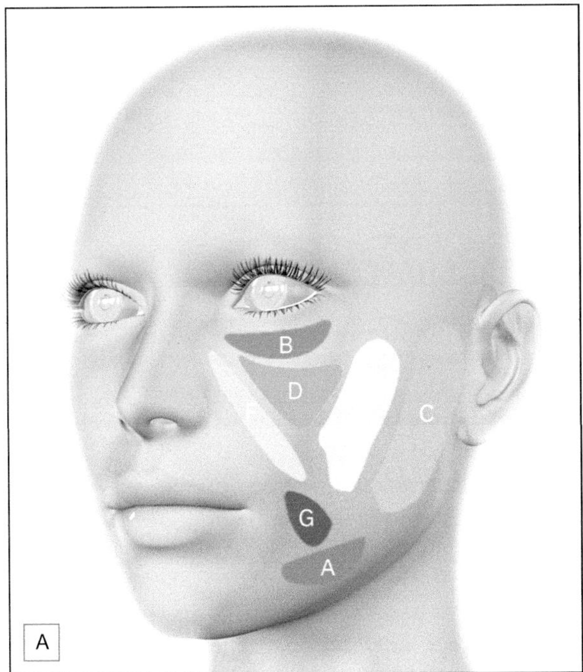

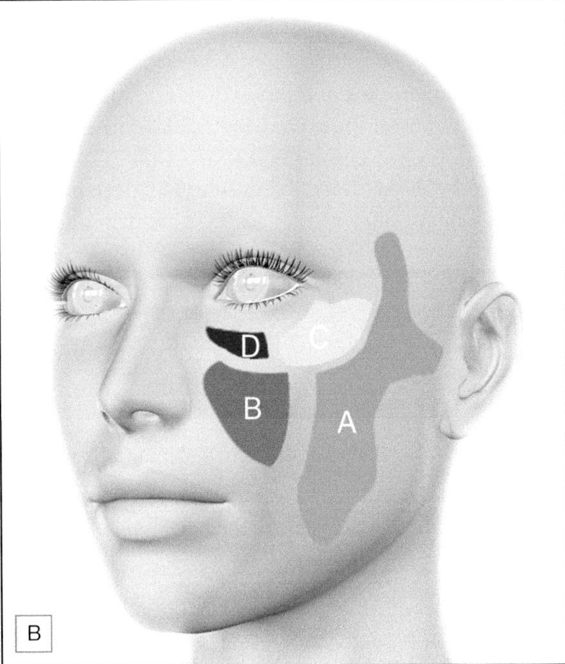

Fig. 3.5 Diagram of facial fat compartments. (A) Superficial fat compartments: *A*, Inferior jowl fat. *B*, Infraorbital fat. *C*, Lateral cheek fat. *D*, Medial cheek fat. *E*, Middle cheek fat. *F*, Nasolabial fat. *G*, Superior jowl fat. (B) Deep fat compartments: *A*, Buccal fat. *B*, Deep medial cheek fat. *C*, Lateral suborbicularis oculi fat. *D*, Medial suborbicularis oculi fat.

migration and fat diminution, there results an alteration in the facial shape, with the loss of the inverted triangle and the resultant squaring of the face. The major retaining ligaments, such as the mandibular and zygomatic ligaments, do not significantly change in length over time, simply in their orientation, due to the shifts in the locations of their osseous attachment points. The zones of the face and facial proportions are an effortless balance in youth and when optimal features are at work. With age, or poorly developed features, comes a burden on retaining ligaments, as volumes shift, sag, or migrate, exaggerating the deep folds of the face.

PEARL 7 Most major retaining ligaments induce deep facial grooves, as the face cascades forward and rotates inward with age.

The facial fat compartments are bilayered, with a superficial and deeper set (Table 3.1). The deeper fat pads allow sliding of mimetic muscles and muscles of mastication, but with aging, it appears that the midfacial fat compartments migrate medially with an inferior shift within the individual compartments. This has led to the popularization of a deeper injection, augmenting the deep system and reinflating the superficial fat pads, allowing better support and projection. Overall, the cutaneous, bony, and adipose changes that lead to an aging face can also project emotions that are undesirable and unintended by the individual. For example, deep glabellar furrows can project anger, hollowed tear troughs can signal the feelings of fatigue and sadness, and laxity in the jawline, along with poor structural definition, typically project dourness or weakness. These are particularly significant when coupled with the typical perioral aging changes of down-turning, narrowing, and lip inversion; these create a sense of sourness and bitterness, expressions that tend to repel rather than attract.

As such, treating the aging face not only addresses its pure aesthetic appearance but also the intangible emotions it elicits.

TABLE 3.1 Superficial and Corresponding Deep Fat Compartments of the Face

Superficial Fat Compartments	Deep Fat Compartments
Nasolabial	Deep medial cheek (medial component)
Superficial medial cheek	Deep medial cheek (lateral component)
Middle cheek	Buccal
Lateral temporal cheek	Lateral suborbicularis oculi (SOOF)
Infraorbital	Medial suborbicularis oculi (SOOF)

Deep compartments may be more prone to atrophy with age, whereas superficial ones tend to hypertrophy

PEARL 8 Facial fat compartments have deep and superficial elements, with the deeper ones particularly prone to atrophy and migration with aging.

Replenishing atrophic compartments aids facial rejuvenation. As an example, deflation of the deep periorbital fat pad with age induces a V-shaped concavity between the medial eyelid and cheek area, opening up the inferior orbital hollows, and a more obvious transition between the lid and cheek. Deep augmentation of the medial suborbicularis fat pads or deep medial cheek fat pad using a deep supra-periosteal injection often improves this tear trough deformity.

PEARL 9 The facial shape seen from the front is ideally an oval in youth, independent of ethnicity in females, and a sharp angular shape, more base-heavy in males.

FACIAL SHAPES

There are many facial shapes that should be pleasing, even at times arresting, from any angle; for example, the sweep of the cheek may be best appreciated from an oblique pose and the projected aspects from a lateral one.

We will start from the anteroposterior (AP) view, as this is the view we see most commonly in the mirror and when in conversation. It should not be forgotten that photographic capture and posing are not usually front-on but various shades of a side-on pose. When looking at the face head-on, volume is important for the outline, contours, shape, symmetry, and the width of the features.

Facial shape is an essential aspect underpinning attractiveness, the appearance of youth, and gender

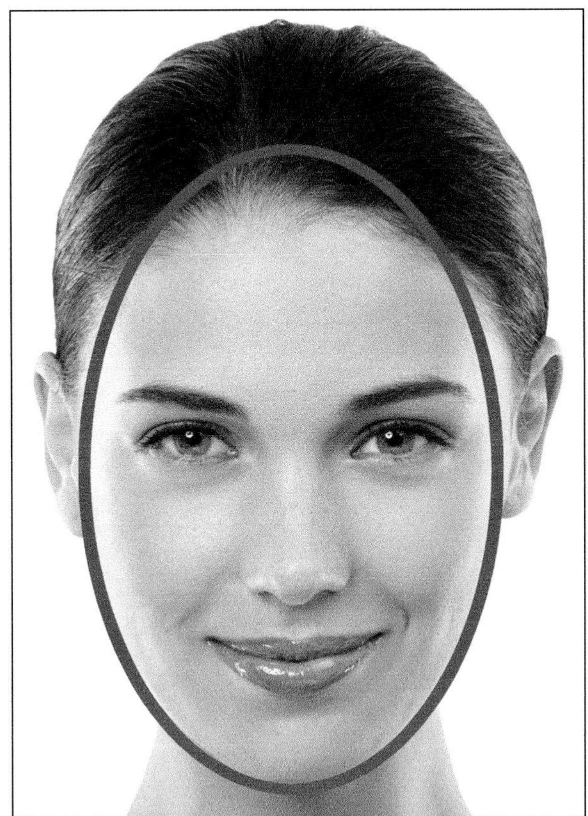

Fig. 3.6 Facial features sitting on oval outline.

identification. In the female, looking at the face front-on, the facial outline ideally approximates a smooth oval. This oval is a combination of bony skeleton, overlain by soft tissues. The oval line should begin at the forehead and curve rather seamlessly around the outside of the face, through the temple, outer cheek, preauricular area, angle of the jaw, jawline, and all the way to the chin. The edge of each of these features should sit on the line of the oval, neither falling short of nor projecting past the oval's edge (Fig. 3.6).

PEARL 10 The oval outline of the attractive female face should pass seamlessly, touching on the temple, cheek, jaw angle, and jawline, through to the chin.

This facial shape is a very similar beauty consideration across all ethnicities and is a strong determinant of age perception. Variations have been termed "heart shaped," or "betel leaf," but these may be variations in the upper half of the oval rather than a difference to the intrinsic oval face. Not all agree with this stance, but most agree that the female facial shape should be wider in the upper half, tapering to a point at the chin, with no particular angular sharpness. Squaring of the face begins soon after a female's peak of maturation, around the age of 25 years, with a more rapid progression into middle age and older years. This masculinizes the face, generally perceived to be less attractive in a woman.

In youth, a fatter face is acceptable, with an evening out of the fat compartments and support provided by retaining ligaments. Weight gain, however, may affect these compartments, which are prone to age-related hypertrophy, resulting in facial squaring and plentiful folds, which are not aesthetically ideal.

A square male face is acceptable, even desirable, but this squareness must have certain characteristics. In the upper face, adequate bizigonial distance is required, with the male facial shape most defined in the lower half, requiring strong masseteric volume and jaw angle (Fig. 3.7). What is not desirable are jowls or excess volume posterior to the masseters overlying the parotids.

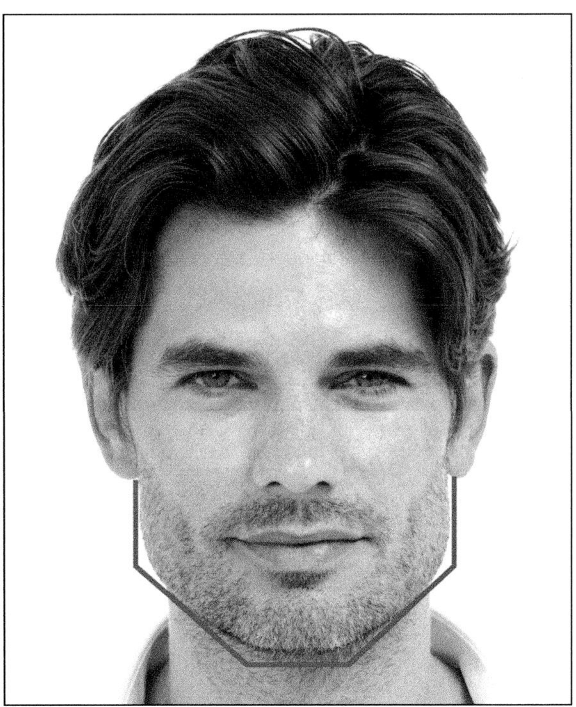

Fig. 3.7 Strong masseteric volume and jaw angle in a male face.

A strong, well-defined jawline and a sculpted, square chin are the features of the ideal, masculine, facial shape for maximal attractiveness.

PEARL 11 Attractive female faces are much wider in the mid and upper face than the lower face, whereas attractive males tend to possess greater lower face volume.

SYMMETRY

Symmetry appears to be our visual clue to the outward show of ideal genetics.

Although symmetry may refer to any aspect of beauty, such as surface irregularities or facial movement peculiarities, it is the differential volume effects that detract most from the perceived beauty of an individual's face.

In one study, only 6 of the 21 subjects were symmetrical across their upper face (bizigonial distance) and only 4 were symmetrical across the lower face (angle of the jaws). Only 3 out of 21 appeared symmetrical across both the upper and lower face. These subjects were taken from some of the objectively most beautiful females in current and past history—film stars, models, and pageant winners.

PEARL 12 Very few people, even very beautiful people, have facial symmetry.

IDEAL PROPORTIONS OF BEAUTY

We now understand that to have a well-proportioned face is a major step toward beauty. The ancient Greeks believed that all beauty was mathematical, and one of the more robust concepts is the golden ratio. This ratio is a mathematical construct fixed at 1.618:1.

In geometry, it is a linear relation in which the smaller length is to the larger length as the larger length is to the complete line. It defines ratios we commonly find appealing in nature, architecture, the human body, and faces. This ratio has been applied to the many aspects integral to the attractive face, and it has helped us understand what truly defines facial beauty.

Swift and Remington explored these Phi concepts to illustrate how best to rejuvenate the face in an approach termed "beautiphication."

It is counterintuitive that a two-dimensional line has been so extensively used to assess facial beauty and to correct proportionality, as the latter represents a three-dimensional concept. The vertical heights of the upper and lower lips, the relationship of eye width to the width across the malar ridges, and the relative proportions of the nose and the teeth are measured by this two-dimensional line, yet represent volume, which is, by definition, three-dimensional.

Division of the face into thirds horizontally, and fifths vertically, is another useful construct for facial assessment and treatment planning. It is most likely that an inbuilt and subliminal sense of mathematical analysis is at work in all of us when assessing beauty. Proportionality is a very strong, yet quiet, aesthetic undercurrent, creating the elusive harmony and balance that pleases and attracts; it is one of the pillars of beauty.

MATURITY INDICATORS

Gender selection is a hard-wired, innate attraction to a particular gender type. The soft-sloping ogee curves in females and the strong angles of males are volume indicators of the attainment of sexual maturity associated with estrogen and testosterone, respectively.

On a more localized level, the human face is meant to be predictable, devoid of volume imperfections. One of the most common, local, volume abnormalities our patients face is atrophic scars. This is so disfiguring to some that it is a source of depression and suicidal ideation. It deeply offends the patient cosmetically and is a frequent cause for seeking treatment. Volume correction in this instance of atrophic scarring has been a neglected aspect in treatment (Fig. 3.8).

PEARL 13 The oval facial shape transcends ethnicity and is the cornerstone of universal beauty, with differences lying more in an individual's intrinsic features.

FACIAL VOLUME, BEAUTY, AND ETHNICITY

Initially, researchers believed that different cultures adhere to different styles of beauty, but this may be erroneous. Darwin espoused that there is no universal standard of beauty; however, much of the research since

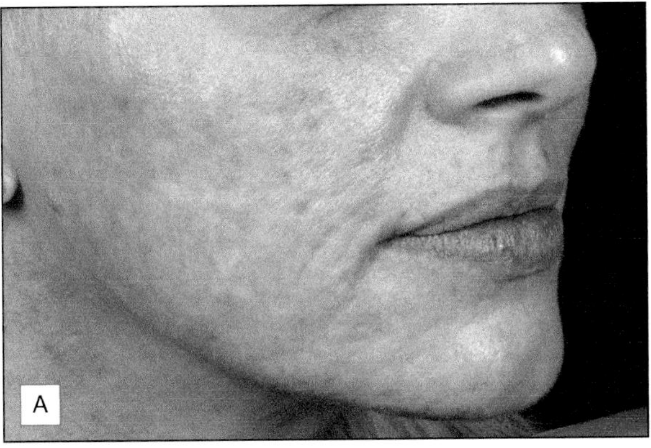

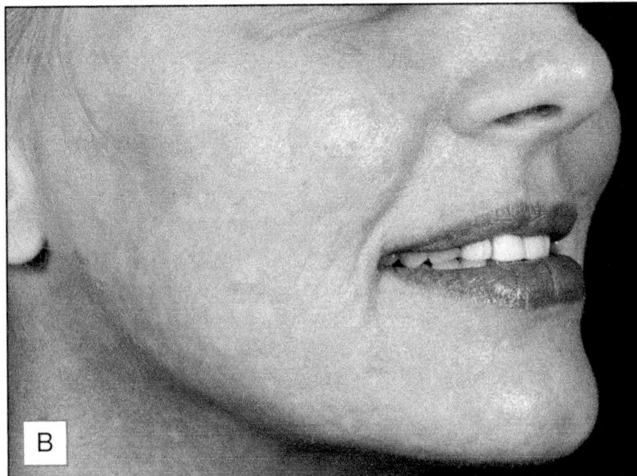

Fig. 3.8 Acne scarring before (A) and after (B) volume treatment.

the 1970s contradicts this and suggests a more universal standard of beauty.

Does our ideal face shape vary with ethnicity? Is an oval facial shape something to which women of any ethnicity can and might aspire? It is probable that a smoothly contoured, oval-shaped perimeter to a woman's face is the cornerstone of universal beauty and, similarly, that an angular face with lower-facial prominence, a defined jawline, a strong square chin, a large nose, and heavy horizontal brows are fundamentals in men.

SO WHERE DO THE DIFFERENCES LIE?

The strengths and weaknesses of the ethnicities are more obvious in the intrinsic features of the face—the nose, lips, cheeks, eyes, brows, and chin—and the way in which they project from the face.

These structures are emphasized in White and Indian people, but poorly projected in East Asian and African people. Lip projection varies amongst ethnicities. Although the upper lip is often quite full in East Asian females, the lower lip tends to be slightly less developed. Lips of White people may be more volume deficient, whereas in West Asian, African, and Hispanic peoples, the proportions and size more often conform to optimal ratios and size.

A consensus group issued a number of statements with regard to East Asian versus White aesthetics. Quoting from that study:

- "Beautiful people of all races show similarity in facial characteristics while retaining distinct ethnic features.
- Asians are not a homogeneous group but rather comprise many varied ethnic origins, with each group having its own unique facial characteristics.
- Treatment to achieve aesthetic changes in Asians should not be viewed as an attempt at Westernization, but rather the optimization of Asian ethnic features, in the same way that Westerners who receive lip enhancement, lateral malar enhancement, or skin tanning are not trying to 'Easternize' their appearance as they attempt to make up for their intrinsic ethnicity-associated structural weaknesses."

These statements may be extrapolated to describe the universality of beauty, with each racial or ethnic group exhibiting greater strength in certain volume-related characteristics than other groups. White people may have more anterior projection of facial features, the midface, and lower face, whereas East Asian and African populations may have more facial width intrinsically. In each group, benefit can be achieved by maximizing good structural characteristics, while improving common structural deficiencies typical of their ethnicity. Truly beautiful people of any ethnicity show the strong points of the group but may be outliers with regard to that group's deficiencies. In terms of volume, an oval facial shape in females and a square, angular face in men are truly youthful and attractive in any ethnicity.

CONCLUSIONS

The appreciation of beauty is a basic, universal and innate skill, which likely has survival value, both for the individual and the human species. The reward is personal safety and security and extends to protecting the sanctity of our current gene pool. A major principle upon which we judge facial beauty is the selective placement of volume. It guides us, assisting in the recognition of one another, especially in the distinction of age and gender for mate selection. The differences in volumetric distribution between males and females and the volume shifts occurring from childhood to maturity are strong indicators of sexual maturity. Beauty in the guise of optimal facial shape, symmetry, sweeping curves in a young adult female, angles and sharpness in a young male, proportions of the face, and the relationship amongst the features relies on volume distribution. Aging distorts the flow of this volume, creating compartmentalization and cascading volume shifts caught up by the retaining ligaments of the face. Volume is integral to every aspect of our understanding of facial beauty. However, there remains an elusive mystery to this most intriguing of concepts, which is dynamic, sublime, subtle and exquisite in its nuances, and defies measure, despite all our attempts. Ultimately, though, the energetic life force emanating from humans is often perceived as the real source of true beauty, and that entity, ethereal by nature, lies entirely in the eye of the beholder.

FURTHER READING

Alam, M., & Dover, J. S. (2001). On beauty: evolution, psychosocial considerations, and surgical enhancement. *Arch Dermatol, 137*(6), 795–807.

Alghoul, M., & Codner, M. A. (2013). Retaining ligaments of the face: review of anatomy and clinical applications. *Aesthet Surg J, 33*(6), 769–782.

Baig, M. A. (2004). Surgical enhancement of facial beauty and its psychological significance. *Ann R Australas Coll Dent Surg, 17*, 64–67.

Baig, M. A. (2004). Surgical enhancement of facial beauty and its psychological significance. *Ann R Australas Coll Dent Surg, 17*, 64–67.

Bonati, L. M., & Jagdeo, J. (2020). A new era of care for the lesbian, gay, bisexual, and transgender community. *Dermatol Clin, 38*(2), xiii–xiv.

Borelli, C., & Berneburg, M. (2010). "Beauty lies in the eye of the beholder"? Aspects of beauty and attractiveness. *J Dtsch Dermatol Ges, 8*, 326–330.

Buggio, L., Vercellini, P., Somigliana, E., Viganò, P., Frattaruolo, M. P., & Fedele, L. (2012). "You are so beautiful": behind women's attractiveness towards the biology of reproduction: a narrative review. *Gynecol Endocrinol, 28*, 753–757.

Cappelle, T., & Fink, B. (2013). Changes in women's attractiveness perception of masculine men's dances across the ovulatory cycle: preliminary data. *Evol Psychol, 11*, 965–972.

Chatterjee, A., Thomas, A., Smith, S. E., & Aguirre, G. K. (2009). The neural response to facial attractiveness. *Neuropsychology, 23*, 135–143.

Claes, P., Walters, M., Shriver, M. D., et al. (2012). Sexual dimorphism in multiple aspects of 3D facial symmetry and asymmetry defined by spatially dense geometric morphometrics. *J Anat, 221*, 97–114.

Cristel, R. T., Dayan, S. H., Akinosun, M., & Russell, P. T. (2021). Evaluation of selfies and filtered selfies and effects on first impressions. *Aesthet Surg J, 41*(1), 122–130.

Dion, K., Berscheid, E., & Walster, E. (1972). What is beautiful is good. *J Pers Soc Psychol, 24*, 285–290.

Dutton D. TED talk. 2010. http://www.ted.com/talks/denis_dutton_a_darwinian_theory_of_beauty.html. Accessed July 29, 2016.

Eagly, A. H., Ashmore, R. D., Makhijani, M. G., & Longo, L. C. (1991). What is beautiful is good, but...: a meta-analytic review of research on the physical attractiveness stereotype. *Psychol Bull, 110*, 109–128.

Fink, B., & Neave, N. (2005). The biology of facial beauty. *Int J Cosmet Sci, 27*, 317–325.

Fisher, M. L., & Voracek, M. (2006). The shape of beauty: determinants of female physical attractiveness. *J Cosmet Dermatol, 5*, 190–194.

Fitzgerald, R., & Rubin, A. G. (2014). Filler placement and the fat compartments. *Dermatol Clin, 32*(1), 37–50. https://doi.org/10.1016/j.det.2013.09.007.

Gierloff, M., Stöhring, C., Buder, T., Gassling, V., Açil, Y., & Wiltfang, J. (2012). Aging changes of the midfacial fat compartments: a computed tomographic study. *Plast Reconstr Surg, 129*, 263–273.

Glassenberg, A. N., Feinberg, D. R., Jones, B. C., Little, A. C., & Debruine, L. M. (2010). Sex-dimorphic face shape preference in heterosexual and homosexual men and women. *Arch Sex Behav, 39*, 1289–1296.

Golle, J., Mast, F. W., & Lobmaier, J. S. (2014). Something to smile about: the interrelationship between attractiveness and emotional expression. *Cogn Emot, 28*, 298–310.

Goodman, G. J. (2006). Acne and acne scarring—the case for active and early intervention. *Aust Fam Phys, 35*, 503–504.

Goodman, G. J. (2012). Treating scars: addressing surface, volume and movement to optimize results, part 1: Mild grades of scarring. *Dermatol Surg*. https://doi.org/10.1111/j.1524-4725.2012.02434.x.

Goodman, G. J. (2012). Treating scars: addressing surface, volume and movement to optimize results, part 2: more severe grades of scarring. *Dermatol Surg*. https://doi.org/10.1111/j.1524-4725.2012.02439.x.

Goodman, G. J. (2015). The oval female facial shape—a study in beauty. *Dermatol Surg, 41*, 1374–1382.

Goodman, G. J., Halstead, M. B., Rogers, J. D., et al. (2012). A software program designed to educate patients on age-related skin changes of facial and exposed extrafacial regions: the results of a validation study. *Clin Cosmet Investig Dermatol, 5*, 23–31.

Hogan, P. C. (2013). Literary aesthetics: beauty, the brain, and Mrs. *Dalloway. Prog Brain Res, 205*, 319–337.

Jefferson, Y. (2004). Facial beauty—establishing a universal standard. *Int J Orthod Milwaukee, 15*, 9–22.

Kane, M. (2015). Commentary on the oval female facial shape—a study in beauty. *Dermatol Surg, 41*, 1384–1388.

Liew, S., Wu, W. T., Chan, H. H., et al. (2020). Consensus on changing trends, attitudes, and concepts of Asian beauty. *Aesthetic Plast Surg, 44*(4), 1186–1194.

Little, A. C., Jones, B. C., & DeBruine, L. M. (2011). Facial attractiveness: evolutionary based research. *Philos Trans Roy Soc B, 366*, 1638–1659.

Little, A. C., & Perrett, D. I. (2011). Facial attractiveness. In R. A. Adams Jr.,, N. Ambady, K. Nakayama, & S. Shimojo (Eds.), *The Science of Social Vision* (pp. 164–185). Oxford: Oxford University Press.

Lu, Y., Wang, J., Wang, L., Wang, J., & Qin, J. (2014). Neural responses to cartoon facial attractiveness: an event-related potential study. *Neurosci Bull, 30*, 441–450.

Magro, A. M. (1999). Evolutionary-derived anatomical characteristics and universal attractiveness. *Percept Mot Skills, 88*(1), 147–166.

Mendelson, B., & Wong, C. (2012). Changes in the facial skeleton with aging: implications and clinical applications in facial rejuvenation. *Aesth Plast Surg, 36*(4), 753–760.

Patel, U., & Fitzgerald, R. (2010). Facial shaping: beyond lines and folds with fillers. *Drugs Dermatol, 9*, s129–s137 (8 suppl ODAC Conf Pt 2).

Penton-Voak, I. S., & Morrison, E. R. (2011). Structure, expression and motion in facial attractiveness. In A. J. Calder, G. Rhodes, M. H. Johnson, & J. V. Haxby (Eds.), *The Oxford Handbook of Face Perception* (pp. 653–672). New York, NY: Oxford University Press.

Postma, E. (2014). A relationship between attractiveness and performance in professional cyclists. *Biol Lett, 10*, 20130966.

Ramanadham, S. R., & Rohrich, R. J. (2015). Newer understanding of specific anatomic targets in the aging face as applied to injectables: superficial and deep facial fat compartments—an evolving target for site-specific facial augmentation. *Plast Reconstr Surg, 136*(5 suppl), 49S–55S. https://doi.org/10.1097/PRS.0000000000001730.

Rhodes, G., Yoshikawa, S., Clark, A., Lee, K., McKay, R., & Akamatsu, S. (2001). Attractiveness of facial averageness and symmetry in non-western cultures: in search of biologically based standards of beauty. *Perception, 3*, 611–625.

Rhodes, G. (2006). The evolution of facial attractiveness. *Ann Rev Psychol, 57*, 199–226.

Rohrich, R. J., Ghavami, A., Constantine, F. C., Unger, J., & Mojallal, A. (2014). Lift-and-fill face lift: integrating the fat compartments. *Plast Reconstr Surg, 133*(6), 756e–767e. https://doi.org/10.1097/01.prs.0000436817.96214.7e.

Samson, N., Fink, B., & Matts, P. J. (2010). Visible skin condition and perception of human facial appearance. *Int J Cosmet Sci, 32*, 167–184.

Schacht, A., Werheid, K., & Sommer, W. (2008). The appraisal of facial beauty is rapid but not mandatory. *Cogn Affect Behav Neurosci, 8*(2), 132–142.

Shome, D., Vadera, S., Male, S. R., & Kapoor, R. (2020). Does taking selfies lead to increased desire to undergo cosmetic surgery. *J Cosmet Dermatol, 19*(8), 2025–2032.

Smith, C. U. (2005). Evolutionary neurobiology and aesthetics. *Perspect Biol Med, 48*, 17–30.

Sui, J., & Liu, C. H. (2009). Can beauty be ignored? Effects of facial attractiveness on covert attention. *Psychon Bull Rev, 16*, 276–281.

Swift, A., & Remington, K. (2011). BeautiPHIcation™: a global approach to facial beauty. *Clin Plast Surg, 38*, 347–377.

Thayer, Z. M., & Dobson, S. D. (2010). Sexual dimorphism in chin shape: implications for adaptive hypotheses. *Am J Phys Anthropol, 143*, 417–425.

Wan, D., Amirlak, B., Rohrich, R., & Davis, K. (2014). The clinical importance of the fat compartments in midfacial aging. *Plast Reconstr Surg Glob Open, 1*(9). https://doi.org/10.1097/GOX.0000000000000035, e92 (eCollection 2013).

Wang, J. V., Rieder, E. A., Schoenberg, E., Zachary, C. B., & Saedi, N. (2020). Patient perception of beauty on social media: Professional and bioethical obligations in esthetics. *J Cosmet Dermatol, 19*(5), 1129–1130.

Werheid, K., Schacht, A., & Sommer, W. (2007). Facial attractiveness modulates early and late event-related brain potentials. *Biol Psychol, 76*, 100–108.

Whitehead, R. D., Ozakinci, G., & Perrett, D. I. (2012). Attractive skin coloration: harnessing sexual selection to improve diet and health. *Evol Psychol, 10*, 842–854.

Wong, C. H., & Mendelson, B. (2015). Newer understanding of specific anatomic targets in the aging face as applied to injectables: aging changes in the craniofacial skeleton and facial ligaments. *Plast Reconstr Surg, 136*(5 suppl), 44S–48S. https://doi.org/10.1097/PRS.0000000000001752.

Xu, Y., Lee, A., Wu, W. L., Liu, X., & Birkholz, P. (2013). Human vocal attractiveness as signaled by body size projection. *PLoS One, 8*, e62397.

Yokoyama, T., Noguchi, Y., Tachibana, R., Mukaida, S., & Kita, S. (2014). A critical role of holistic processing in face gender perception. *Front Hum Neurosci, 8*, 477.

Zhang, H., Teng, F., Chan, D. K., & Zhang, D. (2014). Physical attractiveness, attitudes toward career, and mate preferences among young Chinese women. *Evol Psychol, 12*, 97–114.

Zhao, M., & Hayward, W. G. (2010). Holistic processing underlies gender judgments of faces. *Atten Percept Psychophys, 72*, 591–596.

4

Introduction to Temporary Fillers: Pros and Cons

Adam K. Brys, Kimberly Butterwick, and Sue Ellen Cox

SUMMARY AND KEY FEATURES

- Temporary fillers are composed of biodegradable materials, including hyaluronic acid, calcium hydroxyapatite, and poly-L-lactic acid. The physical properties of temporary fillers vary and subsequently can have substantially different aesthetic applications.

These uses of temporary fillers have expanded beyond their initial introduction as rhytid-reducing products.

- The numerous pros of temporary fillers readily outweigh the cons, explaining their emergence and widespread popularity among consumers. Nevertheless, injectors should understand the capabilities, advantages, risks, and limitations associated with temporary fillers.

INTRODUCTION

Overwhelmingly, temporary fillers are safe and effective treatments that patients deem worthwhile. The latter is supported by the continuously increasing popularity of filler injections, with millions of injections performed worldwide on an annual basis. The American Society for Dermatologic Surgery 2019 Member Survey shows a 78% increase in soft tissue filler treatments in an 8-year span. It follows almost by definition that the pros must outweigh the cons. Nevertheless, prior to attempting to achieve a specific cosmetic outcome with an individual patient, the pros and cons of temporary fillers must be considered to ensure that an aesthetically successful outcome can realistically and safely be achieved.

HISTORY OF TEMPORARY FILLERS

The invention of the syringe in 1844 allowed the initial use of filling agents for cosmetic purposes as early as the 19th century. Paraffin and autologous fat were the first agents described, but popular use was severely limited by the common occurrence of adverse events and a general lack of efficacy. It was not until the 1980s that the US Food and Drug Administration (FDA) approved multiple bovine collagen products for use as facial fillers and these techniques began to emerge as acceptable, albeit not mainstream, treatments. Despite their approval, filler injection remained cumbersome and complex, with multiple barriers preventing their widespread adoption among consumers, such as the need for harvesting autologous

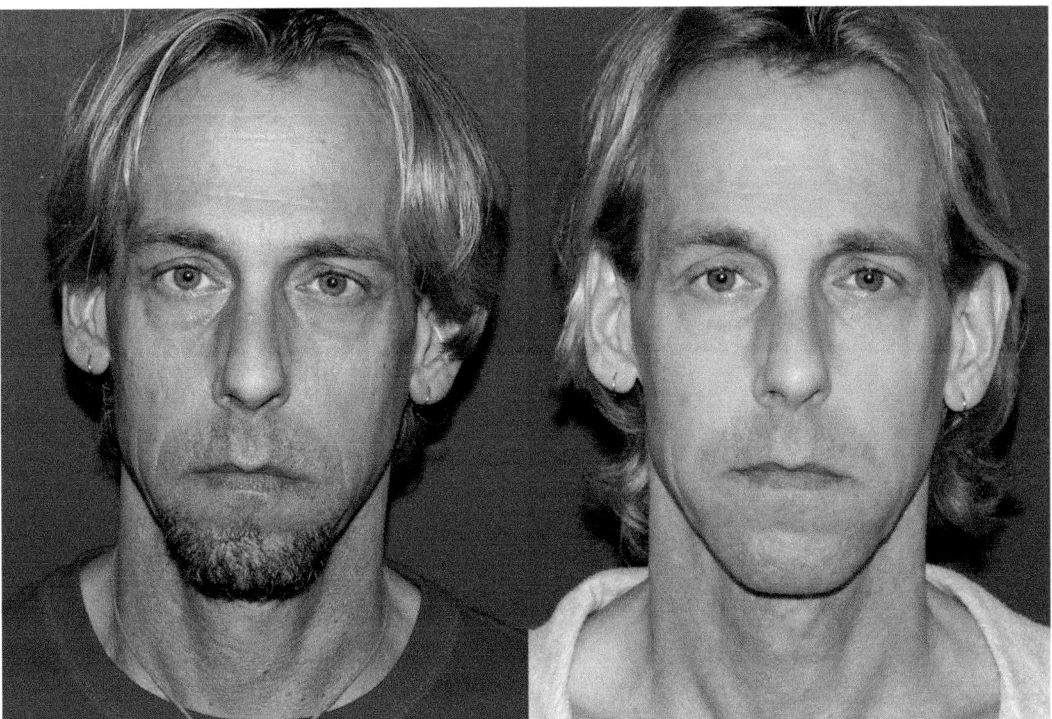

Fig. 4.1 Before *(left)* and 4 years after *(right)* ongoing treatment with poly-L-lactic acid injections. Three vials were injected during the first year of treatment, with one vial injected annually thereafter.

fat or preprocedural allergy testing in the case of bovine collagen. In 2003, the introduction of biocompatible and manufacturable hyaluronic acid (HA), a temporary filler, ushered in the modern era of filler injections.

OVERALL VALUE OF TEMPORARY FILLERS

Aesthetic improvement is the primary indication for temporary filler injection. Given the influence of physical appearance on critical measures important to all individuals—quality of life, mood, relationships, and even the likelihood of gainful employment or accruement of social capital from a young age—the use of noninvasive procedures to modify aesthetic features should not be marginalized. Indeed, there are now increasing objective data supporting the positive impact of temporary filler injections on not only physical appearance but also self-esteem, mood, and quality of life. In a study of patients treated with poly-L-lactic acid (PLLA) and calcium hydroxylapatite (CaHA) for antiretroviral-induced lipoatrophy, significant improvements in both physical tissue status (measured as total subcutaneous thickness) and in mental health, depressive symptoms, and social functionality were observed (Fig. 4.1). In another study of patients treated with HA fillers, improvements in quality of life and self-esteem were similarly noted.

USES OF TEMPORARY FILLERS

Temporary fillers were initially introduced as agents serving primarily to fill rhytids and replete age-related volume loss. Relative to permanent fillers, there are robust data to support the applications of temporary fillers for these purposes. Specific studies support their efficacy in the correction of moderate to severe wrinkles and folds, including for use in the nasolabial folds, the perioral region, as well as the dorsal hands. As a result, there is a preponderance of experience demonstrating that temporary fillers can achieve target endpoints and provide patient satisfaction with regard to volume restoration and rhytid reduction.

Lip augmentation is among the best studied and most popular applications of temporary filler (Fig. 4.2). Unlike many permanent fillers, HA fillers integrate smoothly and can be used for submucosal implantation in the lips without the creation of palpable abnormalities. A 2018 study comparing two HA products for lip enhancement demonstrated that approximately 86% of patients felt more attractive following injections, with improvement attained in more than 70% of patients as assessed by blinded evaluations.

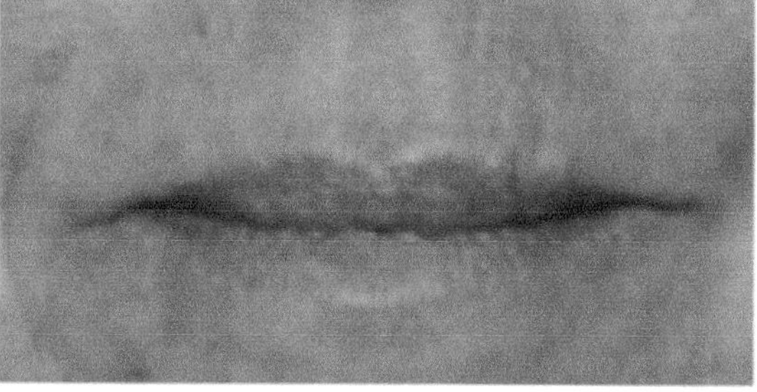

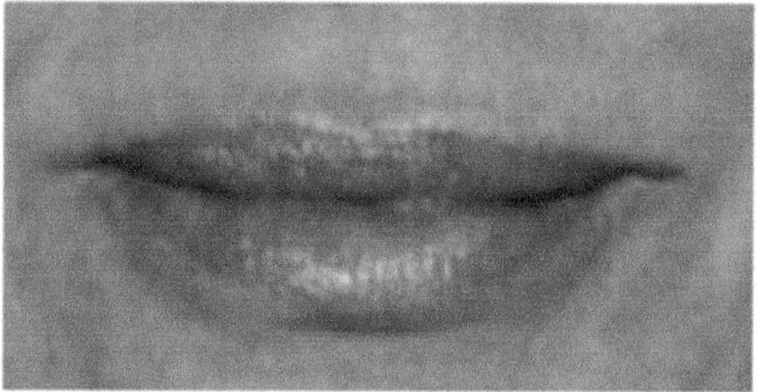

Fig. 4.2 Before *(top)* and after *(bottom)* injection of 0.2 cc of small particle hyaluronic acid (HA) to the vermillion and 1.0 cc of highly cohesive HA filler to the body of the upper and lower lips.

Given the quantity of experience with temporary fillers as well as the variability in their individual rheologic properties, it is not surprising that experienced injectors have expanded the applications of temporary fillers multifariously over the past two decades. Today, temporary fillers allow experienced injectors to address more complex aesthetic concerns in both older and younger patients. In addition to reversing age-related changes, temporary fillers can be used to correct defects, augment tissues, enhance beautifying features, and modify facial shape altogether. For example, the natural aesthetic features of the various facial shapes (oval, angular, heart shaped, and round) can be modified with temporary filler injection to subtly improve appearance. With attention to a patient's baseline facial shape, an experienced injector can choose injection sites that harness the inherent strengths and mitigate inherent weaknesses of each facial shape.

Experienced injectors report numerous uses for temporary fillers for facial shaping. Chin injections can be offered to patients with recessed chins or class II retrognathic occlusion for aesthetic considerations, while lateral jawline injections can restore the youthful appearance of the lower face and jawline (Fig. 4.3). Recently, two HA fillers have been FDA approved for chin augmentation.

Overly narrow, rounded, or square face shapes can be subtly contoured to increase proportionality to achieve

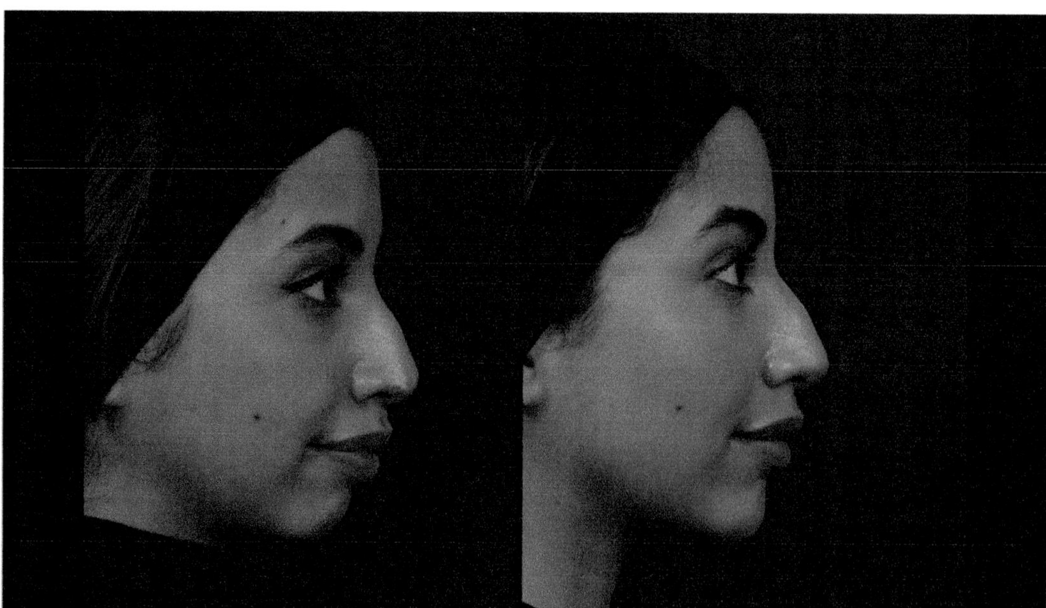

Fig. 4.3 Before *(left)* and after *(right)* injection of 2 mL of hyaluronic acid filler to the chin, pogonium and angle of the mandible. (Photo courtesy of Sue Ellen Cox, MD.)

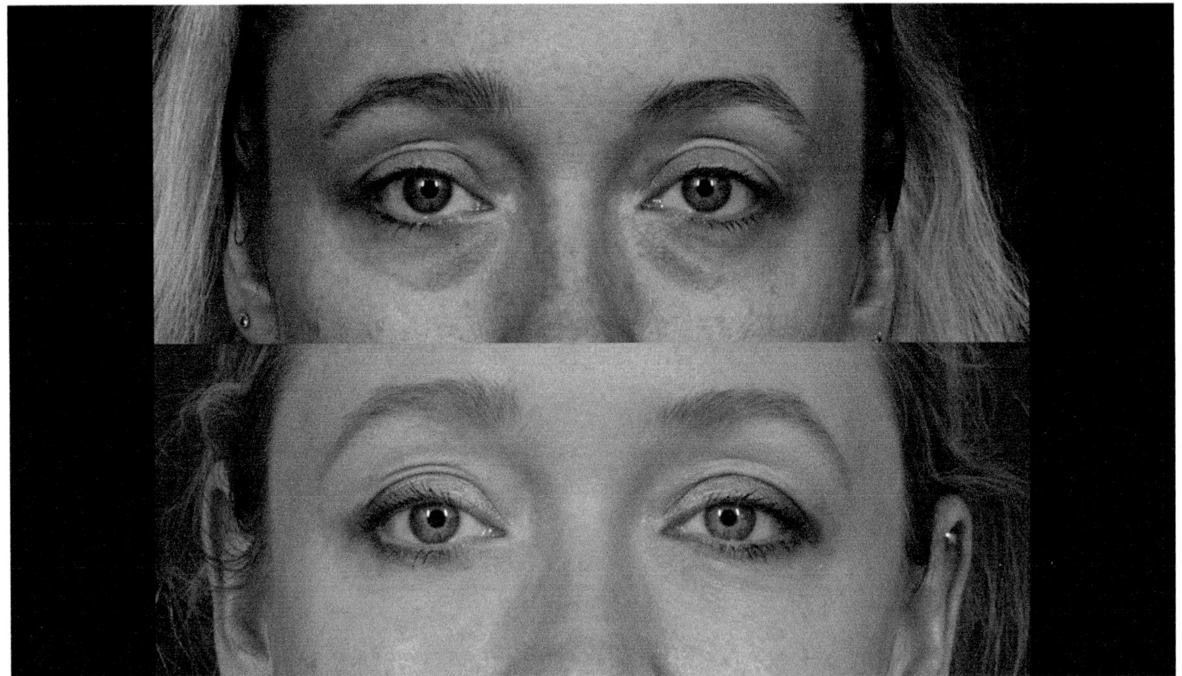

Fig. 4.4 Before *(top)* and after *(bottom)* injection of 2 mL of filler to the tear troughs. (Photo courtesy of Sue Ellen Cox, MD.)

aesthetically preferable norms. Temples and tear troughs are also commonly treated off-label uses and have been studied to improve facial shape and erase shadows (Fig. 4.4). Other defects, such as en coup de sabre morphea, have also been corrected using temporary fillers (Fig. 4.5). Off-the-face off-label uses for temporary fillers include areas such as the arms, chest neck, and buttocks (Fig. 4.6). It is notable that in nearly all novel applications of filler use, results from temporary fillers are the first to be reported in the literature.

PROPERTIES OF TEMPORARY FILLERS

As a molecule naturally present in humans, HA offers high natural levels of biocompatibility and low levels of antigenicity compared to other fillers. Compared to bovine collagen-containing products such as permanent fillers containing polymethylmethacrylate (e.g., Bellafill), hypersensitivity to HA fillers is 10 to 30 times less common. Hypersensitivity reactions to calcium hydroxyapatite and PLLA are similarly uncommon given their inert and biocompatible properties. Thus, preprocedural allergy testing is unnecessary, making these products more easily deliverable to the consumer.

To resist immediate degradation by naturally occurring hyaluronidase, cross-linking of HA products is necessary. The degree and type of cross-linking determine many properties of HA filler, such as deformability (G'), viscosity, and duration of effect. Largely due to differences in cross-linking, the many FDA-approved HA fillers can have varying properties and, depending on these, may be ideally suited to injections in certain anatomic locations. As a result, using temporary fillers alone, an experienced injector can more appropriately tailor product selection to both the desired treatment outcomes and the movement in each area (i.e., using different products for the lip injections than for perioral or temporal fossae injections). The availability of multiple FDA-approved injectables with properties that can vary slightly or drastically is a distinct advantage over permanent products.

While temporary fillers by definition require repeat injections, their duration of action can be relatively long lived depending on product selection as well as anatomic site of injection. For example, products placed in the tear troughs may produce a noticeable effect for longer periods of time than similar products placed in the lips. The biostimulatory effects of fillers, particularly

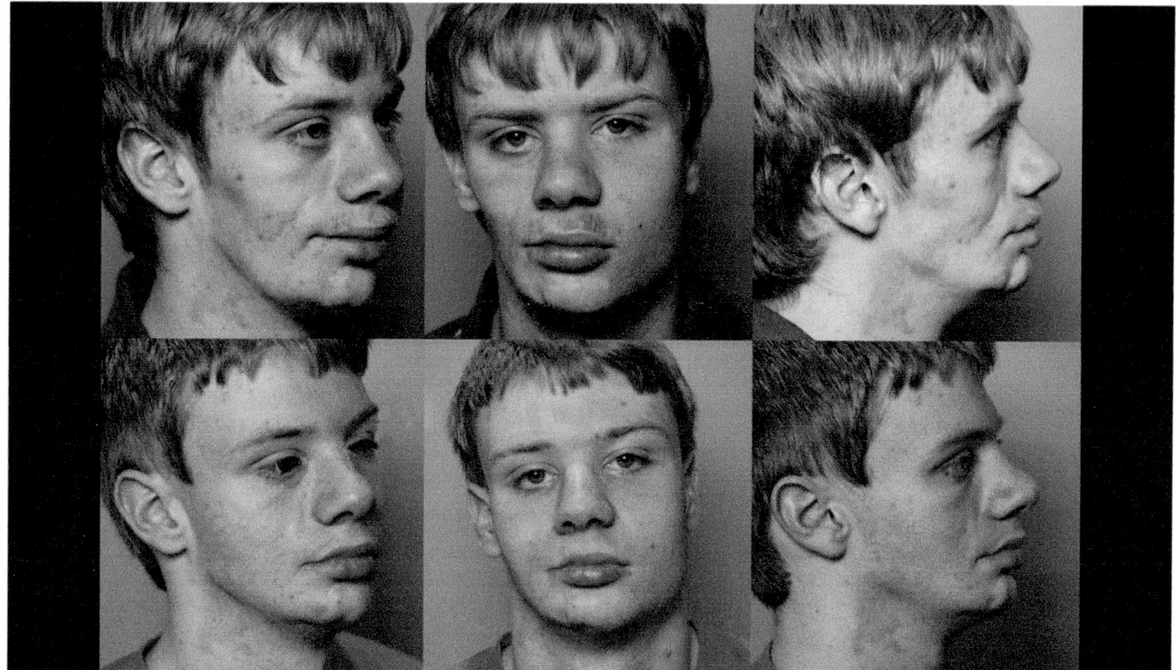

Fig. 4.5 Before *(top)* and after *(bottom)* treatment of hemifacial atrophy with 18.2 mL of calcium hydroxylapatite to the right side of face, jawline and submalar area and 1.0 mL of hyaluronic acid filler to the right lower eyelid, chin, and nasolabial fold over the course of 12 months. (Photo courtesy of Sue Ellen Cox, MD.)

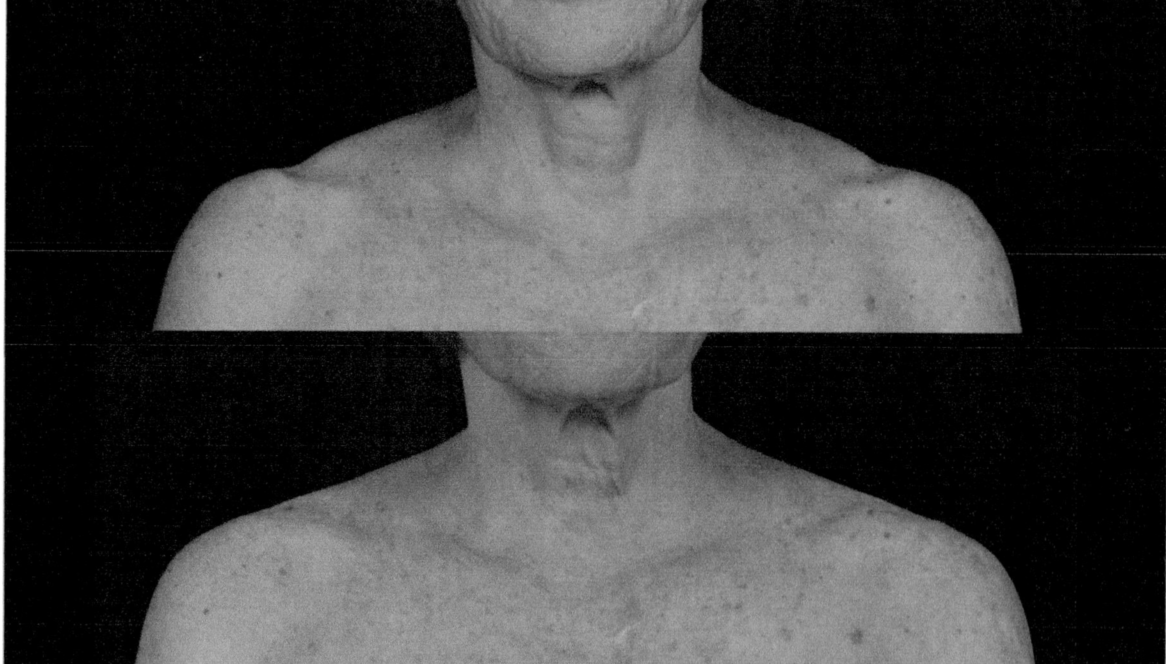

Fig. 4.6 1.5 cc of calcium hydroxylapatite to each shoulder to correct depression caused by heavy handbags. (Photo courtesy of Sue Ellen Cox, MD.)

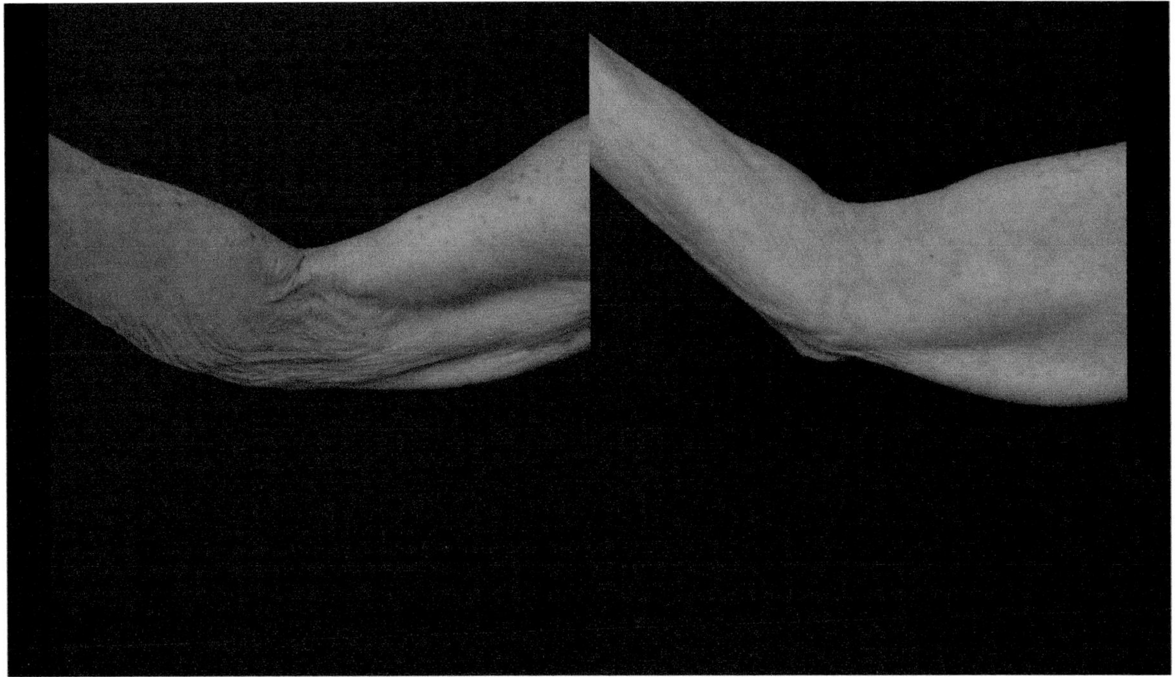

Fig. 4.7 Before *(left)* and after *(right)* treatment with 6 mL of calcium hydroxylapatite mixed 1:2 for skin laxity.

CaHA and PLLA, can lead to longer-term local production of collagen at the injection sites (Fig. 4.7). As a whole therefore, temporary fillers may have durations of action that last anywhere from 6 to 18 months or longer.

Although they eventually do require repeat treatment, which can be seen as a distinct disadvantage compared with permanent filler products, this is at the same time an advantage because it allows for the injector to modify their treatment approach based on the natural aging process of the patient, the patient's changing aesthetic priorities, changes in body weight over time, and changes in societal expectations for beauty. In the modern era, rapid changes in technology, such as the popularity of "selfie" photographs or the rapid adaptation of videoconferencing, can have profound impacts on patients' priorities, and temporary fillers inherently allow for these adjustments.

Moreover, HA products have the added benefit of reversibility with hyaluronidase, adding an additional layer of safety in the event of complications. While this has reported therapeutic value in the treatment of arterial embolization, it is also of benefit in the event of nodule formation, overfilling, or an otherwise dissatisfied patient. Notably, there is recent evidence to support the potential use of sodium thiosulfate for dissolution of nodules resulting from calcium hydroxyapatite injections. In comparison, nodule formation in the case of permanent fillers occurs later, potentially complicating diagnosis, and treatment options are generally limited to nonspecific therapies such as observation, systemic or local corticosteroids, intralesional antimitotic agents, or excision.

ADDITIONAL ADVANTAGES OF TEMPORARY FILLERS

Perhaps the greatest advantage of temporary fillers is their noninvasive nature, with almost immediate gratification following the procedure. This allows patients to avoid altogether many of the complications associated with surgery, such as surgical recovery (downtime), scars, and the risks of anesthesia. Other risks, such as bleeding, wound infection, dehiscence, keloid, or hypertrophic scar formation, are substantially lower. Unlike surgery or permanent filler treatment, hyaluronidase injection or time itself can more readily reverse results in those patients who are dissatisfied with their results. Additionally, in comparison to alternative noninvasive modalities such as laser resurfacing, temporary filler injection is safe in all skin colors, as the risk of postinflammatory pigmentary alteration is negligible. Temporary filler injections are advantageous in these treatments in that they can be performed in a stepwise manner until a desired outcome is achieved, allowing more flexibility in the precise positioning of a product. Apart from being reversed if a patient is dissatisfied, there are many inherent advantages to injectable products that are temporary in nature. Not only does this allow for patients to optimize their filler experience with time, as mentioned earlier, but also temporary fillers can provide age-appropriate results, and these can be modified as the patient ages. This is in contrast to permanent fillers or surgery, which does not necessarily evolve with the patient's age-related changes and aesthetic priorities.

SAFETY OF TEMPORARY FILLERS

Temporary filler injections have known risks. These risks vary from mild, short-term concerns such as pain, swelling, and ecchymosis to more severe complications including hypersensitivity reaction, infection, and vascular occlusion with consequent cutaneous necrosis or blindness. Prior to treatment with any injectable filler, the patient and provider must both be aware of these risks and how they can vary based on application (e.g., lip augmentation versus nonsurgical rhinoplasty). As temporary fillers become further commoditized procedures, injectors may have increasing needs to educate patients and correct misconceptions related to safety. This is particularly important as one study demonstrated that incomplete informed consent was the most common factor in litigation related to filler use.

In the hands of experienced injectors, these risks are reproducibly low for temporary fillers. Over a decade spanning from 2007 to 2017, the US FDA Manufacturer and User Facility Device Experience (MAUDE) Database cataloged only 5024 reports of adverse events despite an estimated 18 million filler injections performed during this time. Although most complications were reported from temporary fillers, temporary fillers also represented the overwhelming majority of products used during this time. In a recent study of 370 dermatologists, the rate of intravascular occlusion—the most feared complication of temporary filler injection—was 1 occlusion per 6410 1-mL syringes. This risk was further reduced to 1 in 40,882 when cannulas were used for injections. Importantly, experienced injectors (>5 years in practice) had 70.7% lower odds of occlusion than inexperienced injectors. Despite these datasets, the precise frequency of adverse events related to temporary filler injection is unknown and likely substantially underestimated as no universal reporting mandates exist.

Relative to other injectables, there is a long track record of safety for temporary fillers. Both PLLA and CaHA have been approved by the FDA for treatment of HIV-associated facial lipoatrophy since 2004 and 2006, respectively. In the case of PLLA, one study of 15,665 injections demonstrated the following rates of complication: bleeding, 3.4%; bruising, 2.3%; nodules, 5.7%; granuloma, 0.3%; discoloration, 0.2%; and skin hypertrophy, 0.1%. In these data, only a single treatment resulted in cutaneous necrosis, supporting an overall conclusion of safety.

DISADVANTAGES OF TEMPORARY FILLERS

Although temporary fillers have achieved mainstream acceptance and have maintained a track record of overall safety, they are not without limitations or potential disadvantages. Prior to commencing treatment with a filler, the injector and the patient must understand that fillers are ultimately neither bone nor soft tissue and that certain results such as drastic facelifts or dramatic changes to bony or cartilaginous structures may not be possible with temporary filler injections. If certain endpoints are demanded by the patient, an injector must know when a referral for a more traditional plastic surgery approach is necessary.

In the minds of many consumers however, the primary disadvantage of filler injections is their relative cost. At the time of writing, the cost of treatment with a single cubic centimeter of filler (i.e., a single syringe) approximates the price of 1 cc (~20 g) of gold. Given that five syringes of filler together are equivalent to 1 teaspoon of liquid, multiple syringes are often needed to achieve aesthetically impactful changes for patients requesting overall rejuvenation. Unlike permanent filler or plastic surgery, results from a single injection generally last on the order of 6 to 18 months, depending on the specific product and the location of treatment. This affords flexibility with regard to changing injection strategies with time; however, it also necessitates more frequent and regular evaluation and injection. While a single treatment with temporary filler costs less than more invasive treatments, such as plastic surgery, with time, the overall cost to maintain outcomes increases manifold. The resulting expense for a treatment that is by definition temporary excludes a substantial portion of potentially interested patients. In combination with advances in technology that decrease manufacturing costs and improve product quality, an increase in competition between the rapidly proliferating number of products available on the market will hopefully result in more affordable temporary fillers.

Despite the costs, in many locales, temporary fillers have increasingly become a commodity. Unlike many more invasive procedures, treatment with temporary filler in the United States and elsewhere is not limited to a group of specially trained physicians. Procedures can therefore be performed by injectors with highly variable levels of experience and often relatively low educational barriers to entry into the market. Less experienced injectors may incentivize patients with lower costs, further commoditizing these procedures. Although commoditization may make temporary filler injections more popular among the public, it also may result in patients with unrealistic expectations and misconceptions of the relatively high level of experience necessary to adequately perform these injections. While limited, there is recent evidence in the literature to support increased safety of temporary filler injections by more experienced physicians who perform these treatments more regularly. Beyond safety, injections performed by less experienced providers can easily look "overdone" or "overfilled" (Fig. 4.8). Our image-conscious culture is rife with examples of unnatural lip volumes, overly dramatic zygomatic prominences, and other caricatured features disproportionately resulting from temporary filler. Although these concerns are real, there are few data to support the extent of training and experience required for aesthetically successful and safe temporary filler injections.

It has long been presumed that consumers of cosmetic procedures and injectable products may have higher rates of body dysmorphia. A 2021 study suggests that addictive tendencies are evident among a significant percentage of patients undergoing more than one minimally invasive cosmetic procedure. While concerning, the prevalence of these tendencies in the overall

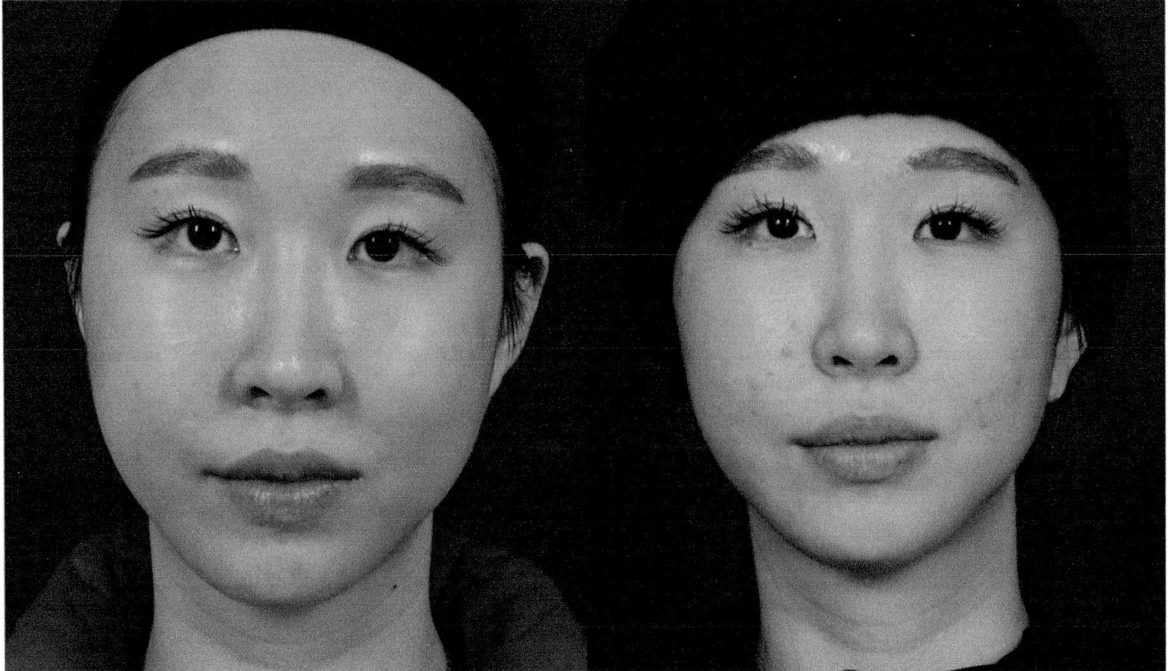

Fig. 4.8 Patient overfilled from dermal filler treatment performed in South Korea *(left)*. Dissolved with 240 units of Hylenex *(right)*. (Photo courtesy of Sue Ellen Cox, MD).

population is unclear. Further, a study specifically examining women undergoing neurotoxin or temporary filler injection did not demonstrate an association with body dysmorphia. While additional evidence is clearly needed to better delineate the relationship between filler injections and body dysmorphia, injectors should remain vigilant and continue to screen all patients for body dysmorphia or possible addiction to cosmetic procedures. Perhaps most relevant to injectors is the natural tendency of patients to demonstrate "Perception Drift," whereby correcting the patient's initial concerns (e.g., augmenting the mid-face with filler injection) establishes a new baseline appearance for the patient and allows previously ignored concerns (e.g., lip volume loss) to become more apparent.

CONCLUSIONS

Temporary fillers have evolved substantially since their initial introduction to the modern cosmetic market. The numerous products now available allow experienced injectors to address a plethora of aesthetic concerns. There is mounting evidence supporting their safety, efficacy, and overall impact. Experience remains vital to obtaining reproducible and satisfying results. Although the advantages of temporary filler overwhelmingly outweigh the disadvantages, limitations remain. The best results can be obtained by integrating temporary fillers into a complementary arsenal of other treatments, including neurotoxins, light and energy-based devices, as well as surgical procedures.

FURTHER READING

Plastic Surgery Statistics Report. (2018). In: Surgeons ASoP, ed. www.plasticsurgery.org. ASPS National Clearinghouse of Plastic Surgery Procedural Statistics.

Alam, M., Hughart, R., Geisler, A., et al. (2018). Effectiveness of low doses of hyaluronidase to remove hyaluronic acid filler nodules: a randomized clinical trial. *JAMA Dermatol*, *154*(7), 765–772.

Alam, M., Kakar, R., Dover, J. S., et al. (2021). Rates of vascular occlusion associated with using needles vs cannulas for filler injection. *JAMA Dermatol.*, *157*(2), 174–180.

Braz, A., & Eduardo, C. C. P. (2020). The facial shapes in planning the treatment with injectable fillers. *Indian J Plast Surg.*, *53*(2), 230–243.

Cohen, J. L., Biesman, B. S., Dayan, S. H., et al. (2015). Treatment of hyaluronic acid filler-induced impending necrosis with hyaluronidase: consensus recommendations. *Aesthet Surg J.*, *35*(7), 844–849.

de Aquino, M. S., Haddad, A., & Ferreira, L. M. (2013). Assessment of quality of life in patients who underwent minimally invasive cosmetic procedures. *Aesthetic Plast Surg.*, *37*(3), 497–503.

Duracinsky, M., Leclercq, P., Herrmann, S., et al. (2014). Safety of poly-L-lactic acid (New-Fill®) in the treatment of facial lipoatrophy: a large observational study among HIV-positive patients. *BMC Infect Dis.*, *14*, 474.

Durairaj, K. K., Devgan, L., Lee Bs, A., et al. (2020). Poly-L-lactic acid for gluteal augmentation found to be safe and effective in retrospective clinical review of 60 patients. *Dermatol Surg.*, *46*(suppl 1), S46–S53.

Goldie, K., Peeters, W., Alghoul, M., et al. (2018). Global consensus guidelines for the injection of diluted and hyperdiluted calcium hydroxylapatite for skin tightening. *Dermatol Surg.*, *44*(suppl 1), S32–S41.

Gordon, R. A., Crosnoe, R., & Wang, X. (2013). Physical attractiveness and the accumulation of social and human capital in adolescence and young adulthood: assets and distractions. *Monogr Soc Res Child Dev.*, *78*(6), 1–137.

Graivier, M. H., Bass, L. M., Lorenc, Z. P., Fitzgerald, R., Goldberg, D. J., & Lemperle, G. (2018). Differentiating nonpermanent injectable fillers: prevention and treatment of filler complications. *Aesthetic Surg J.*, *38*(suppl_1), S29–S40.

Hilton, S., Sattler, G., Berg, A. K., Samuelson, U., & Wong, C. (2018). Randomized, evaluator-blinded study comparing safety and effect of two hyaluronic acid gels for lips enhancement. *Dermatol Surg.*, *44*(2), 261–269.

Jiang, B., Ramirez, M., Ranjit-Reeves, R., Baumann, L., & Woodward, J. (2019). Noncollagen dermal fillers: a summary of the clinical trials used for their FDA approval. *Dermatol Surg.*, *45*(12), 1585–1596.

Kontis, T. C., & Rivkin, A. (2009). The history of injectable facial fillers. *Facial Plast Surg.*, *25*(2), 67–72.

Moradi, A., Shirazi, A., & David, R. (2019). Nonsurgical chin and jawline augmentation using calcium hydroxylapatite and hyaluronic acid fillers. *Facial Plast Surg.*, *35*(2), 140–148.

Povolotskiy, R., Oleck, N., Hatzis, C., & Paskhover, B. (2018). Adverse events associated with aesthetic dermal fillers: a 10-year retrospective study of FDA data. *Am J Cosmetic Surg.*, *35*(3), 143–151.

Rayess, H. M., Svider, P. F., Hanba, C., et al. (2018). A cross-sectional analysis of adverse events and litigation for injectable fillers. *JAMA Facial Plast Surg.*, *20*(3), 207–214.

Rullan, P. P., Olson, R., & Lee, K. C. (2020). The use of intralesional sodium thiosulfate to dissolve facial nodules from calcium hydroxylapatite. *Dermatol Surg.*, *46*(10), 1366–1368.

Scharschmidt, D., Preiß, S., Brähler, E., Fischer, T., & Borkenhagen, A. (2017). Body experience and self-esteem after minimally invasive skin rejuvenation: study of female patients using botulinum toxin A and/or dermal fillers. *Hautarzt.*, *68*(12), 959–967.

Shah, P., Rangel, L. K., Geronemus, R. G., & Rieder, E. A. (2021). Cosmetic procedure use as a type of substance-related disorder. *J Am Acad Dermatol.*, *84*(1), 86–91.

Sivek, R., & Emer, J. (2014). Use of a blunt-tipped microcannula for soft tissue filler injection in the treatment of linear scleroderma (en coup de sabre). *Dermatol Surg.*, *40*(12), 1439–1441.

Sola, C. A., & Fabi, S. G. (2019). Perception drift. *Dermatol Surg.*, *45*(12), 1747–1748.

Vanaman Wilson, M. J., Jones, I. T., Butterwick, K., & Fabi, S. G. (2018). Role of nonsurgical chin augmentation in full face rejuvenation: a review and our experience. *Dermatol Surg.*, *44*(7), 985–993.

van Rozelaar, L., Kadouch, J. A., Duyndam, D. A., Nieuwkerk, P. T., Lutgendorff, F., & Karim, R. B. (2014). Semipermanent filler treatment of HIV-positive patients with facial lipoatrophy: long-term follow-up evaluating MR imaging and quality of life. *Aesthet Surg J.*, *34*(1), 118–132.

5

Restylane Filler Product Family

Margo Lederhandler and Rhoda S. Narins

SUMMARY AND KEY FEATURES

- The Restylane filler family is a safe, reliable class of injectable fillers that have low potential for allergic response.
- These fillers are not permanent and thus ideal to use for treatment-naïve patients and for injectors of all levels because they can be easily dissolved with hyaluronidase.
- The type of injection technique selected should be based on anatomic site and on injector skill.
- Common areas for injection include the cheeks, followed by the nasolabial folds, chin, and lips. More advanced injection sites on the face include the infraorbital hollows, temples, and jawline, and nonfacial areas include the neck, décolletage, dorsal hands, earlobes, and body sites of unwanted laxity such as upper inner arms and knees.
- Optimal depth of filler placement, which varies by site and goals of correction, and amount of volume replacement required are the key components to consider prior to product selection.
- Restylane family fillers can be layered on top of each other or on top of other semipermanent fillers.
- Hyaluronic acid (HA) fillers can last from 3 to 18 months or longer, depending on location and amount of product previously injected; they last for longer in areas of low mobility and shorter in areas of greater movement.
- Postoperative sequelae, namely, edema and bruising, commonly last only a few days.
- Cannulas can be used to inject HA fillers and result in decreased bruising as well as decreased risk of occlusion.

INTRODUCTION

The use of an exogenous material to augment soft tissue can be traced back to Neuber in 1893, who used fat transplanted from the arms to correct facial defects. Since that time, substances used to volumize the face have changed rapidly and include both biodegradable and nonbiodegradable products. The Restylane family is a class of nonpermanent, biodegradable fillers with an average duration of action of 6 to 12 months, with demonstrated effect up to 18 months or longer at certain sites. This chapter will review the current Restylane products available in the US marketplace and provide injection tips for the most common facial areas injected. Patient preparation, potential complications, as well as advice on how to manage patient expectations will be discussed.

BACKGROUND

Restylane injectable fillers are commonly used to correct moderate to severe facial lines, restore volume loss that occurs during the natural course of aging, and augment natural volume to achieve desired cosmesis. Since the US Food and Drug Administration (FDA) approval of Restylane in December 2003, the Restylane injectable market has continued to expand, along with the hyaluronic acid (HA) filler market in general. According to the American Society for Dermatologic Surgery (ASDS), there were approximately 1.6 million soft tissue filler injections performed in 2019 alone by ASDS members, which represents an increase in 78% over the last 8 years. This does not include procedures performed by plastic surgeons or other aesthetic practitioners. Moreover, the recent COVID-19 pandemic has led to an even larger boom in injectables, in light of increased work from home and video conferencing. When it comes to filler selection, knowing where to place these fillers is as important as understanding the subtle differences between their rheologic and physicochemical properties. In general, Restylane injectables are safe, confer a soft look, are predictable in their volumizing capacity, and, crucially, are easily reversible with hyaluronidase.

BASIC SCIENCE

HA, or hyaluronan, is an anionic, hydrophilic, nonsulfated glycosaminoglycan that is abundant in human connective tissue. As one of the chief components of the extracellular matrix, HA stabilizes intercellular structures and forms part of the fluid matrix in which collagen and elastic fibers become embedded. With age, HA concentration in the skin decreases, resulting in reduced dermal hydration, which manifests as an increase in lines and folds. In addition, excessive exposure to ultraviolet B rays causes cells in the dermis to stop producing HA. In its natural form, HA has a half-life of 1 to 2 days and is metabolized by the liver to carbon dioxide and water. As a compound, it can absorb up to 1000 times its molecular weight in water; its mechanism of action as a filler is mainly through hydration. In a large immunogenicity study, nonanimal stabilized HA (NASHA) products did not elicit cellular or humoral responses in 98% of participants, suggesting that these products are not commonly allergenic or immunogenic. However, hypersensitivity reactions have rarely been reported, such as acute angioedema within minutes after injection of HA filler in the lips.

There are several important factors, known as the rheologic and physicochemical properties, in the formulation of HA filler products that determine how the product will function (Table 5.1). The HA molecule is stabilized with cross-linked hydroxyl groups. It is this cross-linking that confers longevity and mechanical strength to the product in the skin. Cross-linking and concentration of HA are key in determining the filler's rheologic properties—elastic modulus (G'), viscous modulus (G''), tan δ (G''/G'), and complex modulus (G^*)—and physicochemical properties—gel fluid uptake (or swelling factor [SwF]) and gel cohesion. Briefly, G' represents the ability of the filler to rebound to its original shape when acted on by dynamic forces, with a higher G' typically signifying a firmer product. G'' represents the filler's viscosity or resistance to dynamic forces, whereby a higher G'' gel is often thicker and requires more force to eject. Tan δ (G''/G') is the proportion of viscosity to elasticity. G^* represents the ability of the filler to resist deformation, which for most HA fillers is comparable to G'. SwF is a marker of gel hydration status, or how much the gel will expand when binding water, whereby a gel with higher SwF is further from equilibrium and will take up more fluid after injection. SwF is not to be confused with tissue swelling. Lastly, gel cohesion represents the filler's dissociation rate, such that a highly cohesive gel dissociates less readily and has

TABLE 5.1 Rheologic and Physicochemical Properties of Restylane Filler Products

Product trade name	HA (mg/mL)	G′	G″	Tan δ	G* (Pa)	SwF (mL/g)
Restylane Refyne	20	47	7	0.16	48	9.7
Restylane Kysse	20	156	12	0.07	156	7.2
Restylane Defyne	20	260	16	0.06	260	6.4
Restylane Silk	20	344	79	0.23	353	2.7
Restylane	20	544	99	0.18	553	2.8
Restylane Lyft	20	545	69	0.13	549	2.8

G' is elastic modulus; G'', viscous modulus; tan δ, G''/G'; and G^*, complex modulus.
HA, Hyaluronic acid, *SwF*, swelling factor.

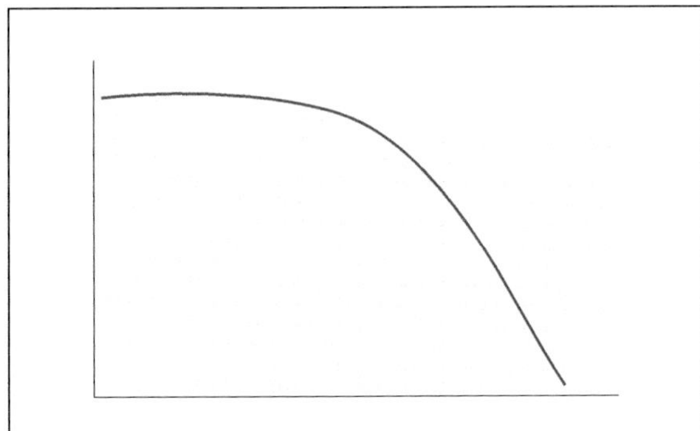

Fig. 5.1 Conceptual degradation curve of nonanimal stabilized hyaluronic acid fillers. Note that the line is not linear, which correlates to the cross-linking agents used to stabilize the filler in the skin. Free hyaluronic acid has a half-life of 1 to 2 days in human skin.

greater ability to lift. Table 5.1 delineates the rheologic and physicochemical properties of all of the Restylane products available in the US marketplace. An understanding of these properties, discussed in greater depth in Chapter 4, is crucial for the injector in product selection, as certain products are better suited than others when it comes to anatomic site and depth of placement.

Owing to the structural matrix of HA filler products, the degradation curve of implanted HA is not linear. Rather, the product retains its effect until the structural complex around the HA molecule is broken down. Once the unbound HA is exposed, efficacy is then lost (Fig. 5.1). As a result, patients will often suddenly notice a change in their appearance rather than experience a gradual loss over time. In addition, patients sometimes feel they look worse after HA injection than they did prior to it; however, this is more of a function of selective memory. For this reason, taking preinjection photographs is important. As with natural hyaluronan, HA fillers can be quickly dissolved with the enzyme hyaluronidase in the case of adverse events or unwanted filler. It has been demonstrated that filler products with greater number of HA cross-linking bonds and greater concentration of HA take longer to dissolve with hyaluronidase.

CHOOSING THE RIGHT RESTYLANE FILLER PRODUCT

The Restylane filler family is divided into two classes based on HA cross-linking technology, NASHAs and XpresHAn. The NASHAs include Restylane, Restylane-L, Restylane Lyft, and Restylane Silk. The XpresHAn products on the US market include Restylane Refyne and Restylane Defyne. The main difference between commercially available Restylane products on the current US market is the firmness, or G′, of the product, and SwF. The NASHAs have a higher G′ and lower SwF compared with the XpresHAn products, which have relatively lower G′ and higher SwF. The higher the G′, the more firm, less elastic, stiffer the product and the longer it lasts in tissue (Table 5.1). The NASHAs' higher G′ enables greater lift and they are therefore often injected at deeper planes (subcutaneous and supraperiosteal), whereas the XpresHAn products, with their lower G′, have greater SwF and greater cohesivity. It is postulated that higher cohesivity gels have greater intradermal integration. Lower G′ products, as they are softer, are more often indicated for more superficial injection planes and can be layered on top of higher G′ products. Lower G′ fillers can also be placed in deeper planes, although greater quantity is required to achieve the desired effect.

When selecting a Restylane product based on anatomic location, the authors have several recommendations (Table 5.2). For areas necessitating greater correction or lift, such as along zygomatic and malar cheeks, jawline, and temples, the authors prefer higher G′ products, such as Restylane Lyft or Restylane-L. Restylane-L may also be used with great results for lip augmentation, and in a patient desiring a cost effective, one-syringe treatment of multiple sites, Restylane-L is a great option. For lip augmentation where greater support is desired, Restylane-L is the authors' preferred filler. However, for a softer, generally plumper lip, Restylane Kysse is a wonderful option. The authors rarely use Restylane Silk with Restylane Kysse now on the market.

For the infraorbital hollows that necessitate greater correction, the authors often choose Restylane-L, with optimal placement in the supraperiosteal plane. The greater G′ of Restylane-L enables more lift here. For patients with infraorbital hollows that are less deep, or when the superficial skin has a thin appearance, a lower G′ product, such as Restylane Refyne, is a nice choice due to better dermal integration. However, this product has greater swell factor; therefore, caution in not overcorrecting should be taken. Incorrect product selection, incorrect technique of filler placement, filler migration, and blockage of lymphatic drainage, among other reasons can all lead to unwanted effects in this

TABLE 5.2 **US Restylane Filler Product Indications and Author Recommendations**

Product trade name	US product indicated injection sites and depth	Authors' tips and pearls
Restylane Defyne	• Moderate to severe, deep facial wrinkles and folds, such as nasolabial folds (mid-to-deep dermis) • Chin augmentation (subcutaneous and/or supraperiosteal)	• The authors like to use this product to correct nasolabial folds and marionette lines and augment the chin.
Restylane Kysse	• Lip augmentation (submucosal) • Correction of upper perioral rhytids and philtral column (mid-dermis to subcutaneous)	• The authors find this product to be very natural looking and ideal for lip augmentation and perioral correction.
Restylane	• Moderate to severe facial wrinkles and folds, such as nasolabial folds (mid-to-deep dermis) • Lip augmentation (submucosal)	• As Restylane is now formulated with lidocaine (Restylane-L), the authors do not use this product much anymore.
Restylane-L	• Moderate to severe facial wrinkles and folds, such as nasolabial folds (mid-to-deep dermis) • Lip augmentation (submucosal)	• This is a great "all-around" filler for the patient who prefers to purchase one syringe for multiple sites. • This is a nice product for the infraorbital hollow.
Restylane Lyft	• Moderate to severe facial folds and wrinkles, such as nasolabial folds (deep dermis to superficial subcutis) • Cheek augmentation and correction of age-related midface contour deficiencies (subcutaneous to supraperiosteal) • Volume deficit in dorsal hand (subcutaneous)	• The authors love this product for areas necessitating greater correction such as cheeks, temples, jawline, chin, severe nasolabial folds, and dorsal hand.
Restylane Refyne	• Moderate to severe facial wrinkles and folds, such as nasolabial folds (mid-to-deep dermis)	• This is a great, soft product that integrates well and is ideal in areas of thin skin or for shallower folds. • The authors like this for the nasolabial folds. • Some providers also like this product for the infraorbital hollows; however, caution should be taken due to swell factor. • This is an ideal product for layering in the superficial planes above filler placed more deeply.
Restylane Silk	• Lip augmentation (submucosal) • Correction of upper perioral rhytids and philtral column (mid-to-deep dermis)	• The authors do not use Restylane Silk much anymore since the advent of Restylane Kysse.

All products are premixed with lidocaine, except for Restylane.

sensitive area, which, to the less advanced injector's eye, may be difficult to recognize as filler complications. With Restylane-L in this region, the injector should be aware that because this is a particle filler, when the product metabolizes several years after placement, the product imbibes a lot of water and some patients may experience superficial edema. If this occurs, the product should be dissolved with hyaluronidase and, if the patient desires, new filler may be placed in the appropriate plane.

For correction of moderate to deep wrinkles and folds, such as nasolabial folds and marionette lines, the authors like Restylane Defyne, as this intermediate G′ product integrates well into the dermis and is not evident upon facial animation. Restylane-L, although not the ideal choice here, may be used in the patient who desires cost effectiveness and minimal syringe number. Restylane Defyne was recently FDA approved for chin augmentation, and the authors like this product, as well as the higher G′ products, Restylane Lyft and Restylane-L, for the chin. For correction of mild to moderate degree nasolabial folds and marionette lines, or other fine lines, Restylane Refyne works quite well due to the lower G′ and dermal integration.

Additionally, it should be noted that not all of the HA in a given filler is cross-linked. Some is free, fragmented, or only lightly cross-linked so that the gel can actually flow out of the syringe with ease. As discussed previously, the cross-linking is what confers longevity to the product, and this does vary within and between brands. In addition to cross-linking, it is worth mentioning that not all HA products are packaged in the fully hydrated state. Due to SwF, volume is created via hydration, and for this reason, patients will often look better or more filled 24 hours after treatment with products like Restylane, which are not completely saturated in the syringe. With that in mind, it is prudent not to overcorrect when using Restylane products.

PATIENT EVALUATION

Prior to injection with any filler, a careful patient history should be obtained. Pertinent items to note in this history include a history of herpes simplex virus, pregnancy or breastfeeding, history of keloid formation, presence of any autoimmune disease, and allergy to lidocaine because most of the fillers now come premixed with lidocaine. A medication history should include use of multivitamins, fish oil, vitamin E, blood thinners, aspirin, ibuprofen, and *Gingko biloba* because all of these can predispose the patient to bruising. Unless medically necessary, the patient should be advised to discontinue these medications 14 days prior to treatment. In addition, alcohol use within 48 hours of injection can cause an increase in bruising tendency. The authors recommended that patients avoid dental procedures 2 weeks prior to and after obtaining filler.

With the recent COVID-19 pandemic and advent of novel vaccines, new data have come to light concerning vaccine side effects as related to injectable filler. In the Moderna mRNA-1273 vaccine trial, 3 subjects out of 15,184 who received at least one dose of the vaccine developed facial or lip swelling in areas of injectable filler placement, while this did not occur for any subjects in the placebo group. The ASDS has released guidance on SARS-CoV-2 mRNA vaccine side effects in injectable filler patients and recommend that patients already treated with fillers should not be discouraged or precluded from receiving vaccines of any kind. Similarly, patients who have had vaccines should not be precluded from receiving injectable fillers in the future. These injectable filler vaccine-related adverse events are rare, temporary, and often responsive to oral corticosteroids and intralesional hyaluronidase and have seen a success in case reports with oral angiotensin-converting enzyme (ACE) inhibitors such as lisinopril. The authors recommend similar timing with regard to getting the SARS-CoV-2 mRNA vaccine as with dental procedures, waiting 2 weeks on either end of filler placement to obtain the vaccine, and most importantly, counseling the patient on this possible side effect so they know to return promptly to the office if this occurs.

If the patient has had fillers in the past, it is recommended that the physician document how long ago, where the fillers were placed, and if the patient was satisfied with the results. Additionally, the prior filler administered should be noted. Adverse reactions have been described in case reports of patients and in murine models where different consecutive fillers were injected at the same site. In addition to history, preinjection photography is a must. These authors prefer at least three views: frontal and left and right side at an oblique angle. If a patient is having a specific area corrected, a close-up picture of that area is also advisable. Informed consent must be obtained, and the patient should be aware of the financial cost of the procedure prior to opening the first syringe. We also advise that baseline facial asymmetry be discussed with the patient and noted in the chart. From a physician standpoint, it is important to inform your malpractice coverage carrier of your intention to use fillers because many uses are considered off-label.

PATIENT PREPARATION

Patients should be asked to remove their makeup, and the areas to be injected should be cleansed with alcohol or a skin-cleansing solution that does not stain the skin, such as chlorhexidine, which is highly effective. However, chlorhexidine can have severe consequences because it is ototoxic and toxic to the cornea, even with inadvertent minimal splash exposure. If injecting near the eye or ear, povidone-iodine is the preferred antiseptic and is both safe and effective. If there are any areas of infection, injection should be deferred. If the area is to be marked, these authors recommend using a white eyeliner pencil, an erasable marker, or povidone-iodine. Use of gentian violet can create a tattoo if the needle is inserted through the marked line. Patients should be in a seated or semireclined position to maximize comfort, while allowing the skin to drape naturally. It is not advisable to have the patient lie down because this can distort the natural contours of the face. Hair should be pulled back with a headband or covered and pulled back with a surgical bonnet. The physician may decide to use a topical or local anesthetic prior to injection. If a topical anesthetic is used, this should be completely removed prior to injection and the area cleansed. Depending on the topical anesthetic and duration of application, hyperemia of the skin can occur and may lead to increased bleeding at injection sites.

In this time of COVID, the authors ask patients to remove their mask for full facial evaluation and also treatment. Even if just treating parts of the face, for example the temples, the authors find it important to view the entire face for ideal balance when injecting filler. Of course, the injector must feel comfortable, and we recommend wearing appropriate personal protective equipment.

> **PEARL 1** If using a custom-formulated topical anesthetic, such as Betacaine Lidocaine Tetracaine (BLT), be sure to monitor the amount of surface area that is covered with the medication because toxicity can result with high concentrations of anesthetic over large surface areas.

PHYSICIAN PREPARATION

A note that includes a detailed facial diagram is helpful to document precisely where filler is placed, and labels from each syringe used should be put in the patient chart for traceability. One should also anticipate adverse events, so we recommend that any physician who is using Restylane products carry hyaluronidase in case of intraarterial occlusion or if the product needs to be dissolved rapidly, nitropaste in the event of purple dusky discoloration upon injection, and juice and crackers in the event a patient has a vasovagal episode. An emergency plan of action should be in place, especially if occlusion happens in an area that could affect vision. If the decision is made to use a topical numbing medication prior to injection, topical steroids should also be kept on hand in the event of an allergic contact reaction. Lastly, it is helpful to have aluminum chloride at concentrations of 20% or higher available in the event of excessive bleeding at a needle insertion point, although most bleeding can be stopped with pressure alone.

INJECTION TECHNIQUES

Several injection techniques exist for the addition of HA fillers to the face and depend mainly on the area of the face that is to be augmented. Table 5.3 delineates the recommended injection techniques by facial area and Chapter 32 of this book discusses filler injection techniques in detail.

> **PEARL 2** The injection technique should vary according to the region of the face, the depth and tissue plane of the injection, and also on the rheologic and physicochemical properties of the Restylane filler being used. Although fanning and cross-hatching provide excellent structural support and enhance volume, they can lead to increased bruising. Similarly, the serial puncture technique allows for more precise microdroplet placement of filler but can be painful for the patient. A blunt-tipped cannula minimizes bruising, pain, and edema and decreases vascular occlusion risk (Video 5.1).

TABLE 5.3 Recommended Injection Technique by Facial Area

Area	Technique[a]
Nasolabial folds	Serial puncture, threading, fanning, or cross-hatching
Marionette lines	Fanning, cross-hatching, or depot
Jawline and jowls (prejowl sulcus and chin)	Serial puncture, depot, or linear threading
Cheeks	Fanning, depot, or cross-hatching
Lips—vermilion border	Linear threading
Lips—tubercles	Serial puncture

[a]Sharp needle or blunt-tipped cannula may be used in any location.

SITE-SPECIFIC TREATMENT STRATEGIES

Nasolabial Folds

Correction of the nasolabial fold is an FDA-approved on-label indication for the majority of Restylane filler products and is the most common site for correction with Restylane fillers. It is important when assessing the nasolabial fold to note the presence or absence of a heavy cheek. If the cheek has dropped substantially, or if the patient is overweight with substantial contribution to the fold from the inferomedial cheek, the fold will be very deep and several syringes of Restylane product will be required before a noticeable result is achieved. If this is the case, consider volumizing the cheek in the area of the zygoma prior to any filler in the fold. This will result in an overall lifting and pulling of the skin back to its original physiologic position. For the deep fold itself, the cross-hatch technique is the best one to use, or one may consider layering a Restylane product over another product that is placed in deeper tissue (e.g., Restylane Refyne over Restylane Lyft). For shallow to medium folds, Restylane-L, Restylane Refyne, or Restylane Defyne (depending on depth) alone can suffice and the fanning technique can be used, starting at the inferior pole. In this case, cheek augmentation is not necessary. Whether to start from the superior or inferior portion of the pole is a matter of physician preference. At the completion of injection, place a gloved thumb on top of the fold and two fingers on the inside of the mouth on the other side of the fold. Gently mold the product to make sure that no nodules or bumps are present. HA fillers are malleable and can be molded after injection.

It is important to remember basic anatomy when injecting the nasolabial folds. The nasal artery runs near the ala, so it is critical when injecting the superior portion of the nasolabial fold that one pulls back on the syringe plunger to make sure no flash of blood is seen. Injecting slowly with small aliquots or the use of a cannula helps to avoid accidental intraarterial injection. The authors typically prefer the use of a cannula in this location for that very reason.

PEARL 3 If you see multiple lines lateral to the nasolabial fold, resist the urge to fill them because they are usually due to dynamic movement. Filling each line may improve their appearance at rest, but they will appear as cords upon animation, unless a low G′ product such as Restylane Defyne is used.

Marionette Lines

With time, the area below the oral commissure hollows, pulls down the corners of the mouth, creating marionette lines, and contributes to jowls. The loss of volume is due to structural bone changes that occur with age; principally, as a person ages, the maxilla and chin grow away from the face and bone resorption decreases maxillary and mandibular height. Along with skin laxity, the result is a sagging appearance of the lower face that responds well to filler use. This location is especially susceptible to bruising after filler injection, and it is important to massage the area after injection to prevent lumps. Because of the need for structural support, the fanning or cross-hatch technique is recommended, as is the use of an intermediate G′ product that integrates well into the dermis, such as Restylane Defyne, or for greater correction, Restylane Lyft or Restylane-L. Typically, 0.5 mL is adequate to volumize each infraoral hollow, although larger amounts are needed to volumize the lower face.

PEARL 4 Although most patients can tolerate injection into the nasolabial folds, the marionette lines tend to be more sensitive. Consider a mental nerve block, which will anesthetize not only this area but also portions of the lower lip. Use 0.2 mL of plain lidocaine 1% and inject in the sulcus next to the second premolar. This injection pain can be reduced with a 15-s application of benzocaine 20% (Hurricane gel) to the mucosa prior to injection.

Jowls

Fat and soft tissue descent along the mandible obscures the bony definition of the jaw, which is considered a hallmark of the youthful face. HA fillers can be used to fill in the prejowl sulcus, thereby minimizing the appearance of the jowls. Filler is placed directly against the mandible and molded in a downward sweeping motion with the fingers around the jawline. The best technique to use for this is either a depot or linear threading. Placement of filler in the jowl area not only gives the illusion of a stronger bone line but also creates a relative tucking of the excess skin in the submental area. Caution should be taken not to masculinize the jaw by squaring the shape in a woman. Restylane Lyft is recommended for this treatment.

PEARL 5 In elderly patients, the mental nerve is particularly exposed in this area of the face because it is covered only by thin platysma and skin. Therefore, to prevent nerve injury from the needle tip, be sure to stay in the upper subcutaneous or dermis, which is higher than in other parts of the face, owing to the thin skin in the jowl area.

Cheeks

With age, the orbicularis oculi muscle loses both its tone and ability to act as a sling around the orbital rim. Subsequently, descent of the orbicularis and malar soft tissue complex prevails. Aging of the midface is dominated by descent of these malar fat pads, resulting in a loss of convexity and a flattened or even concave appearance of the cheeks. Filling the cheeks may result in softening of the nasolabial folds but requires injection in a deep subcutaneous or fascial plane. If using Restylane products, more than one syringe may be needed. It is important when injecting in this area that the patient be asked to smile so that the physician does not inadvertently create a chipmunk appearance in the patient. It is important to fan or cross-hatch injections and blend the cheeks back toward the temple so that the person does not appear to have implants at rest.

Anatomically one must keep in mind bony structure and face shape as related to race and gender. It is also important to have a discussion with the patient with regard to the hollow below the zygoma because many people want fuller cheeks but do not want to lose this line of definition on the face. Layering filler in this area is successful, as is use of more viscous HA products.

Infraorbital Region

The tear trough or infraorbital hollow is a special area most responsive to a HA filler. Small aliquots are placed deeply below the orbicularis muscle, along the orbital rim with a linear threading technique. For the infraorbital hollows that necessitate greater correction, the authors often choose Restylane-L, with optimal placement in the supraperiosteal plane. The greater G′ of Restylane-L enables more lift here. For patients with infraorbital hollows that are less deep, or the superficial skin has a thin appearance, a lower G′ product, such as Restylane Refyne, is preferable due to better dermal integration. Care must be taken not to overfill this area because it may lead to eyelid edema and nodularity. Postinjection SwF can also lead to lymphatic obstruction.

PEARL 6 Although it is possible to fill the cheeks through an intraoral approach, caution should be used, owing to the resident bacteria present in oral flora. A biofilm can be created, which can lead to severe complications. These authors recommend a transcutaneous approach when using HA or any other filler products.

Lips

By the second decade of life, lip volume has reached full thickness in both men and women and starts decreasing by the mid-30s. In addition to the lips themselves, the vermilion border tends to thin, the corners of the mouth begin to slope downward, and fine lines appear on the upper and lower cutaneous lip, which over time elicit the complaint of "lipstick bleeding." The philtral ridge should not be overlooked either because this flattens with the elongation of the cutaneous upper lip. Keep in mind that the philtral ridge is not a vertical ridge but rather angles slightly toward the columella from each apex of the cupid's bow, so restoration should be shaped accordingly. Injection of the lips is a staged process and is preferably performed with Restylane Kysse rather than the more viscous HA products, although Restylane-L is also commonly used. Prior to Restylane Kysse approval, Restylane Silk was commonly used here. A recent study comparing Restylane Kysse to Juvederm Volbella found that significantly less Restylane Kysse product was needed to obtain the same results, subject satisfaction, and duration of treatment.

An infraorbital nerve block and mental nerve block may be considered for patient comfort, but it should be noted that it is important to work quickly after these blocks because the numbing will distort the position of the patient's lips. In addition, expect significant swelling, and more bleeding and bruising in this area than in other parts of the face, which can cause a physician to overcorrect one area in response to edema rather than actual volume change. It is important to note any baseline asymmetry in the lips, as well as the presence of any scars, which can make filling more difficult. Lip injections of HA are placed in three planes: (1) volume filling submucosal within the lip muscle, (2) linear threading of the vermillion line, and (3) superficial injection of rhytides. The vermillion injection gives contour, shape, and lift to the lip. Identify the white roll at the border of the lip, and, starting at the corner of the mouth, Insert the needle and use a linear-threading technique to inject into the white roll in an anterograde fashion. Repeat on the other side, making sure to fill to the apex of cupi"s bow. Great caution should be taken not to breach the vermilion border or to overfill the border, as doing so can lead to the unwanted duck-lip appearance. After crisping of the vermilion border (which by default will evert the lip and create the appearance of fullness), consider a droplet injection into each of the two tubercles of the upper and lower lips to give a more pronounced pout.

It is important to note that the natural lip ratio varies with ethnicities. In White people, the lower lip is naturally fuller than the upper lip, with an ideal ratio of upper lip to lower lip being 1:1.6, which is based on the concept of the Fibonacci proportion. In skin of color, on the other hand, the upper lip and lower lip are usually of similar proportion. This should be discussed with the patient so that, once filling of the upper lip is complete, the patient understands if some product should be added to the lower lip to maintain the ideal ratio. Although it is important to inform patients of the traditional ratios and offer expert guidance, with today's social media-heavy culture, injectors should be aware of current trends that patients may desire which can break the traditional proportion norms.

POSTTREATMENT CARE AND COMPLICATION MANAGEMENT

In general, Restylane fillers are safe, effective, and easy to use. Complications are generally limited to edema and bruising. After injection, patients are advised to ice the area for up to 10 minutes in every hour. Reusable ice packs can be given to the patient, or they can use a bag of frozen peas, which is easy to mold over the area. In the lips, patients are encouraged not to purse their lips or fold them on top of each other, which may cause product movement in the first 6 hours. For lip augmentation, the authors often give 20 to 30 mg of oral prednisone for the patient to take either that day or the following morning to reduce swelling. The following day, patients are advised to expect additional edema as hydration occurs. This may result in a feeling of soreness, which can be relieved with acetaminophen. Bruising can occur up to 72 hours after treatment. Anecdotally, *Arnica forte* can be used to prevent bruising, but no definitive evidence exists to suggest that this is always successful. The Tyndall effect is possible if the product is placed too superficially, as are nodules or lumps. The only way to correct this is to dissolve the product with hyaluronidase, keeping in mind that this will deplete some native HA in the epidermal matrix as well. Repeat injection should be delayed for 1 week after use of hyaluronidase. Other complications, such as vascular occlusion and nodules, are possible but rare. Extra care is needed for injections of the nose, glabella, and forehead, where the risk of intraarterial injection is high and cases of blindness have been reported. In the case of intraarterial occlusion, Restylane fillers are quite easy to dissolve with hyaluronidase. A multidisciplinary task force for the ASDS recently published evidence-based guidelines for the prevention and treatment of adverse events with injectable filler.

If an entire syringe of product is not used on a patient, some physicians store the product at room temperature or in the refrigerator for up to 6 months, carefully labeling the product with the patient's name. Because a physician cannot guarantee sterility of the product after it has been injected, we do not recommend this approach. However, if one is to do so, the authors recommend uncapping the used needle, expressing any gel remaining in the hub, and replacing either the original cap or a new needle prior to storage to minimize any chance of growth of skin flora from the used needle tip.

CONCLUSIONS

The Restylane family of injectable fillers is a great choice for injectors of all levels and for treatment of all patients. The range of products available in the marketplace is fairly diverse and, once implanted, creates reproducible results with ease. Additionally, Restylane products are more cost effective than some of the other HA fillers available on the US market. The success of these fillers is as dependent on the injectable as it is on the injector and proper technique.

FURTHER READING

American Society for Dermatologic Surgery Survey on DermatolAmerican Society for Dermatologic Surgery Survey on Dermatologic Procedures. Report of 2019 Procedures. December 2020.

Alam, M., Kakar, R., Dover, J. S., et al. (2021). rates of vascular occlusion associated with using needles vs cannulas for filler injection. *JAMA Dermatol.*, *157*(2), 174–180.

Avram, M., Bertucci, V., Cox, S., Jones, D., & Mariwalla, K. (2020). *Guidance Regarding SARS-CoV-2 mRNA Vaccine Side Effects in Dermal Filler Patients.* https://www.asds.net/Portals/0/PDF/secure/ASDS-SARS-CoV-2-Vaccine-Guidance.pdf.

Bachmann, F., Erdmann, R., Hartmann, V., Becker-Wegerich, P., Wiest, L., & Rzany, B. (2011). Adverse reactions caused by consecutive injections of different fillers in the same facial region: risk assessment based on the results from the Injectable Filler Safety study. *J Eur Acad Dermatol Venereol.*, *25*(8), 902–912.

Bellew, S. G., Carroll, K. C., Weiss, M. A., & Weiss, R. A. (2005). Sterility of stored nonanimal, stabilized hyaluronic acid gel syringes after patient injection. *J Am Acad Dermatol.*, *52*(6), 988–990.

Brody, H. J. (2005). Use of hyaluronidase in the treatment of granulomatous hyaluronic acid reactions or unwanted hyaluronic acid misplacement. *Dermatol Surg.*, *31*(8 pt 1), 893–897.

Carruthers, A., Carey, W., De Lorenzi, C., Remington, K., Schachter, D., & Sapra, S. (2005). Randomized, double-blind comparison of the efficacy of two hyaluronic acid derivatives, Restylane perlane and hylaform, in the treatment of nasolabial folds. *Dermatol Surg.*, *31*(11 pt 2), 1591–1598. discussion 1598.

Carruthers, J., & Carruthers, A. (2003). A prospective, randomized, parallel group study analyzing the effect of BTX-A (Botox) and nonanimal sourced hyaluronic acid (NASHA, Restylane) in combination compared with NASHA (Restylane) alone in severe glabellar rhytides in adult female subjects: treatment of severe glabellar rhytides with a hyaluronic acid derivative compared with the derivative and BTX-A. *Dermatol Surg.*, *29*(8), 802–809.

Cohen, J. L. (2008). Understanding, avoiding, and managing dermal filler complications. *Dermatol Surg.*, *34*(suppl 1), S92–S99.

Day, D. J., Littler, C. M., Swift, R. W., & Gottlieb, S. (2004). The wrinkle severity rating scale: a validation study. *Am J Clin Dermatol.*, *5*(1), 49–52.

Edsman, K., Nord, L. I., Ohrlund, A., Larkner, H., & Kenne, A. H. (2012). Gel properties of hyaluronic acid dermal fillers. *Dermatol Surg.*, *38*(7 pt 2), 1170–1179.

Fagien, S., Bertucci, V., von Grote, E., & Mashburn, J. H. (2019). Rheologic and physicochemical properties used to differentiate injectable hyaluronic acid filler products. *Plast Reconstr Surg.*, *143*(4), 707e–720e.

Flynn, T. C., Sarazin, D., Bezzola, A., Terrani, C., & Micheels, P. (2011). Comparative histology of intradermal implantation of mono and biphasic hyaluronic acid fillers. *Dermatol Surg.*, *37*(5), 637–643.

Hamilton, R. G., Strobos, J., & Adkinson, N. F., Jr. (2007). Immunogenicity studies of cosmetically administered nonanimal-stabilized hyaluronic acid particles. *Dermatol Surg.*, *33*(suppl 2), S176–S185.

Hanke, C. W., Rohrich, R. J., Busso, M., et al. (2011). Facial soft-tissue fillers conference: assessing the state of the science. *J Am Acad Dermatol.*, *64*(4 suppl), S66–S85. e61–136.

Hexsel, D., Soirefmann, M., Porto, M. D., Siega, C., Schilling-Souza, J., & Brum, C. (2012). Double-blind, randomized, controlled clinical trial to compare safety and efficacy of a metallic cannula with that of a standard needle for soft tissue augmentation of the nasolabial folds. *Dermatol Surg.*, *38*(2), 207–214.

Hilton, S., Sattler, G., Berg, A. K., Samuelson, U., & Wong, C. (2018). Randomized, evaluator-blinded study comparing safety and effect of two hyaluronic acid gels for lips enhancement. *Dermatol Surg.*, *44*(2), 261–269.

Hirsch, R. J., Cohen, J. L., & Carruthers, J. D. (2007). Successful management of an unusual presentation of impending necrosis following a hyaluronic acid injection embolus and a proposed algorithm for management with hyaluronidase. *Dermatol Surg.*, *33*(3), 357–360.

Jones, D. H., Fitzgerald, R., Cox, S. E., et al. (2021). Preventing and treating adverse events of injectable fillers: evidence-based recommendations from the American Society for Dermatologic Surgery Multidisciplinary Task Force. *Dermatol Surg.*, *47*(2), 214–226.

Juhasz, M. L. W., Levin, M. K., & Marmur, E. S. (2017). The kinetics of reversible hyaluronic acid filler injection treated with hyaluronidase. *Dermatol Surg.*, *43*(6), 841–847.

Kablik, J., Monheit, G. D., Yu, L., Chang, G., & Gershkovich, J. (2009). Comparative physical properties of hyaluronic acid dermal fillers. *Dermatol Surg.*, *35*(suppl 1), 302–312.

Lederhandler, M. B. D., Anolik, R., & Geronemus, R. G. (2021). The rise and fall of the pale puffy lower eyelid pillow. *J Drugs Dermatol.*, *20*(4), 475–476.

Leonhardt, J. M., Lawrence, N., & Narins, R. S. (2005). Angioedema acute hypersensitivity reaction to injectable hyaluronic acid. *Dermatol Surg.*, *31*(5), 577–579.

Lorenc, Z. P., Ohrlund, A., & Edsman, K. (2017). Factors affecting the rheological measurement of hyaluronic acid gel fillers. *J Drugs Dermatol.*, *16*(9), 876–882.

Lupo, M. P., Smith, S. R., Thomas, J. A., Murphy, D. K., & Beddingfield, F. C., III. (2008). Effectiveness of Juvederm Ultra Plus dermal filler in the treatment of severe nasolabial folds. *Plast Reconstr Surg.*, *121*(1), 289–297.

Matarasso, S. L., Carruthers, J. D., Jewell, M. L., & Restylane, Consensus G. (2006). Consensus recommendations for soft-tissue augmentation with nonanimal stabilized hyaluronic acid (Restylane). *Plast Reconstr Surg.*, *117*(3 suppl), 3S–34S.

Monheit, G. D., Baumann, L. S., Gold, M. H., et al. (2010). Novel hyaluronic acid dermal filler: dermal gel extra physical properties and clinical outcomes. *Dermatol Surg.*, *36*(suppl 3), 1833–1841.

Munavalli, G. G., Knutsen-Larson, S., Lupo, M. P., & Geronemus, R. G. (2021). Oral angiotensin-converting enzyme inhibitors for treatment of delayed inflammatory reaction to dermal hyaluronic acid fillers following COVID-19 vaccination—a model for inhibition of angiotensin II-induced cutaneous inflammation. *JAAD Case Rep., 10*, 63–68.

Narins, R. S., & Bowman, P. H. (2005). Injectable skin fillers. *Clin Plast Surg., 32*(2), 151–162.

Narins, R. S., Brandt, F. S., Dayan, S. H., & Hornfeldt, C. S. (2011). Persistence of nasolabial fold correction with a hyaluronic acid dermal filler with retreatment: results of an 18-month extension study. *Dermatol Surg., 37*(5), 644–650.

Narins, R. S., Coleman, W. P., 3rd, Donofrio, L. M., et al. (2010). Improvement in nasolabial folds with a hyaluronic acid filler using a cohesive polydensified matrix technology: results from an 18-month open-label extension trial. *Dermatol Surg., 36*(suppl 3), 1800–1808.

Narins, R. S., Jewell, M., Rubin, M., Cohen, J., & Strobos, J. (2006). Clinical conference: management of rare events following dermal fillers–focal necrosis and angry red bumps. *Dermatol Surg., 32*(3), 426–434.

Nayfeh, T., Shah, S., Malandris, K., et al. (2021). A systematic review supporting the American Society for Dermatologic Surgery guidelines on the prevention and treatment of adverse events of injectable fillers. *Dermatol Surg., 47*(2), 227–234.

Ohrlund, J. A., & Edsman, K. L. (2015). The myth of the "biphasic" hyaluronic acid filler. *Dermatol Surg., 41*(suppl 1), S358–S364.

Solish, N., Bertucci, V., Percec, I., Wagner, T., Nogueira, A., & Mashburn, J. (2019). Dynamics of hyaluronic acid fillers formulated to maintain natural facial expression. *J Cosmet Dermatol., 18*(3), 738–746.

Sorensen, E. P., & Council, M. L. (2020). Update in soft-tissue filler—associated blindness. *Dermatol Surg., 46*(5), 671–677.

Steinsapir, K. D., & Woodward, J. A. (2017). Chlorhexidine keratitis: safety of chlorhexidine as a facial antiseptic. *Dermatol Surg., 43*(1), 1–6.

Stocks, D., Sundaram, H., Michaels, J., Durrani, M. J., Wortzman, M. S., & Nelson, D. B. (2011). Rheological evaluation of the physical properties of hyaluronic acid dermal fillers. *J Drugs Dermatol., 10*(9), 974–980.

Tran, C., Carraux, P., Micheels, P., Kaya, G., & Salomon, D. (2014). In vivo bio-integration of three hyaluronic acid fillers in human skin: a histological study. *Dermatology., 228*(1), 47–54.

6

Juvéderm Family

Rohit Kakar, Laurel M. Morton, and Nowell Solish

SUMMARY AND KEY FEATURES

- The Juvéderm family of fillers comprises a collection of commercially available hyaluronic acid fillers that utilize proprietary cross-linking technology designated as Hylacross and Vycross.
- The Hylacross collection includes Juvéderm Ultra and Juvéderm Ultra Plus.
- The Hylacross fillers are homogenous smooth gels distinguished by their adequate lifting capacity and durability.
- The Vycross collection includes Juvéderm Voluma, Juvéderm Vollure, Juvéderm Volbella, Juvéderm Volite, and Juvéderm Volux.
- The Vycross fillers are homogenous smooth gels characterized by their improved duration, host tissue integration, and malleability.
- Vycross fillers have been reported to result in rare inflammatory reactions weeks to years following injection.

INTRODUCTION

Hyaluronic acid (HA) dermal fillers are primarily utilized to enhance facial anatomy and correct volume deficits that predominantly result from facial aging. In general, HA fillers are effective, safe, and reversible, resulting in widespread usage globally. Over 84% of the 2.7 million soft tissue injections performed in 2019 were HA based. Of these injections, the Juvéderm family of HA fillers are the most broadly used, commercially available HA products in the world. They represent advancements in proprietary cross-linking technology that provide varying degrees of smoothness, lift, and moldability. This chapter will discuss the defining biophysical characteristics and clinical utility of each Juvéderm filler currently available, which include Juvéderm Ultra, Juvéderm Ultra Plus, Voluma, Vollure, Volbella, Volite, and Volux.

THE JUVÉDERM FAMILY OF FILLERS

Hylacross and Vycross Technology

The first Juvéderm HA filler was approved in Europe and Canada in 2000 and by the US Food and Drug Administration (FDA) in 2006. The HA is derived from *Streptococcus equi* bacteria and does not contain animal proteins. A proprietary cross-linking technology, designated Hylacross, was employed to generate a smooth homogenous product using a higher concentration of HA (24 mg/mL) and a greater duration of effect than other products available at the time of release (Fig. 6.1). The high concentration and high cohesivity of these agents resulted in increased durability and lifting capacity, respectively. The HA used is predominantly high-molecular- weight HA. Compared to the technology used by the Restylane products, Hylacross agents are comprised of cross-linked HA that is produced as monophasic

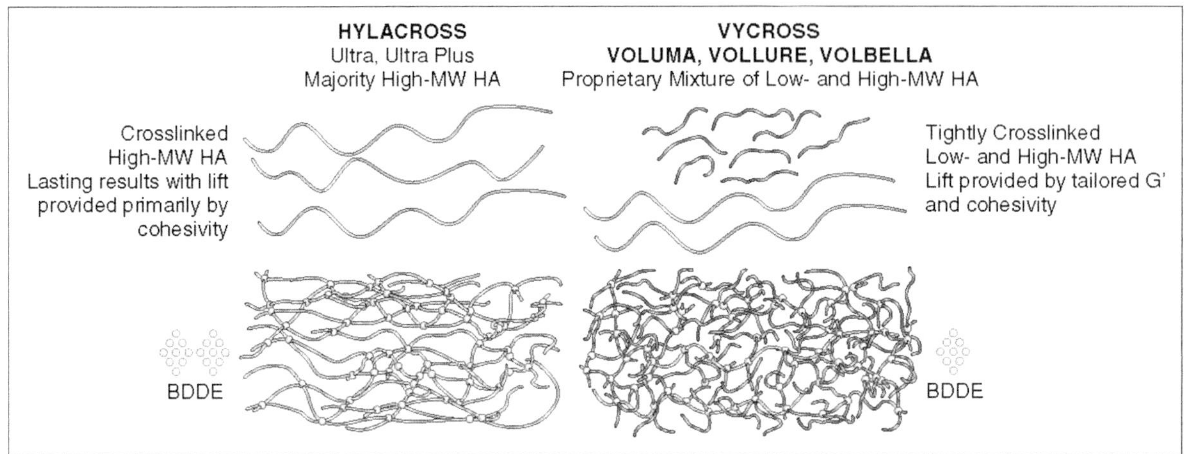

Fig. 6.1 Crosslinking of Hylacross and Vycross.

gels and are not passed through sizing screens/sieves. As a result, the Hylacross products are not as granular in consistency as the Restylane products, which can be visualized when magnified. Currently, two Hylacross formulations are commercially available: Juvéderm Ultra and Juvéderm Ultra Plus, which are differentiated only by their cross-linking (6% vs. 8%, respectively). These products are more hydrophilic than the Vycross products.

The Vycross collection of fillers utilize a different technology to blend high- and low-molecular-weight HA to produce a more efficiently cross-linked and smooth homogeneous gel that balances cohesivity and G′. The cross-linking agent, 1,4-butanediol diglycidyl, allows for more efficient and tight binding using a lower HA concentration, which results in improved duration (resistance to degradation) and less swelling due to less space being available for water uptake. With optimization of gel properties, different Vycross products can be used for different planes of injection, anatomic location, and specific indications. In addition, compared to Hylacross fillers, the lower cohesivity of the Vycross agents allows for malleability. The Vycross collection of fillers includes Juvéderm Voluma (20 mg/mL), Juvéderm Vollure (17.5 mg/mL), Juvéderm Volbella (15 mg/mL), Juvéderm Volite (12 mg/mL), and Juvéderm Volux (25 mg/mL). With this range of products and their individual properties, an injector may employ the entire Vycross platform to tailor the lift and spread to address treatment needs.

Each product within the Juvéderm family of fillers is noncytotoxic, nonirritant, nontoxic, nonsensitizing, sterile, biodegradable, nonpyrogenic, viscoelastic, clear, and colorless.

Hylacross: Juvéderm Ultra and Juvéderm Ultra Plus

The original formulation of Juvéderm was FDA approved in 2006 for the treatment of facial wrinkles and folds. Thereafter, an additional clinical trial revealed that the effects of one treatment may endure for up to 12 months, resulting in a label extension by the FDA in 2007. In 2010, the XC Juvéderm products, which contain 0.3% lidocaine, received FDA approval. Most recently, FDA approval for lips was granted in October 2015. Currently, the Hylacross products commercially available include Juvéderm Ultra and Juvéderm Ultra Plus, both with an HA concentration of 24 mg/mL, but differing percentages of cross-linking (6% vs. 8%, respectively). They are both available in XC formulations, where the added lidocaine does not appear to affect rheology but improves patient comfort (Table 6.1).

Juvéderm Ultra XC is available in a 1.0-mL syringe packaged with a 30-gauge needle. It has a G′ of 207 Pa and a cohesivity of 97 gmf. The duration of effect is up to 9 months. It is best suited for moderate depressions/wrinkles and lip definition. In the authors' experience, Juvéderm Ultra XC's softer consistency allows for its utility in a variety of anatomic sites, especially periorally, at the nasolabial fold, and within the lips (Fig. 6.2). When treating nasolabial folds, the authors have found that patients often return for reinjection before the 12-month duration reported.

TABLE 6.1 **Indications and Rheologic Properties of Hyaluronic Acid Dermal Fillers**

Filler	Indication	HA Concentration	G′ (@ 5 Hz, Pa)	Cohesivity (gmf)
Juvéderm Ultra XC	Filling any medium-sized depressions of the skin via mid-dermis injection, as well as for lip definition	24 mg/mL	207	97
Juvéderm Ultra Plus XC	Mid and/or deep depression of the skin via mid and/or deep dermis injection, as well as for lip definition and enhancement	24 mg/mL	244	108
JuvédermVolux	Restore and create volume of the face	25 mg/mL	665	93
Juvéderm Voluma XC	Restore volume of face	20 mg/mL	353	35
Juvéderm Vollure with lidocaine	Treatment of nasolabial folds	17.5 mg/mL	317	24
Juvéderm Volbella with lidocaine	Enhancement of the lips and perioral lines	15 mg/mL	274	18
Juvéderm Volite	Filling of fine lines and for the improvement of skin quality	12 mg/mL	166	12

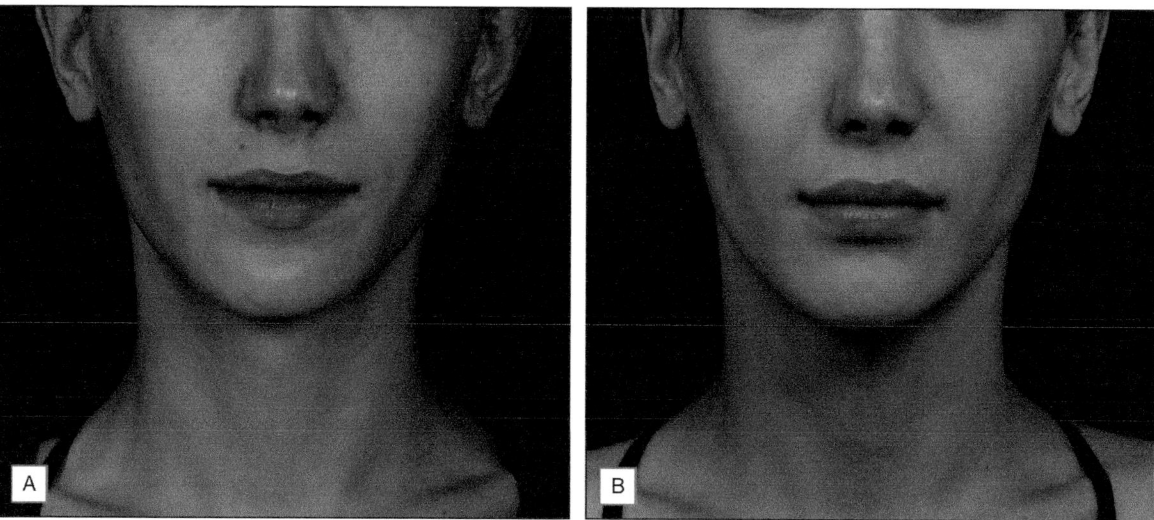

Fig. 6.2 A young woman treated in the lips with Juvéderm Ultra and Juvéderm Voluma in the cheeks, chin, and mandible. (A) Image of patient prior to treatment. (B) Image of patient following treatment.

Juvéderm Ultra Plus XC is also available in a 1.0-mL syringe, packaged with a 27-gauge needle. The product has a G′ of 244 and a cohesivity of 108 gmf. The effective duration is up to 12 months. Juvéderm Ultra Plus XC is best used for correction of mid-to-deep depressions, addition of volume, lip definition, and lip enhancement. Compared to Juvéderm Ultra XC, the authors have found Juvéderm Ultra Plus XC to be useful where there exists slightly more volume loss and additional lift is needed.

PEARL 1 Although delayed hypersensitivity reactions have been reported with Vycross fillers, the entirety of the collection provides the ability to lift, volumize, and improve skin appearance at varying anatomical sites and planes with improved duration and reduced swelling.

Vycross: Juvéderm Voluma, Vollure, Volbella, Volite, and Volux

Juvéderm Voluma. Juvéderm Voluma was the first Vycross product released, receiving FDA approval for correction of midfacial volume deficit (MVD) in October 2013. The pivotal multicenter, single-blind, randomized controlled trial demonstrated both good outcomes and safety profiles. It later received FDA approval for chin augmentation in June 2020. The formulation consists of an HA concentration of 20 mg/mL, G′ of 353, a cohesivity of 35 gmf, and water uptake of 227%. It is commercially available in 1.0-mL syringes packaged with a 27-gauge needle. It may also be used with a 25-gauge needle or cannula.

With the aforementioned properties, Voluma's foremost utility lies in its ability to provide structural volume. As its FDA approved indication suggests, it is especially useful for treating volume loss in the midface. The medial, malar, and apex portions of the cheek are suitable zones of treatment with Voluma, but gender considerations should always be taken into account (Video 6.1). Further, in the authors' experience, treatment of these areas also appears to address nasolabial folds by providing lift. In general, when injecting Voluma, it is typically best to inject subcutaneously and supraperiosteally so as to avoid visibility of the product. In addition, it is advisable to assess the patient in different positions as one is injecting (oblique, profile, head tilting down) so as to create naturally appearing contours and avoid a "done" appearance.

Voluma may also be used to enhance structural support to the chin, as evidenced by its most recent FDA approval. A significant amount of product may be needed to achieve the desired aesthetic result and one must also be mindful of the gender considerations inherent to treating this area. Further, although not FDA approved, Voluma has been used at the angle of the jaw and along the jawline in both genders. By providing projection and definition to the chin and jaw, a more youthful appearance to the lower face is achievable.

When compared to the Hylacross fillers, the lower cohesivity, good integration into host tissue, decreased water uptake, and extended duration distinguish Voluma. The lower cohesivity allows for high initial malleability, and the high HA concentration combined with the tighter crosslinking decreases water uptake, which results in minimal postinjection swelling following product deposition. Therefore, the product can be molded, yet maintain a high lift capacity that is not temporarily altered after injection. In addition, Voluma appears to easily integrate into host tissue, resulting in a more natural aesthetic result during movement (Fig. 6.3). The higher crosslinking and high HA concentration contribute to Voluma's long duration of approximately 2 years; however, the authors have found that patients typically return for retreatment before the 2-year mark.

Following Voluma's introduction, blending of the product with plain lidocaine was performed by some clinicians to adjust its use to different applications, which possibly resulted in the impetus to develop Vollure and Volbella. Via blending, HA concentration can affect the properties of the filler, resulting in a softer, less elastic, and less viscous agent that does not produce as much lift and may enhance tissue integration. However, following the introduction of other Vycross products, this practice is no longer as common.

Juvéderm Vollure. Juvéderm Vollure contains an HA concentration of 17.5 mg/mL, a G′ of 317 Pa, and a cohesivity of 24 gmf. In 2017, it received FDA approval for the treatment of moderate to severe facial wrinkles and folds with a duration up to 18 months. It is indicated for injection into the deep dermis or subdermally. Several studies have demonstrated Vollure's safety, efficacy, and subject satisfaction in the treatment of nasolabial folds. It is commercially available in 1.0-mL syringes that are packaged with a 30-gauge needle.

In the authors' experience, and as indicated by the aforementioned studies, Vollure is a particularly effective product for improving the perioral region. It can be used to provide support to both the upper and lower perioral regions, softening the nasolabial folds and marionettes and restoring structure to atrophic areas created by aging. Vollure is similarly suitable for gentle improvement of deeper lines of the cheek and forehead. The authors have also utilized the product for lip definition and enhancement, contouring of the nasal dorsum and tip, forehead/brow volumization, and restoration of earlobe structure in proximity to perforations created from piercing.

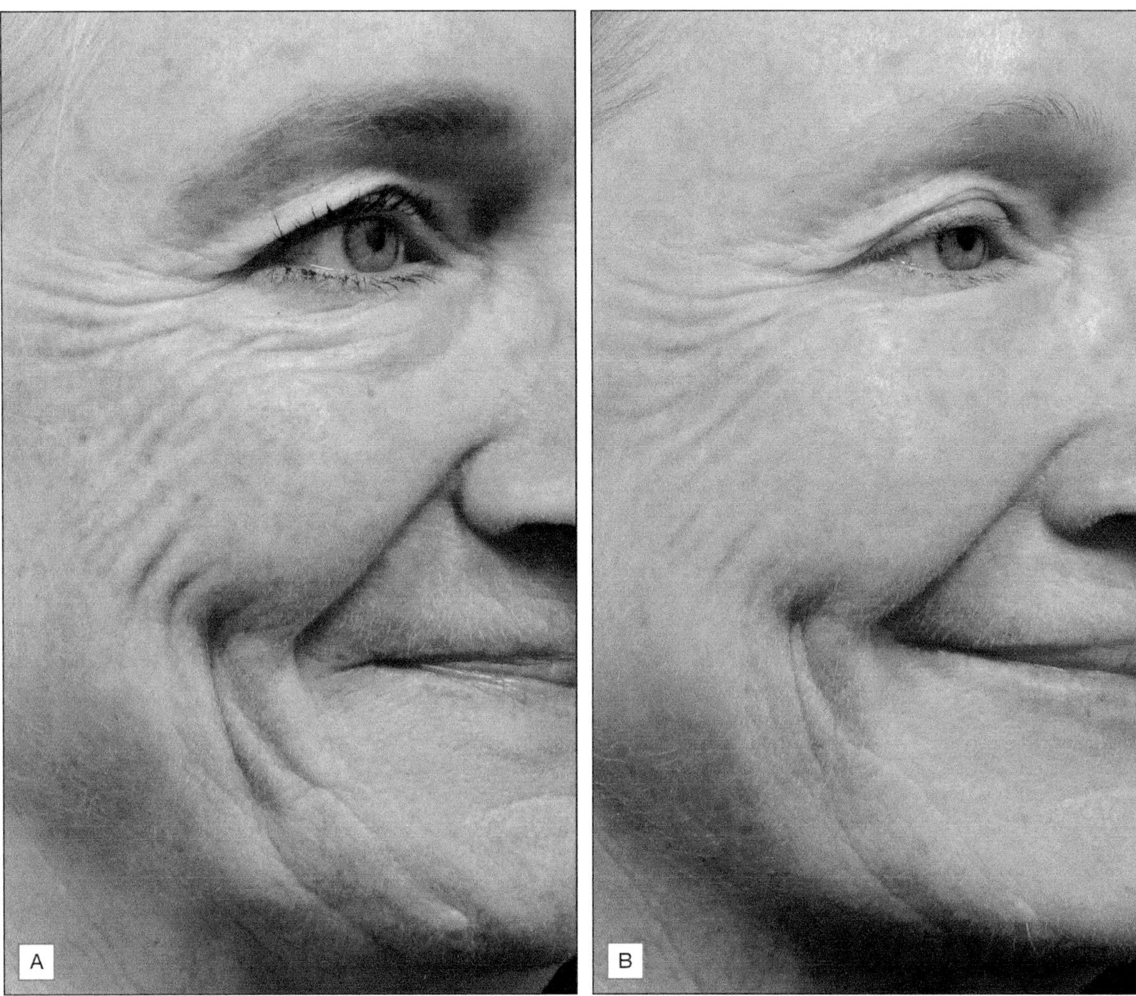

Fig. 6.3 A female patient treated with Voluma is shown in animation in both the before (A) and after (B) photographs to demonstrate the natural appearance of this correction and improvement in skin quality.

> **PEARL 2** Juvéderm Voluma is an excellent volumizer that can provide lift and structure to tissue.
> Juvéderm Vollure is more appropriate for filling of deeper lines and lip definition. Juvéderm Volbella is best suited for treating finer lines and creating softer volumization, especially periorally.

Juvéderm Volbella. Juvéderm Volbella is a soft product with a HA concentration of 12 mg/mL, a G′ of 274 Pa, and a cohesivity of 18 gmf. It received FDA approval in 2016 for enhancement of the lips and perioral lines. Volbella is recommended for injection into the superficial or mid-dermis, lip mucosa, or submuscular/preperiosteal layer. It is commercially available in 0.55-mL and 1.0-mL syringes that are packaged with 30-gauge and 32-gauge needles. Volbella lasts for approximately 9 to 12 months.

Volbella's utility primarily resides in its ability to improve the lower face. In particular, it can provide subtle enhancement and hydration to the lips, by softly rejuvenating and plumping without much adding considerable lift or volumization (Videos 6.2 and 6.3). Volbella is also able to spread and integrate well, making it useful for softening perioral lines as well as other superficial lines on the face, including the glabella, forehead, lateral canthus, cheek, and neck (Fig. 6.4).

Juvéderm Volite. Juvéderm Volite is a newer HA filler with a HA concentration of 12.0 mg/mL, a G′ of 166 Pa,

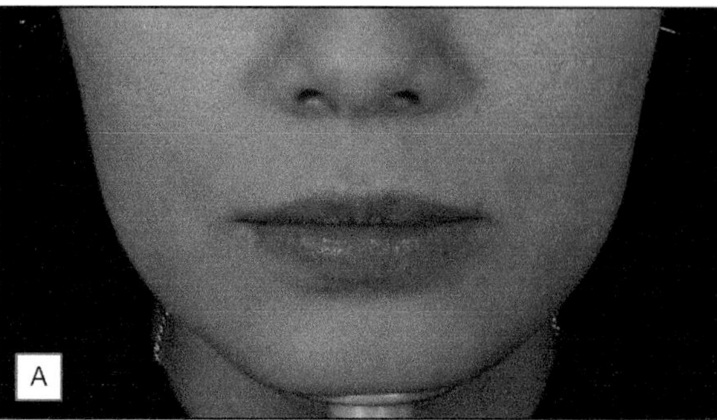

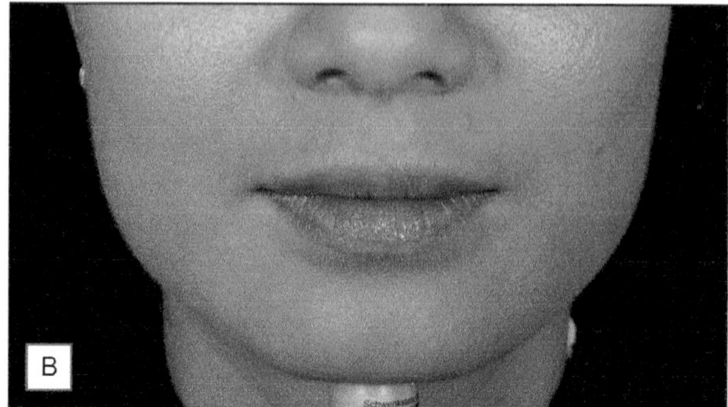

Fig. 6.4 Juvéderm Volbella and Vollure used in conjunction to treat the lips for an optimal aesthetic result. (A) Image of patient prior to treatment. (B) Image of patient following treatment.

and a cohesivity of 12 gmf. It launched in 2017 in Europe as a filler for superficial cutaneous depressions (fine lines) and for the improvement of skin quality characteristics, such as elasticity and hydration. Although not yet approved for use in the United States, it is commercially available in Europe and Canada in 1.0-mL syringes that are packaged with 32 G needles.

Several published studies have demonstrated Volite's efficacy. Through analysis of digital photography, Cavallini et al. objectively established Volite's ability to visibly better skin texture. Similarly, Niforos et al. found improvements in responder ratings of skin deformation, hydration, and smoothness as well as fine lines following two to three treatments with median total volumes of 3.9 mL at the initial and 2.6 mL at repeat treatment(s). Nakab et al. has possibly substantiated these findings via observation of improvements in skin quality biomarkers following injection of the product into living human explants. Specifically, increases in collagen density, fibrillin-1 AQP3 expression, and acidic glycosaminoglycan content were identified.

A recent expert panel of 12 international clinicians assembled by Allergan has established consensus guidelines for patient selection, injection technique, anatomic treatment regions, and pre-/postinjection management recommendations based on experience with Volite. When selecting patients, it was advised Volite would be most suitable for patients with early signs of aging, lower grade acne scarring, dry skin, and younger patients with mild photodamage and concerns about skin appearance. However, it was noted that most patients can typically expect improvements in skin appearance regardless of age, sex, or ethnicity following injection. The panel advised when treating patients with Volite that the product be administered via microdepot injections into the deep dermis generally with 0.5 cm to 1.0 cm spacing, but this may be customized based on patient's degree of roughness, photodamage, and rhytides. The target areas of injection were identified as the malar, perioral, neck, and décolletage based on skin characteristics. Although the consensus did not include the forehead due to its unique sebaceous properties, the investigators state that clinical data have demonstrated utility for Volite's use in the treatment of forehead lines. The authors have found the product is also useful for mild tear trough correction as well as superficial perioral and periocular lines.

Juvéderm Volux. Juvéderm Volux is the latest addition to the Vycross collection. It was launched in Europe in 2019 as a product for restoring and volumizing the face, particularly the chin and jaw area, for up to 18 to 24 months. Volux has a HA concentration of 25.0 mg/mL, a G' of 665 Pa, and a cohesivity of 93 gmf. Implantation depth is advised at the subcutaneous or supraperiosteal planes. Although not yet approved for use in the United States, it is commercially available in Europe and Canada in 1.0-mL syringes that are packaged with 27 G needles.

With a significantly high G' and high cohesivity, Volux has excellent lifting capacity. Two pivotal trials have indicated that Volux is safe and effective for restoration of the chin and jaw with improvements in chin projection and subject satisfaction. The total median treatment volumes were 2.28 mL and 3.43 mL in the individual studies. Both studies found significant changes in the glabella-subnasal pogonion angle and satisfaction scores.

PEARL 3 Juvéderm Volite is best used for improving skin quality and texture. Juvéderm Volux has the highest G′ and cohesivity of all the Vycross agents, making it excellent for volumizing the chin and jawline.

ADVERSE EVENTS: IDENTIFICATION, MANAGEMENT, AND AVOIDANCE

Although Hylacross and Vycross products have been used for over a decade with a relatively good safety profile, avoiding and managing adverse events related to filler is paramount for all injectors utilizing these injectables. While possible with any dermal filler and less commonly with Hylacross products, delayed inflammatory nodule formation following the use of Vycross products, in particular, has been reported in the literature and observed anecdotally by the authors. However, these occurrences appear uncommon as a recent chart reviews of Voluma-related delayed adverse events (DAEs) and of Volbella-related DAEs both found incidence rates of 1% per patient.

Common side effects of injection include erythema, edema, ecchymoses, and nodules. Following injection, erythema and edema are expected and routine. The amount of edema can vary based on the filler type selected, instruments utilized, and injection technique employed. Nodules can be formed purposefully as a result of technique and then compressed to create specific aesthetic outcomes, but also unexpectedly.

Nodules that occur immediately or soon after placement are defined as immediate. Immediate nodules are commonly the result of accumulated filler, or less commonly migration, and typically present as a painless, nonvisible lump. Treatment typically consists of massage for redistribution or hyaluronidase. In contrast, nodules that occur more than 30 days after placement are considered to be DAEs. It appears that there are at least two different types of delayed nodules: painless small nodules called delayed-onset nodules and delayed or late inflammatory nodules that typically present as a tender nodule, cyst, or plaque, months to years after injection.

Delayed-onset nodules respond to a combination of monthly hyaluronidase and intralesional corticosteroids over several months. The cause remains unknown.

The etiology of DAEs appears multifactorial but is not yet clear. Currently, an immunologic stimulus prior to the presentation of a DAE appears involved, such as a flu-like or bacterial illness, dental procedure, pregnancy, or increased personal stress. Further, a seasonal variation has been noted with an increased frequency between October and January, which is typically cold and flu season. In addition, the composition of Vycross itself may play a role as the presence and/or physiologic degradation of low-molecular-weight HA into intermediate- sized fragments are proinflammatory. Other evidence suggests that contaminants introduced during the manufacturing of low-molecular-weight HA may be responsible for this proinflammatory effect. Beyond this, a bacterial infection or formation of a biofilm have also been implicated. Biofilms result in a low grade infection resistant to antibiotics and the immune system.

The authors have found several effective treatment options when a DAE occurs. These include a 5- to 14-day course of systemic corticosteroids, often 30 mg of prednisone once-daily in the morning. Intralesional triamcinolone may also be injected. An antibiotic, such as doxycycline or clarithromycin, can be added as well. It is important to note that higher doses of hyaluronidase are required to break down Vycross products due to greater cross-linking. If the nodule is fluctuant, incision and drainage may be needed to obtain cultures and antibiotic sensitivities. Of note, in the aforementioned chart review of DAEs occurring with Voluma, some resolved with no intervention in approximately 6 weeks; thus, watchful waiting may be considered. In addition, nodule formation was not a contraindication to future retreatment with Vycross products in these patients.

As with all injectables, prevention of adverse events is key. We strongly encourage maintaining a properly antiseptic injection environment to reduce bacterial contamination from *Cutibacterium acnes* or other skin-surface bacteria. The authors advise appropriately cleansing the skin with alcohol or surgical scrub. In addition, some practitioners consider it prudent to avoid injection within 2 weeks of dental work, upper respiratory tract infection, or vaccination.

PEARL 4 If a delayed inflammatory nodule develops, oral prednisone and/or intralesional triamcinolone are effective treatment options. Hyaluronidase may also be used if recalcitrant to prednisone. Dosing of hyaluronidase may depend on degree of cross-linking.

CONCLUSIONS

With significant advances in cross-linking technology, the Juvéderm family of HA fillers are the most extensively utilized commercially available HA products worldwide. With smooth consistencies and efficacious outcomes, the Hylacross and Vycross fillers are able to provide results for nearly every age-related deficit. The Hylacross products, Juvéderm Ultra and Ultra Plus, have and continue to be used for treatment of the lips, nasolabial folds, and marionettes for approximately 15 years. The Vycross products are used to provide lift, volumize, and improve skin appearance in various regions of the face. For volumization and lift, Voluma or Volux may be most appropriate. If a softer lift is desired, especially periorally, Vollure would be the product of choice. Volbella can provide hydration and subtle plumping of the lips as well as delicate filling of lines, and if improvement in overall skin texture is desired, Volite may be useful. However, no matter the product used, all clinicians must be aware of the adverse events that can occur and how to appropriately avoid and manage these situations.

FURTHER READING

American Society of Plastic Surgeons. Cosmetic plastic surgery statistics: cosmetic procedure trends. (2019). https://www.plasticsurgery.org/documents/News/Statistics/2019/plastic-surgery-statistics-full-report-2019.pdf. Accessed February 28, 2021.

Baeva, L. F., Lyle, D. B., Rios, M., Langone, J. J., & Lightfoote, M. M. (2014). Different molecular weight hyaluronic acid effects on human macrophage interleukin 1b production. *Journal of Biomedical Materials Research Part A, 102*, 305–314.

Beleznay, K., Carruthers, J. D., Carruthers, A., Mummert, M. E., & Humphrey, S. (2015). Delayed-onset nodules secondary to a smooth cohesive 20 mg/mL hyaluronic acid filler: cause and management. *Dermatologic Surgery, 41*(8), 929–939.

Bhojani-Lynch, T. Late-onset inflammatory response to hyaluronic acid dermal fillers. *Plastic and Reconstructive Surgery Global Open, 5*, e1532.

Cavallini, M., Papagni, M., Ryder, T. J., & Patalano, M. (2019). Skin quality improvement with VYC-12, a new injectable hyaluronic acid: objective results using digital analysis. *Dermatologic Surgery, 45*(12), 1598–1604.

Christensen, L., Breiting, V., Bjarnsholt, T., et al. (2013). Bacterial infection as a likely cause of adverse reactions to polyacrylamide hydrogel fillers in cosmetic surgery. *Clinical Infectious Diseases, 56*, 1438–1444.

Dayan, S., Maas, C. S., Grimes, P. E., Beer, K., Monheit, G., Snow, S., Murphy, D. K., & Lin, V. (2020). Safety and effectiveness of VYC-17.5L for long-term correction of nasolabial folds. *Aesthetic Surgery Journal, 40*(7), 767–777.

Dong, Y., Arif, A., Olsson, M., et al. (2016). Endotoxin free hyaluronan and hyaluronan fragments do not stimulate TNF-a, interleukin-12 or upregulate co-stimulatory molecules in dendritic cells or macrophages. *Scientific Reports, 6*, 36928.

Eccleston, D., & Murphy, D. K. (2012). Juvéderm(®) Volbella™ in the perioral area: a 12-month prospective, multicenter, open-label study. *Clinical Cosmetic Investigation Dermatology, 5*, 167–172.

Goodman, G. J., Swift, A., & Remington, B. K. (2015). Current concepts in the use of Voluma, Volift, and Volbella. *Plastic Reconstructive Surgery, 136*(suppl 5), 139S–148S.

Humphrey, S., Jones, D. H., Carruthers, J. D., Carruthers, A., Beleznay, K., Wesley, N., Black, J. M., Vanderveen, S., & Minokadeh, A. (2020). Retrospective review of delayed adverse events secondary to treatment with a smooth, cohesive 20-mg/mL hyaluronic acid filler in 4500 patients. *Journal of the American Academy of Dermatology, 83*(1), 86–95.

Jiang, D., Liang, J., & Noble, P. W. (2011). Hyaluronan as an immune regulator in human diseases. *Physiological Reviews, 91*, 221–264.

Jones, D., & Murphy, D. K. (2013). Volumizing hyaluronic acid filler for midface volume deficit: 2-year results from a pivotal single-blind randomized controlled study. *Dermatologic Surgery, 39*, 1602–1611.

Jones, D., Tezel, A., & Borrell, M. (2010). In vitro resistance to degradation of hyaluronic acid dermal fillers by ovine testicular hyaluronidase. *Dermatologic Surgery, 36*, 804–809.

Juvéderm Ultra Directions for Use. (2016). Pringy France: Allergan Inc.

Juvéderm Ultra Plus Directions for Use. (2016). Pringy France: Allergan Inc.

Levy, P. M., De Boulle, K., & Raspaldo, H. (2009). A split-face comparison of a new hyaluronic acid facial filler containing pre-incorporated lidocaine versus a standard hyaluronic acid facial filler in the treatment of naso-labial folds. *Journal of Cosmetic and Laser Therapy, 11*(3), 169–173.

Lyle, D. B., Breger, J. C., Baeva, L. F., et al. (2010). Low molecular weight hyaluronic acid effects on murine macrophage nitric oxide production. *Journal of Biomedical Material Research Part A, 94*, 893–904.

Mansouri, Y., & Goldenberg, G. (2015). Update on hyaluronic acid fillers for facial rejuvenation. *Cutis, 96*(2), 85–88.

Monheit, G., Beer, K., Hardas, B., Grimes, P. E., Weichman, B. M., Lin, V., & Murphy, D. K. (2018). Safety and effectiveness of the hyaluronic acid dermal filler VYC-17.5L for nasolabial folds: results of a randomized, controlled study. *Dermatologic Surgery, 44*(5), 670–678.

Nakab, L., Hee, C.K., Guetta, O. Improvements in skin quality biological markers in skin explants using hyaluronic acid filler VYC-12L. *Plastic and Reconstructive Surgery Global Open*, *8*(3), e2723.

Niforos, F., Ogilvie, P., Cavallini, M., Leys, C., Chantrey, J., Safa, M., Abrams, S., Hopfinger, R., & Marx, A. (2019). VYC-12 injectable gel is safe and effective for improvement of facial skin topography: a prospective study. *Clinical, Cosmetic and Investigative Dermatology*, *12*, 791–798.

Ogilvie, P., Benouaiche, L., Philipp-Dormston, W. G., Belhaouari, L., Gaymans, F., Sattler, G., Harvey, C., & Schumacher, A. (2020). VYC-25L hyaluronic acid injectable gel is safe and effective for long-term restoration and creation of volume of the lower face. *Aesthetic Surgery Journal*, *40*(9). NP499–NP510.

Ogilvie, P., Sattler, G., Gaymans, F., Belhaouari, L., Weichman, B. M., Snow, S., Chawla, S., Abrams, S., & Schumacher, A. (2019). Safe, effective chin and jaw restoration with VYC-25L hyaluronic acid injectable gel. *Dermatologic Surgery*, *45*(10), 1294–1303.

Ogilvie, P., Thulesen, J., Leys, C., Sykianakis, D., Chantrey, J., Safa, M., Figueiredo, V., Heydenrych, I., Cavallini, M., Langeland, E. K., & Wetter, A. (2020). Expert consensus on injection technique and area-specific recommendations for the hyaluronic acid dermal Filler VYC-12L to treat fine cutaneous lines. *Clinical, Cosmetic and Investigative Dermatology*, *13*, 267–274.

Pinsky, M. A., Thomas, J. A., Murphy, D. K., et al. (2008). Juvederm vs. Zyplast Nasolabial Fold Study Group. Juvederm injectable gel: a multicenter, double-blind, randomized study of safety and effectiveness. *Aesthetic Surgery Journal*, *28*, 17–23.

Raspaldo, H., De Boulle, K., & Levy, P. M. (2010). Longevity of effects of hyaluronic acid plus lidocaine facial filler. *Journal of Cosmetic Dermatology*, *9*, 11–15.

Sadeghpour, M., Quatrano, N.A., Bonati, L.M., Arndt, K.A., Dover, J.S., Kaminer, MS. (2019). Delayed-onset nodules to differentially crosslinked hyaluronic acids: comparative incidence and risk assessment. *Dermatologic Surgery, 45*(8), 1085–1094.

Sattler, G., Philipp-Dormston, W. G., Van Den Elzen, H., Van Der Walt, C., Nathan, M., Kolodziejczyk, J., Kerson, G., & Dhillon, B. (2017). A prospective, open-label, observational, postmarket study evaluating VYC-17.5L for the correction of moderate to severe nasolabial folds over 12 months. *Dermatologic Surgery*, *43*, 238–245.

Shumate, G., Chopra, R., Jones, D., Messina, D. J., & Hee, C. K. (2018). In vivo degradation of crosslinked hyaluronic acid fillers by exogenous hyaluronidases. *Dermatologic Surgery*, *44*, 1075–1083.

Termeer, C., Benedix, F., Sleeman, J., et al. (2002). Oligosaccharides of hyaluronan activate dendritic cells via toll-like receptor 4. *Journal of Experimental Medicine*, *195*, 99–111.

Termeer, C. C., Hennies, J., Voith, U., et al. (2000). Oligosaccharides of hyaluronan are potent activators of dendritic cells. *Journal of Immunology*, *165*, 1863–1870.

7

The Belotero Family

Berthold Rzany

SUMMARY AND KEY FEATURES

- Belotero is a commonly used group of hyaluronic acid fillers.
- It is cross-linked with 1,4-butanediol diglycidyl ether (BDDE), forming a cohesive and polydensified matrix (CPM).
- There are several products of various thicknesses in the Belotero line, some with and others without lidocaine. These include Belotero Volume, Intense, Balance, and Soft.
- Good clinical data (e.g., data from at least one randomized controlled trial) have been published for Belotero Balance (formerly Belotero Basic) and Belotero Volume.
- In a 6-month study of nasolabial folds filling. Belotero Balance demonstrates at least a one-grade improvement at the end of the study.
- After treatment of the cheeks with Belotero Volume, about one half of the patients still showed at least a one-grade improvement after 18 months.
- The Belotero family of products has a good safety profile.

INTRODUCTION

Hyaluronic acid (HA)–based dermal fillers are currently the most popular, nonpermanent injectable materials available for the correction of age-related changes of the face for wrinkles, folds, and volume loss. HA fillers derive from bacterial fermentation from a specific *Streptococcus* strain (*Streptococcus equi*), a bacterium nonpathogenic in humans. Because natural HA does not persist in tissues for more than 24 hours, it needs to be chemically stabilized by cross-linking techniques. Most hyaluronic-based fillers, such as the Belotero brand, are stabilized by 1,4-butanediol diglycidyl ether (BDDE).

DIFFERENTIATION OF HYALURONIC ACID FILLERS

How do we differentiate HA fillers? Outside the United States, a multitude of injectable fillers, specifically HA fillers, are available. However, most of them are not based on good randomized controlled trials (RCTs). Without good-quality RCTs, it is difficult to give guidance on the efficacy and safety for these products. The Belotero family discussed in this chapter has several well-done RCTs.

METHODS

For this chapter, a Medline search was performed with the aim to identify clinical trials on the Belotero family of fillers. To reduce bias, only larger randomized controlled clinical trials and case series were included in this overview.

THE BELOTERO FAMILY

Belotero is produced and distributed by Merz Pharmaceuticals (Raleigh, NC). The stabilizer is BDDE, and according to the manufacturer, two cross-linking processes are used, leading to a cohesive and polydensified matrix (CPM), which is supposed to ease injection while maintaining long-lasting results. Belotero offers several different formulations: Belotero Soft (superficial), Balance (formally known as Basic), Intense, and Volume (deep). The HA concentration differs between the products from 20 mg/mL (Belotero Soft), 22 mg/mL (Belotero Balance), 25.5 mg/mL (Belotero Intense), to 26 mg/ml (Belotero Volume). The Belotero products come with and without lidocaine.

Evidence

There are two randomized controlled clinical trials of Belotero Balance in the treatment of nasolabial folds (NLFs) and upper lips lines, respectively. There was one randomized controlled clinical trial on Belotero Volume for the treatment of the malar area. There were two large German case series, one focusing on Belotero Balance and one on Belotero Intense

Randomized Controlled Trials

The aim of the first trial was to compare the safety and effectiveness of Belotero Balance with that of bovine collagen (likely Zyplast; name not provided) in the correction of moderate to severe NLFs in a split-face study. This is a standard study design for a filler product when approaching the US market. The study included 118 patients who were randomized to receive Belotero Balance and bovine collagen on contralateral sides of the face. NLF severity was measured using the 5-point Wrinkle Severity Rating Scale (WSRS). As expected, compared with bovine collagen, Belotero Balance was doing better at weeks 8 ($P = .009$), 12 ($P = .001$), 16 ($P = .001$), and 24 ($P = .001$). There were no significant differences between the two groups in the proportion of adverse events considered related to the injection site procedure. Most adverse events were mild to moderate in severity and resolved within 7 days

The Butterwick trial focused on the upper lip lines. Here, Belotero Balance was compared with Juvéderm Ultra (Allergan/AbbVie, Irvine CA). Although the authors saw a better performance for Juvéderm Ultra, the objective Lip Wrinkles Score did show quite similar results between both products (Table 7.1).

The Kerscher and Prager trial performed a randomized split face study of volume augmentation of the malar area. The patients received 2 mL of Belotero Volume (CPM-26) to one cheek and 2 mL of Juvéderm Voluma (VYC-20) on the contralateral cheek. A total of 46 patients, mostly female, were included in the study. Noninferiority could be proven for Belotero Volume in comparison to Juvéderm Voluma at 3 months. Patients were followed up for 18 months. At this time point, 51% of the scores was still improved by at least one grade for both sides.[4] No difference in safety was reported between the two products.

Case Series

The Narins RCT was extended by an 18-month open-label extension phase. Of the 118 patients, 94 were reinjected with Belotero Balance, to both sides at various time points and followed for a maximum of an additional 72 weeks (96 weeks with the 24 weeks). The severity of the NLFs showed an improvement from baseline on both sides of the face. The mean change from baseline was greater on the side of the face injected with Belotero Balance than on the contralateral side injected with bovine collagen. The mean Global Aesthetic Improvement Scale (GAIS) scores, as assessed by the treating physician, were between 2 (improved) and 3 (much improved) at all time points. Only one (2.9%) related adverse event (hematomas on both sides of the face) was documented.

There was one further case series on Belotero Balance on NLFs with a follow-up of 6 months. In this case series by Dirting et al., 114 subjects with moderate to severe NLFs were treated with Belotero Balance. After 6 months, 81% of 109 subjects who finished the 6-month study showed at least a one-point improvement on the WSRS for NLFs. Adverse events were mild, with acute erythema and swelling in approximately 70% of patients. In another case series from Hevia et al. on the correction of the infraorbital hollow, Belotero Balance was demonstrated to be efficacious and safe.

For Belotero Intense, a large case series comprising 149 patients can be found. In contrast to the previous trials, patients could be treated in several areas at the same time. However, follow-up was limited to only 3 months. Efficacy was measured by the WSRS (5-point score) and GAIS. Most treated folds were NLFs (83.9%), followed by Marionette lines (32.9%) and melolabial folds (20.8%). Mean WSRS improved significantly by 1.9 points from initially 3.98 to 2.07 (12 weeks). Satisfaction was described as either good or excellent by 94% of the patients. Most common adverse events were acute erythema (63.8%), swelling (52.3%), and pain (49%) (Note that at that time Belotero Intense did not contain lidocaine). These adverse events generally appeared on the treatment day and resolved over time (Table 7.2).

TABLE 7.1 Randomized Clinical Trials on Belotero Products

Reference	Products	Randomized/ blinded	Area assessed	Duration of study	No of patients	Objective outcome criteria	Comments
Narins et al. (2010)	Belotero compared with bovine collagen	Y/evaluator blinded	NLF	6 months	118 (92.6% females)	5-point WSRS	Belotero is safe and effective and superior to bovine collagen at 6 months.
Butterwick et al. (2015)	Juvéderm Ultra vs. Belotero Balance	Y/evaluator blinded	Perioral lines	6 months	132 (99% females)	4-point Perioral Lines Severity Scale, SGA (Subjects Global Assessment of Change)	Juvéderm Ultra shows pretty very similar effects compared to Belotero (Note that the authors see some superiority of Juvéderm Ultra).
Kerscher et al. (2017) Prager et al. (2017)	Belotero Volume (CPM-26) vs. Juvéderm Voluma	Y by cheek, elevator blinded	Moderate to severe sunken upper cheeks (MAS)	Up to 18 months, main outcome after 3 months	45	One grade improvement on MAS upper cheek scale	Noninferiority could be demonstrated for CPM-26, and safety was comparable between both products.

NLF, Nasolabial fold; *WSRS*, Wrinkle Severity Rating Scale.

TABLE 7.2 Case Series on Belotero Products

Reference	Products	Randomized/ blinded	Area assessed	Duration of study	No of patients	Objective outcome criteria	Comments
Dieting et al. (2008)	Belotero Balance	No/no	Nasolabial fold	6 months	114 (92.4% female)	5-point WSRS	This was a multicenter study. Product was assessed as efficacious and safe.
Narins et al. (2010)	Belotero Balance	No/no	Nasolabial fold	18 months	95 (92.6% females)	5-point WSRS	This is an extension study from the RCT from Narins et al. (2010). At baseline, all subjects received Belotero Balance.
Pavicic et al. (2011)	Belotero Intense	No/no	Nasolabial folds, marionette lines, melolabial folds, cheeks, lips and chin	3 months	149 (88.9% females)	5-point WSRS, GAIS	A real-life study with multiple areas treated, NLF and marionette lines were treated mostly with 83.9% and 32.9%, respectively.
Hevia et al. (2014)	Belotero Balance	No/blinded evaluator; however, the sequence of treatment not blinded	Infraorbital hollow	10 months	46 (38 females)	5-point FWS	Product was efficacious and safe.

FWS, Facial Wrinkle Scale; *GAIS*, Global Aesthetic Improvement Scale; *NLF*, nasolabial fold; *RCT*, randomized controlled trial; *WSRS*, Wrinkle Severity Rating Scale.

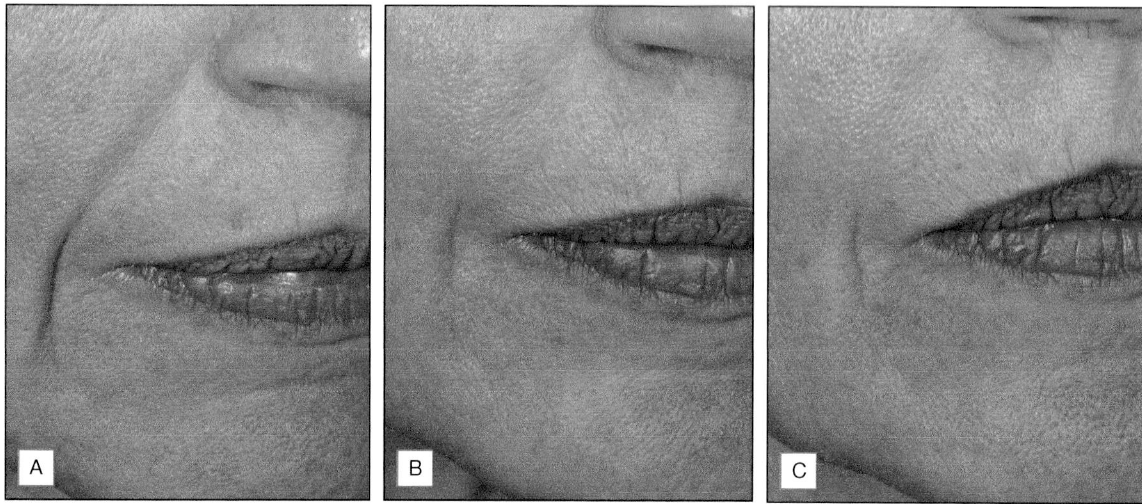

Fig. 7.1 (A) Patient (56 years old) at baseline. (B, C) 14 days and 182 days after a single injection of 1 mL Belotero Intense, respectively.

Rare Adverse Events

The Belotero family is a safe group of HA fillers. Only one granulomatous reaction has been reported to our knowledge.

Clinical Impressions

The nice thing with the Belotero family is that they come in not too many different products With three major products (either with or without lidocaine), I can nearly treat every indication using Belotero Volume/ Intense for deeper injections and Belotero Balance for more superficial indications (Figs. 7.1A–C and 7.2A–C). Belotero Balance is very soft and integrates nicely in the injected area. It is one of my favorite products for infraorbital hollows because it can be easily molded in. Merz does not have a specific lip product. Usually, Belotero Balance or Belotero Intense is injected in the lip area (Video 7.1). In some countries, these products have been named for the indication Belotero Lips Shape (Belotero Intense) and Belotero Lips Contour (Belotero Balance) coming with 0.6 mL instead of 1 mL volume. For lip augmentation, compared with other products, Belotero Balance is softer but on the other hand might not last as long for this very movable indication.[3]

CONCLUSIONS

Belotero Balance and Belotero Volume have been demonstrated to be effective and safe HA products for the correction of NLFs and volume loss of the cheek. For the correction of lip lines, Belotero Balance seems to be comparable if not quite as effective as Juvéderm Ultra Smile. Belotero Balance has been shown in a case series to be effective and safe for the correction of the infraorbital hollow. In another case series, Belotero Intense has been shown to be effective and safe for various deep lines and wrinkles.

ACKNOWLEDGMENT

Martina Kerscher, Heike Buntrock, and Vanessa Hartmann contributed to the chapter of an earlier edition of the book that served as a basis for this chapter.

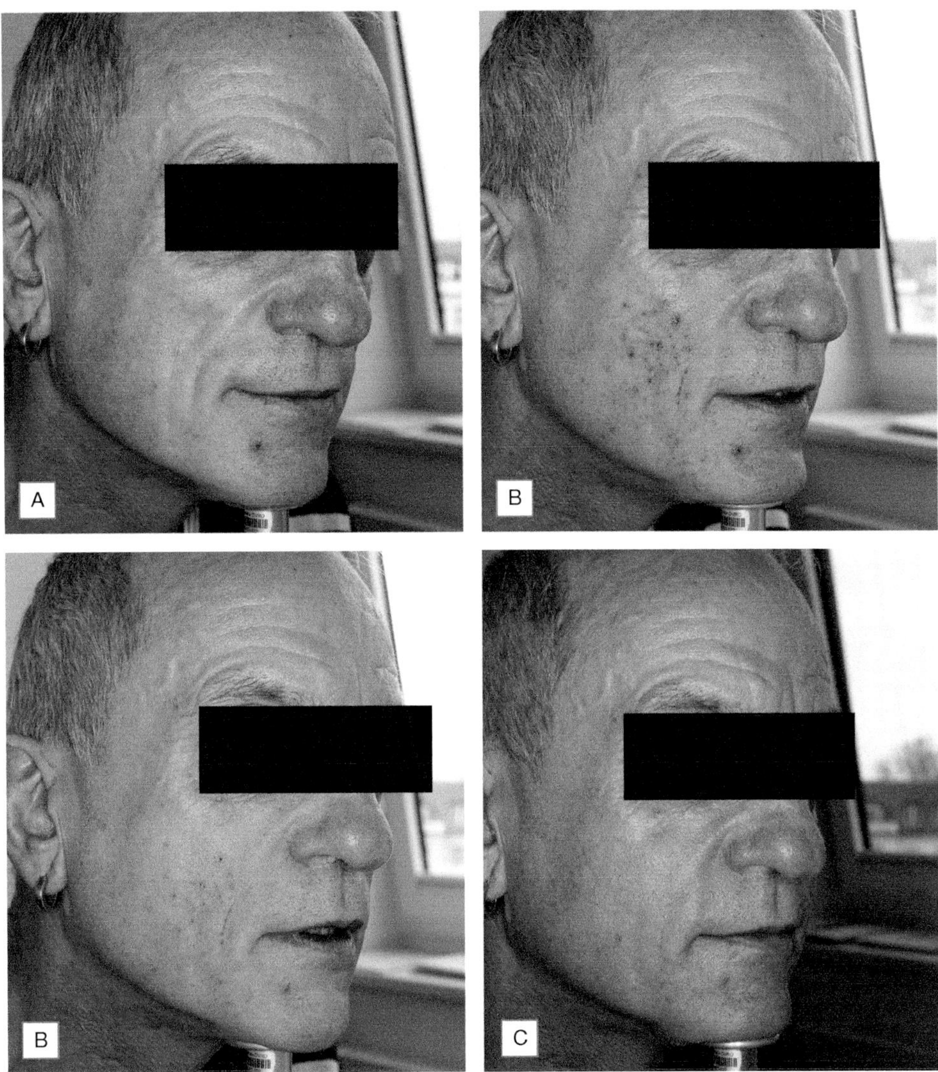

Fig. 7.2 (A) Patient (58 years old) with drug-induced lipoatrophy at baseline. (B, C) Immediately and 2 weeks after 2 mL of Belotero Volume and 2 mL Belotero Intense per site. As the injections were done by needle, the little entry points can be seen immediately after the injection.

FURTHER READING

Butterwick, K., Marmur, E., Narurkar, V., et al. (2015). HYC-24L demonstrates greater effectiveness with less pain than CPM-22.5 for treatment of perioral lines in a randomized controlled trial. *Dermatologic Surgery*, *41*(12), 1351–1360.

Dirting, K., Lampe, H., Wolters, M., et al. (2008). Hyaluronsäurefiller zur Korrektur der Nasolabialfalten—Ergebnisse einer klinischen Studie [Hyaluronic acid filler for correction of nasolabial grooves—results of a clinical study]. *Journal of the German Society of Dermatology*, *6*(suppl 2), S10–S14.

Gandy, J., Bierman, D., & Zachary, C. (2017). Granulomatous reaction to Belotero Balance: a case study. *Journal of Cosmetic Laser Therapy*, *19*(5), 307–309.

Hevia, O., Cohen, B. H., & Howell, D. J. (2014). Safety and efficacy of a cohesive polydensified matrix hyaluronic acid for the correction of infraorbital hollow: an observational study with results at 40 weeks. *Journal of Drugs in Dermatology*, *13*, 1030–1036.

Kerscher, M., Agsten, K., Kravtsov, M., & Prager, W. (2017). Effectiveness evaluation of two volumizing hyaluronic acid dermal fillers in a controlled, randomized, double-blind, split-face clinical study. *Clinical Cosmetic Investigative Dermatology*, *10*, 239–247.

Narins, R. S., Coleman, W., Donofrio, L., et al. (2010). Nonanimal sourced hyaluronic acid-based dermal filler using a cohesive polydensified matrix technology is superior to bovine collagen in the correction of moderate to severe nasolabial folds: results from a 6-month, randomized, blinded, controlled, multicenter study. *Dermatologic Surgery*, *36*(suppl 1), 730–740.

Narins, R. S., Coleman, W. P., 3rd, Donofrio, L. M., et al. (2010). Improvement in nasolabial folds with a hyaluronic acid filler using a cohesive polydensified matrix technology: results from an 18-month open-label extension trial. *Dermatologic Surgery*, *36*(suppl 3), 1800–1808.

Pavicic, T. (2011). Efficacy and tolerability of a new monophasic, double-crosslinked hyaluronic acid filler for correction of deep lines and wrinkles. *Journal of Drugs in Dermatology*, *10*, 134–139.

Prager, W., Agsten, K., Kravtsov, M., & Kerscher, P. M. (2017). Mid-face volumization with hyaluronic acid: injection technique and safety aspects from a controlled, randomized, double-blind clinical study. *Journal of Drugs in Dermatology*, *16*(4), 351–357.

Rayess, H. N., Svider, P. V., Hanba, C., et al. (2018). A cross-sectional analysis of adverse events and litigation for injectable fillers. *JAMA Facial Plast Surgery*, *20*(3), 207–214.

8

Resilient Hyaluronic Acid (RHA®) Fillers

Conor J. Gallagher and Joely Kaufman

RHA BASIC SCIENCE AND MANUFACTURING

Resilient Hyaluronic Acid (RHA) is the name given to a collection of hyaluronic acid (HA) products manufactured by Teoxane SA (Geneva, Switzerland) and marketed in the United States by Revance Therapeutics Inc. (Nashville, TN, USA). First introduced to the European market in 2015, the RHA gels were designed to address the current and future needs of health care practitioners and consumers. Treatment with dermal fillers has evolved over time, from an early focus on the direct filling of bothersome static facial lines and folds to a more contemporary view that the treatment approach should be based on an understanding of the three-dimensional anatomic changes that underlie the appearance of the static lines and, furthermore, the selection of products that are designed to complement the face, not only at rest but also, most importantly, in animation.

The prime directive in the design of the RHA collection of products was to create gels that fulfilled two needs, that is, had desirable physical characteristics that enabled a high degree of clinical effectiveness and, at the same time, were highly dynamic, moving seamlessly with facial animation. To create such gels, Teoxane aimed to minimize alteration to the HA chains, limiting tethering of the HA due to crosslinking and minimizing degradation of the HA chains during the manufacturing process.

This unique RHA manufacturing process, termed "Preserved Network Technology" (PNT), begins with exclusively high-molecular-weight HA chains. However, in PNT, the standard butanediol diglycidyl ether (BDDE) crosslinking process has been modified in several ways, including reducing the crosslinking temperature and optimizing other reaction conditions to minimize HA chain degradation during crosslinking and, thus, minimizing the amount of BDDE crosslinking required to create optimal gel characteristics. The end result has been to create RHA gels with extractable HA chains of approximately 600 kD in length (i.e., approximately two to four times the length of the HA chains typically found in similar analyses of other cohesive HA gels) and substantially lower chain modification with BDDE (1.9%–4.0% crosslinking) than other cohesive gels. In preserving the HA chain length and minimizing rigid crosslinkers, the RHA gels rely on the intrinsic three-dimensional nature of the gel network and more dynamic, noncovalent intramolecular bonds to provide the gel structure, extensibility, and cohesivity.

The RHA collection encompasses a range of four products (RHA 1–4) designed to provide progressively increasing levels of tissue support. As will be described later, these products exhibit physical characteristics designed to allow them to be placed more superficially than other products in their class without fear of the product bunching or of an unnatural appearance on facial animation. RHA 1 is formulated with 15 mg/mL HA, approximately 1.9% crosslinked, and designed for placement in the most superficial tissue planes. RHA 2 through 4 contain 23 mg/mL HA and are differentiated by their degree of crosslinking, with RHA 2 being 3.1% crosslinked, RHA 3 being 3.6% crosslinked, and RHA 4 being 4.0% crosslinked. All products in the RHA collection contain 0.3% lidocaine for patient comfort.

RHA 2, 3, and 4 have a unique US Food and Drug Administration indication for the treatment of "dynamic wrinkles and folds," reflective of the design intent to create a product range that can adapt and integrate with facial movement. In the United States, RHA 2 and 3 are indicated for placement in the mid to deep dermis and are ideal for the treatment of moderate facial wrinkles or folds, whereas RHA 4 is indicated for placement in the deep dermis or superficial subcutaneous planes. However, the physical properties of RHA 4 are such that it can provide support for deep fat pad reflation in areas such as the midface and, given its dynamic properties, can be layered in the superficial plane to provide contour or refill depleted superficial fat pads. This sits in contrast to other products designed for deep placement, which are often palpable or visible upon animation when placed superficially.

RHA GEL PROPERTIES

The purpose of evaluating and quantifying the physical characteristics of HA gels is to provide some comparative guidance to clinicians as to how the products will behave in tissue. Although a highly precise science, the interpretation of these values has become fraught over the years, with much energy spent on debating the merits and clinical relevance of such measures as G' (commonly referred to as "gel firmness" or "gel elasticity") and gel cohesivity. In evaluating RHA, Teoxane focused on the measurement of the physical characteristics most relevant to contemporary gels, that is, the ability to provide an appropriate amount of lift for the area the gel is designed for and the ability of the gels to provide support in the dynamic environment of the face. G' and cohesivity, although calculable for RHA products, are point measurements and not reflective of dynamic performance. To appropriately characterize the RHA gels, it was necessary to expand the rheologic toolbox. G' can be extended to examine the ability of the gel to maintain its G' under progressively increasing deformations in an effort to model the ability of the gel to better preserve its integrity and physical characteristics and, therefore, tissue support during dynamic facial motion. In all product categories, the RHA gels sustain their G' across a greater range of dynamic motion. This can be quantified as dynamic strength, or the product of the G' value and the amount of deformation force that the gel can withstand without breaking down (Fig. 8.1).

A second relevant tool used to assess dynamic performance of HA gels is an assessment of the ability of a product to undergo steady progressive deformation without losing its structure (i.e., its ability to stretch). This measure provides a comparative evaluation of the ability of a gel to adapt to stresses due, for instance, to tissue stretching. Fig. 8.1 illustrates the relative stretch scores for the Superficial, Utility, and Structural classes of HA products. It can be observed that, in each class, the RHA products exhibit a greater degree of stretch than other products. These data help affirm that the design goal of creating highly dynamic products has been met and, when translated to clinical practice, suggests that RHA products can confidently be placed in the more mobile superficial planes.

CLINICAL TRIAL EXPERIENCE

The safety and effectiveness of RHA 2, 3, and 4 have been demonstrated in 15-month pivotal trials conducted in the United States. These comparative, split-face trials demonstrated the noninferiority of RHA 2 and 3 to Juvéderm® Ultra XC for the treatment of moderate or severe nasolabial folds (Fig. 8.2), whereas RHA 4 was found to be noninferior to Restylane® Lyft, again in the treatment of nasolabial folds. In the RHA 4 study, a statistically significant difference in mean wrinkle severity improvement favoring RHA 4 was observed at all evaluated time points (Fig. 8.3). In each of these studies, more than 78% of subjects in the RHA treatment arm maintained at least a 1-point improvement over baseline at the 15-month final time point. As in most dermal filler studies, a touch up was permitted at week 2 after the initial treatment, and although re-treatment was permitted after 24 weeks in each of the studies, by week 36, only 6.1% of RHA 2 patients and 8.5% of RHA 3 patients had qualified for and received re-treatment, with 10.3% of RHA 4 patients receiving re-treatment at week 36 compared with 13.8% of Restylane Lyft patients. In general, the RHA products were well tolerated, and the common treatment site reactions were similar in nature and frequency to the comparators. Furthermore, no delayed-onset treatment-related adverse events were reported.

A smaller, 18-month comparative study was conducted in Europe that compared RHA 2 to Juvéderm

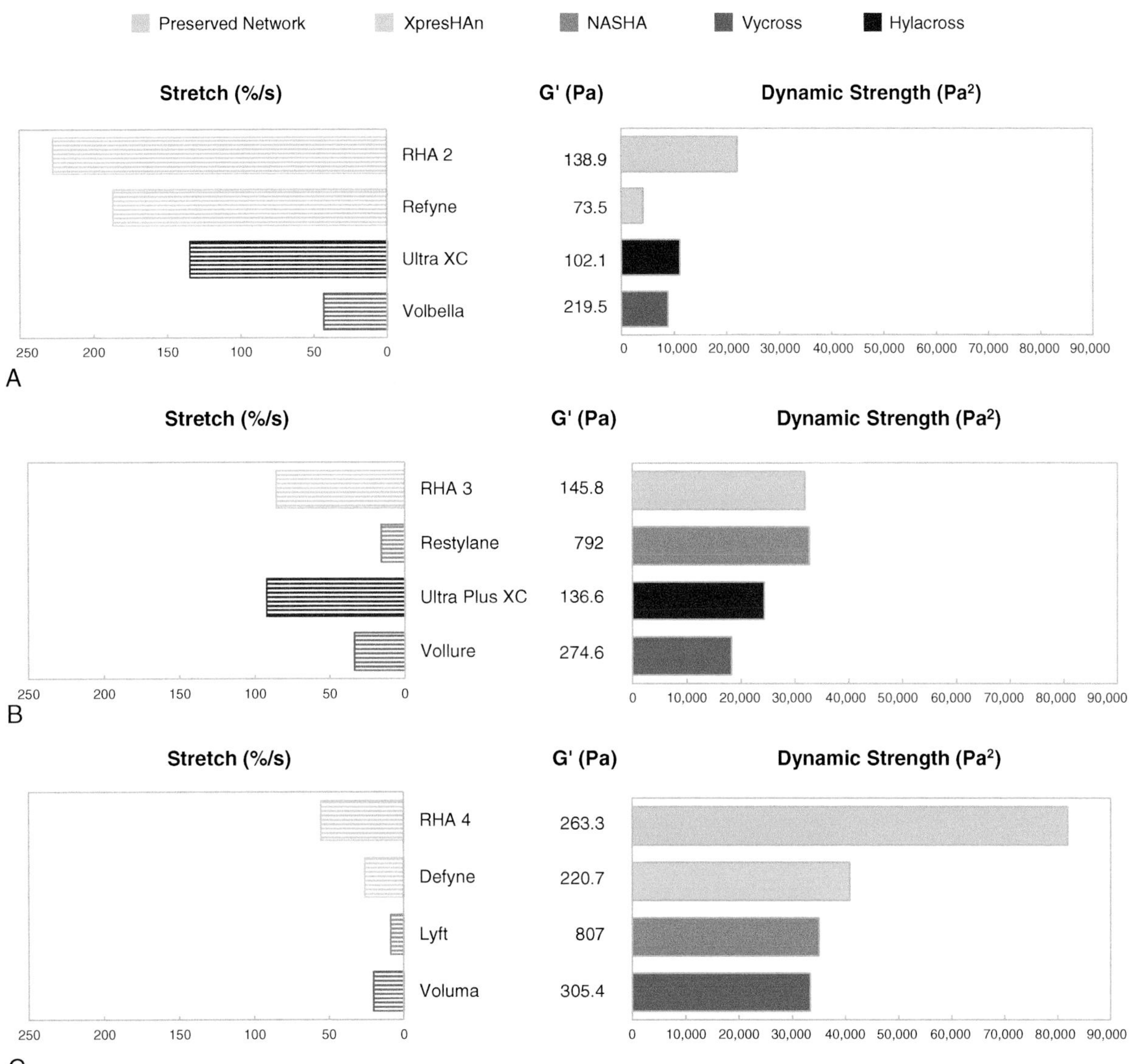

Fig. 8.1 Elasticity measurements (G'), dynamic strength scores, and stretch scores for (A) more superficial fillers, (B) utility fillers, and (C) deeper fillers. The dynamic strength measures the ability to maintain physical integrity over a range of stresses or deformations, while the stretch score measures the ability to deform or adapt to movement. *RHA*, Resilient Hyaluronic Acid.

Volift/Vollure, RHA 3 to Juvéderm Ultra XC, and RHA 4 to Teosyal® Ultra Deep, a non-RHA product from Teoxane. The RHA-treated nasolabial folds received slightly less volume than the comparators, yet the studies found no statistically significant differences in the treatment effects between RHA and the comparator products, with the exception of RHA 4, which showed significantly better effectiveness over Ultra Deep at the 15-month time point.

RHA 1 has been studied in a randomized blinded study on perioral lines, with a no-treatment control group. In this 52-week study, 80.7% of subjects were responders at the primary time point (week 8) by the blinded evaluator and 66% maintained at least a 1-grade

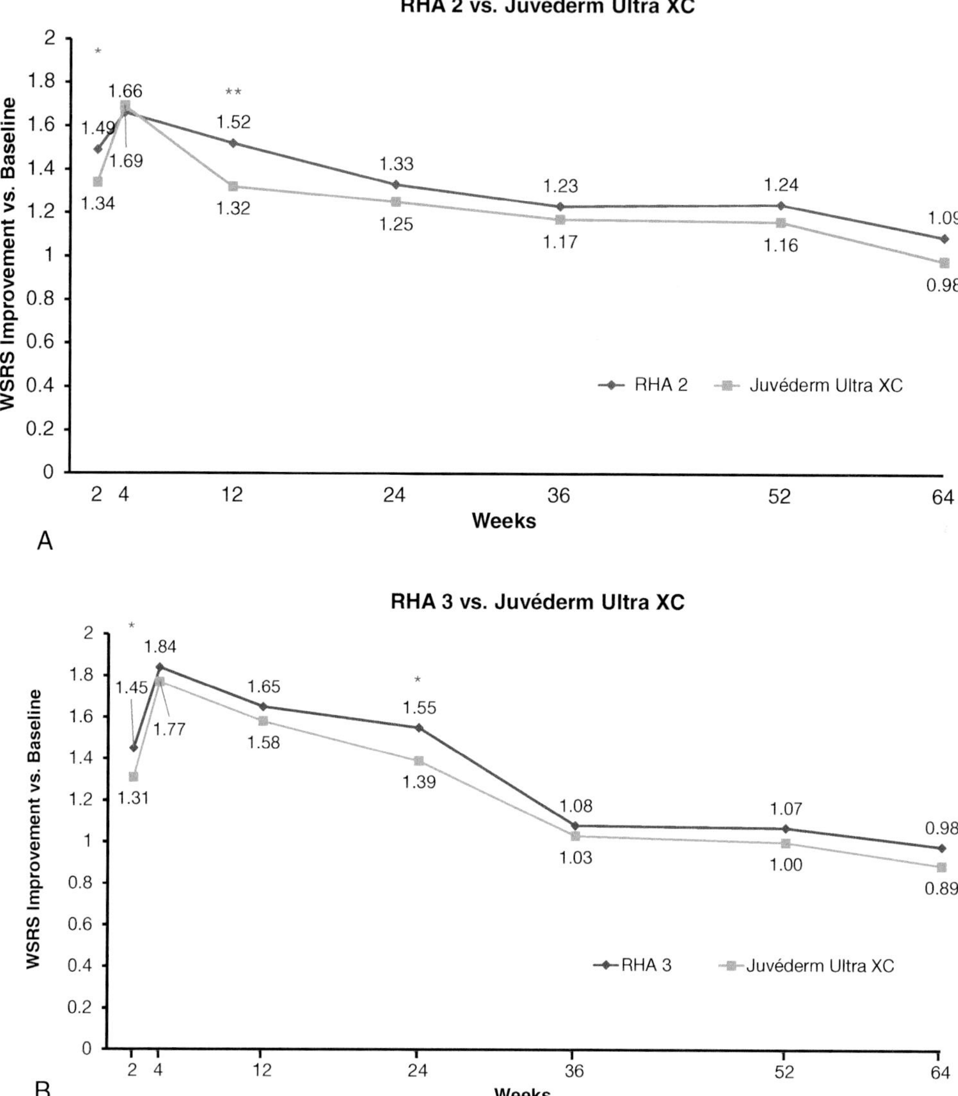

Fig. 8.2 Treating investigator assessment of the evolution over 15 months of mean WSRS scores in nasolabial folds in subjects treated with (A) RHA 2/Juvéderm Ultra XC and (B) RHA 3/Juvéderm Ultra XC. Results from a within-subject (split-face) clinical trial. *$P < .05$; ** $P < .001$. Data are from the per-protocol population. *RHA*, Resilient Hyaluronic Acid; *WSRS*, Wrinkle Severity Rating Scale. (From Monheit, G., Kaufman-Janette, J., Joseph, J.H., Shamban, A., Dover, J.S., Smith, S. (2020). Efficacy and safety of two Resilient Hyaluronic Acid fillers in the treatment of moderate-to-severe nasolabial folds: a 64-week, prospective, multicenter, controlled, randomized, double-blinded, and within-subject study. *Dermatologic Surgery, 46*(12), 1521–1529. © 2020 by the American Society for Dermatologic Surgery, Inc. Published by Wolters Kluwer Health, Inc. All rights reserved.)

improvement in perioral rhytid severity at the 52-week visit. Satisfaction with the treatment outcome was reported by 91.8% of patients at week 4 and 88.3% at the 52-week visit. In this study, the most common treatment-related adverse events were lumps and bumps/contour irregularities (17%), which may be to be expected considering the superficial (intradermal) placement of the product; firmness (11.0%); and injection site bruising (10.5%). No delayed-onset nodules were reported in these clinical trials.

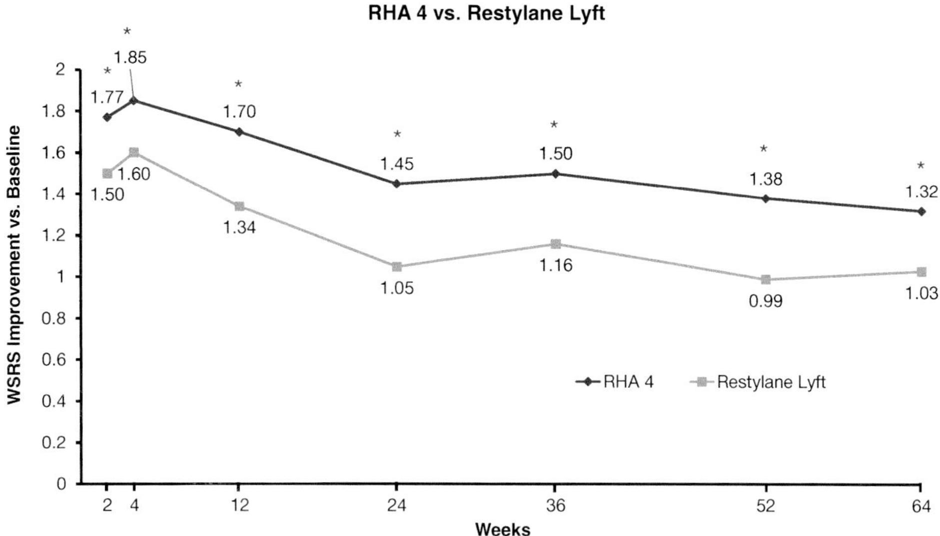

Fig. 8.3 Treating investigator assessment of the evolution over 15 months of mean WSRS scores in nasolabial folds in subjects treated with RHA 4/Lyft. Results from a within-subject (split-face) clinical trial. $*P \leq .001$. Data are from the per-protocol population. *RHA*, Resilient Hyaluronic Acid; *WSRS*, Wrinkle Severity Rating Scale. (From Kaufman-Janette, J., Taylor, S.C., Cox, S.E., Weinkle, S.H., Smith, S., Kinney, B.M. (2019). Efficacy and safety of a new Resilient Hyaluronic Acid dermal filler, in the correction of moderate-to-severe nasolabial folds: a 64-week, prospective, multicenter, controlled, randomized, double-blind and within-subject study. *Journal of Cosmetic Dermatology, 18*(5), 1244–1253; licensed under CC BY 4.0.)

CLINICAL EXPERIENCE

The RHA products have been in clinical use in the United States since 2020 and globally since 2015. During this time, real-life experience has been acquired, allowing health care practitioners to better understand the utility of these HA products. The current approach to facial rejuvenation with HA fillers favors a multiplane approach to address both deep and superficial volume loss. Experienced injectors have adopted the new approach to rejuvenation of being a multidimensional full-facial treatment. With high G'/inelastic filler products, deep placement allows for structural support while hiding the firm filler. When these products are placed in the more superficial planes, they often become visible with facial animation. In addition, when these types of fillers were placed in the superficial nasolabial fold, it resulted in an unnatural pushing up of the fold into the medial cheek. Certainly, in highly mobile areas, there is a demand for fillers that look and feel more natural.

Injection techniques with a more dynamic filler are slightly different than with an inelastic filler. Dynamic fillers can be placed in all planes, including the more superficial fat pads and dermal layers, without being visible on animation. This has allowed for the filling of areas that previously might not have been approachable with stiffer HA fillers. Those areas include the lateral cheek hollow, preauricular spaces, and superficial lateral smile lines. These areas have previously been difficult to improve with an inelastic HA filler due to the lack of stretch, which can result in an unnatural bulging of product with animation. An elastic product that can maintain its structure despite the repetitive movements seen with facial animation allows for a more natural and durable aesthetic outcome.

In the midface, RHA can be used for both superficial and deep injections laterally and medially. This is especially useful in thinner faces and in patients desiring a more natural cosmetic result, where product can be used in a tapering method from the zygoma all the way to the mandible. In addition, although structural support via a periosteal approach at the lateral zygoma is important to facial lifting, injection into the more superficial layers is crucial for the correction of facial contour and improvement of the nasolabial folds and marionette lines. A filler that can combine dynamic strength and stretch is an important addition to the armamentarium of tools in facial aesthetics. In our clinical practice, RHA has become very popular for use in this multilayer injection approach.

FURTHER READING

Faivre, J., Gallet, M., Tremblais, E., Trévidic, P., & Bourdon, F. (2021). Advanced concepts in rheology for the evaluation of hyaluronic acid-based soft tissue fillers. *Dermatologic Surgery*, *47*(5), e159–e167.

Kaufman-Janette, J., Taylor, S. C., Cox, S. E., Weinkle, S. H., Smith, S., & Kinney, B. M. (2019). Efficacy and safety of a new Resilient Hyaluronic Acid dermal filler, in the correction of moderate-to-severe nasolabial folds: a 64-week, prospective, multicenter, controlled, randomized, double-blind and within-subject study. *Journal of Cosmetic Dermatology*, *18*(5), 1244–1253.

Monheit, G., Kaufman-Janette, J., Joseph, J. H., Shamban, A., Dover, J. S., & Smith, S. (2020). Efficacy and safety of two Resilient Hyaluronic Acid fillers in the treatment of moderate-to-severe nasolabial folds: a 64-week, prospective, multicenter, controlled, randomized, double-blinded, and within-subject study. *Dermatologic Surgery*, *46*(12), 1521–1529.

Rzany, B., Converset-Viethel, S., Hartmann, M., et al. (2019). Efficacy and safety of 3 new Resilient Hyaluronic Acid fillers, crosslinked with decreased BDDE, for the treatment of dynamic wrinkles: results of an 18-month, randomized controlled trial versus already available comparators. *Dermatologic Surgery*, *45*(10), 1304–1314.

Salti, G., & Rauso, R. (2015). Facial rejuvenation with fillers: the dual plane technique. *Journal of Cutaneous Aesthetic Surgery*, *8*(3), 127–133.

Sundaram, H., Shamban, A., Schlessinger, J., Kaufman-Janette, J., Joseph, J. H., Lupin, M., Draelos, Z., Carey, W., Smith, S., & Eaton, L. (2022). Efficacy and safety of a new resilient Hyaluronic Acid Filler in the correction of moderate-to-severe dynamic perioral rhytides: a 52-week prospective, multicenter, controlled, randomized, evaluator-blinded study. *Dermatologic Surgery*, *48*(1), 87–93.

Teoxane. Directions for use for RHA 2, RHA 3, and RHA 4. https://www.accessdata.fda.gov/cdrh_docs/pdf17/P170002C.pdf. Accessed June 6, 2021.

Calcium Hydroxylapatite Ultradilute, HA Dilution

Steven Krueger, Bassel H. Mahmoud, Ada Regina Trindade de Almeida, and David M. Ozog

INTRODUCTION

Calcium hydroxylapatite (CaHA; Radiesse, Merz North America, Raleigh, NC) is an opaque, white-colored filler consisting of CaHA microspheres (25–45 μm in diameter) suspended in an aqueous carboxymethylcellulose carrier gel. The synthetic CaHA microspheres are smooth in shape, uniform in size, and composed of minerals (calcium and phosphate) that occur naturally in human bone and teeth, making them physiologically inert and biocompatible. The particles are resorbed and eliminated naturally through the body's normal metabolic and excretory processes.

The two-staged mechanism of action of CaHA involves volume replacement and subsequent biostimulation. The carrier gel provides an initial volume augmentation and then gradually dissipates, while CaHA microspheres stimulate the endogenous production of collagen and elastin through fibroblast activation. Animal studies have demonstrated neocollagenesis beginning as early as 4 weeks posttreatment and continuing for at least 12 months. A histological study of patients receiving supraperiosteal injections of CaHA demonstrated peak concentrations of newly formed type III collagen at four months, while type I collagen predominated at 9 months, consistent with the process of natural neocollagenesis. Elastin expression and angiogenesis also increased, suggesting that dermal remodeling was accompanied by improved nutrient supply to the skin. It is through these mechanisms that CaHA filler provides sustained aesthetic improvement long after implantation.

In 2006, CaHA received US Food and Drug Administration (FDA) approval for correction of moderate to severe facial lines and folds and correction of soft tissue loss from HIV lipoatrophy. An indication for correcting volume loss in the dorsal hands was approved in 2015. Since then, several other body areas have been treated off-label with good effect. This chapter will briefly discuss the use of CaHA as a volumizing filler and then focus primarily on the increasingly popular off-label use of dilute and hyperdilute CaHA as a biostimulatory agent.

CaHA AS A VOLUMIZER

For over a decade, CaHA has been used undiluted or slightly diluted to provide immediate correction of soft-tissue volume loss. This is followed by a biostimulatory effect resulting in tighter and thicker skin. The effects have been shown to last for 15 months on average, and in some cases 30 months or more. Longevity varies depending on treatment location, injection technique, and patient age and metabolism.

CaHA has one of the highest viscosities among the available dermal fillers, which prevents migration in areas without significant muscle movement. It also has a high elasticity (G'), providing it with high lifting capacity. These properties make CaHA well suited for facial volume correction in multiple layers depending on the treatment location. Supraperiosteal implantation of undiluted product provides deep volume restoration, while subcutaneous implantation of slightly diluted product provides contour reconstruction, and superficial dermal implantation of highly diluted product provides skin tightening. When used for volumizing, CaHA can immediately correct creases and hollows (Video 9.2). It can be applied to all areas of the face except the glabella, periorbital area, and lips. Injection techniques and experience have been published for facial areas including the forehead, temples, zygomatic cheeks, jawline, and chin, among others. The ability of CaHA to create angled contours has also made it a popular filler for men. While the amount injected may vary by location, the correction ratio for CaHA is approximately 1:1, so overcorrection should be avoided.

CAHA AS A BIOSTIMULATORY AGENT

More recently, CaHA has been increasingly used off-label in a dilute (1:1, i.e., 1.5 mL of product plus 1.5 mL of diluent) or a hyperdilute (≥ 1:2, i.e., ≥ 3 mL of diluent) form to provide dermal rejuvenation without tissue volumization. Hyperdilution causes the carboxymethylcellulose gel to become dispersed, resulting in little or no volumizing effect, while the CaHA microspheres stimulate long-term tissue remodeling. This allows for a more superficial injection over a larger treatment area. Dilutions up to 1:6 (1.5 mL of CaHA product to 9 mL of diluent) have been shown to stimulate collagen and elastin. However, it is not yet clear yet whether neocollagenesis or neoelastogenesis is optimized by a specific ratio. The ideal CaHA dilution should be titrated based on skin thickness and tissue laxity to ensure smooth product placement. One syringe (1.5 mL) of CaHA is typically used to treat an area of 100 to 300 cm^2, but this may vary based on local anatomical features.

To properly dilute CaHA, a LuerLock syringe containing diluent is connected to the original product syringe through a transfer adaptor in a sterile mixing environment. Up to 1.5 mL of 2% lidocaine with or without epinephrine has been used for its anesthetic effect to dilute CaHA, but bacteriostatic saline solution can be added if higher dilutions are required. The syringes should be large enough to accommodate the total volume of filler plus diluent. At least 20 passes between the two syringes should be performed to adequately mix their contents. The final mixture should be injected immediately after reconstitution since components separate quickly, especially with higher dilutions. The physician injector, rather than an assistant, should perform his/her own dilution procedure.

Two separate expert panels provide consensus guidelines detailing the safe and effective use of dilute and hyperdilute CaHA. Both emphasize that the goal is to deliver a thin, smooth, and uniform coating of product at an appropriate depth. This can be achieved with a fanning injection technique or parallel, serial retrograde linear threads in the deep dermal or subdermal plane. Superficial placement of less diluted CaHA can result in unwanted product visibility, especially in areas of thin or darker skin. Massaging the injected area helps to evenly distribute the final product.

Needles (27–30 gauge) or cannulas (22–25 gauge) may be used for injection. Needles allow for extreme precision of movement and deep injection, but can cause more trauma and placement of material at multiple anatomic levels. Cannulas are less traumatic and allow for the placement of product within the desired tissue plane over large areas. Approximately 0.1 or 0.1 to 0.2 mL aliquots are typically deposited with each pass when using a needle or cannula, respectively.

One panel recommends two to three sessions performed at 1- to 2-month intervals for an optimal skin tightening effect, while another recommends one to three sessions during the first year followed by maintenance injections every 12 to 18 months thereafter. Based on data suggesting that the highest deposition of new collagen and elastin occurs approximately 4 months after injection, the latter group recommends follow-up at 3 to 4 months after the initial treatment with reinjection as needed. The use of higher dilutions in certain body areas may necessitate more frequent evaluation and additional treatment sessions.

Addition of Hyaluronic Acid

Hyaluronic acid (HA) has also been added to CaHA filler as a mixture to compensate for the unexpected early volume loss that may occur due to rapid absorption of the carrier gel. In one study, 1 mL of HA and 0.5 mL of lidocaine were added to 1.5 mL of CaHA filler, and the mixture maintained constant volume with high patient satisfaction. A recently introduced PEGylated HA-CaHA filler (Stimulate, MatexLab SA, Lugano, Switzerland) has demonstrated significant stimulation of type III collagen fibers. At present, literature is limited on this combination.

The following sections will discuss recommended techniques for administering dilute or hyperdilute

CaHA for the purpose of dermal rejuvenation in specific body locations.

Face

Dilute and hyperdilute CaHA can provide dermal rejuvenation in the mid and lower face, serving as an adjunct to volumizing fillers in this location. It is generally not used superficially in the forehead or temporal areas. For facial treatments, the preferred dilution is 1:1. This ratio has been shown to improve atrophic acne scars when used in combination with microfocused ultrasound with visualization (MFU-V). Dilutions up to 1:3 may be used for more superficial product placement in areas of thin skin or greater laxity. One syringe to the entire face or to each side of the face is typically sufficient for one treatment. Entering the skin perpendicular to the course of major vessels reduces the risk of vascular complications.

In a recent study, injections of hyperdilute CaHA in a 1:2 ratio safely and effectively decreased aging severity scores of the mid and lower face four months posttreatment. Noninvasive imaging demonstrated collagen remodeling and increased vascularization, and high patient satisfaction scores were achieved.

Neck and Décolletage

Although the use of CaHA in the neck and décolletage is off label, it has been shown to improve skin quality and promote skin tightening. In one study, subjects with skin laxity received linear subdermal injections (beginning laterally and moving medially towards the midline) of CaHA diluted to varying degrees with bacteriostatic saline based on skin thickness: 1:2 for normal skin, 1:4 for thin skin, and 1:6 for atrophic skin. Immunohistochemical analysis demonstrated significant increases in collagen, elastin, and angiogenesis up to 7 months after treatment. Skin elasticity and pliability (evaluated by cutometry) and dermal thickness (evaluated by ultrasound) also improved significantly. The procedure was well tolerated with high subject and investigator satisfaction scores. Patients with only mild tissue laxity or excess skin in the neck derive the most benefit. Because the skin of the neck is thin and adherent to the underlying platysma, the use of cannulas is recommended to reduce the risk of product visibility and nodule formation that results from injections that are too superficial. Products can be delivered by cannula via retroinjection with three to five entrance points or by needle via the linear-threading technique. Dilutions of 1:2 to 1:4 are typically used according to the patient's skin thickness. One syringe is typically sufficient for each treatment of the neck.

In the décolletage, hyperdilute CaHA is recommended in ratios of 1:2 to 1:3 for patients with mild laxity and/or photodamage, while a ratio of 1:4 can be used for those with more significant atrophy (Video 9.2). Between 0.5 and 1 syringe is typically sufficient for one treatment of the décolletage, multiple sessions may be required for maximum effect, and follow-up should occur 6 to 9 months posttreatment.

Buttocks and Thighs

When used alone or in combination with other treatments, CaHA injections can significantly improve skin contour irregularities of the buttocks and thighs. Because changes in the skin's fibrous structure contribute to worsening of cellulite, the aim is to improve the strength and elasticity of the dermis and superficial fascia. One study demonstrated a significant improvement in skin laxity and cellulite appearance when CaHA (diluted 1:1 with 2% lidocaine) was delivered using a microdroplet fanning technique with a 25-gauge cannula immediately after MFU-V. Ninety days after the procedure, there was a nearly 50% improvement in the cellulite severity scale, high subject satisfaction scores, and histologic evidence of neocollagenesis.

For treatment of skin laxity and surface irregularities of the buttocks, CaHA can be used in dilutions ranging from 1:1 to 1:6 depending on the dermal thickness. Products can be delivered using a cannula with a fanning or asterisk-shaped injection technique or using a needle with a linear-threading technique over the contour of the buttocks, prioritizing the upper and lateral regions. A cross-hatching technique using lower dilutions (1:1 or 1:2) can be used for cellulite dimples. One syringe of CaHA per buttock is typically sufficient for each session. Three treatments administered at 3- to 4-month intervals may be required to achieve a maximum effect.

When used to improve skin quality over the thighs, CaHA can be used in dilutions ranging from 1:1 to 1:4 according to the degree of laxity. This treatment is ideal for patients with mild surface irregularities and limited skin laxity without excess fat. Fanning or asterisk-shaped injections can be performed with a cannula over multiple entry points. Some recommend a "rasping" technique whereby stiff cannulas are used to scrape the underside of the dermis. A needle can also be used with a linear-threading technique. Treatments should target the inner and posterior thigh areas, with one syringe per region per session. Given the large treatment area, vigorous massage must be performed postprocedurally to ensure smooth product dispersion. The risk of bruising is higher in this area due to the presence of varicose veins.

Stretch Marks

Striae distensae are characterized by disordered collagen and reduced elastin fibers leading to dermal atrophy. In a study of subjects with red or white atrophic striae, an increase in the quality and quantity of dermal collagen and elastin was found in areas treated with a combination of CaHA diluted 1:1 with 2% lidocaine, microneedling, and topical ascorbic acid. The loss of dermal tissue can be filled using a combined deep subdermal and intradermal microbolus ("string of pearls") technique consisting of 0.05 mL aliquots of product deposited at each point along the center of the stria. Alternatively, one to two linear strands of CaHA can be injected in a retrograde threading fashion using 0.5 mL per strand. A superficial injection resulting in a yellowish discoloration due to product visibility may actually lend a more natural appearance to white striae. CaHA should be injected into striae until a palpable depression can no longer be appreciated, followed by vigorous massage to smooth the filler material.

Abdomen

One study found that injecting CaHA using a body vectoring technique induced significant reductions in skin flaccidity and increased skin density and thickness in the abdomen 5 weeks after a single treatment, but the product was not hyperdiluted. A case series of female patients receiving subdermal injections of CaHA diluted 1:4 with saline solution across the abdominal wall (via linear-threading technique along Langer's lines) demonstrated a 27% increase in dermal thickness. This increase was associated with high patient and physician satisfaction scores.

Contour irregularities of the abdomen typically require correction of deeper volume deficits before dilute or hyperdilute CaHA can be layered more superficially. Products can be distributed across the four abdominal quadrants using a cannula with a fanning, asterisk-shaped, or cross-hatching technique. Needles can also be used with a linear-threading technique (Fig. 9.1 and Video 9.1), which is well suited for the periumbilical region. The dilution can range from 1:1 to 1:4. Generally, when treating large areas, each 1.5-mL syringe of CaHA can treat an area of 100 cm^2 (10×10 cm). Using a dilution ratio of 1:1, 3 mL of total solution would therefore be able to treat the umbilical area, whereas 6 mL may be required to treat larger abdominal areas. One syringe each may be sufficient for treating the upper and lower abdomen, respectively. Follow-up should occur 6 to 9 months posttreatment. A synergistic effect can be achieved when combining CaHA injections with other skin-tightening therapies, such as radiofrequency, ultrasound, or laser devices.

Arms

Hyperdilute CaHA is an effective treatment for patients with mild skin laxity in the upper arms (Fig. 9.2). Treatment improves the appearance of skin crepiness and laxity, especially in patients younger than 50 years of age. In one study of subjects receiving CaHA injections to the upper arms (1.5 mL/arm/visit) over two monthly sessions, significant improvement was observed in skin quality (flaccidity and volume distribution) 4 months after the second treatment, but the product was not hyperdiluted. In a case series of female patients receiving subdermal injections of CaHA diluted 1:2 with normal saline and 2% lidocaine into the upper arms, cutometry measurements demonstrated a progressive increase in skin elasticity up to 3 months after a single treatment. This increase was associated with high patient and physician satisfaction scores. One method of treatment involves injecting the circumferential upper arm with two syringes (3 mL) of CaHA diluted 1:2 with lidocaine and saline (9 mL total of solution) into the immediate subdermal plane with a fanning technique. Another technique requires only 0.5 to 1 syringe to be distributed along the inner arm using a cannula with two to four fanning retroinjections. Dilution ratios of 1:1 to 1:4 may be used depending on the local skin thickness. The addition of lidocaine may improve patient comfort in this area because the upper arm skin is generally more sensitive than other areas.

Injection of CaHA diluted 1:2 using a retrograde fanning technique with a cannula has been shown to effectively treat actinic purpura on the forearms. It is theorized that the filler causes total dermal recovery in aged skin, providing protection to dermal vessels.

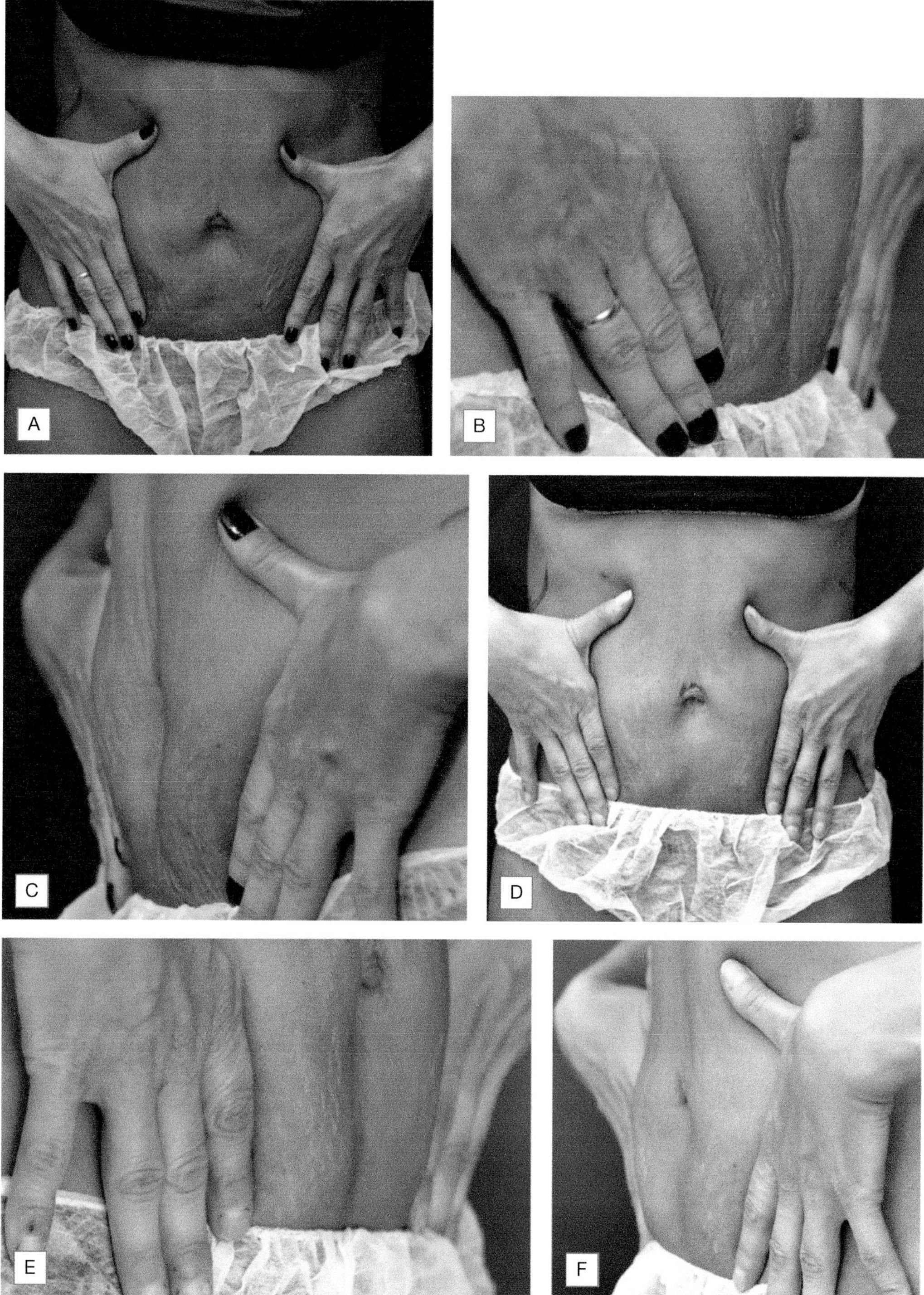

Fig. 9.1 A 42-year-old female presented with abdominal skin laxity (A–C). Thirty days after one treatment session with two syringes of calcium hydroxylapatite hyperdiluted in a 1:2 ratio, a significant tightening effect was noted (D–F). (Courtesy of Dr. Almeida.)

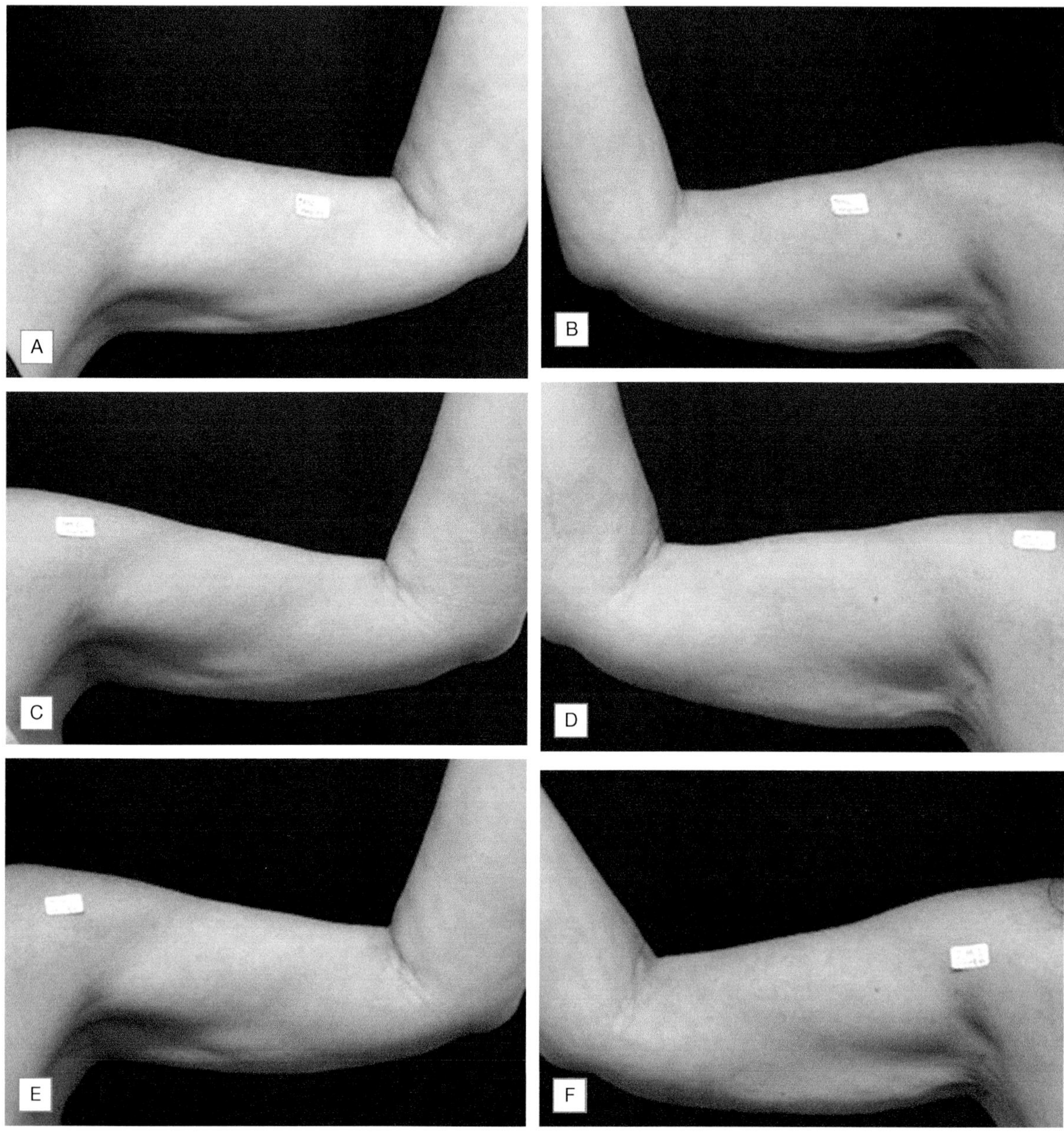

Fig. 9.2 A 59-year-old female presented with arm skin laxity (A–B). After one treatment session with one syringe per arm of calcium hydroxylapatite hyperdiluted in a 1:2 ratio, a progressive tightening effect was appreciated at 60 days (C–D) and 15 months (E–F). (Courtesy of Dr. Almeida.)

Hands

Aging of the hands is characterized mainly by skin thinning and fat reduction between the metacarpal bones, which increase the visibility of underlying tendons and veins. Dilute CaHA injection was first described as an approach to hand augmentation in 2007. In 2015, CaHA became the first filler approved by the FDA for correcting volume loss in the dorsal hands. Since then, its use in this location has been described with varying dilutions, delivery techniques, and injection planes (Figs. 9.3 and 9.4). The dilution process allows for the injected bolus to be easily massaged between the

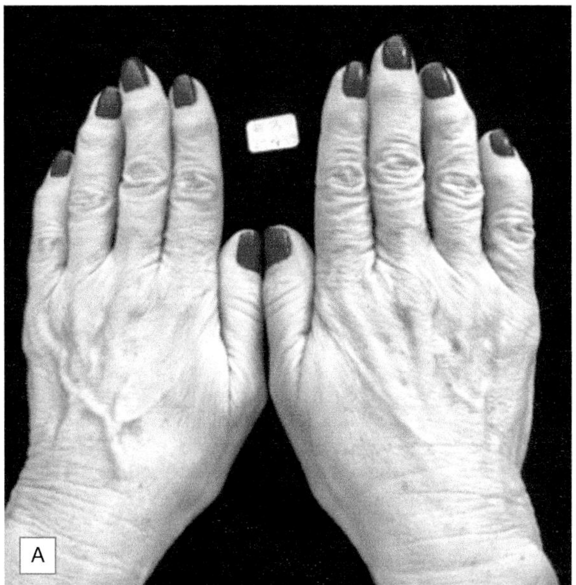

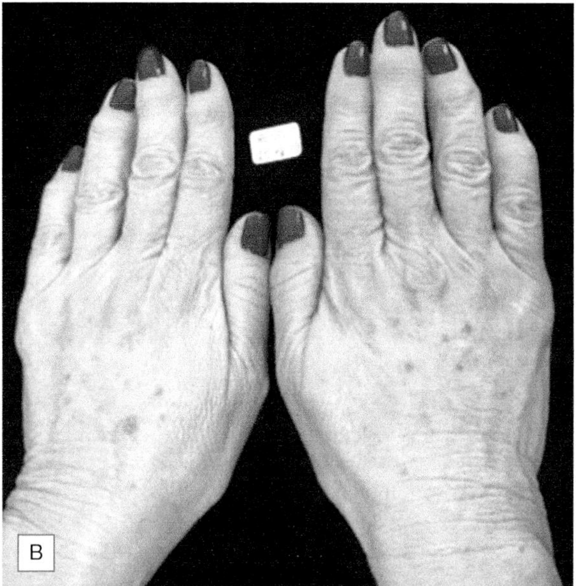

Fig. 9.3 A female presented with skin aging of the hands (A). Improvement due to reduced visibility of tendons and veins is appreciated immediately after injection of one-half syringe per hand of calcium hydroxylapatite hyperdiluted in a 1:2 ratio (B). A 25 G cannula was used to ensure correct product placement in the superficial plane. (Courtesy of Dr. Almeida.)

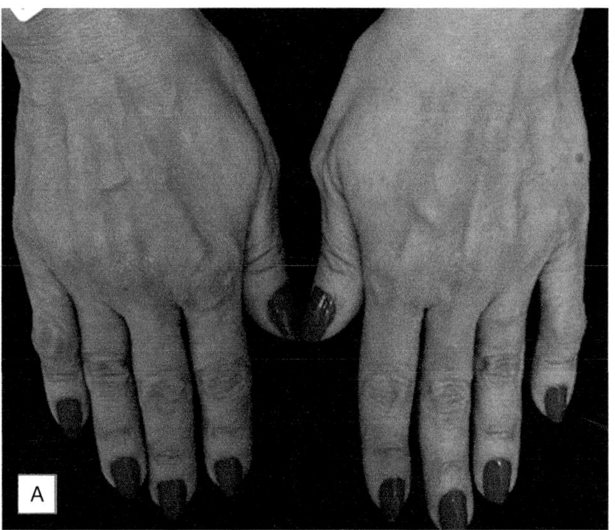

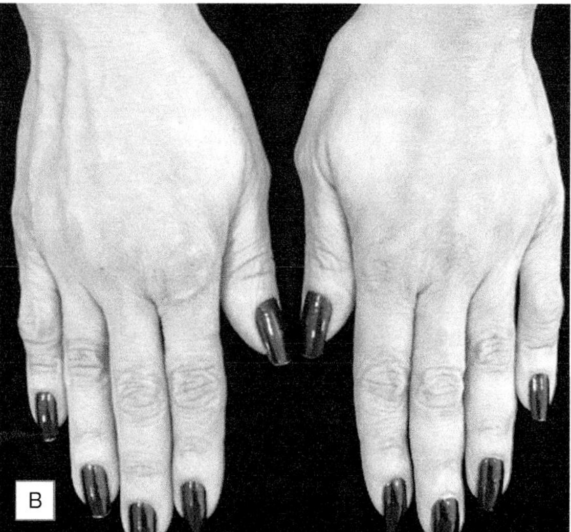

Fig. 9.4 A female with skin aging of the hands before (A) and 2 months after (B) injection of one-half syringe per hand of calcium hydroxylapatite hyperdiluted in a 1:2 ratio. Reduced visibility of tendons and veins give the hands a more youthful appearance. (Courtesy of Dr. Almeida.)

metacarpal spaces, reduces the pain of injection, and decreases postprocedural edema, bruising, and nodule formation. The deep fat lamina of the hands that lies near veins and tendons can be easily accessed with a needle and is a safe and effective depth for hand rejuvenation with CaHA. However, some experts believe that a more superficial, subdermal injection using a cannula leads to better outcomes and a lower risk of damage to underlying structures. A review of 220 hand rejuvenation procedures suggested that proximal-to-distal fanning injections accessing the superficial lamina with a cannula are associated with fewer adverse events (AEs). In a study of 15 women, CaHA diluted 1:1 with 2% lidocaine was found to improve the skin quality (including aging grades, viscoelasticity measures, and total collagen density) of aging hands 6 months after treatment. There was no substantial difference in the results between a previously described tenting technique (consisting of small bolus injections into the intermetacarpal deep fat lamina with a 27-gauge needle after pinching the overlying skin to form a "tent") and a superficial lamina technique (consisting of subdermal injections with a 25-gauge cannula in a fanning distribution through two proximal punctures). However, slightly higher patient satisfaction and a lower risk of AEs favor the use of cannulas in this area. The correct plane of injection is identified relative to the dorsal hand veins: movement of the needle/cannula visualized above the veins indicates a superficial lamina injection, while movement visualized below the veins indicates a deep lamina injection. A study of 114 subjects receiving CaHA injections with a needle using the tenting technique at a lower dilution (1.5 mL CaHA in 0.26 mL of 2% lidocaine) for hand volumization also resulted in significant improvement by 3 months that was maintained through 12 months. However, this study demonstrated a high prevalence of AEs. Despite normal postprocedural hand function tests, 15% of subjects reported loss of sensation and 48% reported difficulty performing activities. A greater dilution may therefore be a safer option when the primary goal is improvement of the skin quality rather than volumization of the dorsal hands. The average patient will require one syringe per hand of CaHA diluted 1:1 for one treatment.

Knees and Elbows

Although there are no clinical studies to date, some experts believe that the local aged appearance of the knees and elbows can be improved with CaHA injections. Treatment is suggested mainly for the region located just superior to the patella or the elbow and can be performed via fanning retroinjections with cannulas or linear threading with needles using one syringe per session per area (half per side). Dilutions can range from 1:1 to 1:4. It is unclear if product migration can occur in these highly active areas.

SAFETY CONSIDERATIONS

After over 15 years of clinical experience, multiple publications have demonstrated the long-term safety and tolerability of CaHA fillers. As with all soft tissue fillers, transient local reactions such as ecchymosis, edema, erythema, pain, and itching have been noted to varying extents. These should not be classified as true filler-specific AEs, but rather as injection-site reactions due mainly to skin trauma from the volume and technique of injection rather than the CaHA filler material itself. Their incidence can therefore be decreased by following appropriate treatment protocols.

In a 2017 review of 21 peer-reviewed articles including over 5000 treatments with CaHA, there was a 3% incidence of filler-specific AEs. These consisted most commonly of nodules (96%), followed by persistent inflammation or swelling (2%), persistent erythema (1%), and overcorrection (1%). The incidence of AEs was highest for lip treatments (9.4%). No infections/biofilms, abscesses, hypersensitivity reactions, product migrations or dislocations, calcifications, granulomas, or other serious AEs were reported in the included studies.

Injection-Site Reactions

The injection-related AEs mentioned previously are generally mild and resolve spontaneously within a few hours to weeks. Bruising can be minimized by slowly injecting small aliquots of product, using blunt cannulas, and limiting the number of skin punctures using linear-threading or fanning techniques. Ideally, all blood-thinning medications should be stopped 1 week prior to injection if possible. The degree of postprocedural edema can be intense, but the application of ice immediately after treatment is generally sufficient to reduce swelling.

The patient should refrain from massaging or manipulating the treatment area for at least 24 hours, as this can disturb the position of the filler. Care should also be taken to minimize excessive sun or heat exposure for 24 hours or until swelling and redness resolve. Some experts instruct patients to stay upright for the remainder of the day and sleep with their head elevated to reduce edema. To minimize the risk of infection, the injector should clean the treatment site with a topical disinfectant, wear gloves, use a new syringe for each subject, and use sterile equipment. Prophylactic valacyclovir can be considered when treating the perioral area in patients with a history of herpes infections.

Pain

Injection-related pain can be managed with the application of ice or other cooling systems, topical anesthetic creams, local infiltration of anesthetic (taking care to limit the total volume injected to prevent tissue distortion), or regional nerve blocks. As previously discussed, up to 1.5 mL of lidocaine can also be combined with CaHA to enhance patient comfort.

Immunological

Because CaHA is considered biocompatible, preprocedural sensitivity testing is not required. The smooth, spherical shape of the microspheres also reduces the risk of a granulomatous reaction. No significant immunological reactions have been reported after implantation.

Nodules

Nodules are by far the most common AE associated with CaHA filler, observed in approximately 3% of treatments in one large-scale review. Given the inert nature of CaHA, nodules are much more likely to result from particle accumulation than from a granulomatous inflammatory response. Foreign body reactions have been reported in only a handful of case reports in over a decade of use. Nodules have been shown to occur most commonly in dynamic facial areas, such as the lips and periorbital area, likely due to product agglomeration from muscle contractions. Avoiding these areas should therefore significantly decrease the risk of nodule formation. Higher dilutions of CaHA likely reduce the risk of nodule formation from product accumulation similar to the reduction seen in higher dilutions of poly-L-lactic acid.

Experts suggest that early nodules arising within 2 weeks postinjection are likely due to technical mishaps (e.g., overfilling or injecting too superficially) and may be treated with intralesional injection of saline or sterile water, vigorous massage, aspiration, or fractional laser therapy. Late nodules are likely due to dislocated or accumulated product material or a foreign body reaction. They typically resolve without intervention given the biodegradable nature of the CaHA microspheres. Resolution after intralesional corticosteroid injection may suggest a granulomatous reaction. Excision has also been described, but this option should be utilized only as a last resort.

Radiographic Safety Concerns

Based on x-ray and computed tomographic (CT) scans of patients treated with facial CaHA injections, one study determined that the product poses no overt radiographic safety concerns. CaHA filler was clearly visible on CT scans performed immediately postinjection but did not obscure underlying structures. The authors concluded that it is unlikely that CaHA depots would be confused with radiographic abnormalities. Only residual amounts of CaHA were observed 12 months postinjection, confirming that the aesthetic effect lasts longer than the product. In addition, the study found no evidence of osteogenesis or product migration after CaHA was implanted in the deep dermis or subcutaneous plane. No calcification or osteogenesis has been reported in the literature, likely due to the fact that progenitor cells for osteogenesis do not exist in soft tissue.

Skin of Color

In a study of 100 subjects with Fitzpatrick skin types IV to VI who received CaHA filler in the nasolabial folds, no reports of keloid formation, hypertrophic scarring, dyspigmentation, or other clinically significant AEs were recorded up to 6 months posttreatment. Postinflammatory hyperpigmentation developed in two subjects with Fitzpatrick skin type III when CaHA was used to treat striae, but the dyspigmentation resolved after 1 month of treatment with a whitening cream (Kligman's formula).

FURTHER READING

Amselem, M. (2016). Radiesse(®): A novel rejuvenation treatment for the upper arms. *Clinical, Cosmetic and Investigational Dermatology*, *9*, 9–14. https://doi.org/10.2147/CCID.S93137.

Bass, L. S., Smith, S., Busso, M., & McClaren, M. (2010). Calcium hydroxylapatite (Radiesse) for treatment of nasolabial folds: Long-term safety and efficacy results. *Aesthetic Surgery Journal*, *30*, 235–238. https://doi.org/10.1177/1090820X10366549.

Bertucci, V., Solish, N., Wong, M., & Howell, M. (2015). Evaluation of the Merz Hand Grading Scale after calcium hydroxylapatite hand treatment. *Dermatologic Surgery*, *41*(suppl 1), S389–S396. https://doi.org/10.1097/DSS.0000000000000546.

Busso, M., & Applebaum, D. (2007). Hand augmentation with Radiesse (calcium hydroxylapatite). *Dermatologic Therapy*, *20*(6), 385–387. https://doi.org/10.1111/j.1529-8019.2007.00153.x.

Carruthers, A., Liebeskind, M., Carruthers, J., & Forster, B. B. (2008). Radiographic and computed tomographic studies of calcium hydroxylapatite for treatment of HIV-associated facial lipoatrophy and correction of nasolabial folds. *Dermatologic Surgery*, *34*(suppl 1), S78–S84. https://doi.org/10.1111/j.1524-4725.2008.34247.x.

Casabona, G., & Marchese, P. (2017). Calcium hydroxylapatite combined with microneedling and ascorbic acid is effective for treating stretch marks. *Plastic and Reconstructive Surgery. Global Open*, *5*(9), e1474. https://doi.org/10.1097/GOX.0000000000001474.

Casabona, G., & Pereira, G. (2017). Microfocused ultrasound with visualization and calcium hydroxylapatite for improving skin laxity and cellulite appearance. *Plastic and Reconstructive Surgery. Global Open*, *5*(7), e1388. https://doi.org/10.1097/GOX.0000000000001388.

Casabona, G. (2018). Combined use of microfocused ultrasound and a calcium hydroxylapatite dermal filler for treating atrophic acne scars: A pilot study. *Journal of Cosmetic and Laser Therapy*, *20*(5), 301–306. https://doi.org/10.1080/14764172.2017.1406606.

Chang, J. W., Koo, W. Y., Kim, E.-K., Lee, S. W., & Lee, J. H. (2020). Facial rejuvenation using a mixture of calcium hydroxylapatite filler and hyaluronic acid filler. *The Journal of Craniofacial Surgery*, *31*(1), e18–e21. https://doi.org/10.1097/SCS.0000000000005809.

Cogorno Wasylkowski, V. (2015). Body vectoring technique with Radiesse(®) for tightening of the abdomen, thighs, and brachial zone. *Clinical, Cosmetic and Investigational Dermatology*, *8*, 267–273. https://doi.org/10.2147/CCID.S75631.

Coleman, K. M., Voigts, R., DeVore, D. P., Termin, P., & Coleman, W. P. (2008). Neocollagenesis after injection of calcium hydroxylapatite composition in a canine model. *Dermatologic Surgery*, *34*(suppl 1), S53–S55. https://doi.org/10.1111/j.1524-4725.2008.34243.x.

Dallara, J.-M., Baspeyras, M., Bui, P., Cartier, H., Charavel, M.-H., & Dumas, L. (2014). Calcium hydroxylapatite for jawline rejuvenation: Consensus recommendations. *Journal of Cosmetic Dermatology*, *13*, 3–14. https://doi.org/10.1111/jocd.12074.

de Almeida, A. T., Figueredo, V., da Cunha, A. L. G., et al. (2019). Consensus recommendations for the use of hyperdiluted calcium hydroxyapatite (Radiesse) as a face and body biostimulatory agent. *Plastic and Reconstructive Surgery. Global Open*, *7*(3), e2160. https://doi.org/10.1097/GOX.0000000000002160.

Emer, J., & Sundaram, H. (2013). Aesthetic applications of calcium hydroxylapatite volumizing filler: An evidence-based review and discussion of current concepts: (part 1 of 2). *Journal of Drugs in Dermatology*, *12*(12), 1345–1354.

Figueredo, V. O., Miot, H. A., Soares Dias, J., Nunes, G. J. B., Barros de Souza, M., & Bagatin, E. (2020). Efficacy and safety of 2 injection techniques for hand biostimulatory treatment with diluted calcium hydroxylapatite. *Dermatologic Surgery*, *46*(suppl 1), S54–S61. https://doi.org/10.1097/DSS.0000000000002334.

Frank, K., Koban, K., Targosinski, S., et al. (2018). The anatomy behind adverse events in hand volumizing procedures: Retrospective evaluations of 11 years of experience. *Plastic and Reconstructive Surgery*, *141*, 650e–662e. https://doi.org/10.1097/PRS.0000000000004211.

Goldie, K., Peeters, W., Alghoul, M., et al. (2018). Global consensus guidelines for the injection of diluted and hyperdiluted calcium hydroxylapatite for skin tightening. *Dermatologic Surgery*, *44*(suppl 1), S32–S41. https://doi.org/10.1097/DSS.0000000000001685.

Goldman, M. P., Moradi, A., Gold, M. H., et al. (2018). Calcium Hydroxylapatite Dermal filler for treatment of dorsal hand volume loss: Results from a 12-month, multicenter, randomized, blinded trial. *Dermatologic Surgery*, *44*(1), 75–83. https://doi.org/10.1097/DSS.0000000000001203.

Graivier, M. H., Bass, L. S., Busso, M., Jasin, M. E., Narins, R. S., & Tzikas, T. L. (2007). Calcium hydroxylapatite (Radiesse) for correction of the mid- and lower face: Consensus recommendations. *Plastic and Reconstructive Surgery*, *120*, 55S–66S. https://doi.org/10.1097/01.prs.0000285109.34527.b9.

Kadouch, J. A. (2017). Calcium hydroxylapatite: A review on safety and complications. *Journal of Cosmetic Dermatology*, *16*(2), 152–161. https://doi.org/10.1111/jocd.12326.

Lapatina, N. G., & Pavlenko, T. (2017). Diluted calcium hydroxylapatite for skin tightening of the upper arms and abdomen. *Journal of Drugs in Dermatology*, *16*(9), 900–906.

Lemperle, G., Morhenn, V., & Charrier, U. (2003). Human histology and persistence of various injectable filler substances for soft tissue augmentation. *Aesthetic Plastic Surgery*, *27*(5), 354–366. discussion 367. https://doi.org/10.1007/s00266-003-3022-1.

Loghem, J. V., Yutskovskaya, Y. A., & Philip Werschler, W. (2015). Calcium hydroxylapatite: Over a decade of clinical experience. *The Journal of Clinical and Aesthetic Dermatology*, *8*(1), 38–49.

Marmur, E. S., Phelps, R., & Goldberg, D. J. (2004). Clinical, histologic and electron microscopic findings after injection of a calcium hydroxylapatite filler. *Journal of Cosmetic and Laser Therapy*, *6*(4), 223–226. https://doi.org/10.1080/14764170410003048.

Marmur, E. S., Taylor, S. C., Grimes, P. E., Boyd, C. M., Porter, J. P., & Yoo, J. Y. (2009). Six-month safety results of calcium hydroxylapatite for treatment of nasolabial folds in Fitzpatrick skin types IV to VI. *Dermatologic Surgery*, *35*(suppl 2), 1641–1645. https://doi.org/10.1111/j.1524-4725.2009.01311.x.

Pavicic, T. (2013). Calcium hydroxylapatite filler: An overview of safety and tolerability. *Journal of Drugs in Dermatology*, *12*(9), 996–1002.

Rovatti, P. P., Pellacani, G., & Guida, S. (2020). Hyperdiluted calcium hydroxylapatite 1: 2 for mid and lower facial skin rejuvenation: Efficacy and safety. *Dermatologic Surgery*, *46*(12), e112–e117. https://doi.org/10.1097/DSS.0000000000002375.

Souza, G. P., & Serra, M. S. (2018). Treatment of actinic purpura with calcium hydroxyapatite. *Surgical and Cosmetic Dermatology*, *10*,355–358.https://doi.org/10.5935/scd1984-8773.20181041201.

Yutskovskaya, Y., Kogan, E., & Leshunov, E. (2014). A randomized, split-face, histomorphologic study comparing a volumetric calcium hydroxylapatite and a hyaluronic acid-based dermal filler. *Journal of Drugs in Dermatology*, *13*(9), 1047–1052.

Yutskovskaya, Y. A., & Kogan, E. A. (2017). Improved neocollagenesis and skin mechanical properties after injection of diluted calcium hydroxylapatite in the neck and décolletage: A pilot study. *Journal of Drugs in Dermatology*, *16*(1), 68–74.

Zerbinati, N., Rauso, R., Protasoni, M., et al. (2019). Pegylated hyaluronic acid filler enriched with calcium hydroxyapatite treatment of human skin: Collagen renewal demonstrated through morphometric computerized analysis. *Journal of Biological Regulators and Homeostatic Agents*, *33*(6), 1967–1971. https://doi.org/10.23812/19-250-L.

10

Poly-L-Lactic Acid

Daniel Yanes, Rebecca Fitzgerald, Shannon Humphrey, and Katie Beleznay

SUMMARY AND KEY FEATURES

- Gradual, subtle, and natural results with a long duration (> 2 years) are achievable with poly-L-lactic acid (PLLA).
- Thorough facial analysis of changes in all structural tissues will enhance site-specific augmentation of volume loss and enhance outcomes.
- PLLA has been increasingly used off label for soft tissue augmentation and improvement of skin laxity in a number of off-face areas, including décolleté, arms, abdomen, and buttocks.
- The amount of product used at one session is determined by the amount of surface area to be treated at that session. The final volumetric correction is determined by the number of treatment sessions.
- Proper technique in the preparation and injection of this biostimulatory agent will minimize adverse events.
- As experience has been gained with this product and techniques have evolved, it has been found to be a safe and effective product with predictable and reproducible results.

INTRODUCTION

Poly-L-lactic acid (PLLA) is a biocompatible and biodegradable synthetic polymer that stimulates collagen production. The currently commercially available forms, Sculptra (Sinclair Pharmaceuticals) and Sculptra Aesthetic (Galderma Laboratories, Fort Worth, TX), were approved by the US Federal Drug Administration (FDA) for the treatment of human immunodeficiency virus (HIV)-associated lipoatrophy in 2004 and "correction of shallow to deep nasolabial fold contour deficiencies and other facial wrinkles using a deep dermal grid pattern injection" in 2009. Since that time, PLLA has been increasingly used off-label for soft tissue augmentation both on and off the face (i.e., buttocks), as well as for improvement of skin laxity (face, décolleté, arms, and abdomen).

PLLA provides gradual, subtle, and natural results with a lasting duration. The approach to treatment with PLLA involves replacing volume by considering a three-dimensional (3D) perspective rather than focusing on individual lines and folds. Proper patient selection and assessment, as well as attention to technique in the preparation and injection of the material, will minimize adverse events and optimize results.

PATIENT SELECTION, EXPECTATIONS, AND SATISFACTION

The gradual results seen with PLLA (usually about 4 weeks after treatment) may not make this the optimal choice for someone looking for an immediate "quick fix" for an upcoming event; however, it is an excellent choice for those wanting subtle, long-lasting results. In the studies used to gain initial FDA approval, almost 80% of patients treated still saw full correction at 25 months (the cutoff time for the study).

Recall that the initial global experience with PLLA was in the HIV-positive population as well as in older cosmetic patients, most of whom required a fair amount of product and multiple treatment sessions to achieve the desired outcome. We now recognize this as an issue of patient selection, not product selection. Older and emptier faces require more product of any kind to achieve correction. Patients who require significant volume need to be corrected with PLLA in a gradual progressive manner over multiple treatment sessions. Treatments are usually administered at 4- to 6-week intervals. Younger or fuller-faced patients may respond well and need less product and fewer treatment sessions. A longer interval between treatment sessions may be prudent for younger or fuller-faced patients who require less volume. This difference is illustrated in the patient cases seen in Figs. 10.1–10.4. The video accompanying this chapter demonstrates treatment of a 41-year-old patient with aging changes superimposed on congenital skeletal hypoplasia (Video 10.1).

PATHOPHYSIOLOGY OF THE AGING FACE: STRUCTURAL AND MORPHOLOGIC

Current thinking conceptualizes the soft tissues of the face as a concentric arrangement of five basic layers, which consist of (1) skin, (2) subcutaneous fat, (3) the musculoaponeurotic layer, (4) areolar tissue, including facial ligaments and facial spaces, and (5) the periosteum and deep muscular fascia. The facial retaining ligaments pass through all layers to bind the skeleton to the superficial fascia (a composite of layers 1–3).

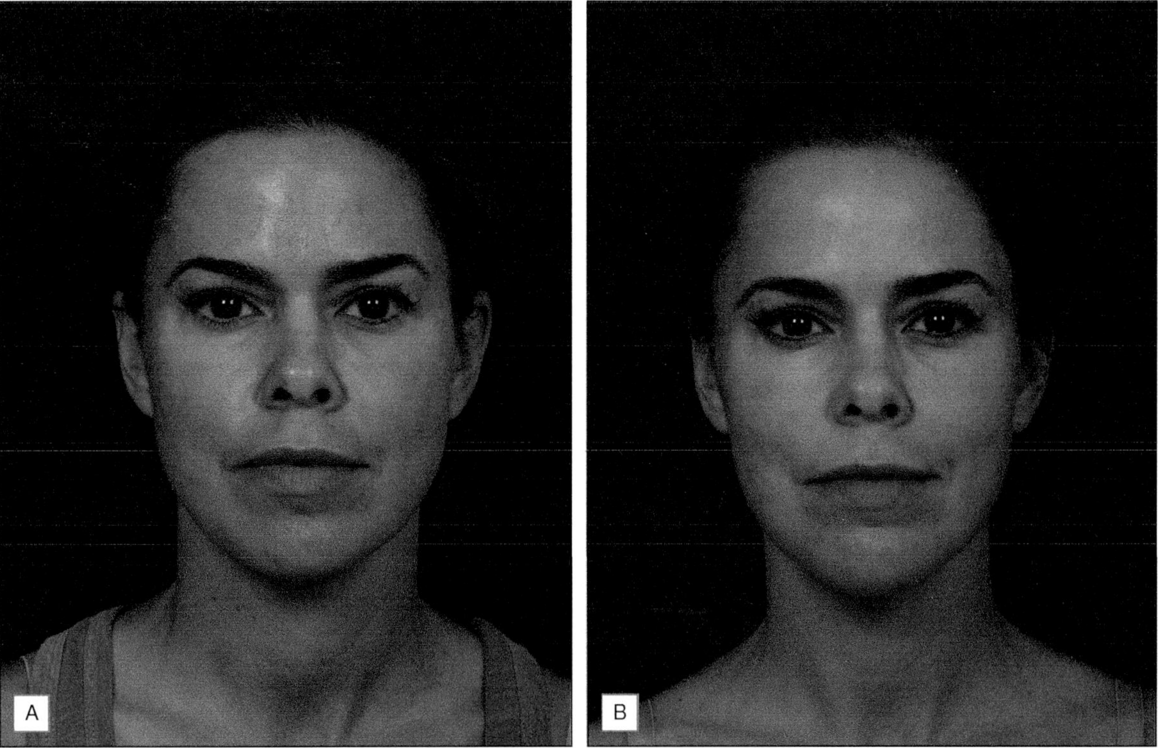

Fig. 10.1 A 41-year-old patient with aging changes superimposed on congenital skeletal hypoplasia before (A) and 4 weeks after (B) two vials of poly-L-lactic acid used panfacially as demonstrated with narration in the video provided for this chapter. Neuromodulater was used in the glabella. Note the increased brow projection, bizygomatic width, and improvement in perioral support giving an improved phi ratio to the lower third of the face. Note also the ovalization of the facial shape as well as improvement in skin quality. See the accompanying video for treatment of this patient.

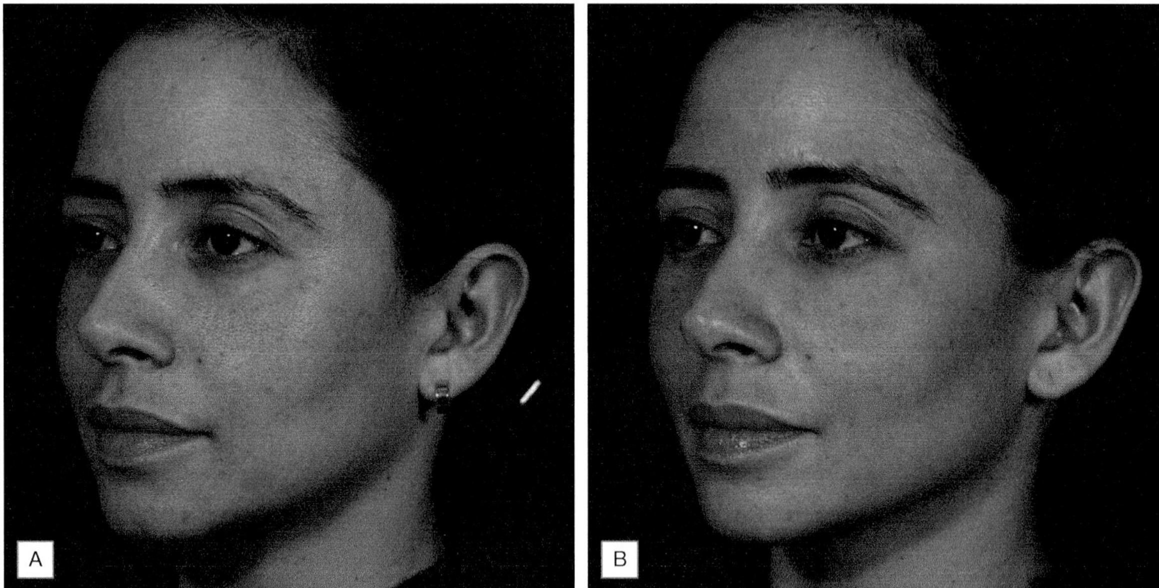

Fig. 10.2 A 38-year-old patient before (A) and 3 months after (B) two vials of poly-L-lactic acid done in one session. The product was placed supraperiosteally along the supraorbital rim, medial maxilla, pyriform aperture, zygoma, and mandible. The product was also placed in the temporal lateral cheek, deep medial cheek, and submentalis fat compartments. Note the effacement of the early shadowing in the nasojugal fold and pre-jowl sulcus leading to sharper definition of the cheeks and jawline.

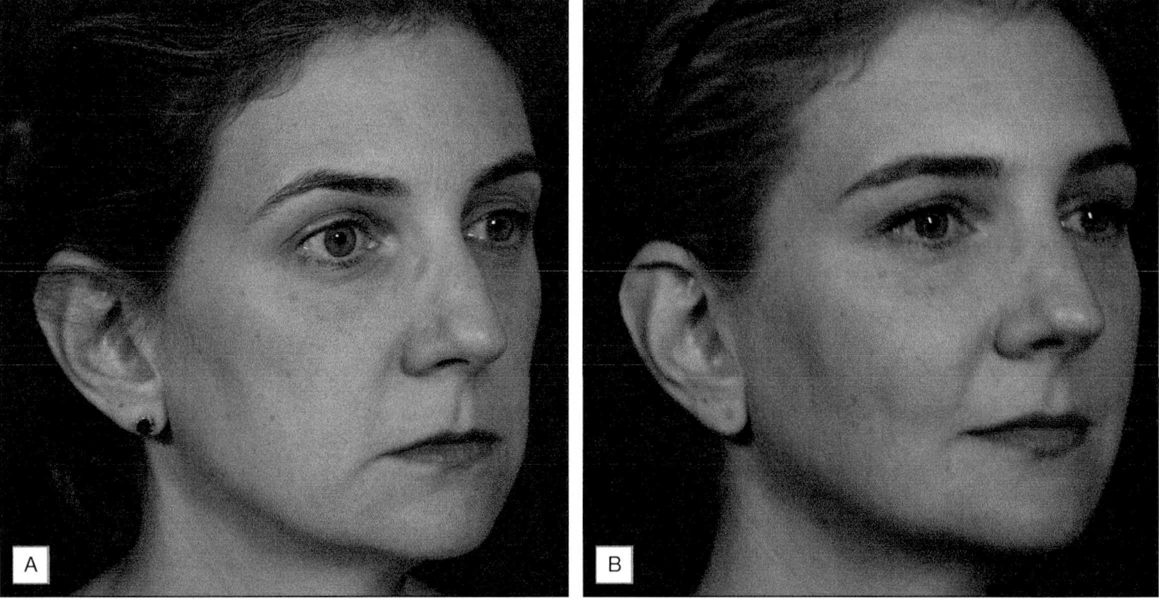

Fig. 10.3 A 38-year-old patient before (A) and 6 months after (B) poly-L-lactic acid two vials per session, three sessions spaced 1 month apart. Note the improvement in the anterior projection and convexity of the face as well as in skin quality. This athletic patient presented with significant loss of volume in her facial fat and therefore required more sessions than most patients her age.

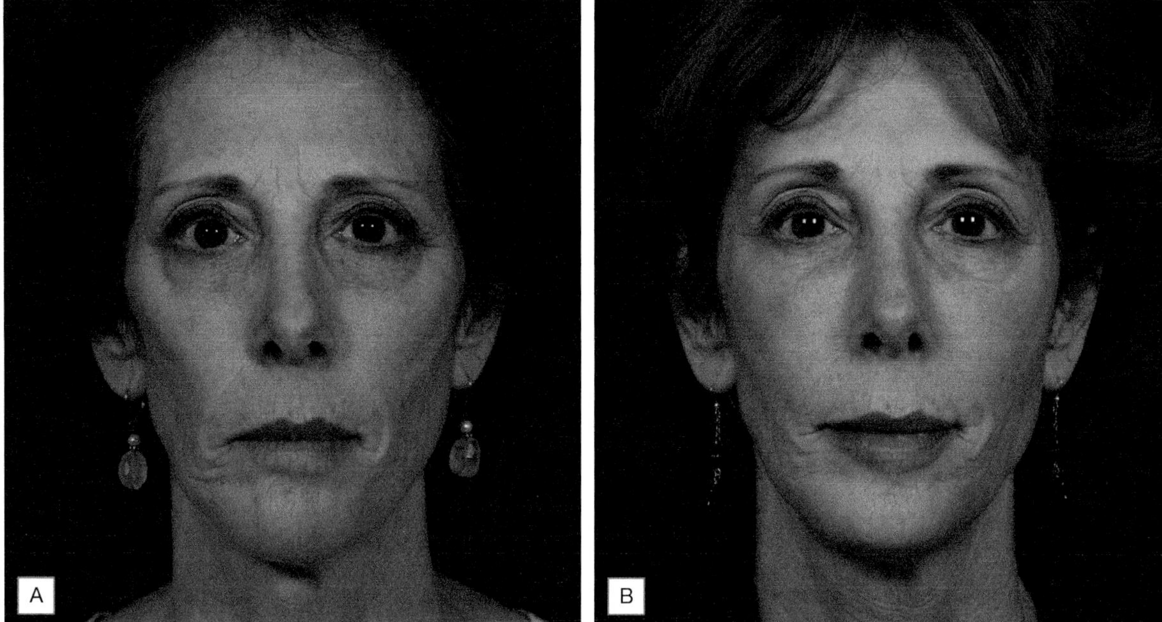

Fig. 10.4 A 59-year-old patient before (A) and 6 months after (B) poly-L-lactic acid (PLLA) three vials per session, two sessions spaced 1 month apart. PLLA was placed supraperiosteally along the supraorbital rim, anterior maxilla, pyriform aperture, and mandible and in fat compartments in the temple, cheek, and chin. Hyaluronic acid and neuromodulator were placed around the eyes and lips with the initial treatment. Note the ovalization and increased anterior convexity of her face as well as the improvement in skin quality.

Aging leads to loss or redistribution of volume in the bony substructure and fat compartments of the face, which may occur in conjunction with loss of elasticity of the skin that envelops it. The facial retaining ligaments often become more visible with aging or fat loss. These changes dictate the morphology of the face in terms of its shape, proportions, and 3D topography. Recognizing where these structures are changing, as well as how that affects neighboring tissues, enhances our ability to address them with site-specific corrections to achieve optimal, natural-looking results. Obviously, this knowledge is in a constant state of evolution.

It is now widely accepted that significant changes occur in specific regions of the facial skeleton with advancing age and these changes in bony structure affect soft tissue position. The most significant changes have been documented in the glabellar, orbital, maxillary, and pyriform angles as well as in the height and width of the orbital and pyriform aperture as seen in Fig. 10.5. Rohrich and Pessa first performed multiple cadaver studies utilizing dye sequestration to show that subcutaneous fat exists in both superficial and deep compartments in 2007. A few years later, Geirloff et al. collaborated this finding using 3D computed tomography and radiopaque dye. Facial fat compartments are illustrated in Fig. 10.6. We now recognize that changes in the volume and position of these fat compartments contribute to the changes in facial contour seen with aging—for example, the contribution of the temporal and lateral superficial fat compartments in the overall oval shape of the face, as well as the role of the midfacial deep cheek compartments in the anterior projection of the midface and the development (or effacement) of nasojugal and nasolabial folds. Mendelson and Wong have done extensive work implicating the important role that the facial ligaments play in the characteristic changes seen in the aging face.

Fig. 10.7 illustrates the location of the "line of ligaments," which delineate the relatively mobile anterior face from the relatively immobile lateral face. Treatment in this lateral facial area (i.e., temple and lateral cheek), as well as supraperiosteal treatment along the lateral zygoma, may serve to lift the cheeks and the jawline.

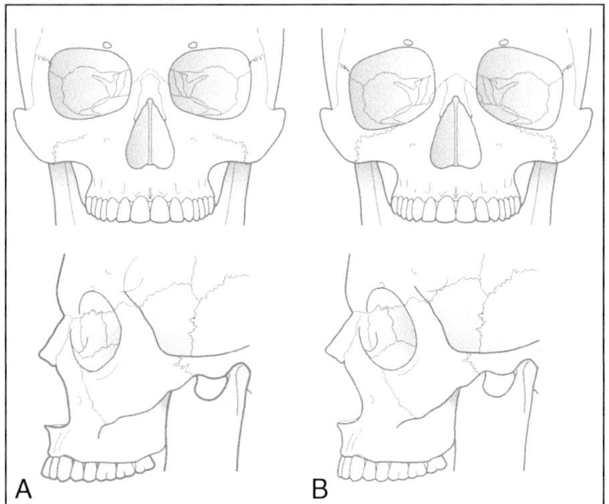

Fig. 10.5 A pictorial summary of age-related changes to the mid-face skeleton. (A) Features of a youthful skull include a malar eminence, infraorbital rim, and pyriform aperture that are positioned anterior and vertical in the sagittal plane. The orbital aperture is small with a horizontally positioned inferior orbital rim. (B) Older patients have a retroclined malar eminence, infraorbital rim, and pyriform aperture compared with that of young patients. The orbital aperture area is increased secondary to progressive curve distortion of the orbital rim superomedially and inferolaterally.

No two faces are exactly the same. Additionally, although the sequence of events as we age is somewhat predictable, the pace of these events is individualized. A deeper understanding of the contributions of all structural layers to facial morphology will help us assess each individual face with greater precision.

PRODUCT AND MECHANISM OF ACTION

PLLA is supplied in a glass vial containing 367.5 mg powdered PLLA microparticles along with sodium carboxymethylcellulose (a suspending agent used to maintain even distribution) and mannitol (to enhance solubility of the product). Prior to use, it is reconstituted with sterile water for injection (SWFI) to form a suspension, which is then left to "hydrate" for at least 2 hours as per the FDA-approved label.

The microparticles of PLLA measure 40 to 63 μm in diameter. This size means that the particles are large enough to avoid phagocytosis by dermal macrophages and cannot pass through capillary walls, but are small enough to be injected with needles as fine as 26 gauge (G).

Once injected, PLLA induces a subclinical inflammatory response, followed by encapsulation of the particles, and subsequent fibroblast proliferation and collagen formation. Goldberg et al. showed a statistically significant 33.7% increase in mean level of type I collagen 6 months after PLLA injection ($p = 0.03$). In addition, increases in type I and type III collagen were seen in 79% and 72% of patients, respectively. PLLA acts differently from traditional injectable fillers as new volume is generated in a gradual, progressive manner through fibroplasia. PLLA is gradually degraded and metabolized to CO_2 and H_2O.

EVOLUTION OF METHODOLOGY

The 2004 FDA approval for HIV lipoatrophy (based on early studies) used 3 to 4 mL SWFI. This was increased to 5 mL with the 2009 aesthetic approval, as newer studies with higher dilutions showed a marked decrease in the incidence of undesirable papules. This methodology has gradually evolved over the last decade of clinical practice, leading to the reconstitution most commonly used currently: 8 to 9 mL on-face and 16 mL off-face, as well as a hydration time of 24 to 72 hours. In addition, subcutaneous and supraperiosteal injections are now used more commonly than the "deep dermal grid pattern" approved in 2009.

Very recently, in vitro studies carried out by the manufacturer were found to support the feasibility of immediate use, allowing for the elimination of hydration time. This new change in the reconstitution procedure is contingent upon an acceptable safety profile from ongoing clinical studies nearing completion. This offers potential for the added convenience of an immediate use product. An updated FDA label reflective of these changes (an 8 mL dilution/1 mL lidocaine reconstitution, subdermal injections, and immediate use with elimination of hydration time) has recently been approved.

POLY-L-LACTIC ACID: TECHNICAL CONSIDERATIONS

Proper technique will minimize adverse events and optimize results when using stimulatory agents such as PLLA as outlined later and summarized in Box 10.1.

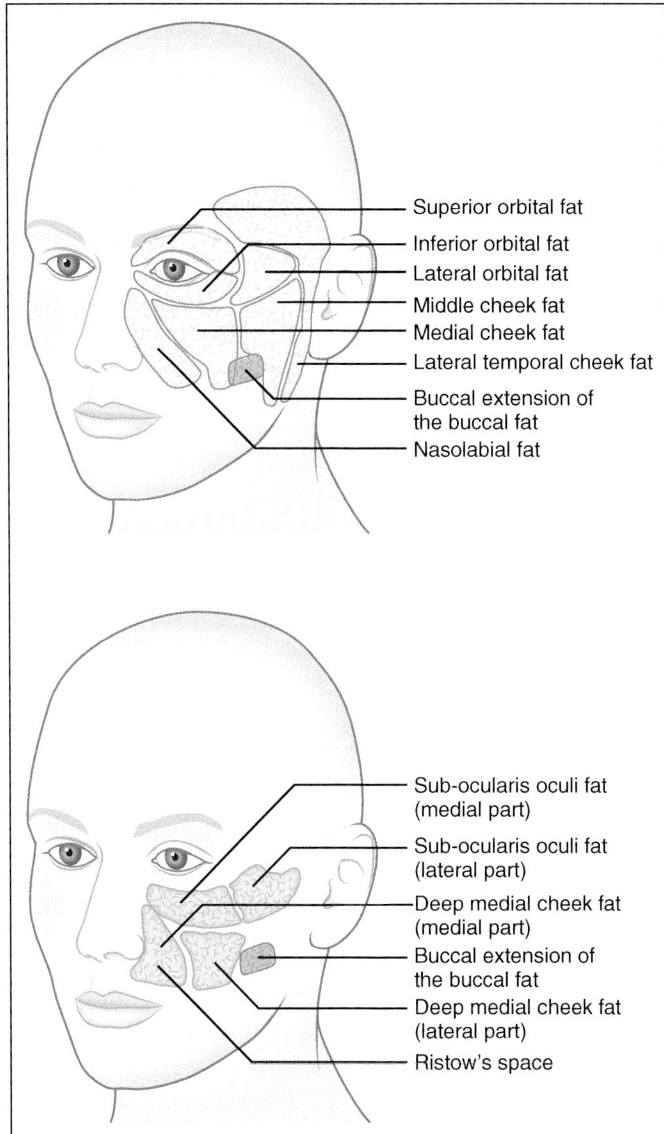

Fig. 10.6 Anatomical relationships of the superficial and deep facial fat compartments. The superficial layer *(yellow)* is composed of the nasolabial fat, the medial cheek fat, the middle cheek fat, the lateral temporal cheek compartment, and three orbital compartments. The deep midfacial fat compartments are composed of the sub-orbicularis oculi fat (medial and lateral parts) and the deep medial cheek fat (medial and lateral parts). Three layers of distinct fat compartments are found laterally to the pyriform aperture, where a deep compartment *(blue)* is located posterior to the medial part of the deep medial cheek fat. The buccal extension of the buccal fat pad extends from the paramaxillary space to the subcutaneous plane. (Modified from Geirloff M, Stohring C, Buder T, et al. Aging changes of the midfacial fat compartments: a computed tomographic study. *Plast Reconstr Surg*. 2012;129(1):263–273.)

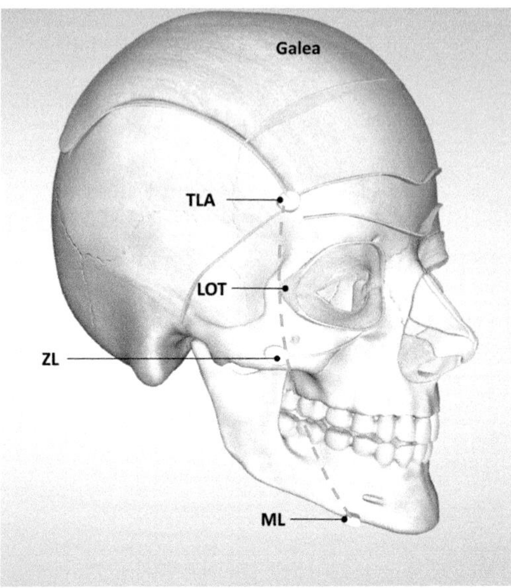

Fig. 10.7 Model of the face showing the major facial ligaments. Note how the ligaments can be aligned into one line located immediately lateral to the lateral orbital rim extending from the temporal crest to the mandible, creating the line of ligaments (indicated in *blue*). *LOT*, Lateral orbital thickening; *ML*, mandibular ligament; *TLA*, temporal ligamentous adhesion; *ZL*, zygomatic ligament. (Adapted with permission from Casabona G, Frank K, Koban KC, et al. Lifting vs volumizing—the difference in facial minimally invasive procedures when respecting the line of ligaments. *J Cosmet Dermatol.* 2019;00:1–7.)

BOX 10.1 Key technical points for achieving optimal outcomes with PLLA.

- Proper preparation and placement are critical. Most problems with this agent stem from global or focal overcorrection ("too much, too soon").
- The product should be evenly suspended immediately prior to each injection as microparticles may precipitate out of suspension.
- Even distribution and appropriate plane of injection of PLLA is key to a desirable outcome.
- Superficial placement leads to visible neocollagenesis.
- Placement in active muscles can lead to clumping of particles and nodules.
- Depositing significant product at one location such as the apex of the "fan" when using a fanning technique can lead to focal papules and nodules.
- Massage should be done immediately postinjection and may be continued for 5 days.

PLLA, Poly-L-lactic acid.

Dilution, Hydration, and Storage

As noted earlier, the most commonly used reconstitution volumes currently are 8 to 9 mL on-face, 16 mL off-face, with a hydration time of 24 to 72 hours. SWFI is recommended for dilution. Traditional reconstitution instructions are to add the SWFI slowly and avoid shaking in order to prevent inadvertent deposition of clumps of dry product on the wall of the vial prior to a period of hydration. The rubber stopper can be removed to add water then replaced using a clean technique. The vial holds less than 10 mL. To achieve the larger dilutions used for off-face injections, the hydrated product can be drawn into a large (i.e., 20 mL) syringe, diluted accordingly, and distributed to smaller 1- to 3-mL syringes via sterile connectors or can be diluted within the individual syringes used to inject just prior to use (i.e., draw up a 1:1 ratio of reconstituted product to SWFI in the syringe, which will be used for injection-mix by swirling the syringe). The hydrated vial can be stored at room temperature for 24 to 72 hours or kept refrigerated for up to 3 to 4 weeks prior to use. Product should be warmed to room temperature prior to injection.

Preparation Prior to Use

Prior to injection, topical anesthetic and/or ice can be applied to the target region. The area should be cleansed thoroughly using topical antiseptics such as 4% chlorhexidine (avoiding eyes and ears) and 70% alcohol immediately prior to injection, as with all filler material.

The vial should be swirled gently, but thoroughly, immediately prior to drawing up the product into syringes for injection to avoid excessive foam and ensure a homogenous suspension. Immediately prior to use, lidocaine 1% to 2% with or without epinephrine can be added to achieve the final dilution (i.e., 8 mL SWFI and 1 mL lidocaine for a final dilution of 9 mL). The lidocaine should be dripped in slowly.

An 18 or 22 G needle may be used to withdraw the suspension into 1- or 3-mL syringes for injection. The rubber stopper can be removed from the vial to facilitate withdrawing the product. Partially filling syringes may be more comfortable for a smaller hand (i.e., 2 mL of product in a 3-mL syringe). Tilt the vial and draw from the bottom to avoid foam, which may cause needle clogging. Any foam present should be expelled from the hub prior to placement of the needle or cannula, which should then be primed prior to use to avoid plugging with tissue upon entry. A 25 or 26 G 1- to 1½-inch needle or 25 G blunt-tipped cannula can be used for injection.

Potentially newer recommendations based on the physicochemical testing and clinical trials noted earlier are still awaiting final determination but are as follows: (1) add 5 mL SWFI and shake vigorously for minute, then (2) add an additional 3 mL SWFI and again shake vigorously for 1 minute, then (3) slowly drip in 1 mL lidocaine, swirl, and use immediately.

Product Amount

The volume (i.e., number of vials) of product used for any single treatment session should be determined by the surface area to be treated at that session, using approximately 0.1 to 0.3 mL/cm for the face. The final volumetric correction is addressed by the number of treatment sessions. This means, for instance, that a very large face with mild volume loss may require three vials injected in only one session, but a small face with severe volume loss may require one to two vials per session over three or more sessions. Off-face areas are most commonly treated with 0.05 to 0.1 mL/cm using a 16 mL dilution; however, there is some variability described in the current literature.

Product Placement

For facial rejuvenation, PLLA is injected deeply in a supraperiosteal location at the temple and along the zygoma, maxilla, and mandible. It may be placed subcutaneously in the midcheek as well. Injections in the preauricular and lateral cheek are done subcutaneously just under the dermis as deeper injections in this area may enter the parotid gland or duct. Fig. 10.8 illustrates site-specific recommendations for facial injection of PLLA. Upon injection, there is an immediate volumizing effect due to the presence of liquid used for reconstitution, which dissipates over 3 to 4 days. The subsequent fibroplasia develops over the next 4 weeks. The injector should massage after every few injections and again at the end of treatment to ensure proper placement of the product. Some recommend that the patient massage the area a few times daily over the next few days, while others feel it has no benefit. Follow the mantra "treat, wait, assess." Patients should receive repeat treatment no sooner than 4 weeks after previous treatment.

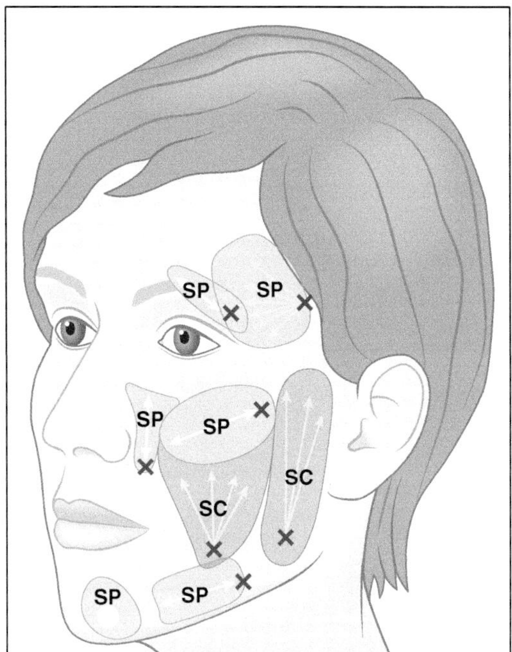

Fig. 10.8 Site-specific recommendations for facial injections of poly-L-lactic acid (PLLA). Potential areas amenable to correction with PLLA are indicated on this model. Recommended points of entry for each anatomic site are marked with a *red X*. Injectable PLLA should be placed supraperiosteally in the temples, lateral brow, zygomatic area, maxillary area, mandibular area, and mental area (*green areas* marked with *SP*). Injectable poly-L-lactic acid should be placed in the subcutaneous fat in the midcheek regions and preauricular area (*purple areas* marked with *SC*). Depending on the anatomic area, recommended techniques include fanning *(yellow arrows)*, retrograde linear threading *(white arrows)*, or depot *(white circle)* injection. (Adapted with permission from Bartus C, Hanke W, Daro-Kaftan E. A decade of experience with injectable poly-l-lactic acid: a focus on safety. *Dermatol Surg*. 2013;39:698–705.)

The product is also used in off-face areas. PLLA injection is a popular nonsurgical approach to gluteal augmentation. The number of vials and sessions needed are dependent on the degree of laxity present and amount of augmentation requested. Combination therapy with skin tightening devices in a thin, fit patient seeking modest improvement in sagging and volume may require less product and sessions than those using monotherapy or needing substantial volume (which may require a high volume of product given over multiple sessions) (Fig. 10.9). The product is injected into the superolateral buttock (often referred to as the "hip dip") using a fanning or linear threading

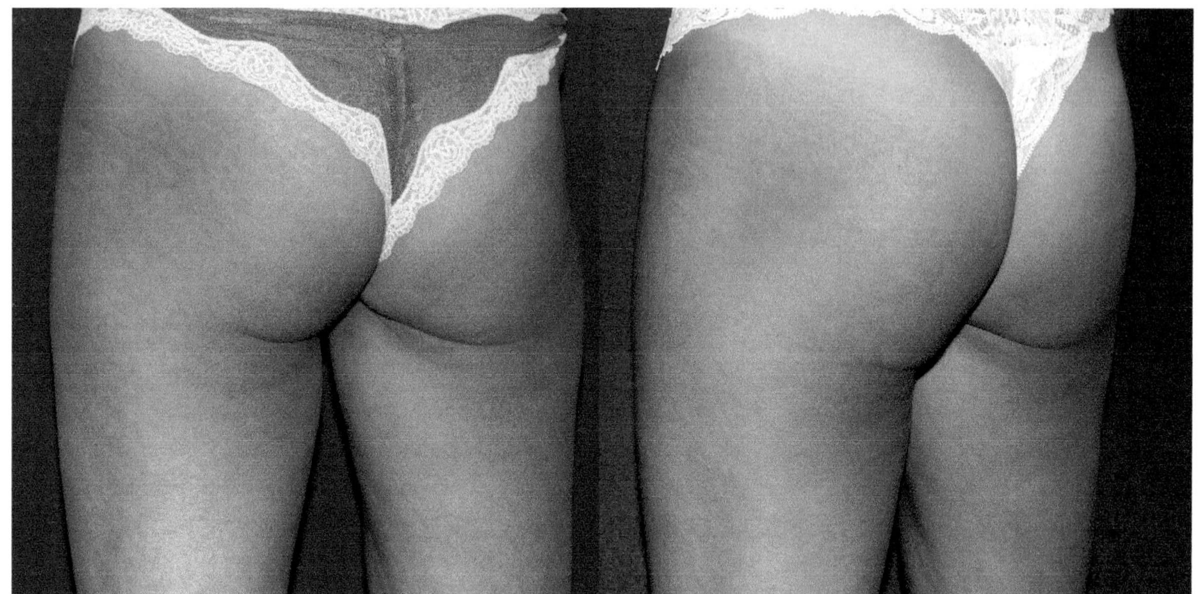

Fig. 10.9 Gluteal augmentation utilizing a combination approach. Patient before *(left)* and 3 months after *(right)* three vials of poly-L-lactic acid to each buttock followed immediately by microfocused ultrasound therapy. (Courtesy of Sabrina Fabi, MD.)

technique, avoiding redisposition of product at the apex of the fan. Injections should be beneath the dermis to avoid nodule formation but must remain superficial to muscle so as to avoid embolization of the underlying gluteal vasculature or trauma to the sciatic nerve, especially when injecting more medially. Injection into the superolateral quadrant of the buttock will help to lift while avoiding complications (Video 10.2).

PLLA has been used successfully in the treatment of skin laxity in the décolleté area, arms, and abdomen. Patients with significant laxity may require multiple sessions (Fig. 10.10, Video 10.3). Upper knees, thighs, and medial ankles have been treated with some improvement. All skin laxity is treated with superficial subcutaneous linear threading or fanning injections. Be aware that papules and nodules have been reported after treatment in the neck and dorsal hands. PLLA has been used successfully in combination with subcision to treat scarring, including acne scarring. Atrophic scarring has been treated with a 16 cc dilution applied topically immediately following fractional erbium laser with some success as well. Fig. 10.11 illustrates site-specific recommendations for nonfacial injection of PLLA.

COMPLICATIONS AND MANAGEMENT

The most common injection-related events are swelling, bruising, erythema, and pain, which typically resolve spontaneously over a short period of time. Other potential complications can be secondary to suboptimal preparation or technique, as well as inflammatory or vascular events. Delaying treatment in an area of active infection or in a patient with active autoimmune disease is recommended.

Papules and nodules result from a focal or global overabundance of product and most commonly stem from suboptimal product reconstitution or placement. Be aware that the product may precipitate out of suspension over time and should be evenly suspended in the syringe immediately prior to injection to avoid uneven distribution. Injection should be in the deep dermal, subcutaneous, or supraperiosteal plane. Superficial injection into the dermis should be avoided as this can lead to visible neocollagenesis seen as lumps and bumps. These are distinct from true clinical granulomas, which are a systemic inflammatory response showing an overabundance of host reaction (e.g., foreign body giant cells), to a relatively small amount of product (Fig. 10.12A). Because this is a systemic response, true

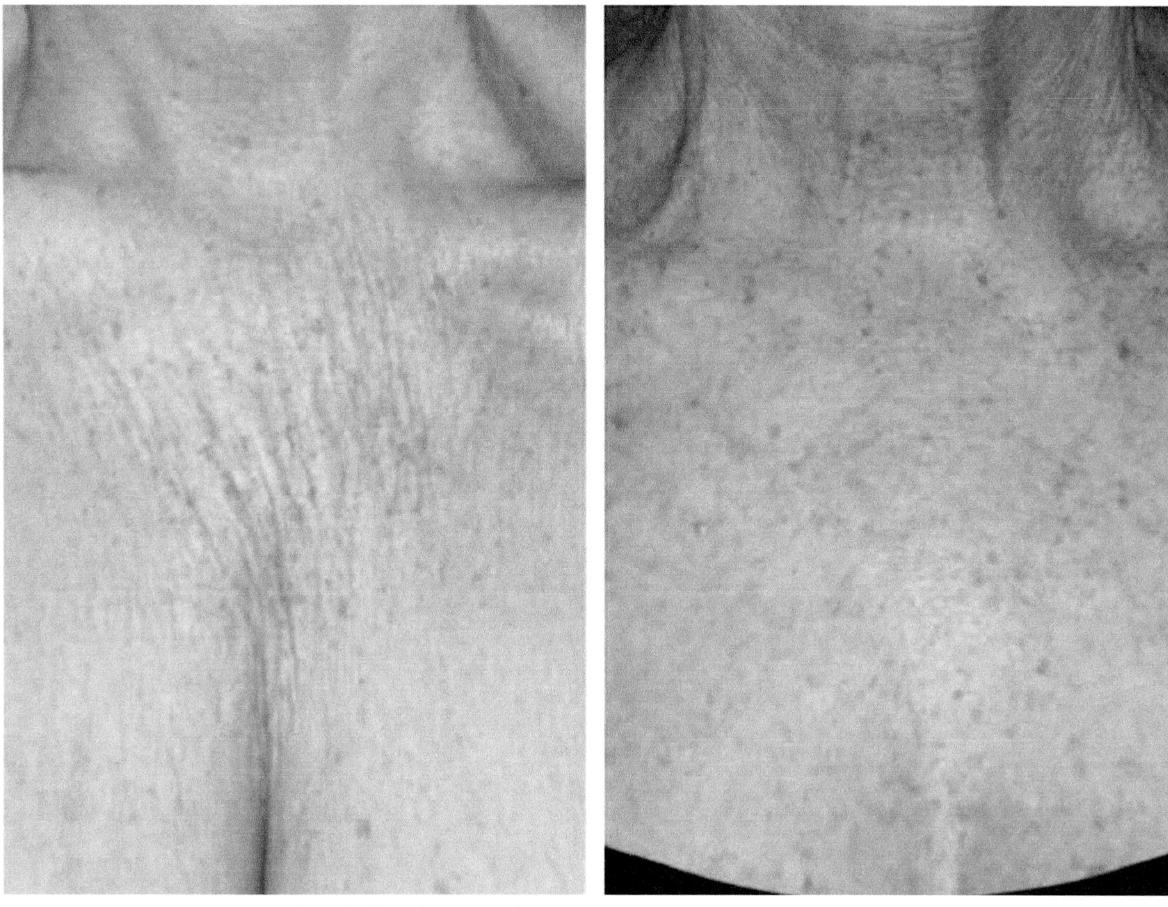

Fig. 10.10 Patient before *(left)* and 2 years after *(right)* poly-L-lactic acid (16 mL dilution) one vial per month for three consecutive months for chest wrinkles and two intense pulsed light treatments for dyschromia. (Reproduced with permission from Vanaman M, Fabi S. Décolletage: regional approaches with injectable fillers plast. *Reconstr Surg*. 2015;136:276S.)

clinical granulomas occur in all treated sites simultaneously, in contrast with papules and nodules, which occur in a limited area. Because true clinical granulomas represent an overabundance of proliferating foreign body giant cells, they respond well to treatment with antimetabolites like 5-fluorouracil (5-FU) or antiinflammatory agents like intralesional corticosteroids (i.e., 0.1 cc of 40 mg/cc Kenalog mixed with 0.9 cc 5-FU 50 mg/cc and no more than 2 cc in one session). This can be injected once a week for 2 weeks, then weekly until resolution. Improvement is usually seen in 2 to 3 weeks. True clinical granulomas have been reported with all currently available commercial fillers and are fortunately rare (0.01%–0.1%). Placement in or through areas of dynamic muscle particularly around the eyes or lips should also be avoided as this can lead to clumping of particles trapped in muscle fibers. Histopathology of these papules or nodules will show an overabundance of product with a few foreign body giant cells (Fig. 10.12B). The presence of these few foreign body giant cells may lead to a histopathologic diagnosis of "granuloma," although these lesions are not, in fact, true clinical granulomas. As papules and nodules represent product, not proliferating cells, they do not respond to treatment with intralesional steroids or 5-FU. In fact, intralesional steroids may make the problem even more visible by causing atrophy around the "bump." This was a common mishap in the early days with this product that is now disappearing due to a wider understanding of the difference between the two. Excision of nodules is an option but

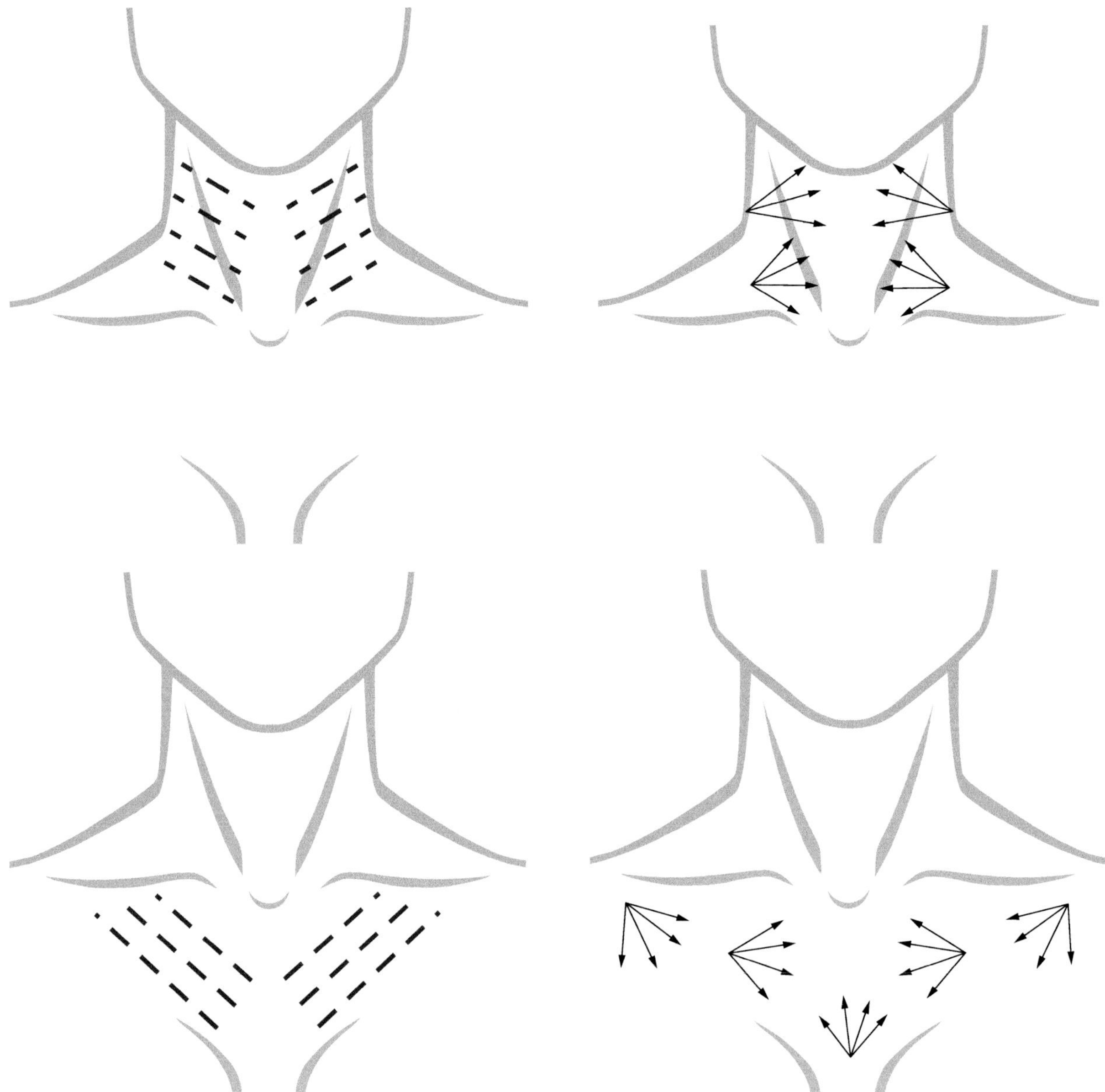

Fig. 10.11 Site-specific recommendations for off-face injections of poly-L-lactic acid utilizing needle or cannula in a linear or fanning pattern. (Modified with permission from Haddad A, Menezes A, Guarnieri C, et al. Recommendations on the use of injectable poly-L-lactic acid for skin laxity in off-face areas. *J Drugs Dermatol* 2019;18(9):929–935.)

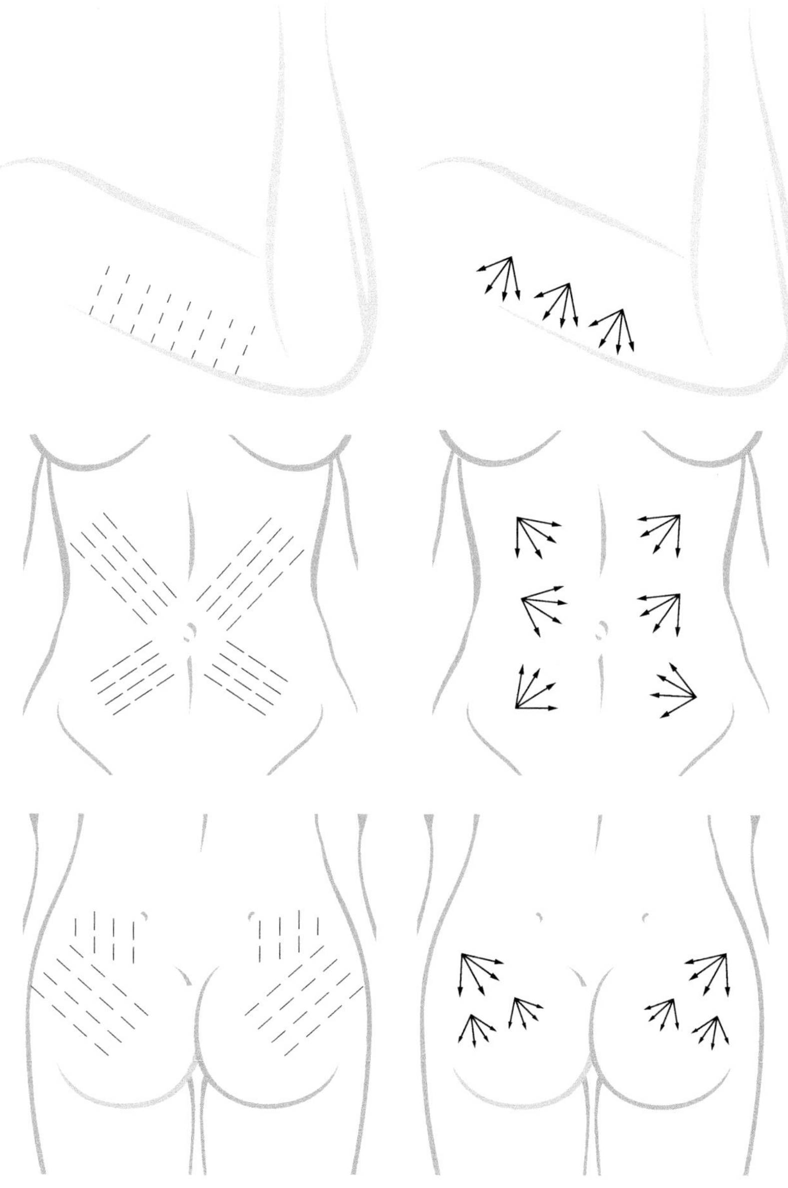

Fig. 10.11, Cont'd

results in a permanent scar. Reassuring the patient that this is a transient process that will resolve spontaneously over time may suffice. Hyaluronic acid filler to camouflage the nodule until it resorbs is a good option. Late-onset (14–24 months) inflammatory nodules have also been described and may represent end-stage degradation of the PLLA product. These can also be treated with injections of steroids or 5-FU but may resolve spontaneously over time.

Vascular complications may occur if the product is inadvertently injected into a blood vessel. This can cause local ischemia and/or skin necrosis. As the product is not dissolvable, supportive therapy such as hyperbaric oxygen can be considered. Blindness secondary to retrograde embolization of product into the ocular vessels, although extremely rare, has been described following injections of all fillers both on- and off-face, highlighting that knowledge and respect of regional

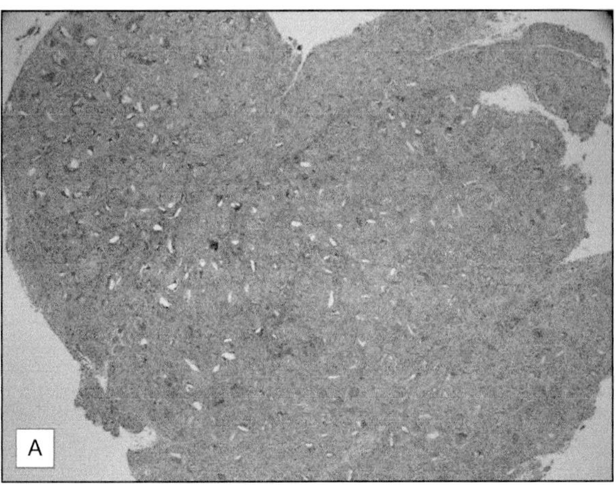

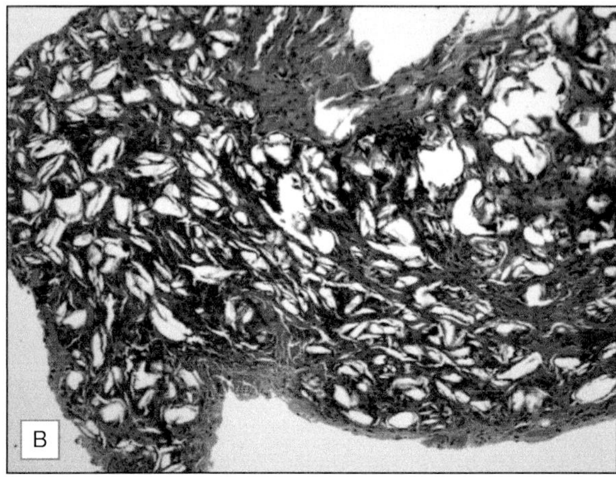

Fig. 10.12 Nodule versus granuloma/low-power histopathology. (A) True granuloma showing an overabundance of host reaction to a small amount of product. (B) Nodule with an overabundance of product trapped in skeletal muscle. (Reproduced with permission from Fitzgerald R, Vleggaar D. Facial volume restoration of the aging face with poly-L-lactic acid. *Dermatol Ther.* 2011;24:2–27.)

anatomy are imperative prior to any filler injection. A reflux maneuver may be carried out prior to each injection to lower the risk intravascular injection, although the reliability of reflux is controversial. Injections should be performed slowly without using excessive pressure. Use of a pump to expedite buttock injections has been described, but the injector should be aware that risk of vascular occlusion has been associated with high injection pressure.

CONCLUSIONS

PLLA is a safe and effective treatment for cosmetic enhancement. By stimulating new collagen, PLLA can restructure the face and gradually restore volume. Optimizing outcomes and minimizing adverse events require awareness and attention to the technical details outlined previously. Careful patient selection and thoughtful facial analysis of changes in all structural tissues will enhance site-specific augmentation and maximize satisfaction.

FURTHER READING

Baumann, K., Alm, J., Norberg, M., & Ejehorn, M. (2020). Immediate use after reconstitution of a biostimulatory poly-L-lactic acid injectable implant. *Journal of Drugs in Dermatology*, *19*(12), 1199–1203.

Casabona, G., Frank, K., Koban, K. C., Freytag, D. L., Schenck, T. L., Lachman, N., Green, J. B., Toni, S., Rudolph, C., & Cotofana, S. (2019). Lifting vs volumizing—the difference in facial minimally invasive procedures when respecting the line of ligaments. *Journal of Cosmetic Dermatology* (Online ahead of print).

Fitzgerald, R., & Vleggaar, D. (2011). Facial volume restoration of the aging face with poly-L-lactic acid. *Dermatologic Therapy*, *24*, 2–27.

Geirloff, M., Stohring, C., Buder, T., Gassling, V., Acil, Y., & Wiltfang, J. (2012). Aging changes of the midfacial fat compartments: A computed tomographic study. *Plastic and Reconstructive Surgery*, *129*(1), 263–273.

Goldberg, D., Guana, A., Volk, A., & Daro-Kaftan, E. (2013). Single-arm study for the characterization of human tissue response to injectable poly-L-lactic acid. *Dermatologic Surgery*, *39*, 915–922.

Haddad, A., Menezes, A., Guarnieri, C., et al. (2019). Recommendations on the use of injectable poly-L-lactic acid for skin laxity in off-face areas. *Journal of Drugs in Dermatology*, *18*(9), 929–935.

Jabbar, A., Arruda, S., & Sadick, N. (2017). Off face usage of poly-L-lactic acid for body rejuvenation. *Journal of Drugs in Dermatology*, *16*(5), 489–494.

Lemperle, G., & Gauthier-Hazan, N. (2009). Foreign body granulomas after all injectable dermal fillers. Part 2. Treatment options. *Plastic and Reconstructive Surgery*, *123*(6), 864–1873.

Lin, M. J., Dubin, D. P., & Khorasani, H. (2020). Poly-L-lactic acid for minimally invasive gluteal augmentation. *Dermatologic Surgery*, *46*(3), 386–394.

Mazzuco, R. (2020). Subcision™ plus poly-l-lactic acid for the treatment of cellulite associated to flaccidity in the buttocks and thighs. *Journal of Cosmetic Dermatology*, *19*(5), 1165–1171.

Mendelson, B., & Wong, C. (2013). *Anatomy of the Aging Face. Section I, Chap 6. Aesthetic Surgery of the Face*. London: Elsevier.

Palm, M., & Goldman, M. (2009). Patient satisfaction and the duration of effect with PLLA: A review of the literature. *Journal of Drugs in Dermatology, 10*, S15–S20.

Palm, M., Mayoral, F., Rajani, A., Goldman, M. P., Fabi, S., Espinoza, L., Andriopoulos, B., & Harper, J. (2021). Chart review presenting safety of injectable PLLA used with alternative reconstitution volume for facial treatments. *Journal of Drugs in Dermatology, 20*(1), 118–122.

Palm, M., Weinkle, S., Cho, Y., LaTowsky, B., & Prather, H. (2021). *A randomized evaluator-blinded, multi-center study to evaluate safety and effectiveness of a biostimulatory poly-L-lactic acid injectable implant after changes in reconstitution*. Presented at: Maui Derm for Dermatologists, Maui, HI.

Rohrich, R., & Pessa, J. E. (2007). The fat compartments of the face: Anatomy and clinical implications for cosmetic surgery. *Plastic and Reconstructive Surgery, 119*, 2219–2227.

Shaw, R., Katzel, E., Koltz, P., et al. (2011). Aging of the facial skeleton: Aesthetic implications and rejuvenation strategies. *Plastic and Reconstructive Surgery, 127*, 374.

Vanaman, M., & Fabi, S. G. (2015). Décolletage: Regional approaches with injectable fillers. *Plastic and Reconstructive Surgery, 136*(5 suppl), 276S–281S.

Vleggaar, D., Fitzgerald, R., Lorenc, Z. P., et al. (2014). Consensus recommendations on the use of injectable poly-L-lactic acid for facial and nonfacial volumization. *Journal of Drugs in Dermatology, 13*(4 suppl), s29–s51.

11

Emervel Family (Now as Restylane Optimal Balance Technology Line Part of the Restylane Family)

Gary D. Monheit and Berthold Rzany

SUMMARY AND KEY FEATURES

- In 2016, the Emervel family has been renamed Restylane to fit better in the portfolio of Galderma.
- Because of the unique optimal balance technology (OBT), it is different from the other Restylane fillers. The Emervel family can be still identified by the blue color of the boxes and brand names with an "e" at the end. The previous name appears as small text on the box.
- The Emervel family comes in several products with and without lidocaine (except for Emervel Touch, now Restylane Fynesse, which is only available without lidocaine).
- The Emervel family is one of the few hyaluronic acid families with good clinical data behind their products.
- The products have been on the market for several years now in Europe and the United States and appear to be efficacious and safe.

INTRODUCTION

Soft tissue filling with hyaluronic acid (HA) began with single-purpose fillers designed and tested for nasolabial folds but subsequently used for multiple facial areas. This began in 2004 with the use and approval of Restylane and was followed rapidly with other HA fillers with similar physical characteristics and rheology. The need for HA filling material that is designed for more than the nasolabial folds coincided with the global approach to treating multiple areas of the face to achieve a natural yet more youthful look sought by our patients. Filling material that will restructure deep facial defects and others that are designed for more superficial defects with a natural appearance stimulates the need for customized filling material for each area. The Emervel family of HA fillers has evolved with specific products designed to treat variable facial indications, including nasolabial folds, marionette lines, perioral lines, cheek folds, tear troughs, and fine dermal wrinkles. Each has specific physical properties and flow characteristics to solve these specific facial problems of aging skin and soft tissue.

As fillers have evolved, the physical characteristics of each family of products have a distinctive composition giving them individual flow characteristics. These modifications make these individual fillers adaptable to various facial areas. The rheology of the filler is related to its formulation, including the source of HA, the concentration of HA, type of cross-linking, degree of cross-linking, particle size, and the manufacturing process.

PHYSICAL PROPERTIES OF THE EMERVEL FAMILY (NOW RESTYLANE OPTIMAL BALANCE TECHNOLOGY FAMILY)

Emervel (Galderma, Lausanne, Switzerland) is a family of five fillers with a range of physical properties designed to accommodate all levels of facial correction. The variables that determine the nature of each product include the following:

1. HA concentration (20 mg/mL)
2. Cross-linking (by 1,4-butanediol diglycidyl ether [BDDE])
3. Calibration (this is the preferred term of the company) or particle size

Because all of the Emervel products maintain the same concentration (20 mg/mL), they vary the degree and type of cross-linking, as well as the three levels of calibration or particle size. This approach to customized filling nature is referred to as "optimal balance technology" (OBT) (Table 11.1). From 2016 on, the Emervel family was integrated in the Restylane brand. For this, several new names were created, making the Emervel brand still distinguishable from the old Restylane brand (Table 11.2).

Calibration is a unique term that is used for this group of fillers and describes the process of processing bulk cross-linked HA into smaller particle sizes to produce optimal size for the area to be treated. This is produced through a "sieving" process for optimal homogenicity. The products with a low cross-linking and with small calibration are designed for superficial injection (e.g., Restylane Fynesse [former Emervel Touch]) as the products with high cross-linking and larger calibration are designed for deeper and more volumetric injections (e.g., Restylane Volyme [former Emervel Volume]). Except for Restylane Fynesse (former Emervel Touch), they are available with and without lidocaine. The calibration particle size and cross-linking determine the differences in the products. BDDE is the reactive cross-linker holding together strands of HA with one end free as a pendant. The degree of cross-linking determines the gel firmness. A firmer gel resists deformation caused by facial movement and has a larger duration but is harder to inject and may be palpable if injected too superficially. The degree of calibration also affects firmness and smaller size is injected easier but will disperse more easily. The superficial gels, Restylane Fynesse (former Emervel Touch) and Restylane Refyne (former Emervel Classic), are thus designed for dermis, while the larger particles are made for deeper and more loosely packed tissue such as subcutaneous tissue (Fig 11.1).

TABLE 11.1 Properties of the Emervel Family (Now Restylane Optimal Balance Technology Family) and Their Clinical Impact

	Calibration	Cross-Linking	Concentration
Benefit	Lifting effect	Firmness	Filler longevity
Adversity	Too big Uneven flow	Implant perceptible with inflammation	Hardness

TABLE 11.2 New and Old Names for the Emervel Family (Now Restylane Optimal Balance Technology Family)

Indication	Old Name	New Name
For very superficial indications, such as fine periocular wrinkles	Emervel Touch	Restylane Fynesse
For medium-sized lines and folds, infraorbital hollow	Emervel Classic	Restylane Refyne[a]
For deeper lines and folds as well as volume deficits	Emervel Deep	Restylane Defyne[a]
For volume substitution, such as cheeks, chin, etc.	Emervel Volume	Restylane Volyme
For lip volume augmentation	Emervel Lip	Restylane Kysee

The Emervel family is now subsummarized under the name of Restylane OBT family. The boxes differ from the Restylane boxes by the blue color and for non-Scandinavians mostly a bit strange appearing names ending with an "e." The previous names appear as a small text at the box.

[a] These products are available in the United States (by 2021).

CLINICAL STUDIES

European and South American Clinical Studies on Emervel

In contrast to the United States, in Europe at that time, generally no clinical trials are required to place

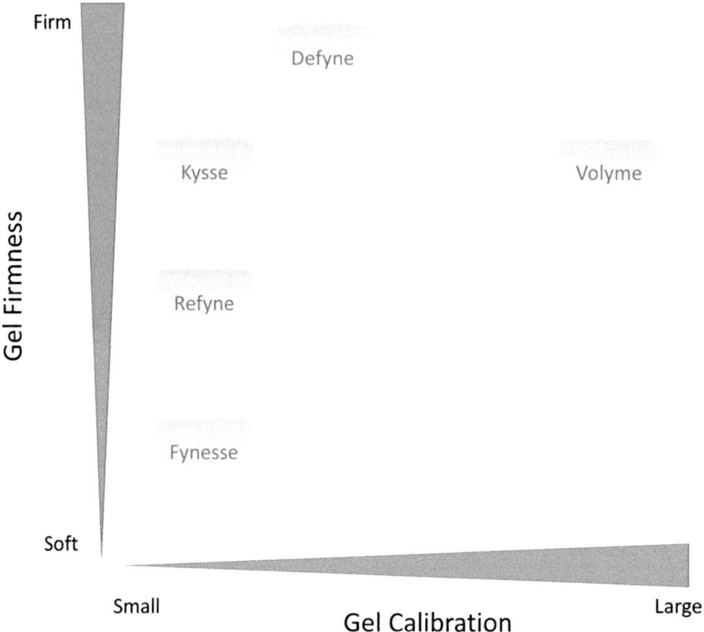

Fig. 11.1 Rheology of hyaluronic acid fillers.

an HA filler on the market. Therefore, it is quite unique that the Emervel family entered the market with several concomitant trials. Two trials were comparative using Restylane products as the benchmark (Table 11.3).

Both trials showed a comparability of the tested products. However, Emervel Deep (now Restylane Defyne) did show a better efficacy compared with Restylane Perlane (now Restylane Lyft).

Three other trials, all case series, focused on real-life scenarios (e.g., treating patients with different members of the Emervel family) (Table 11.4). Results from one trial (the Fresh study trial Rzany et al.) have appeared in several subpublications. These studies do not focus on comparability but more on effectiveness (how is the product working when its use is less restricted) and how safe is the product (usually the numbers of included patients are quite high, which allows also statements on less frequent adverse effects). However, one large trial did only follow up the patients for a couple of weeks.

In addition, a smaller comparative trial has been conducted, comparing Emervel Lips (now Restylane KYSSE) versus Juvéderm Volbella, respectively. Interestingly, the efficacy between the products compared was quite similar (Table 11.5).

United States Clinical Study

The Emervel US study was a multicenter, randomized, evaluator-blinded, intraindividual right–left comparing effectiveness and safety of Emervel Classic (now Restylane Refyne) and Emervel Deep (now Restylane Defyne) to Juvéderm Ultra and Juvéderm Ultra Plus to correct contralateral nasolabial folds.

This was a study for effectiveness: noninferiority versus a comparator. A blinded evaluation assessed safety, and adverse events were assessed by patient and evaluator. The Emervel Classic wrinkle scale was used with a baseline of three (moderate) to four (severe) nasolabial folds. An initial touchup was allowed, if needed, and injected volumes of both fillers were the same.

The results at 6 months showed that the mean changes in wrinkle severity score at 24 weeks were equal. This was true for both studies: Emervel Classic (now Restylane Refyne) versus Juvéderm Ultra and Emervel Deep (now Restylane Defyne) versus Juvéderm Ultra Plus. The adverse event profiles were also similar, as well as patient satisfaction (Table 11.6).

TABLE 11.3 Comparative European Trials With Emervel (for the New Restylane Names, see Table 11.2)

Reference	Products	Randomized/ Blinded	Area Assessed	Duration of Study	No. of Patients	Objective Outcome Criteria	Comments
Ascher et al.[1]	Emervel Deep vs. Restylane Perlane	Y/Y	NLF	6 months	60	5-point WSRS	Emervel Deep provides better efficacy and similar tolerability compared with Restylane Perlane.
Rzany et al.[2]	Emervel Classic vs. Restylane	Y/Y	NLF	18 months	52	5-point WSRS	Emervel Classic provides similar efficacy and better overall tolerability compared with Restylane.

NLF, Nasolabial fold; *WSRS*, Wrinkle Severity Rating Scale.

TABLE 11.4 Case Series With the Emervel Family (for the New Restylane Names, see Table 11.2)

Reference	Products	Randomized/ Blinded	Area Assessed	Duration of Study	No. of Patients	Objective Outcome Criteria	Comments
Rzany et al.[3,4]	Emervel Touch, Classic, Deep, Volume and Lips	Case series, multicenter study (58 physicians), collected between September 2010 and July 2011	At least three of the eight indications (periorbital lines, tear troughs, cheek folds, nasolabial folds, upper lip lines and marionette lines; cheek and lip enhancement)	6 months	77	Lemperle Rating scale (6 points) and Lip Fullness Scale, overall aesthetic improve-ment	At 6 months, 79.7% of participants were satisfied or very satisfied with the durability of the results.[a]
Talarico et al.[11]	Emervel Volume	Case series, multicenter study	At least two indications among the chin, temporal areas, cheeks, cheekbones, jawline, nasolabial fold	18 months	60 subjects	Volume loss scale (4 points), as well as Lemperle Rating scale (6 points), GAIS, Vectra 3D	At 18 months still one-point improvement in 68.3% of patients, 6 patients with nodule formation, mostly mild

Continued

TABLE 11.4 Case Series With the Emervel Family (for the New Restylane Names, see Table 11.2)—cont'd

Reference	Products	Randomized/ Blinded	Area Assessed	Duration of Study	No. of Patients	Objective Outcome Criteria	Comments
Fahri et al.[7]	Emervel Classic, Deep, Volume and Lips	Consecutive case series, multicenter	Nasolabial folds and marionette lines by score—other areas only for treatment (cheek, lips, supramental crease, tear trough)	2–4 weeks	1822	5-point score for nasolabial folds and marionette lines	No long-term data on efficacy and safety are given

[a] Several subpublications came out of this trial, all published in a supplement of the *Journal of Drugs in Dermatology* (e.g., References 3 to 6)
GAIS, Global Aesthetic Improvement Scale.

TABLE 11.5 Comparative Lip Volume Trials With Emervel Lips (for the New Restylane Names, see Table 11.2)

Reference	Products	Randomized/ Blinded	Area Assessed	Duration of Study	No. of Patients	Objective Outcome Criteria	Comments
Hilton et al.[8]	Emervel Lips versus Juvéderm Volbella	Randomized comparative multicenter study	Thin to moderately thick lips	12 months	60 (58 females)	Lip Fullness Grading Scale (LFGS) (5 points)	The improvement in the LFGS was similar. A smaller volume of Emervel Lips was required to achieve similar results.

TABLE 11.6 Comparative US Trials With Emervel (for the New Restylane Names, see Table 11.2)

Products	Randomized/ Blinded	Area Assessed	Duration of Study	No. of Patients	Objective Outcome Criteria	Comments
Emervel Classic Lidocaine versus Juvéderm Ultra (Fagien et al.[9])	Y/Y	NLF	6 months	170	5-point WSRS	Similar efficacy and safety
Emervel Deep Lidocaine versus Juvéderm Ultra Plus (Baumann et al.[10])	Y/Y	NLF	6 months	162	5-point WSRS	Similar efficacy and safety

NLF, Nasolabial fold; *WSRS*, Wrinkle Severity Rating Scale.

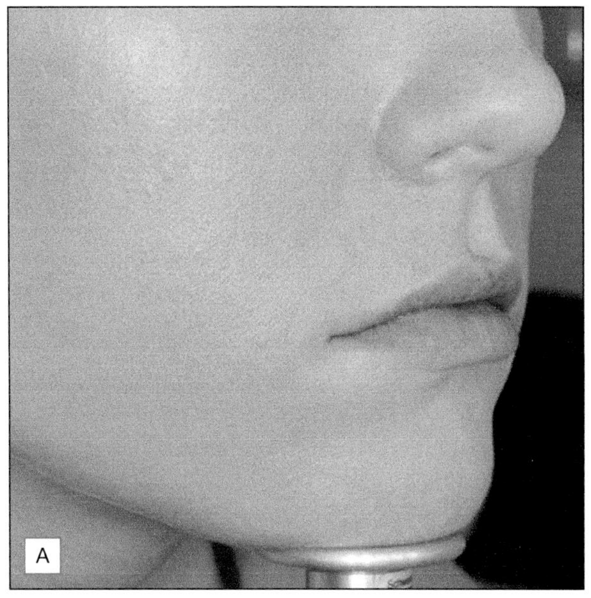

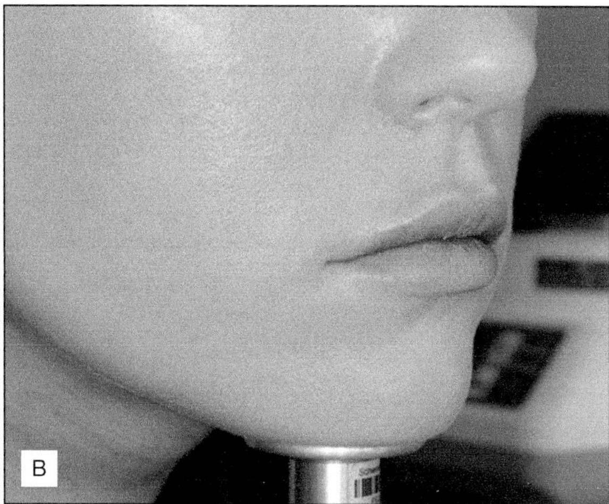

Fig. 11.2 Lips before (A) and 1 week after (B) augmentation with 1 mL Emervel Lips in a 23-year-old patient.

EMERVEL/RESTYLANE OPTIMAL BALANCE TECHNOLOGY PRODUCTS IN CLINICAL PRACTICE—USE OF THE DIFFERENT TYPES IN DIFFERENT AREAS (I.E., NASOLABIAL FOLDS, LIPS, VOLUME FILLING)

The Emervel/Restylane OBT family is quite large, ranging from Restylane Fynesse (former Emervel Touch) for very superficial lines to Restylane Volyme (former Emervel Volume) for deep augmentations. The perioral region is well treated with Restylane Refyne (former Emervel Classic) and Restylane Kysse (former Emervel Lip) targeting the nasolabial folds, marionette lines, and red of lips as well. The key to successful injection in this area is appropriate volumizing of the lips and correction of surrounding areas, which will harmonize the result for a natural youthful effect. It is important that the cosmetic physician blend the result with the full face rather than concentrating on one area alone.

Cheek enhancement can be successfully treated with Restylane Volyme (former Emervel Volume) and/or Restylane Defyne (former Emervel Deep), the firmer products.

Very unique is Restylane Kysse (former Emervel Lips). It is a very good product for augmenting the lip red (Fig. 11.2A,B), specifically in younger patients with few elastosis. In contrast to other products, it is quite firm, so that patients might feel the filler for a couple of weeks after the injection. Some colleagues use Restylane Kysse also for elevating the infraorbital hollows. However, for this indication, also Restylane Fynesse (former Emervel Touch) can be used.

HOW DOES IT COMPARE WITH OTHER HYALURONIC ACID FILLERS IN DIFFERENT AREAS?

There are not a lot of comparative trials between different HA products. Based on the comparative trial of Emervel Deep and Classic (now Restylane Defyne and Refyne), there is not much difference from Restylane Perlane (now Restylane Lyft) and Restylane. In a further study between Emervel Lips (now Restylane KYSSE) and Juvéderm Volbella by Hilton al. (2018), no clinical difference could be noted at least for the 6-month data when looking at efficacy. Concerning other Emervel products, our guess would be that there are no clinically relevant differences when comparing Restylane Fynesse (former Emervel Touch) to, say, Restylane Vital (except for the pain because Restylane Fynesse is not available with lidocaine).

CONCLUSIONS

In summary, the Restylane OBT (former Emervel family) of customized fillers presents five unique HA products designed for facial rejuvenation in various locations of the face and at variable depths. The science, product analysis, and clinical validation all indicate these to be useful products for the cosmetic physician.

FURTHER READING

Ascher, B., Bayerl, C., Brun, P., et al. (2011). Efficacy and safety of a new hyaluronic acid dermal filler in the treatment of severe nasolabial lines—6-month interim results of a randomized, evaluator-blinded, intra-individual comparison study. *Journal of Cosmetic Dermatology*, *10*, 94–98. https://doi.org/10.1111/j.1473-2165.2011.00550.x.

Baumann, L., Weiss, R. A., Grekin, S., et al. (2018). Comparison of hyaluronic acid gel with (HARDL) and without lidocaine (HAJUP) in the treatment of moderate-to-severe nasolabial folds: A randomized, evaluator-blinded study. *Dermatologic Surgery*, *44*(6), 833–840. https://doi.org/10.1097/DSS.0000000000001424.

Cartier, H., Trevidic, P., Rzany, B., Sattler, G., Kerrouche, N., & Dhuin, J. C. (2012). Perioral rejuvenation with a range of customized hyaluronic acid fillers: Efficacy and safety over six months with a specific focus on the lips. *Journal of Drugs in Dermatology*, *11*(suppl 1), s17–s26. PMID:22497040.

Fagien, S., Monheit, G., Jones, D., et al. (2018). Hyaluronic acid gel with (HARRL) and without lidocaine (HAJU) for the treatment of moderate-to-severe nasolabial folds: A randomized, evaluator-blinded, phase III study. *Dermatologic Surgery*, *44*(4), 549–556. https://doi.org/10.1097/DSS.0000000000001368.

Farhi, D., Trevidic, P., Kestemont, P., Emervel French Survey Group, et al. (2013). The Emervel French survey: A prospective real-practice descriptive study of 1,822 patients treated for facial rejuvenation with a new hyaluronic acid filler. *Journal of Drugs in Dermatology*, *12*(5), e88–e93. PMID:23652965.

Hilton, S., Sattler, G., Berg, A. K., Samuelson, U., Wong, C., et al. (2018). Randomized, evaluator-blinded study comparing safety and effect of two hyaluronic acid gels for lips enhancement. *Dermatologic Surgery*, *44*(2), 261–269. https://doi.org/10.1097/DSS.0000000000001282.

Kestemont, P., Cartier, H., Trevidic, P., et al. (2012). Sustained efficacy and high patient satisfaction after cheek enhancement with a new hyaluronic acid dermal filler. *Journal of Drugs in Dermatology*, *11*(suppl 1), s9–s16. PMID:22497039.

Rzany, B., Bayerl, C., Bodokh, I., et al. (2011). Efficacy and safety of a new hyaluronic acid dermal filler in the treatment of moderate nasolabial folds: 6-month interim results of a randomized, evaluator-blinded, intra-individual comparison study. *Journal of Cosmetic and Laser Therapy*, *13*, 107–112. https://doi.org/10.3109/14764172.2011.571699.

Rzany, B., Cartier, H., Kestemont, P., et al. (2012). Full-face rejuvenation using a range of hyaluronic acid fillers: Efficacy, safety, and patient satisfaction over 6 months. *Dermatologic Surgery*, *38*(7 pt 2), 1153–1161. https://doi.org/10.1111/j.1524-4725.2012.02470.x.

Rzany, B., Cartier, H., Kestermont, P., et al. (2012). Correction of tear troughs and periorbital lines with a range of customized hyaluronic acid fillers. *Journal of Drugs in Dermatology*, *11*(suppl 1), s27–s34. PMID:22497041.

Talarico, S., Meski, A. P., Buratini, L., et al. (2015). High patient satisfaction of a hyaluronic acid filler producing enduring full-facial volume restoration: An 18-month open multicenter study. *Dermatologic Surgery*, *41*(12), 1361–1369. https://doi.org/10.1097/DSS.0000000000000549.

12

Autologous Fat

Lauren Duffey Crow

SUMMARY AND KEY FEATURES

- Autologous fat is an ideal filler that provides patients with long-lasting revolumization. With proper patient assessment, planning, and treatment, facial augmentation provides a safe means to restore the youthful contours of the face. The use of autologous nanofat, microfat, and stromal vascular fraction in small grafts placed strategically throughout the soft tissue planes of the face stimulates ongoing regeneration of facial texture, volume, and contour.
- Indications for Autologous Fat Transfer (AFT).
- Patient selection.
- Pre-operative assessment and planning.
- Fat harvesting techniques.
- Graft preparation.
- Graft placement.
- Postoperative considerations and complications.

INTRODUCTION

Autologous fat is an ideal filler for facial rejuvenation as it is relatively abundant and easy to obtain, immunologically compatible, and longer lasting than the available bioengineered injectable products. Autologous fat transfer (AFT) is regarded as an elegant technique to correct volume deficits and aging of the face. It allows for a minimally invasive restoration of soft tissue contour and facial atrophy with precise titration and placement of the patient's own fat. Soft tissue volume loss can result from trauma, scarring, post tumor extirpation, chronic wounds, HIV lipodystrophy, and congenital anomalies. However, the most common cause of soft tissue and bony volume loss in the face is the natural aging process. Facial aging is a multifaceted and dynamic process in which all the structures of facial anatomy play a role. The subcutaneous fat of the face is partitioned into discrete anatomic compartments, and these fat compartments carry variable propensities for age-related volume loss. Additionally, gradual changes in the thickness and elasticity of skin, decreased adherence between the skin and subcutaneous tissue, sagging of the soft tissues, weakening of the facial muscles, and the progressive decrease in the volume of the craniofacial skeleton all contribute to the natural aging process. AFT is a nonimmunogenic and safe means to address facial volume loss.

Although fat grafting is an old technique that can be dated to as early as 1893, it has gained increasing popularity for use in facial and cosmetic surgery. Since the advent of liposuction, adipose tissue is easily obtainable in substantial quantities and yields significant amounts of multipotent cells to be used for transplantation. Harvesting and preparation of fat grafts do not require cell culture and can be performed in-office on the same day as grafting, making the procedure clinically feasible for both patients and physicians.

Since the discovery of adipose-derived stem cells in 2001, there has been increasing research into the clinical applications of these multipotent mesenchymal-derived progenitor cells. Different techniques by which adipose-derived stem cell preparations can be processed, whether as macrofat, microfat, or nanofat, allow for different depths and areas of application within the soft tissue planes of the face. The initial isolated adipose tissue is composed of adipocytes and stromal vascular fraction (SVF) cells, which include adipose stem cells, pre-adipocytes, fibroblasts, vascular endothelial cells, and immune cells. There are now a number of studies and reviews to support the improved survival of fat grafts with the addition of adipose stem cells and SVF cells to enhance survival.

PREOPERATIVE CONSIDERATIONS AND PATIENT SELECTION

The most important factor for achieving excellent results is appropriate patient selection. As with all aesthetic preoperative consultations, it is important to discuss expectations, timelines, and risks and benefits of AFT. Pre- and postoperative photos from five standard angles should be taken to document and display for the patient the volumetric changes associated with the procedure. These include frontal, bilateral lateral, and bilateral oblique views (Fig. 12.1A–C).

The ideal candidate for AFT should have a sufficient fat volume source as well as facial volume loss (thin face with a normal or elevated body mass index). Patients with a low body mass index will not have sufficient fat stores to harvest for transplantation and their fat is programmed to remain lean even after grafting (not giving a robust change). Additionally, patients should remain at a stable weight, as fluctuations in weight will affect fat grafting outcomes. A 10-pound weight loss will diminish the results, while a 10-pound weight gain may cause the patient to appear overly full. Patients below the age of 60 years tend to have better outcomes and require fewer treatments to achieve the desired results. This is thought to be due to the decreased abundance and plasticity of mature stem cells as patients age. As a rule, fat transfer should not be performed in smokers due to the resultant vasoconstriction that will not support the survival of the fat grafts. A patient should be questioned regarding prior trauma or surgical procedures to avoid harvesting fat grafts from sites of increased fibrosis. For patients with a history of eyelid surgery, especially lower eyelid surgery, there is a risk of prolonged lower eyelid edema following AFT, and patients should be counseled about this risk. The surgeon should also elicit a history of cheek or chin implantation as this will prevent placement of fat grafts at the level of the periosteum in these locations.

Patients undergoing AFT should be in stable medical condition. Any patients requiring anticoagulating agents should consult with cardiology or hematology prior to stopping these medications so as to avoid undue risk of clot formation. Because blood is toxic to the fat grafts, anticoagulation must be stopped prior to fat grafting and can be restarted only once an appropriate amount of time has passed postoperatively. Patients are advised to avoid/discontinue aspirin, nonsteroidal anti-inflammatory medications, fish oil, vitamin E, and herbal supplements 2 weeks before and 1 week following treatment. The senior author (SO) recommends supplementation with bromelain 500 mg twice a day on an empty stomach starting 1 week prior to surgery and continued for 1 week postoperatively to help reduce postoperative swelling and bruising.

Patients should be counseled regarding the need for appropriate social and physical downtime. AFT performed under local and tumescent anesthesia, with proper avoidance of blood thinning medications and supplements, usually results in a 7- to 8-day recovery. The risks of AFT include infection, bleeding, vascular occlusion, necrosis, fat cysts, granulomas, and, in rare cases, blindness. Prophylactic antibiotics are not recommended unless the patient has orthopedic or cardiac conditions necessitating prophylaxis.

HARVESTING OF FAT GRAFTS

Selection of the appropriate anatomic area for adipocyte harvesting should be based upon the body habitus of the patient as well as history of previous surgery or trauma. Reviews of AFT have failed to show significant differences in adipocyte survival based upon harvest site.[7] However, most surgeons agree that the ideal harvest site is the outer thigh, due to increased levels of mesenchymal cells and collagen. This area is followed by the flanks and the abdomen in order of preference. However, liposuction within areas of prior surgery should always be avoided, as these sites tend to yield a more bloody or fractured aspirate. The site must have both adequate surface area and subcutaneous thickness as measured by the palm and pinch test to allow for sufficient quantity of fat to be harvested. A palm size area ($\sim 200\,cm^2$) with a pinch thickness of at least 0.25 cm allows for approximately 50 mL of fat graft.[12] The approximate quantity of fat available for harvest at the donor site should be calculated and checked against the fat volume needed for revolumization. Oftentimes, patients have asymmetry of fat on their thighs or flanks; thus, the harvesting process can be used to give a secondary benefit by making the patient more symmetric by removing more fat from the fuller area.

The harvesting site should be marked and prepared with betadine (Fig. 12.2A). Incision points should be

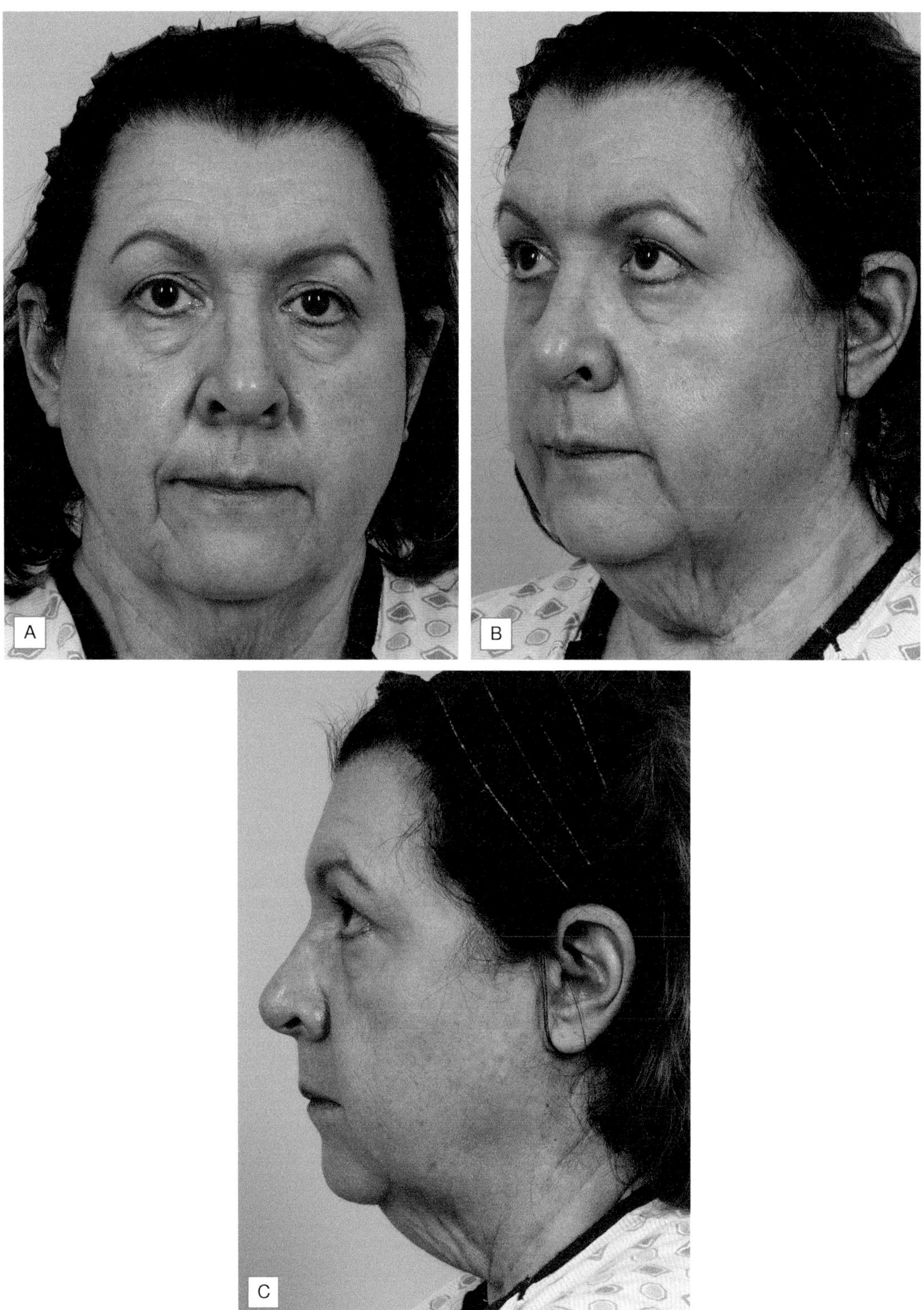

Fig. 12.1 The five standard angles for preoperative photos for AFT, taken from (A) frontal view, (B) bilateral oblique views (right and left), and (C) bilateral lateral views (right and left).

anesthetized with 1% lidocaine with epinephrine, and stab incisions can be made with a No. 15 blade. Tumescent anesthesia consisting of 0.2% tumescent anesthesia solution with 1:500,000 epinephrine should be injected through these incision sites into the donor site. The tumescent solution is administered with a 2-mm infiltrating cannula and a 20-mL syringe in a fanning technique.

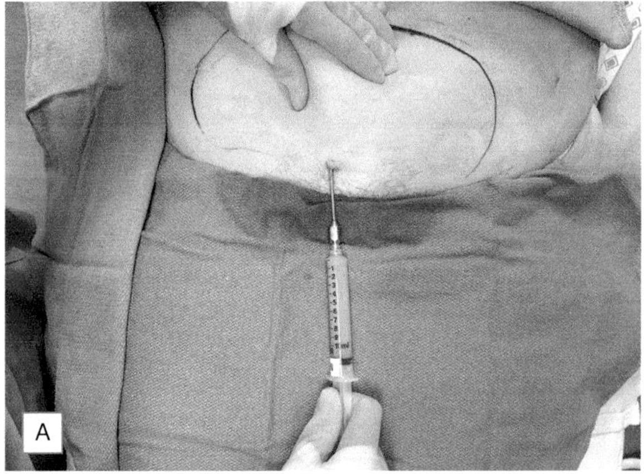

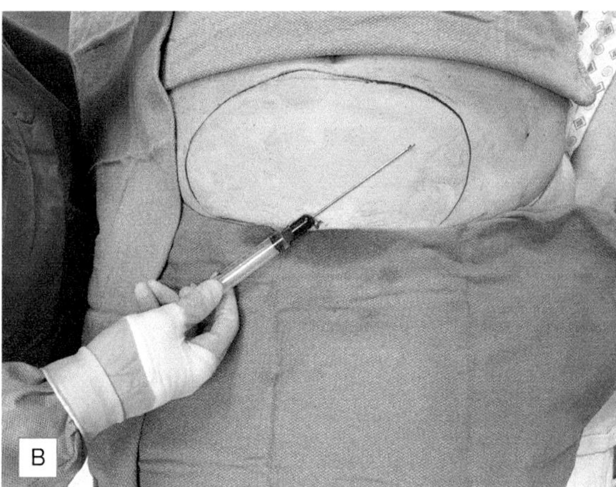

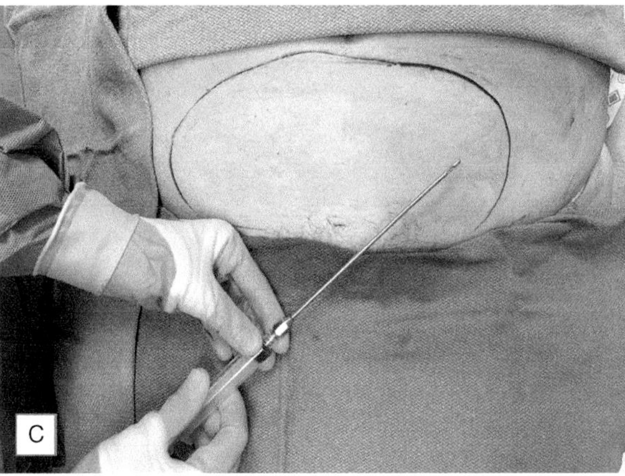

Fig. 12.2 Photographs (A, B, and C) of fat harvesting procedure.

A 10-ml syringe is used for the fat harvesting. Prior to harvesting the fat, 1 mL of 25% albumin (Baxter Pharmaceuticals, Deerfield, IL) should be placed in the syringes to concentrate the fat and restore oncotic pressure. The nanofat should be harvested using a 14-g Carraway Harvester Cannula (Tulip Medical Products, San Diego, CA) (Fig. 12.2B). To harvest the microfat and macrofat grafts, a Byron accelerator cannula (Mentor, Irvine, CA) is used (Fig. 12.2C). Manual suction with 1 to 2 mL suction (< 6 mm Hg) should be used so as to avoid damage to the grafts. Using a gentle, fanning motion, the fat should be gradually collected in the syringes. The filled syringes are inverted and left to decant while the other syringes are filled. Infranatant fluid is expelled and the syringes are topped off again with fat. The incision sites are left open to drain and to heal by secondary intent.

PREPARATION OF GRAFTS

Harvested fat should be centrifuged using a closed system or sterile rotors at no higher than 3000 RPM for about 30 to 60 seconds (Fig. 12.3). This allows for

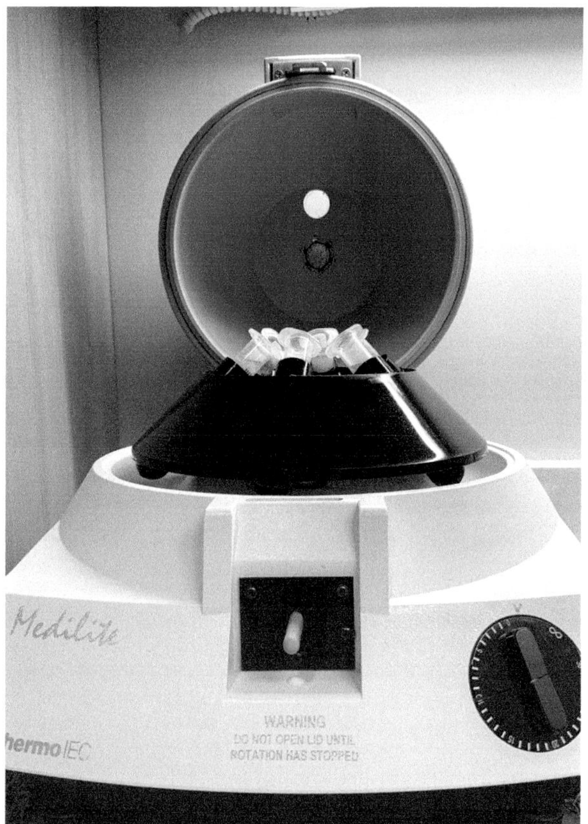

Fig. 12.3 Fat centrifuge.

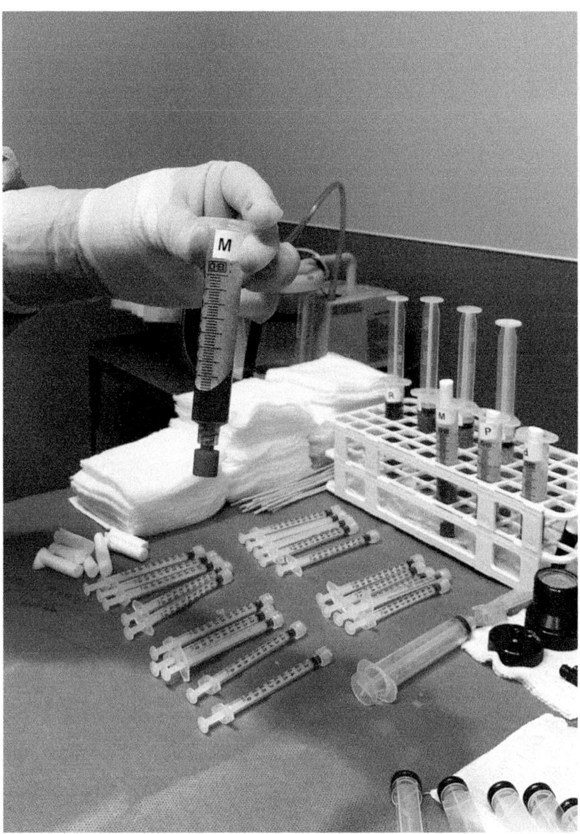

Fig. 12.4 Separation of fat after centrifuge.

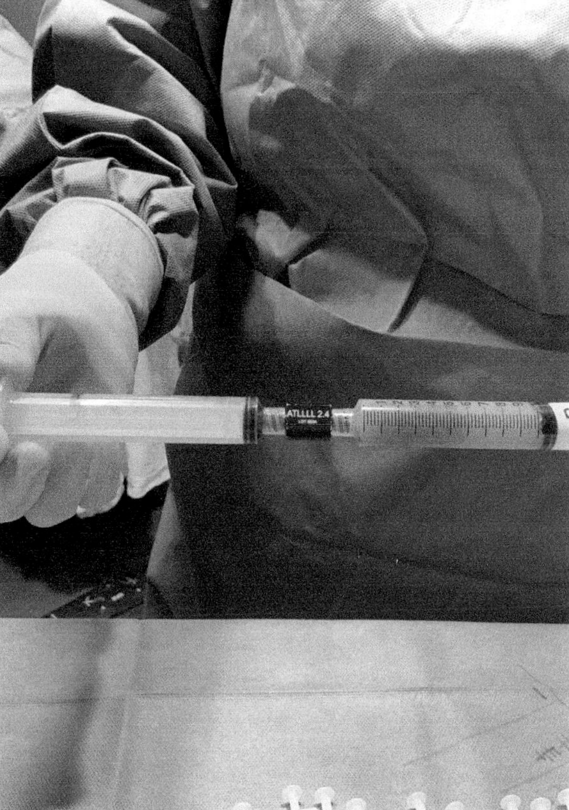

Fig. 12.5 Mechanical processing of nanofat for isolation of adipocyte derived mesenchymal stem cells.

adequate separation of purified fat, concentrated growth factors, and adipose-derived stem cells beneficial to graft retention, while preventing overconcentration and rupture of fat cells. The supernatant is made up of ruptured fat cells and oil and should be wicked from the syringe (Fig. 12.4) using a sterile telfa pad strip or sterile dental rolls. The central part of the centrifuged product is made up of viable adipocytes, stem cells, and growth factors, which will become the fat graft. The infranatant is made up of fluid and can be easily drained from the bottom of the syringe.

Nanofat—Tissue Stromal Vascular Fraction

Nanofat is also referred to as "tissue SVF" (tSVF) in different scientific articles. It implies a mixture of adipocyte-derived stem cells and extracellular matrix cells. To create the nanofat, the fat that was harvested through the Tulip cannula should be micronized and emulsified further. Mechanical processing of nanofat for isolation of adipocyte derived mesenchymal stem cells (AD-MSCs) is performed using the Tulip nanofat system (Tulip Medical Products). First, the fat is passed back and forth through a 2.4-mm luer lock for a total of 20 to 30 passes, followed by a 1.2-mm luer lock for another 20 to 30 passes (Fig. 12.5). The fat will then be pushed through an autologous cellular matrix (ACM) device to filter out the stroma and mature adipocytes while allowing the stem cells to pass through. The micronized fat is pushed through the ACM filter and collected in a syringe with the patient's platelet-rich plasma (PRP). The nanofat will be used in areas of thinner skin to enhance the texture of the skin. Nanofat is not used to volumize an area.

Approximately 1 mL of nanofat or SVF will be added to 9 mL of regular and microfat grafts for stem cell enhancement. Once the fat grafts have been prepared, they should be transferred to 1-mL syringes for injection (Fig. 12.6).

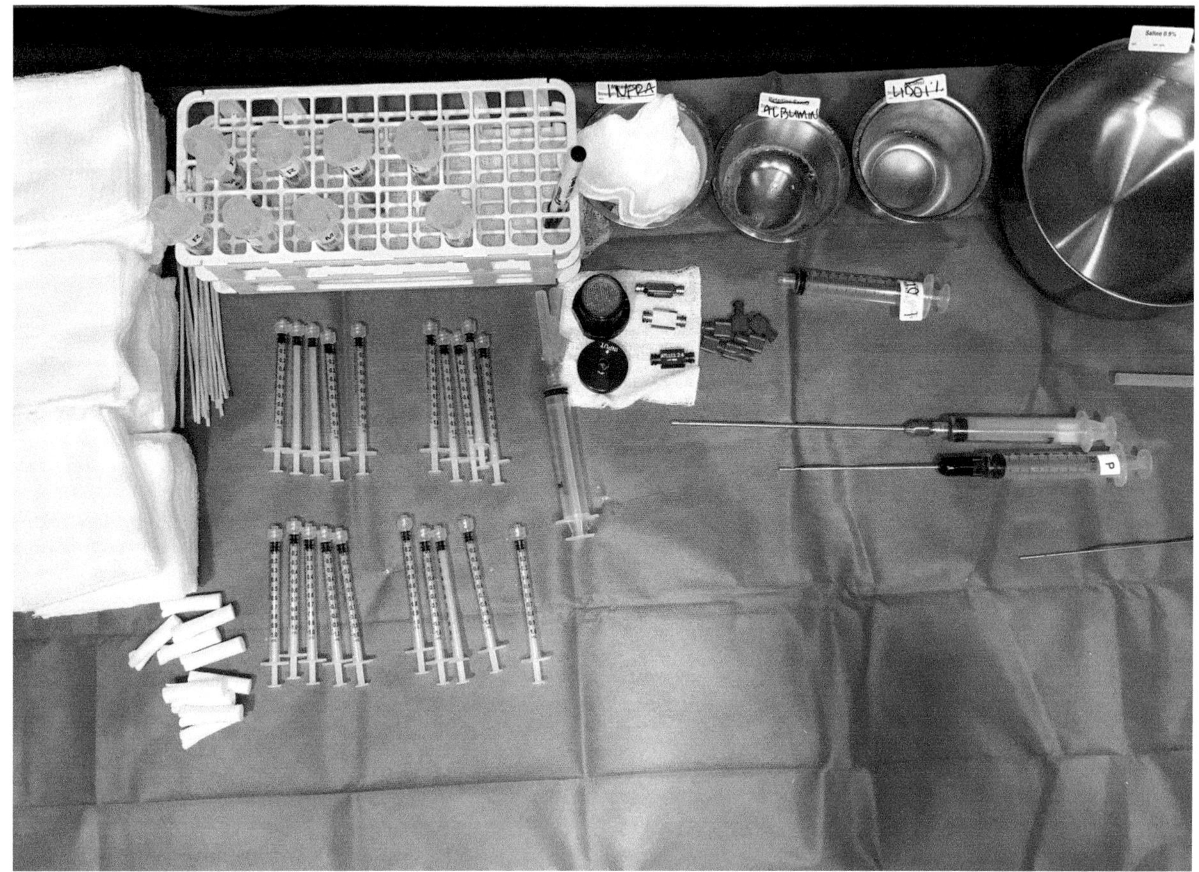

Fig. 12.6 Sterile setup for fat transfer.

GRAFT PLACEMENT

The face should be cleansed thoroughly with 70% alcohol, and preoperative markings should be made to delineate the facial fat compartments designated for revolumization (Fig. 12.7A,B). Upright positioning of the patient during preoperative marking is critical as asymmetry, laxity, and hollowing change with positioning. The markings should be reviewed with the patient prior to the start of the procedure.

Surgical incision points are drawn to accommodate as few access points as possible while still allowing reach and mobility for accurate fat graft placement. This usually involves access points at the midbrow, lateral zygoma, lateral nasolabial fold, and the gonial angle bilaterally (Fig. 12.8). Nerve blocks of the supraorbital, supratrochlear, infraorbital, zygomaticofacial, and mental nerves should be placed with 1% lidocaine with epinephrine according to the desired treatment areas. Proper nerve block placements allow for less tumescent anesthesia to be used to achieve comfort.

Tumescent anesthesia is then injected via a 20-mL syringe connected to a 25-gauge spinal needle to infiltrate the areas of the face not reached by the nerve blocks (Fig. 12.9). Typical volumes of tumescent anesthesia are 15 to 30 mL of 0.2% lidocaine with epinephrine 1:500,000 for the total face.

A 16-gauge No-Kor needle (Becton Dickinson, Franklin Lakes, NJ) is then used to make stab incisions at designated access points (Fig. 12.10). After priming the Coleman II cannula (Mentor, Irvine, CA) (Fig. 12.11) for fat graft placement, care must be taken to ensure that the open port is directed toward the deep tissue. When switching between nanofat and microfat, the cannula should be flushed with normal saline and reprimed.

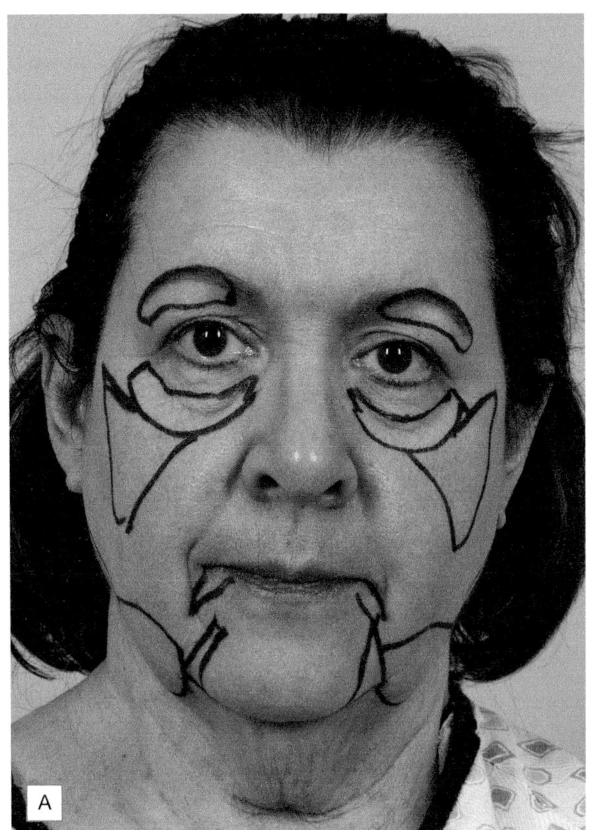

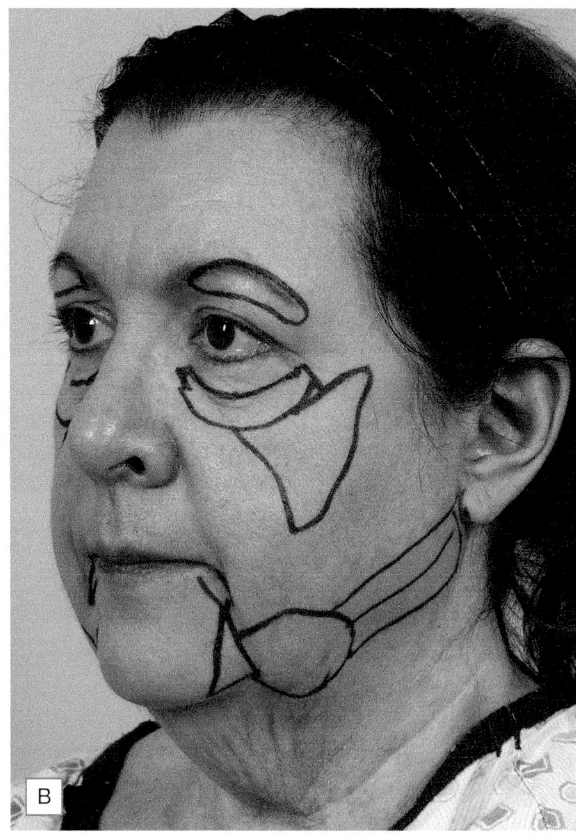

Fig. 12.7 Preoperative markings to delineate the facial fat compartments designated for revolumization.

Fat is injected using 1-mL syringes to avoid large boluses of fat from being injected into tissue. The goal is to deposit aliquots about 0.05 mL in size into various anatomic levels (Box 12.1). This allows the fat to imbibe nutrients from the surrounding tissue until it establishes a vascular supply. Larger aliquots of fat may result in the outer portion of the graft surviving and the central portion becoming necrotic, giving rise to fat cysts. The palm of the injecting hand should be used to provide gentle pressure on the plunger of the syringe so as to inject tiny aliquots of fat. This gives the surgeon greater control than if using one's thumb to push on the plunger.

All fat grafting incision points are sutured with a single, 5-0 fast absorbing gut suture. The incisions are sutured to minimize the risk of infection and to help ensure that the incisions heal in an inconspicuous manner.

Brows

Nanofat (0.5–1 mL) can be placed in the subdermal plane along the eyebrow and orbital rim through an access point at the mid brow (Fig. 12.12A,B). This superficially placed nanofat is used to enhance skin texture and quality and should be injected in a linear threading technique. With microfat, a small amount (1–2 mL) can be added to the fat pad of the superior brow. A small amount of microfat can also be placed under the brow along the periosteum for added lift. This can also be performed in a linear threading manner.

Temples

Temples can be accessed from the lateral zygoma or along the hairline above the zygomatic arch. This allows access to both the temporal fossa as well as to the lower orbital rim. Approximately 2 to 3 mL of microfat is deposited in the subcutaneous tissue using a zigzag placement to avoid linear strands of fat that may become visible. Placement of fat deep to the temporalis muscle is not recommended as the fat may bulge and become apparent during mastication.

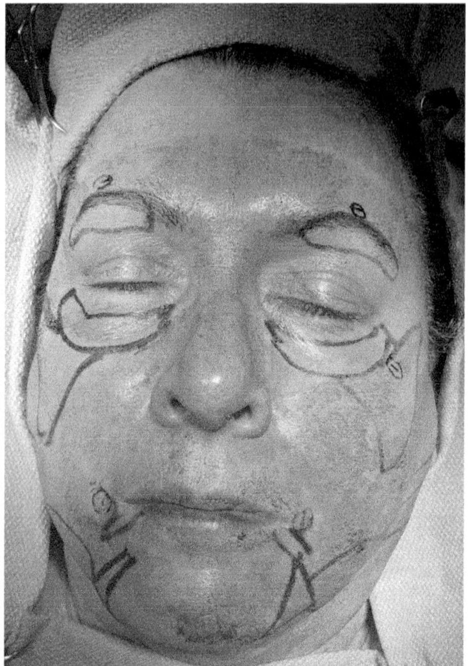

Fig. 12.8 Surgical incision points are drawn to accommodate as few access points as possible while still allowing reach and mobility for accurate fat graft placement. This usually involves access points at the midbrow, lateral zygoma, lateral nasolabial fold, and the gonial angle bilaterally.

Orbital Rim and Tear Trough

Through the lateral orbital rim or mid malar region, nanofat can be injected subdermally to enhance skin quality using nonlinear pattern of placement (Fig. 12.13). Microfat can be injected along the supraperiosteum through a downward pointing cannula in a zigzag motion. This motion is used for injection in areas with thin skin to avoid the formation of linear rolls of visible fat. Patients with thicker skin may benefit from macrofat injection for greater augmentation with less risk of the fat becoming visible. However, the tear trough region is by far the most challenging area to inject. Beginner surgeons are urged to start augmenting cheeks and the lower face until they become comfortable with placing precise quantities of fat in various tissue planes.

Zygoma and Malar Cheeks

Via entry through the lateral zygoma, the cannula can used to place macrofat in small linear aliquots along the periosteum (Fig. 12.14). Approximately 2 to 3 mL of microfat is injected at this location. The cannula is then redirected into the muscular plane and then into the subcutaneous plane, thus giving three different levels of fat grafting to this area. Care must be

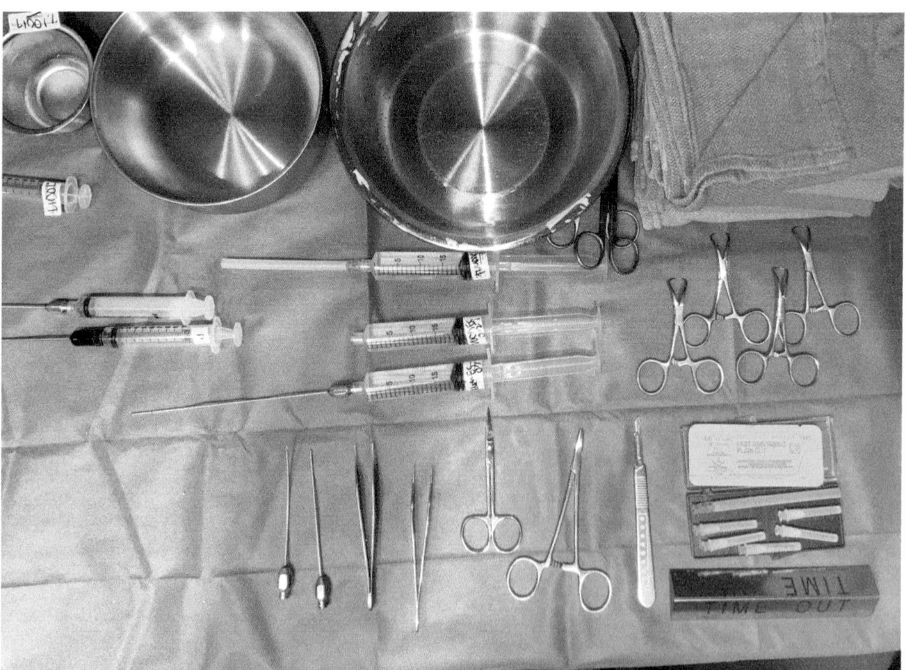

Fig. 12.9 Tumescent anesthesia is injected via a 20-mL syringe connected to a 25-gauge spinal needle to infiltrate the areas of the face not reached by the nerve blocks.

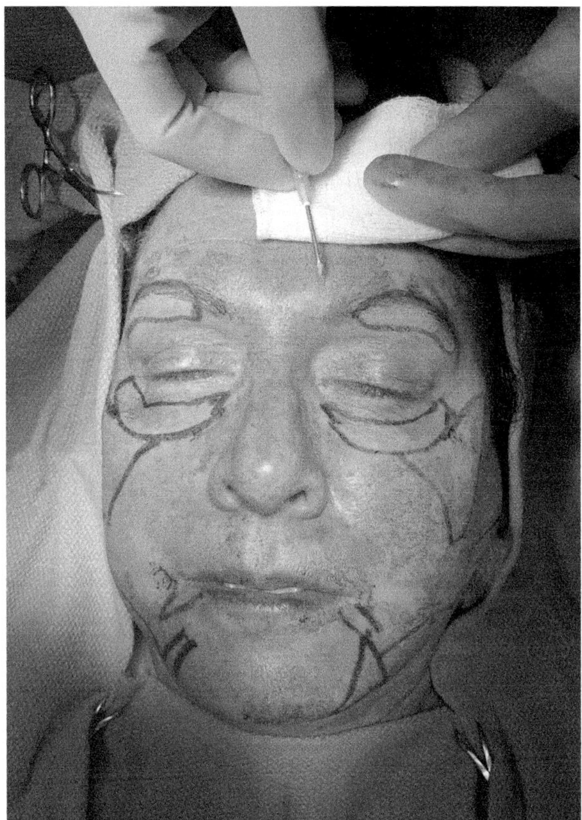

Fig. 12.10 A 16-gauge No-Kor needle (Becton Dickinson, Franklin Lakes, NJ) is then used to make stab incisions at designated access points.

taken to avoid placing too much fat superficially as this can give rise to surface irregularities that can be disfiguring.

Lips

Through the use of an access point just lateral to the oral commissure, the cannula can then be rotated to an upward or downward angle to address both the upper and lower cutaneous lip (Fig. 12.15). The texture and tone of the perioral rhytids can be addressed with the placement of nanofat along the superficial cutaneous lip. Typically, 1 mL of nanofat is placed subdermally in each quadrant around the mouth.

Microfat or macrofat can then be added at a mucosal depth through the same access point at the lateral oral commissure to improve lip volume. Fat should be placed in tiny aliquots with linear threading. Placement of microfat should extend subdermally beyond the vermillion border to provide a smooth transition and further address perioral rhytids. Typically, 1 mL of microfat is placed per quadrant, for a total of 4 mL.

Melolabial Folds

To address the melolabial folds, macrofat can be injected from the lateral zygoma into the subdermal plane using a subcision-like technique. This allows small aliquots of fat to be placed just medial and just under the melolabial fold in a superficial plane. By performing the subcision and placing the fat superficially, one can achieve better effacement of the melolabial fold. The goal is to soften the fold and not to overfill the area. Typically, 1 mL of fat per side is used.

Chin and Melomental Folds

The melomental folds are filled in several planes. At the mandibular border, the fat is placed along the periosteum, intramuscularly, and subdermally. As filling proceeds more cephalad, toward the oral commissures, the fat is placed subdermally as there is no periosteum in this area. This area usually requires 2 to 4 mL per side.

Macrofat can be injected subdermally and at the periosteum to enhance the volume and projection of the chin. Through an entry point along the mandibular border anterior to the mandibular ligament, the lateral zygoma (Fig. 12.16), or through the gonial angle, macrofat can then be injected along the periosteum with a fanning approach to revolumize the medial chin. This area typically requires 3 to 4 mL of macrofat.

Mandible

With aging, the mandible loses both height and width, thus making neck laxity more pronounced. Macrofat can be added through the gonial angle with linear threading to enhance the jawline and address the upward jawline regression observed with aging. Because the skin in this area is thicker, grafts can be placed in a linear fashion. Grafts can be added in multiple planes, including subdermal, intramuscular, and periosteal. The goal of fat grafting in this area is to improve the jawline definition and to lengthen the face. Thus, fat is placed both cephalad and caudad to the mandibular border, allowing for elongation of the face (Fig. 12.17A,B).

Demonstration of facial fat transfer - Video 12.1.

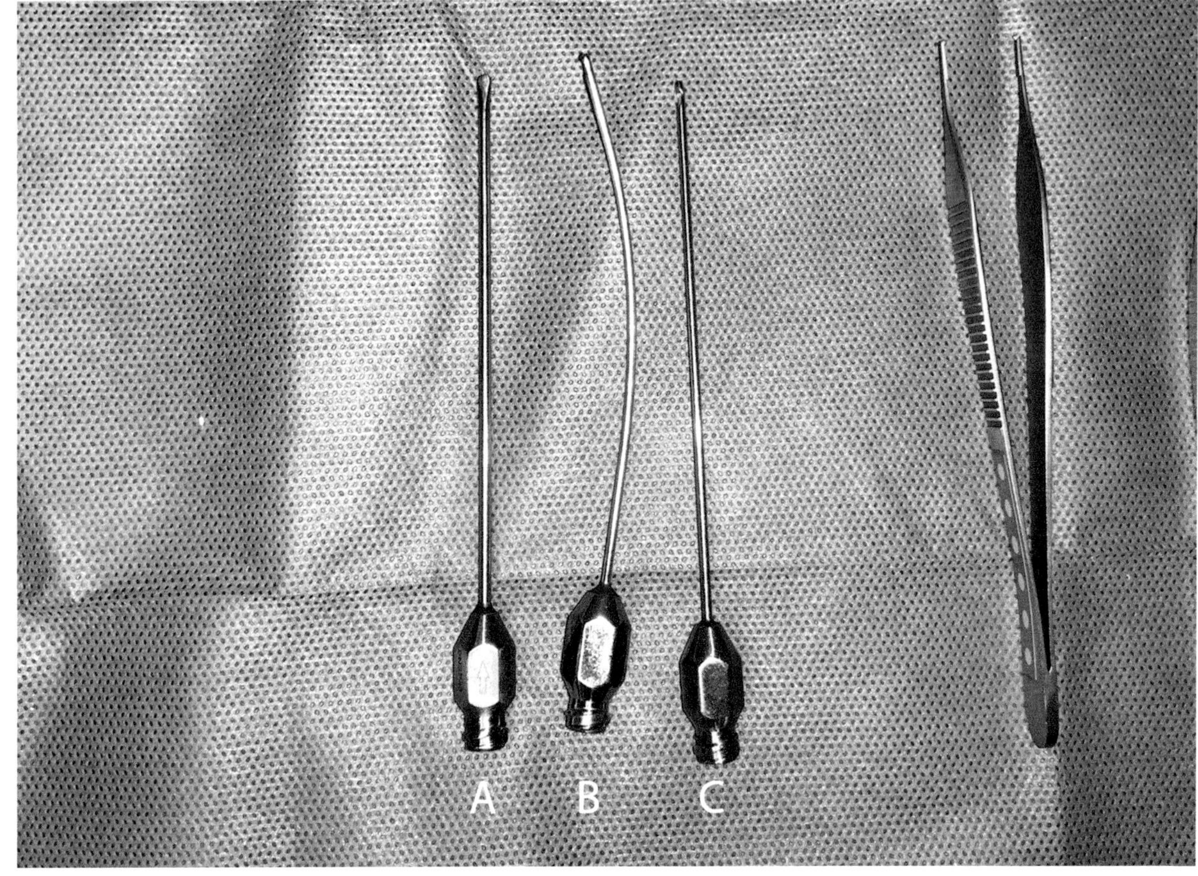

Fig. 12.11 Various micro-fat and nanofat cannulas used for fat transfer.

BOX 12.1 Depth of Fat Graft Placement by Anatomic Location

Anatomic Region	Nanofat	Microfat	Macrofat
Brows[a]	Subdermal plane along eyebrow and orbital rim	Fat pad of the superior brow, periosteum beneath brow	
Temples[a]		Subcutaneous place	
Orbital rim and tear trough[a]	Subdermal plane along eyebrow and orbital rim	Supraperiosteum	
Zygoma and malar cheeks		Supraperiosteum with small linear aliquots, muscular plane, subcutaneous plane	
Lips	Subdermal along the superficial cutaneous lips	Mucosal with small linear aliquots, Subdermal beyond the vermillion border	Mucosal
Melolabial folds			Subdermal with subcision technique
Chin and melomental folds		Periosteal, intramuscular, and subdermal along mandible, then subdermal along the melomental folds	Subdermal and periosteal at the projection of the chin, Periosteal along the medial chin with a fanning technique
Mandible	Subdermal	Subdermal, intramuscular, and periosteal with linear technique	Subdermal, intramuscular, and periosteal with linear technique

[a]Areas that require a zigzag pattern or nonlinear injection technique to avoid formation of visible fat "rolls."

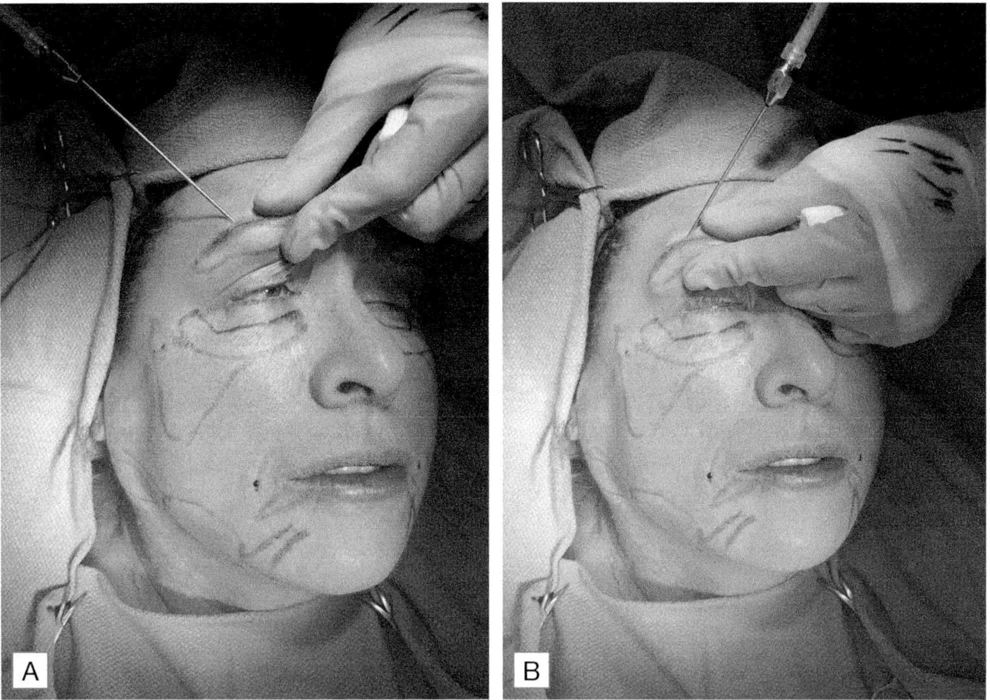

Fig. 12.12 Nanofat (0.5–1 mL) can be placed in the subdermal plane along the eyebrow and orbital rim through an access point at the mid brow.

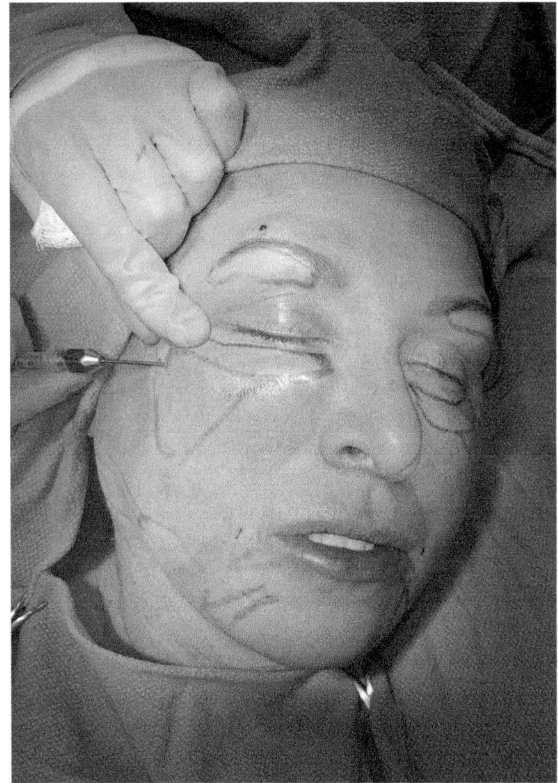

Fig. 12.13 Through the lateral orbital rim or mid malar region, nanofat can be injected subdermally to enhance skin quality using nonlinear pattern of placement.

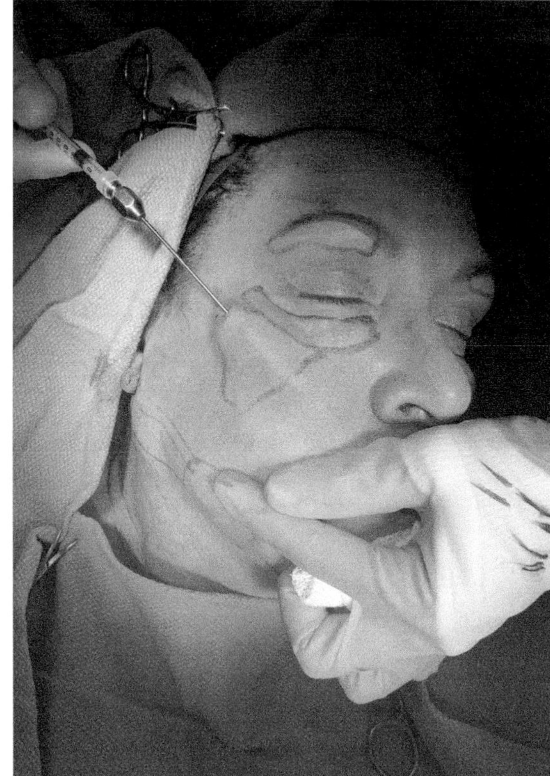

Fig. 12.14 Via entry through the lateral zygoma, the cannula can used to place macrofat in small linear aliquots along the periosteum.

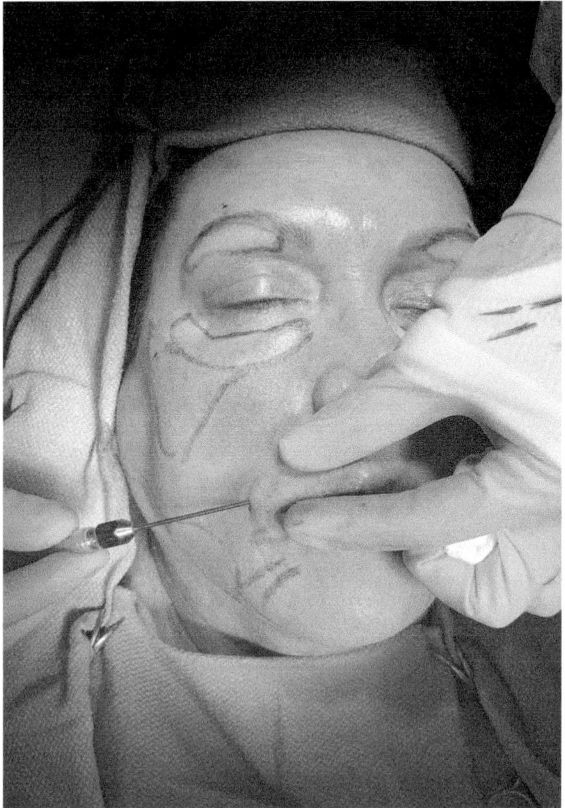

Fig. 12.15 Through the use of an access point just lateral to the oral commissure, the cannula can then be rotated to an upward or downward angle to address both the upper and lower cutaneous lip.

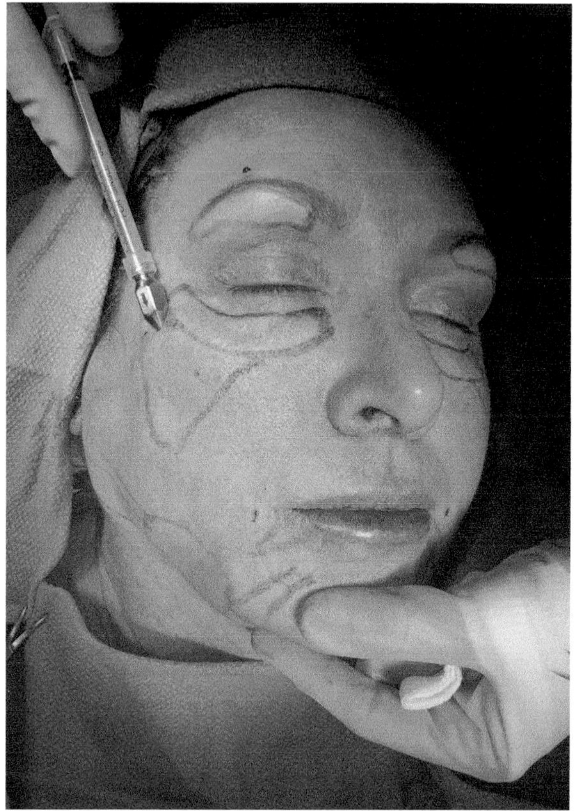

Fig. 12.16 Through an entry point along the mandibular border anterior to the mandibular ligament, the lateral zygoma, or through the gonial angle, macrofat can then be injected along the periosteum with a fanning approach to revolumize the medial chin.

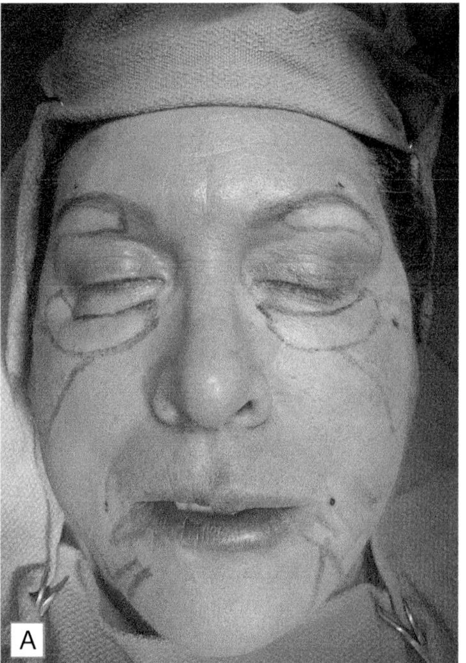

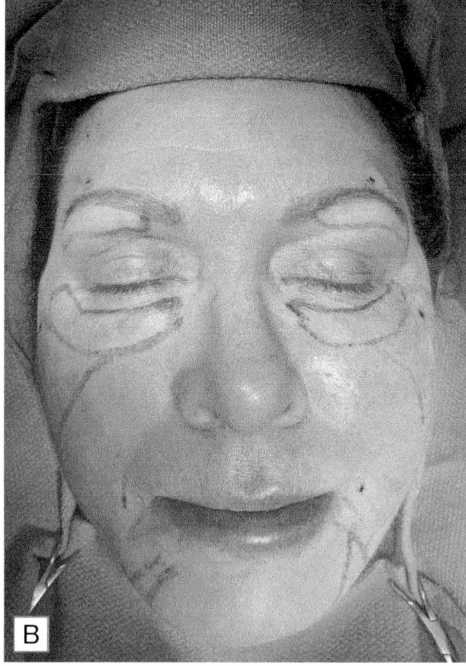

Fig. 12.17 Fat is placed both cephalad and caudad to the mandibular border, allowing for elongation of the face.

POSTOPERATIVE CONSIDERATIONS

Postoperatively, patients should be counseled to expect variable degrees of swelling and bruising, which will develop in the first 24 to 48 hours and will then gradually resolve over the course of 1 to 2 weeks (Fig. 12.18A,B). To ameliorate swelling, patients are instructed to place a cool compress such as a lightweight ice-pack or bag of frozen peas over the face for 5 to 10 minutes every hour while awake during the first 48 postoperative hours. Patients are also encouraged to sleep in a supine position with the head slightly elevated for the first week. If medically required, anticoagulants should restarted at 48 to 72 hours. All other blood-thinning agents (nonsteroidal antiinflammatory drugs [NSAIDs], fish oil) should be held for at least 1 week following AFT to minimize bleeding and graft necrosis.

Patients are able to cleanse the skin of the face on the same day as surgery using distilled water and a gentle cleanser. Patients should not massage the face or scrub excessively. For 2 weeks following AFT, all forms of exercise should be avoided to reduce the risk of shearing the new blood supply forming around the grafts. Patients should be counseled to avoid dental work for 2 weeks following surgery as this has the potential to seed the fat grafts with bacteria. To make the most of expected downtime, patients can consider adding other complementary procedures to the AFT, such as ablative laser resurfacing, chemical peels, blepharoplasty, and/or a facelift.

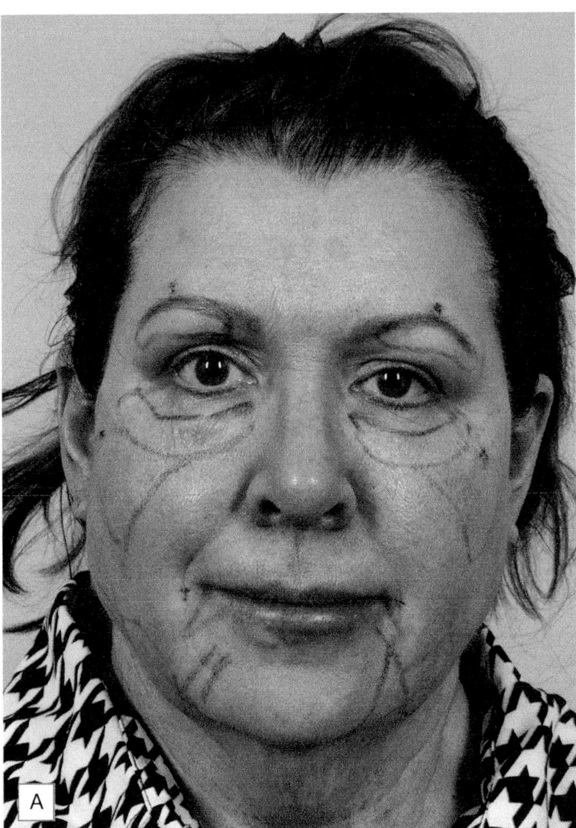

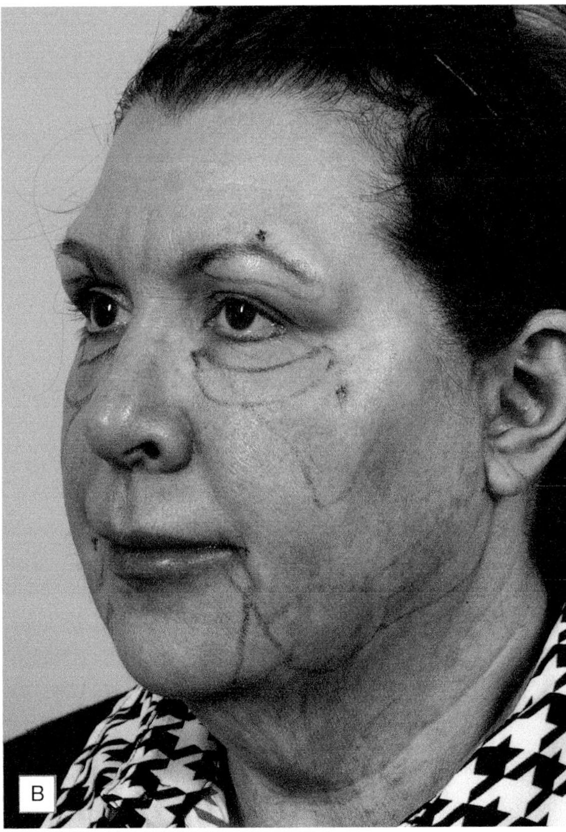

Fig. 12.18 Post-operative swelling and bruising, which will develop in the first 24 to 48 hours.

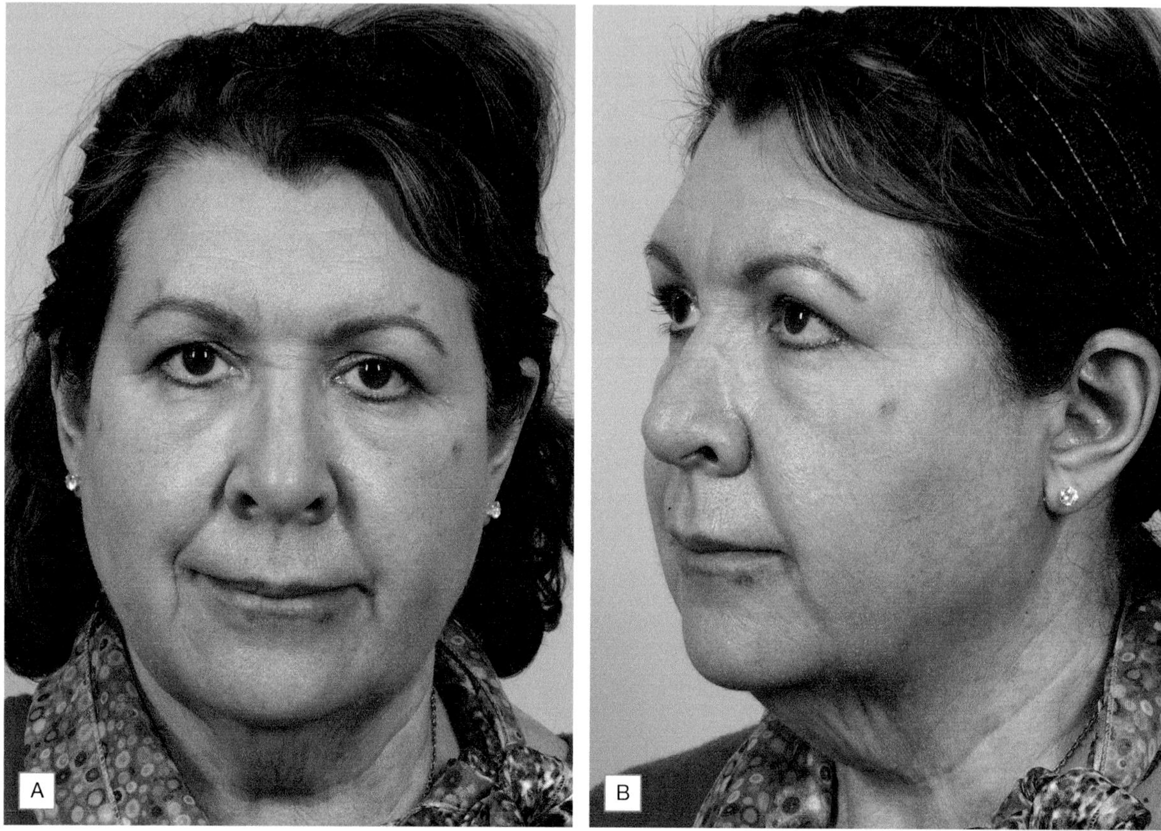

Fig. 12.19 Resolution of post-operative swelling and bruising occurs within the first 1–2 weeks.

The first postoperative visit should be conducted 7 days (Fig. 12.19A,B) following the procedure and followed by a reassessment at 3 months. Patients are informed in writing about what they can expect over the ensuing 6 to 12 months. The first month after AFT, patients will look their best then patients are told to expect some volume loss in the first 3 months as the mature adipocytes die. Apoptosis of these cells signals the preadipocyte cells to begin to proliferate and develop into mature cells. Around 3 to 6 months it may appear that there is not too much change as this is occurring. However, patients should be counseled to expect continued improvement of facial volume over the next 6 to 12 months (Fig. 12.20A–D). The Tonnard method of injecting tiny aliquots of nanofat and microfat has been shown to produce ongoing stem cell differentiation and tissue regeneration that leads to continued improvement of facial volume.[6] After the 4- to 6-month mark, patients can be reevaluated for the need for additional fat grafting.

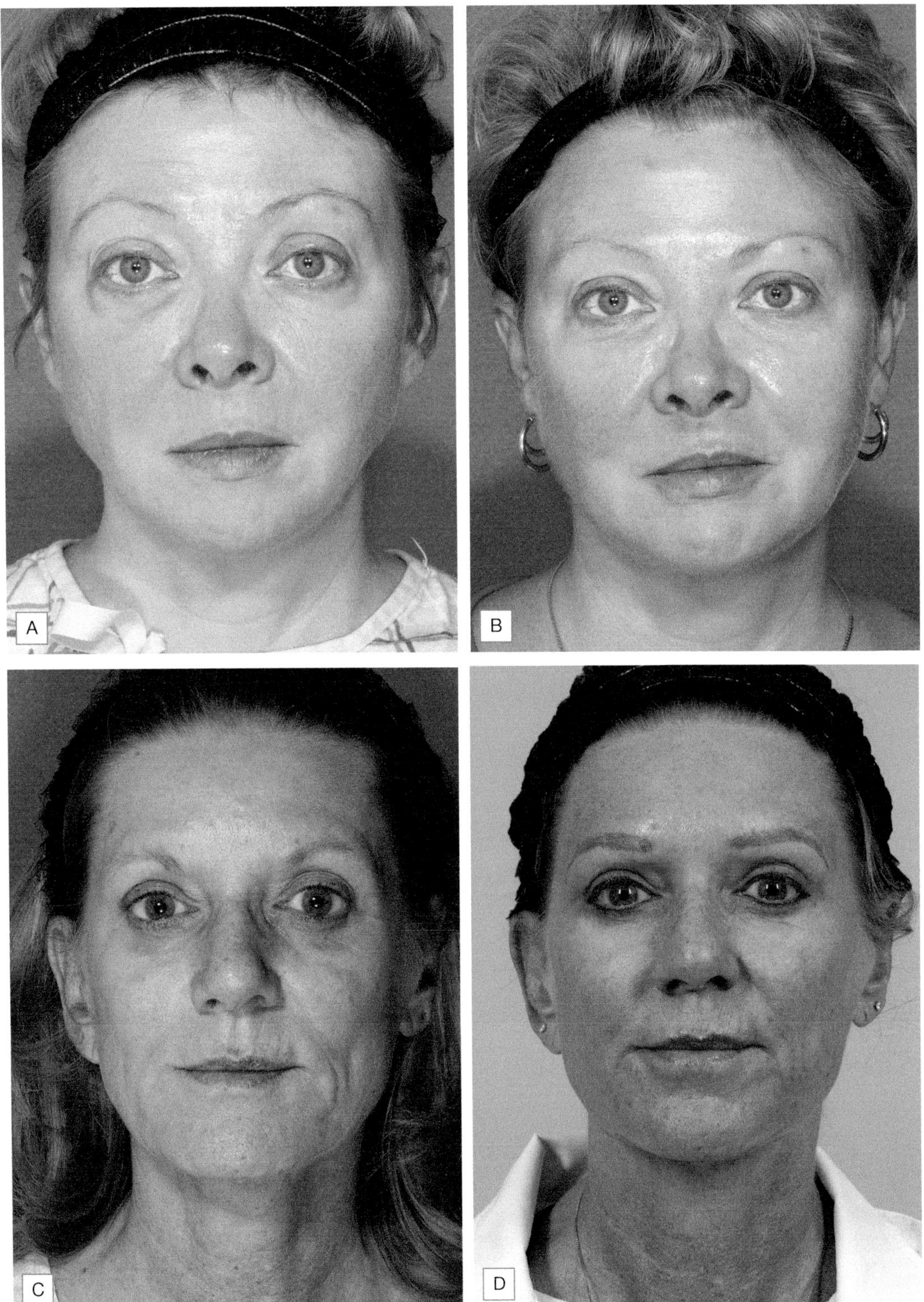

Fig. 12.20 Before (A, C) and After (B, D) pan-facial rejuvenation with fat transfer.

COMPLICATIONS

The most serious complication related to all injectable facial fillers is vascular occlusion, particularly occlusion of vessels supplying orbital structures. The rate of vascular occlusion appears to be slightly higher with injection of fat than with injection of synthetic facial fillers but is most likely due to the use of sharp needles and large syringe sizes to inject the fat in the central face region. In a systematic review of reported cases of vascular occlusion published in 2012, none of the fat-occluded patients recovered any sight. Despite the severity of this complication, it is an overall rare complication. To limit the risks of vascular occlusion and fat embolism, slow retrograde injection at low pressure with constant movement and the use of a blunt-tip cannula attached to a 1-mL syringe are recommended. Small-volume injection also helps to reduce the risk of venous compression.

Donor site complications related to liposuction appear to be minimal, and include pain, swelling, hematoma formation, infection, contour irregularities, paresthesia, hypertrophic scarring, and, rarely, damage to intraperitoneal or intramuscular structures with cannula penetration. In a systematic review of the literature from 2018, the overall complication rate for AFT was reported to be 2.27%. Complications, in order of most frequently reported to least frequently reported, included asymmetry, fat cysts/granulomas, prolonged edema, bleeding, graft hypertrophy, fat necrosis, infection, erythema, telangiectasia, and activation of acne. Asymmetry can be addressed with subsequent AFT or with the addition of other facial fillers. Fat nodules can be resolved or improved with intralesional steroid injections.

Clinicians should also be watchful for complications associated with conscious sedation and general surgical procedures. These complications include lidocaine toxicity, opioid overdose, benzodiazepine overdose, and anaphylactic reactions. Reversal agents and epinephrine should be kept on-hand in case of toxicity.

CONCLUSIONS

Autologous fat is an ideal filler that provides patients with long-lasting revolumization. With proper patient assessment, planning, and treatment, facial augmentation provides a safe means to restore the youthful contours of the face. The use of autologous nanofat, microfat, and SVF in small grafts placed strategically throughout the soft tissue planes of the face stimulates ongoing regeneration of facial texture, volume, and contour.

FURTHER READING

Boureaux, E., Chaput, B., Bannani, S., et al. (2016). Eyelid fat grafting: Indications, operative technique and complications; a systematic review. *Journal of Cranio-Maxillo-Facial Surgery*, *44*(4), 374–380. https://doi.org/10.1016/j.jcms.2015.12.013.

Bourin, P., Peyrafitte, J.-A., & Fleury-Cappellesso, S. (2011). A first approach for the production of human adipose tissue-derived stromal cells for therapeutic use. *Methods in Molecular Biology Clifton NJ*, *702*, 331–343. https://doi.org/10.1007/978-1-61737-960-4_24.

Carruthers, J. D. A., Fagien, S., Rohrich, R. J., Weinkle, S., & Carruthers, A. (2014). Blindness caused by cosmetic filler injection: A review of cause and therapy. *Plastic and Reconstructive Surgery*, *134*(6), 1197–1201. https://doi.org/10.1097/PRS.0000000000000754.

Fitzgerald, R., Graivier, M. H., Kane, M., et al. (2010). Update on Facial aging. *Aesthetic Surgery Journal*, *30*, 11S–24S. https://doi.org/10.1177/1090820X10378696.

Geissler, P. J., Davis, K., Roostaeian, J., et al. (2014). Improving fat transfer viability: The role of aging, body mass index, and harvest site. *Plastic and Reconstructive Surgery*, *134*(2), 227–232. https://doi.org/10.1097/PRS.0000000000000398.

Gornitsky, J., Viezel-Mathieu, A., Alnaif, N., Azzi, A. J., & Gilardino, M. S. (2019). A systematic review of the effectiveness and complications of fat grafting in the facial region. *JPRAS Open*, *19*, 87–97. https://doi.org/10.1016/j.jpra.2018.12.004.

Hamza, A., Lohsiriwat, V., & Rietjens, M. (2013). Lipofilling in breast cancer surgery. *Gland Surgery*, *2*(1), 7–14. https://doi.org/10.3978/j.issn.2227-684X.2013.02.03.

Illouz, Y.-G., & Illouz, Y.-G. (1983). Body contouring by lipolysis: A 5-year experience with over 3000 cases. *Plastic and Reconstructive Surgery*, *72*(5), 591–597. https://doi.org/10.1097/00006534-198311000-0.

Khouri, R. K., Rigotti, G., Cardoso, E., Khouri, R. K., & Biggs, T. M. (2014). Megavolume autologous fat transfer: Part II. Practice and techniques. *Plastic and Reconstructive Surgery*, *133*(6), 1369–1377. https://doi.org/10.1097/PRS.0000000000000179.

Lazzeri, D., Agostini, T., Figus, M., et al. (2012). Blindness following cosmetic injections of the face. *Plastic and Reconstructive Surgery*, *129*(4), 995–1012. https://doi.org/10.1097/PRS.0b013e3182442363.

Lin, J.-Y., Wang, C., & Pu, L. L. Q. (2015). Can we standardize the techniques for fat grafting? *Clinics in Plastic Surgery*, *42*(2), 199–208. https://doi.org/10.1016/j.cps.2014.12.005.

Mashiko, T., & Yoshimura, K. (2015). How does fat survive and remodel after grafting? *Clinics in Plastic Surgery*, *42*(2), 181–190. https://doi.org/10.1016/j.cps.2014.12.008.

Neuber, F. (1893). Fettransplantation Bericht uber die Verhandlungen der Deutscht Gesellsch Chir. *Zentralblatt fur Chirurgie*, *22*, 66.

Rihani, J. (2019). Microfat and nanofat: When and where these treatments work. *Facial Plastic Surgery Clinics of North America*, *27*(3), 321–330. https://doi.org/10.1016/j.fsc.2019.03.004.

Rohrich, R. J., & Pessa, J. E. (2007). The fat compartments of the face: Anatomy and clinical implications for cosmetic surgery. *Plastic and Reconstructive Surgery*, *119*(7), 2219–2227. https://doi.org/10.1097/01.prs.0000265403.66886.54.

Strong, A. L., Cederna, P. S., Rubin, J. P., Coleman, S. R., & Levi, B. (2015). The current state of fat grafting: A review of harvesting, processing, and injection techniques. *Plastic and Reconstructive Surgery*, *136*(4), 897–912. https://doi.org/10.1097/PRS.0000000000001590.

Tonnard, P., Verpaele, A., Peeters, G., et al. (2013). Nanofat grafting: Basic research and clinical applications. *Plastic and Reconstructive Surgery*, *132*, 1017–1026. https://doi.org/10.1097/PRS.0b013e31829fe1b0.

Zuk, P. A., Zhu, M., Mizuno, H., et al. (2001). Multilineage cells from human adipose tissue: Implications for cell-based therapies. *Tissue Engineering*, *7*(2), 211–228. https://doi.org/10.1089/107632701300062859.

13

Introduction to Permanent Fillers: Pros and Cons

Paola Barriera, Shilpi Khetarpal, and Jeffrey S. Dover

SUMMARY AND KEY FEATURES

- Permanent fillers are materials composed of nonabsorbable or permanent materials.
- These agents can provide long-lasting results but carry more potential risk.
- Polymethylmethacrylate and liquid injectable silicone are the only currently available permanent fillers available in the United States.
- Nonbiodegradable fillers can achieve full and long-lasting correction but carry the risk of permanent adverse effects.

INTRODUCTION

In the past 15 years, there has been a dramatic increase in the use of injectable facial fillers for rejuvenation of the aging face. With more than 2.7 million soft tissue filler procedures performed in 2019 in the United States, there has been increasing interests in research and development of both temporary and permanent agents. There is no universally accepted classification for soft tissue fillers; however, they can be classified by their origin—natural animal, synthetic, or natural synthetic. They can be further classified by their longevity: temporary, semipermanent, or permanent. An ideal soft tissue filler is one that is effective; easy and painless to inject; feels natural; is nontoxic, nonreactive, noncarcinogenic, and nonimmunologic; has a low incidence of adverse events; and is long lasting.

The US Food and Drug Administration (FDA) defines permanent fillers as materials that are composed of nonabsorbable or permanent materials. These agents can provide excellent, long-term results but carry more potential risk and require a higher level of injector skill given that complications are more common compared with temporary agents and can be more difficult to resolve. In the United States, the currently available permanent fillers are polymethylmethacrylate (PMMA) and liquid injectable silicone (LIS), but only the former is approved by the FDA for the correction of nasolabial folds and moderate to severe, atrophic, distensible facial acne scars on the cheek in patients over the age of 21 years. Several other agents are available for use outside the United States or are currently being developed (Table 13.1).

TABLE 13.1 Permanent Fillers by Category and Composition

Category	Branded product	Composition
Liquid injectable silicone	Silikon-1000	Purified polydimethylsiloxane polymer
	Adato Sil-ol-5000	Purified polydimethylsiloxane polymer
Other "silicones"	Adulterated and unknown products	Variable and often unknown
Polyalkylimide gels (hydrophilic)	Bio-Alcamid	3% or 4% polyalkylimide gel in 97% or 96% sterile water
Polyacrylamide gels (hydrophilic)	Amazingel	Polyacrylamide gel in sterile water
	Aquamid	2.5% polyacrylamide gel in 97.5% sterile water
Polymethylmethacrylate (hydrophobic)	Arteplast/Artecoll/Artefill	< 20 μm PMMA microspheres in a bovine collagen carrier
	Bellafill	30–50 μm PMMA microspheres in a bovine collagen carrier
Acrylic hydrogel (hydroxyethylmethacrylate/ethylmethacrylate) (hydrophobic)	Dermalive	45–65 μm polygonal fragments acrylic hydrogel (40%) in HA (60%)
	Dermadeep	80–110 μm polygonal fragments acrylic hydrogel (40%) in HA (60%)

HA, Hyaluronic acid; *PMMA*, polymethylmetacrylate.
Prather C.L., Wiest L.G. Modified from *Soft Tissue Augmentation, Complications of Permanent Fillers*. 3rd ed. USA: Elsevier Saunders; 2013.

POLYMETHYLMETHACRYLATE

Bellafill (Suneva Medical, San Diego, CA) is a third-generation PMMA and collagen filler that is an updated version of its predecessor created more than 20 years ago. The original product was never commercially available in the United States (Arteplast/Artecoll); however, a refined version called Artefill was used in the United States. Although these agents were effective, they had a high incidence of foreign body granuloma formation at 2.5%, due to the small PMMA microsphere size (< 20 μm) that provoked a foreign body response due to macrophages digesting these small particles. The latest generation, Bellafill, has 20% larger PMMA microspheres (30 to 50 μm) suspended in a water-based gel containing 3.5% bovine collagen and 0.3% lidocaine. The larger particle size decreases digestion by macrophages and overall immunogenicity; the smoothness and uniformity of the individual microspheres mitigate an inflammatory response; and clumping of the particles is prevented by the viscosity of the bovine collagen that embeds the microspheres evenly in place. Due to the bovine collagen component, the FDA recommends a skin test at least 28 days prior to use because of a 3% rate of collagen hypersensitivity. The collagen component is absorbed 1 to 3 months after injection, and the PMMA microspheres act as a scaffold for the development of autologous type 3 collagen and procollagen-1. This combination of neocollagenesis followed by microencapsulation of PMMA microspheres by fibroblasts in the new tissue provides for long-lasting results. The growth and pattern of new connective tissue mimic a normal wound healing response.

A series of multiple injections are necessary to achieve the optimal outcome. Results can take several months to more than a year after injection. It is essential for the practitioner to take a conservative approach and wait 1 to 3 months between injections, which is the time required for the degradation of the collagen carrier. Although complications with Bellafill are less than with its predecessors, they can still occur. If injections are placed too superficially, nodules, beading, and scarring can occur. Overall, the PMMA–collagen gel dermal filler has demonstrated an excellent safety and effectiveness profile in clinical trials and 12-year postmarketing surveillance data (PMSD). The reported adverse event rate for 754,229 syringes distributed worldwide during this period is 0.11%. However, the underreporting bias characteristic of PMSD often leads to adverse event rates that are lower than those observed in real life. The process of manufacturing and purifying PMMA has played a major role in minimizing adverse events for Bellafill.

The new generation of PMMA has a lower incidence of delayed granuloma formation due to the more uniform and larger size and shape of microspheres. PMMA microsphere size is critical to avoid phagocytosis, and particles less than 20 μm in size cause a foreign body response. The original generation of PMMA agents had granuloma rates of 2.5% at 5 years compared with 1.7% with the latest generation product. In 2006, Bellafill received FDA approval for nasolabial folds and in late 2014 for moderate to severe, atrophic, distensible facial acne scars on the cheeks. The product has strict manufacturing requirements and unique formulation characteristics that make it superior when compared with prior PMMA products. Bellafill is the only PMMA filler manufactured in the United States and uses a more refined collagen carrier matrix derived from bovine collagen sources that come from a restricted herd. The new class of PMMA-based fillers has a longevity greater than 5 years and if injected properly can be safe for its approved indications in the appropriate patient type—one who desires long-lasting correction.

LIQUID INJECTABLE SILICONE

LIS, a highly purified long-chain polydimethylsiloxane trimethylsiloxy terminated silicone oil, is one of the oldest and longest lasting injectable fillers. It received FDA approval in 1959 for intraocular use as retinal stabilizing agents, for retinal tamponade during vitreous surgery. In the 1990s, the FDA approved two new forms of medical-grade, highly purified silicone—Silikon 1000 (Alcon, Fort Worth, TX) and Adato Sil-ol-5000 (Bausch & Lomb, Rochester, NY)—for ophthalmological use related to retinal detachments. Since the enactment of the FDA Modernization Act in 1997, physicians have been allowed to use legally marketed FDA-approved products for an indication that is not in the approved labeling. Thus, an interest in silicone oil as a dermal permanent filler was renewed. Its off-label uses for cosmetic therapy include human immunodeficiency virus (HIV) lipoatrophy, acne scarring, and facial volume enhancement.

Similar to PMMA, LIS induces new collagen production around individual microdroplets in addition to producing a direct volume-filling effect. Complications vary from minor and temporary to serious and permanent. Minor complications include erythema, ecchymoses, and edema at injection sites, which can occur with any soft tissue filler. More serious complications include infection, silicone granuloma formation (weeks to years after placement), ulceration, inflammatory nodules, vascular occlusion, and migration. Many of these complications occur when using contaminated industrial-grade products or improper injection technique. It is recommended that one of the FDA-approved, medical-grade silicone oils—Silikon 1000 or Adato Sil-ol-5000—be used with the microdroplet technique. With this technique, droplets of 0.01-mL aliquots are injected in the subcutaneous fat or deep dermis in the desired locations. Silikon 1000 and Adato Sil-ol-5000 differ in viscosity, which is measured in centistokes (cs). As their names suggest, Silikon has a viscosity of 1000 cs, whereas Adato Sil-ol has a viscosity of 5000 cs. Silicone oil is available from manufacturers in Mexico and South America; however, these formulations can be contaminated and impure, resulting in a high rate of complications. Before the microdroplet technique was developed, LIS was injected in large boluses in a single session, resulting in high rates of migration of the product. Despite potential complications, LIS has many "ideal" qualities for soft tissue filling. It is colorless, odorless, nonvolatile, noncarcinogenic, thermally stable for heat sterilization, and chemically stable at room temperature (allowing for storage for long periods of time); does not have to be reconstituted prior to use; does not require skin testing; and when injected properly looks very natural. If used for the correct indications in the hands of a skilled injector, medical-grade silicone oil is a safe, economic, permanent dermal filler with minimal complications that has been used for more than half a century under the practice of "off-label use of an approved medical device."

OTHER PERMANENT FILLERS

Synthetic facial implants serve a similar purpose to permanent fillers. Most are composed of either silicone or polytetraflurothene (Gore-tex). Downsides of these implants are that they are often visible through the skin (especially with movement), they can become visible as facial anatomy changes, and they also may compress nearby structures.

There are other categories of injectable products available outside the United States or are currently in development. Polyacrylamide hydrogel—Aquamid (Polymekon, Milan, Italy)—is a biocompatible, nonabsorbable hydrogel containing water and cross-linked polyacrylamide that augments soft tissue through a direct, volume-filling effect. Aquamid is available and approved in several European, Middle Eastern, and Asian countries for the treatment of rhytides, facial contouring, and HIV lipoatrophy. Although the studies conducted with Aquamid demonstrate high rates of patient satisfaction, the complication rates are high when compared with the temporary hyaluronic acid (HA) fillers. Side effects include unevenness, nodule formation, and displacement of the gel. Delayed immune mediated events have been reported approximately 10 months after the product had been injected; these include inflamed nodules and pseudoabscesses.

Bio-Alcamid is a 97% hydrophilic polyalkylimide hydrogel that was a permanent filler previously approved for use in Canada for facial contouring and the treatment of HIV-related lipoatrophy. After injection, an inflammatory reaction occurs within 45 to 60 days and leads to a thin fibrous capsule forming around the injected material. It was most commonly used in the malar and lower midface region, and success has also been reported with its use for chin augmentation. Overall, patients reported a high success rate with the product when small amounts were used with each injection session (10 to 30 cm^3 per side). There have been no reports of foreign body granulomas. Unfortunately, the product becomes mobile after approximately 4 years and tracks around the face giving unsightly lumps (Fig. 13.1A,B). Removal can be achieved through tumescent analgesia with puncture and drainage with manual compression over several sessions. In a study with 2000 injections, 12 patients had infections (0.06%), which were all caused by *Staphylococcus* and treated successfully with oral antibiotics and needle aspiration.

IMAGING PATTERNS

Injectable facial fillers are seen as incidental findings on imaging including ultrasound, computed tomography (CT), magnetic resonance imaging (MRI), and positron emission tomography (PET)-CT. Imaging findings vary with the type of dermal filler.

- PMMA. Ultrasound imaging of PMMA-based fillers was previously defined as hyperechoic dots with a minitail reverberation artifact. A recent study found that PMMA-based fillers were associated with a "coarse-grained snowy" pattern, which is characterized by hyperechoic images distributed all over the tissue, associated with posterior echogenic shadow.
- Silicone. Silicone oil ultrasound pattern has been defined as "fine-grain snowfall," which is characterized

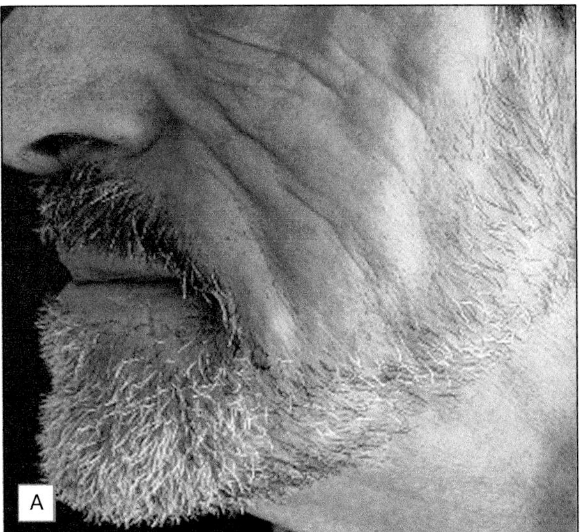

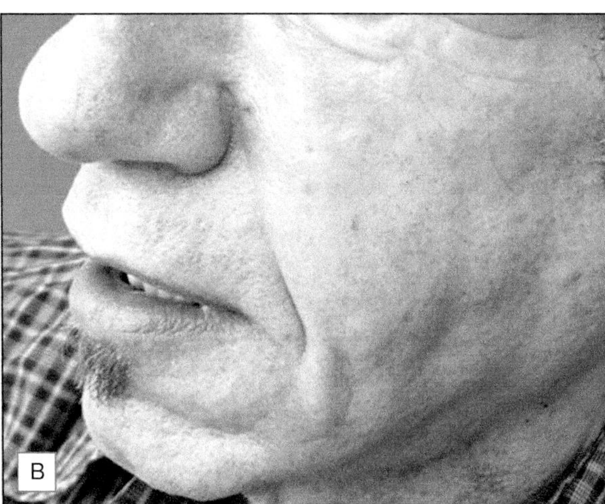

Fig. 13.1 (A and B) Four years after injection with Bio-Alcamid, both patients present with unsightly lumps on the cheeks. (Photos courtesy of Drs. Jean Carruthers and Alastair Carruthers.)

by alternating hyperechoic imaging, with posterior echogenic shadows. The MRI appearance of silicone fillers varies according to viscosity and purity. The low-viscosity silicone oil is slightly hyperintense to water on T1-weighted (T1W) images, iso- or slightly hypointense to water on T2W images, and hyperintense on the "silicone-only" sequence. High-viscosity silicone oil is hypointense on T2W images. A "silicone-only" sequence is designed to suppress all tissues except silicone. On CT, silicone appears slightly hyperdense.

- Polyalkylimide and polyacrylamide hydrogels (PAAGs). PAAG fillers feature a high water content and thus appear hyperintense on T2W and hypointense on T1W sequences. On CT, PAAG appears as a well-defined area of fluid attenuation.

PROS OF PERMANENT FILLERS

The use of medical-grade LIS and PMMA is now supported by a wide array of scientific evidence that shows these permanent fillers can be used safely and effectively by a skilled injector. After correction with these agents, there is no need for maintenance injections, which contribute to additional cost and inconvenience. Bellafill is the only dermal filler FDA approved to treat acne scarring. It is also the only nonresorbable filler approved by the FDA for the correction of nasolabial folds.

CONS OF PERMANENT FILLERS

Unlike permanent fillers, the HA group of injectable agents has a unique characteristic, which is their reversibility with enzymatic digestion with hyaluronidase. Their lack of permanence and ease of correction, with the ability to be dissolved, makes the HA group of fillers attractive to physicians and patients alike. A concern in the use of permanent, synthetic dermal fillers is the safety profile of these long-lasting agents. Many clinicians avoid these agents because of this fear that after the agent has been injected, it cannot be easily removed. Although all fillers have potential side effects, the side effects associated with permanent agents tend to be longer lasting due to continued presence of product. The other concern of permanent fillers is their irreversibility as facial shape changes with age. Nonbiodegradable fillers can achieve full and long-lasting correction but carry the risk of permanent adverse effects.

FURTHER READING

American Society of Plastic Surgeons. (2020). *Plastic Surgery Statistics Report 2019* (online). American Society of Plastic Surgeons. https://www.plasticsurgery.org/documents/News/Statistics/2019/plastic-surgery-statistics-full-report-2019.pdf.

Attenello, N. H., & Maas, C. S. (2015). Injectable fillers: Review of material and properties. *Facial Plastic and Surgery, 31*, 29–34.

Carruthers, J., Carruthers, A., & Humphrey, S. (2015). Introduction to fillers. *Plastic Reconstructive Surgery, 136*(5S), 120S–131S.

Conrad, K., Togerson, C. S., & Gillman, G. S. (2008). Applications of GORETEX implants in rhinoplasty reexamined after 17 years. *Archives of Facial Plastic Surgery, 10*(4), 224–231.

Duffy, D. (2002). The silicone conundrum: A battle of anecdotes. *Dermatologic Surgery, 28*(7), 590–595.

Ellis, D. A. F., & Segall, L. (2007). Review of non-FDA approved fillers. *Facial Plastic Surgery Clinics of North America, 15*(2), 239–246.

Ellis, L., Cojen, J., & High, W. (2012). Granulomatous reaction to silicone injection. *Journal of Clinical Aesthetic Dermatology, 5*(7), 44–47.

Fulton, J., & Caperton, C. (2012). The optimal filler: Immediate and long-term results with emulsified silicone with cross-linked hyaluronic acid. *Journal of Drugs in Dermatology, 11*(11), 1336–1341.

Jones, D. H., Carruthers, A., Brody, H. J., Black, J. M., Humphrey, S., Carruthers, J., Wesley, N. O., Minokadeh, A., et al. (2019). Ten-year and beyond follow-up after treatment with highly purified liquid-injectable silicone for HIV-associated facial lipoatrophy: A report of 164 patients. *Dermatologic Surgery, 45*(7), 941–948. https://doi.org/10.1097/DSS.0000000000001889.

Joseph, J. H. (2015). The case for synthetic injectables. *Facial Plastic Surgery Clinics of North America, 23*(4), 433–445. https://doi.org/10.1016/j.fsc.2015.07.003.

Joseph, J. H., Eaton, L. L., & Cohen, B. R. (2015). Current concepts in the use of Bellafill. *Plastic Reconstructive Surgery, 136*(5S), 171–179.

Lehman, A., Pilcher, B., Roberts, W. E., Schlesinger, T. E., & Vachon, G. (2020). Postmarket experience of polymethylmethacrylate-collagen gel dermal filler. *Dermatologic Surgery, 46*(8), 1086–1091. https://doi.org/10.1097/DSS.0000000000002222.

Lemperle, G., Knapp, T. R., Sadick, N. S., & Lemperle, S. M. (2010). ArteFill permanent injectable for soft tissue augmentation: I. Mechanism of action and injection techniques. *Aesthetic Plastic Surgery, 34*(3), 264–272.

Liu, M. H., Beynet, D. P., & Gharavi, N. M. (2019). Overview of deep dermal fillers. *Facial Plastic Surgery, 35*(3), 224–229. https://doi.org/10.1055/s-0039-1688843.

Mills, D. C., Camp, S., Mosser, S., Sayeg, A., Hurwitz, D., & Ronel, D. (2013). Malar augmentation with a polymethylmethacrylate-enhanced filler: Assessment of a 12-month open-label pilot study. *Aesthetic Surgery Journal, 33*(3), 421–430.

Mundada, P., Kohler, R., Boudabbous, S., Toutous Trellu, L., Platon, A., & Becker, M. (2017). Injectable facial fillers: Imaging features, complications, and diagnostic pitfalls at MRI and PET CT. *Insights into Imaging, 8*(6), 557–572. https://doi.org/10.1007/s13244-017-0575-0.

Narins, R. S., & Cohen, S. R. (2010). Novel polymethylmethacrylate soft tissue filler for the correction of nasolabial folds: Interim results of a 5-year long-term safety and patient satisfaction study. *Dermatologic Surgery, 36*, 766–774.

Nettar, K., & Maas, C. (2012). Facial filler and neurotoxin complications. *Facial Plastic Surgery, 28*(3), 288–293.

Niamtu, J. (2018). Injectable fillers: Lip augmentation, lip reduction, and lip lift. In J. Niamtu (Ed.), *Cosmetic facial surgery* (pp. 569–638). Edinburgh: Elsevier.

Pacini, S., Ruggiero, M., Morucci, G., Cammarota, N., Protopapa, C., & Gulisano, M. (2002). Bio-Alcamid: A novelty for reconstructive and cosmetic surgery. *Italian Journal of Anatomy and Embryology, 107*, 209–214.

Ronan, S. J., Eaton, L., Lehman, A., Pilcher, B., & Erickson, C. P. (2019). Histologic characterization of polymethylmethacrylate dermal filler biostimulatory properties in human skin. *Dermatologic Surgery, 45*(12), 1580–1584. https://doi.org/10.1097/DSS.0000000000001877.

Schelke, L. W., Velthuis, P. J., & van Dijk, M. R. (2018). Polyalkylimide: A nonstable filler over time. *Dermatologic Surgery, 44*(4), 563–567. https://doi.org/10.1097/DSS.0000000000001388.

Urdiales-Gálvez, F., De Cabo-Francés, F. M., & Bové, I. (2021). Ultrasound patterns of different dermal filler materials used in aesthetics. *Journal of Cosmetic Dermatology, 20*(5), 1541–1548. https://doi.org/10.1111/jocd.14032.

Wilson, Y., & Ellis, D. (2011). Permanent soft tissue fillers. *Facial Plastic Surgery, 27*(6), 540–546.

Yamauchi, P. S. (2014). Emerging permanent filler technologies: Focus on aquamid. *Clinical Cosmetic and Investigational Dermatology, 7*, 261–266.

14

Liquid Injectable Silicone

Ardalan Minokadeh, Harold Brody, and Derek Jones

SUMMARY AND KEY FEATURES

- Two forms of highly purified injectable liquid silicone (Silikon-1000 and Adatosil-5000) are US Food and Drug Administration (FDA) approved for intraocular tamponade of retinal detachment.
- Both products may be legally injected off-label for skin augmentation, according to the 1997 FDA Modernization Act.
- Industrial liquid silicone, including "medical-grade" industrial liquid silicone, may contain contaminants that cause granulomatous reactions.
- Industrial-grade liquid silicone should never be injected into the human body.
- Three rules should always be followed when using liquid injectable silicone (LIS) for skin augmentation, as follows:
  - Rule 1: Inject only FDA-approved highly purified liquid silicone.
  - Rule 2: Use only the microdroplet technique.
  - Rule 3: Inject limited amounts of volume at monthly intervals or longer.
- There is much evidence supporting the safety and efficacy of LIS for human immunodeficient virus-associated lipoatrophy. However, late-appearing granulomatous reactions are not infrequent (> 5%), may be managed with intralesional injections of 5-fluorouracil and triamcinolone, but tend to recur.
- With proper protocol, serious adverse events are rare and are usually treatable.
- Given the availability of newer longer-lasting volumizing hyaluronic acid fillers, they can be considered as an alternative for the management of HIV-associated facial lipoatrophy, although they are more expensive. Use of LIS can be considered in disease states where cost benefits outweigh the risk of adverse events.
- Use of small-volume microdroplet LIS in the treatment of acne scarring may be less likely to lead to the development of delayed reactions with persistent lumps.

INTRODUCTION

Physicians and patients continue to strive for the "ideal filler," which would offer consistent, sustained results that remain natural and free of complications over time and that would be biocompatible, safe, cost-effective, and versatile. When injected properly, highly purified liquid injectable silicone (HPLIS) meets the majority of these criteria. However, as with any permanent filler, late-appearing lumps, bumps, and granulomatous reactions may occur. Use of injectable silicone has historically been met with controversy. However, when modern HPLIS was properly injected in small amounts using the microdroplet technique with repeat treatments spaced at least a month apart, physicians have achieved optimal and enduring correction of scars, rhytides, and facial atrophy.

HPLIS may be much less forgiving than temporary fillers and is a potential liability when it is injected incorrectly, results in undesired augmentation, or serves as a nidus for inflammation and infection. Therefore, to achieve good outcomes, experience and precise technique are imperative. Physicians should use HPLIS only after extensive training in proper technique and patient selection. Candidates for treatment should have clear treatment objectives and understand that multiple treatment sessions may be required to achieve optimal correction and that late-appearing (months to many years) inflammatory and granulomatous reactions clinically appearing as nodules or firmness occur more frequently then with most hyaluronic acid fillers.

Patients who desire immediate correction or are uncertain of their treatment goals or are risk-adverse are better treated with temporary fillers rather than HPLIS.

BASIC SCIENCE

Silicon (Si) is a relatively inert element that is essential to humans in small amounts and is second only to oxygen as the most abundant element of the Earth's crust. "Silicone" describes a group of synthetic polymers containing elemental silicon. Polymers in the silicone family may exist in solid, liquid, and gel states, with various chemical, physical, and thermal properties. Silicone polymers also vary with regard to purity, sterility, and biocompatibility. Although various silicone polymers are used for medical use, *polydimethylsiloxane* is the liquid injectable silicone (LIS) used for soft tissue augmentation. The molecular structure of this colorless, odorless, nonvolatile oil consists of repeating dimethylsiloxane units with terminal trimethylsiloxane ends.

The viscosity of a given liquid silicone product is dependent upon the mean number and chain length of the dimethylsiloxane subunits within the polymer, with longer chain molecules conferring a higher viscosity. Viscosity is measured in centistokes (cs), where 1 cs equals the viscosity of water. Current HPLIS is either 1000 cs (similar to the viscosity of honey) or 5000 cs.

Silicones have not been found to be carcinogenic and have demonstrated "an enviable record of safety," according to a 1998 National Science Panel investigating silicone implants, reported by Diamond et al. HPLIS is not altered in vivo, although small amounts may be phagocytized and enter the reticuloendothelial system.

MECHANISM OF ACTION

HPLIS first creates immediate volume enhancement by a direct space-filling effect. Additional filling occurs by the deposition of new collagen via fibroplasia. After injection, a localized inflammatory reaction ensues, consisting of neutrophil migration and some degree of macrophage phagocytic activity, with fibroblasts depositing a thin-walled collagen capsule around the silicone microdroplet. This capsule effectively anchors the microdroplet in place and prevents migration.

Several filler products, both temporary and permanent, were reported by Jones in 2009 to induce collagen fibroplasia as a partial mechanism of action for aesthetic improvement.

Rather than attempting to reach optimal correction in one session, fibroplastic fillers require that smaller amounts of product be injected over several sessions spaced 1 to 2 months apart or longer. This avoids overcorrection by allowing the fibroplastic process adequate time to occur prior to subsequent treatment sessions.

CONTROVERSY

The past several decades have witnessed notable debate regarding the safety of LIS, with both critics and advocates arguing their positions based largely on anecdotal data rather than rigorous trials. The true number of patients treated with liquid silicone available prior to 1990 who have historically experienced treatment success versus significant complications is simply unknown.

A further difficulty in historically analyzing the safety of "silicone" as an augmenting agent is that, apart from the modern, US Food and Drug Administration (FDA)-approved products available since the 1990s, an unknown number of products claiming to be silicone have likely been adulterated, impure, or nonsilicone substances altogether. Although highly purified 1000 and 5000 cs products intended for injection into the human body were FDA approved for human use in the 1990s, various substances masquerading as silicone have been injected for the past 60 years, at times with significant complications, as reported by Delage et al., Baselga and Pujol, and Rapaport et al. Even products labeled as "medical-grade" silicone have not historically been regulated or authenticated. A 1989 analysis by Parel of six "medical-grade" silicone oils commonly used for injection revealed six different products of variable viscosity, each with significant amounts of elemental impurities and low-molecular-weight adulterants that can produce inflammatory and granulomatous reactions.

Critics argue that liquid silicone is an inherently unpredictable implant, fraught with potential complications. Several anecdotal reports of complications, such as cellulitis, nodules, granulomatous reactions, and migration, have been described by the groups previously discussed, although variables, such as product purity, volume, and injection technique, could not be established with certainty. Furthermore, complications were reported by Rapaport et al. to occur as long as 36 years after treatment. Migration of the product to other areas of the body may occur when large boluses of liquid silicone are injected, but this has never been reported when using the microdroplet technique, as in the studies by Duffy in 2005 and Price et al. in 2006.

Advocates posit that HPLIS is extremely safe and beneficial when three rules of injection are strictly followed: (1) use only FDA-approved products intended for injection into the human body, (2) exclusively use the microdroplet technique, and (3) strictly follow a protocol using limited volumes injected over multiple sessions spaced monthly or longer.

Several authors have published excellent safety records of longer-term follow-up on patients treated with liquid silicone. Wallace et al. reported long-term follow-up over 41 years using liquid silicone as a soft tissue substitute for plantar fat loss in more than 1500 patients, with 25,000 recorded silicone injections; they found that the host response to injections consisted of a "banal and stable fibrous tissue formation." Other authors, including Jones et al., Chen et al., Orentreich and Leone, and Hevia, have published multiple reports of their extensive and successful experience with liquid silicone and reiterate that the three principles of product purity, appropriate technique, and proper protocol are imperative for success. Duffy, who has written extensively on the subject, gathers that LIS has been used for soft tissue augmentation worldwide for at least 40 years and hypothetically in at least 200,000 patients in the United States. He cautions that, although pure liquid silicone may be a superior filler for the permanent correction of certain defects, physicians who use it must realize that its misuse, or the use of other materials masquerading as pure silicone, have created "a pervasive climate of distrust and a veritable minefield of extraordinarily unpleasant medico-legal possibilities." Such perceptions reiterate the importance of ongoing trials because they replace anecdotal reports with more rigorously obtained data. Despite 60 years of use, only within the past 12 years have well-designed trials begun with the newer generation of standardized, highly purified products injected according to strict protocol. These studies have so far demonstrated a profile of safety and efficacy in the short-term. However, late-appearing granulomatous reactions manifesting as nodules or firmness around the implant many years after treatment are not uncommon (Jones, 2019). Collection of ongoing objective data and longer-term follow-up are necessary to provide clarity into the true risks and benefits of soft tissue augmentation with modern HPLIS.

INDICATIONS AND PATIENT SELECTION

Although there are currently no FDA-approved cosmetic indications for HPLIS, it may be legally injected off-label for the augmentation of human immunodeficiency virus (HIV)-associated facial lipoatrophy, nasolabial folds, labiomental folds, midmalar depressions, lip atrophy, hemifacial atrophy, acne scarring, other atrophic scarring, age-related atrophy of the hands, corns and calluses of the feet, and healed diabetic neuropathic foot ulcers (see the studies by Orentreich and Jones, Balkin, and Fulton et al.) (Figs. 14.1–14.4). HPLIS is specifically contraindicated for injection into the breast, eyelids, or bound-down scars or injection into an actively inflamed site. Its safety has not been studied in pregnant or breast-feeding women. It should not be injected into patients with chronic bacterial sinusitis, dental caries, or other active bacterial infection or in those who may be predisposed to trauma in the treated area. In addition, HPLIS is not a substitute for surgical lifting, chemical or laser resurfacing, dermabrasion, or treatment of dynamic rhytides with botulinum toxin. The ideal patient is one with appropriate insight into the permanent and off-label nature of LIS, a realistic attitude regarding achievable results, in good physical health, and compliant with recommendations. Patients seeking immediate correction or temporary augmentation should be treated with temporary fillers. Serious consideration by both the patient and the physician must be given to the longevity of results obtained with HPLIS and the real possibility of late-appearing granulomatous reactions appearing years posttreatment as lumps and firmness around the implant. Although permanent fillers may be preferred to temporary fillers owing to their longevity, one must consider the possibility that personal and societal aesthetic

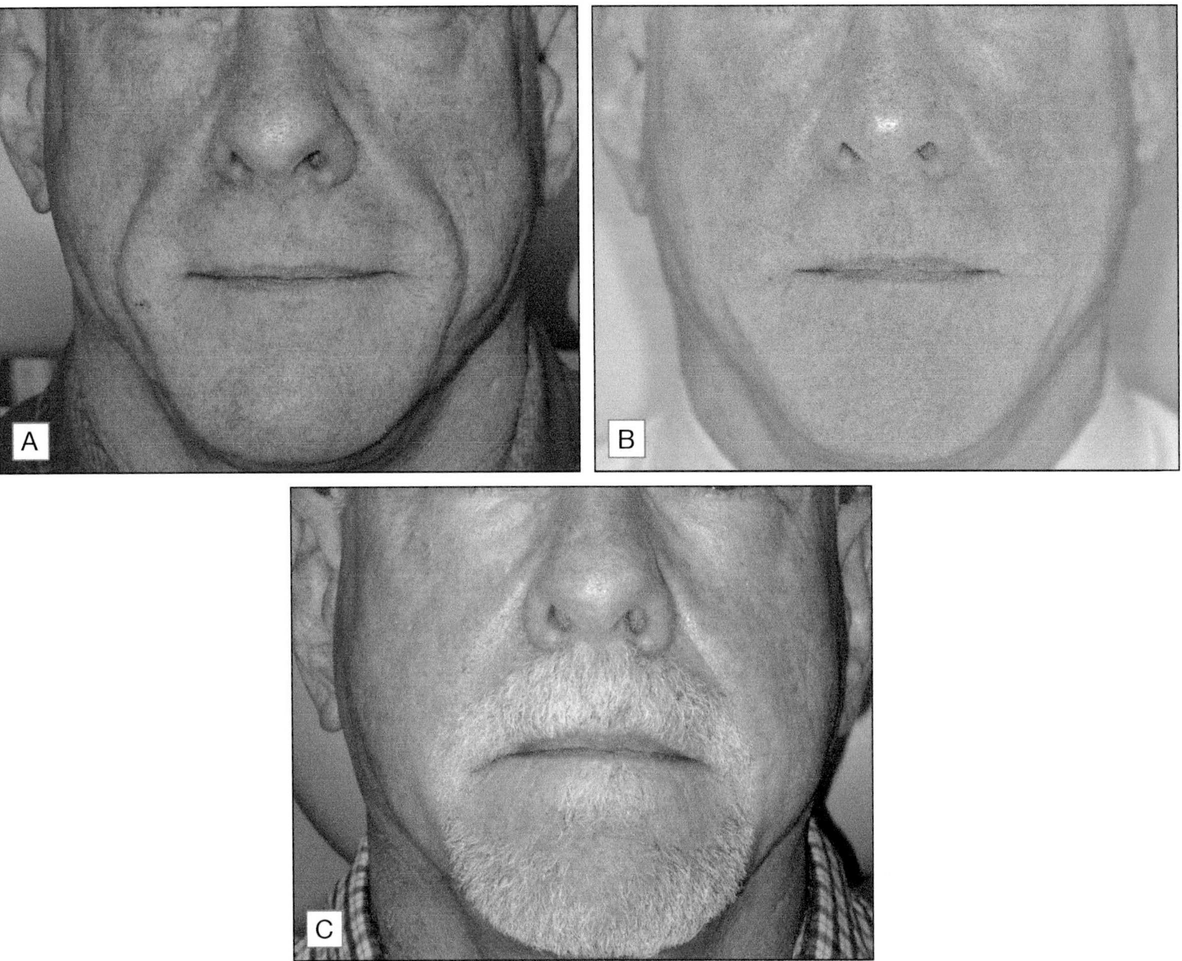

Fig. 14.1 (A) Human immunodeficiency virus (HIV) facial lipoatrophy. (B) After correction with a series of monthly injections with Silikon-1000. (C) Ten-year follow-up.

goals may change over time. Furthermore, an undesirable result will be unlikely to diminish with time and may be difficult to correct.

The previously mentioned indications for HPLIS are also well served by modern, temporary fillers, such as hyaluronic acid, calcium hydroxylapatite, and poly-L-lactic acid. However, over a decade ago, HIV-related facial lipoatrophy (HIV FLA) was an epidemic and HPLIS was, in the authors' view, the most cost-effective option. Those affected were often stigmatized, leading to psychologic distress, social and career impediments, and impaired compliance with HIV medications. Temporary treatment options were limited by excessive cost and necessity of frequent treatments, in a condition for which large volumes and a durable correction are required. The newer longer-lasting volumizing hyaluronic acid fillers may provide an alternative to LIS for HIV FLA with a substantial safety profile, demonstrated in a proof of concept by Hausauer and Jones in 2018.

An open-label pilot trial by Jones et al. published in 2004 evaluated the safety and efficacy of highly purified 1000 cs silicone oil injected by microdroplet technique for the treatment of HIV FLA. Data on 77 patients with a complete correction were analyzed, and it was determined that the volume of silicone, number of treatments, and time required to reach optimal correction were directly related to initial severity of lipoatrophy ($P < .0001$). Supple, even facial contours were routinely restored, with all patients tolerating treatments well. Approximately 3-monthly treatments using 2 mL of

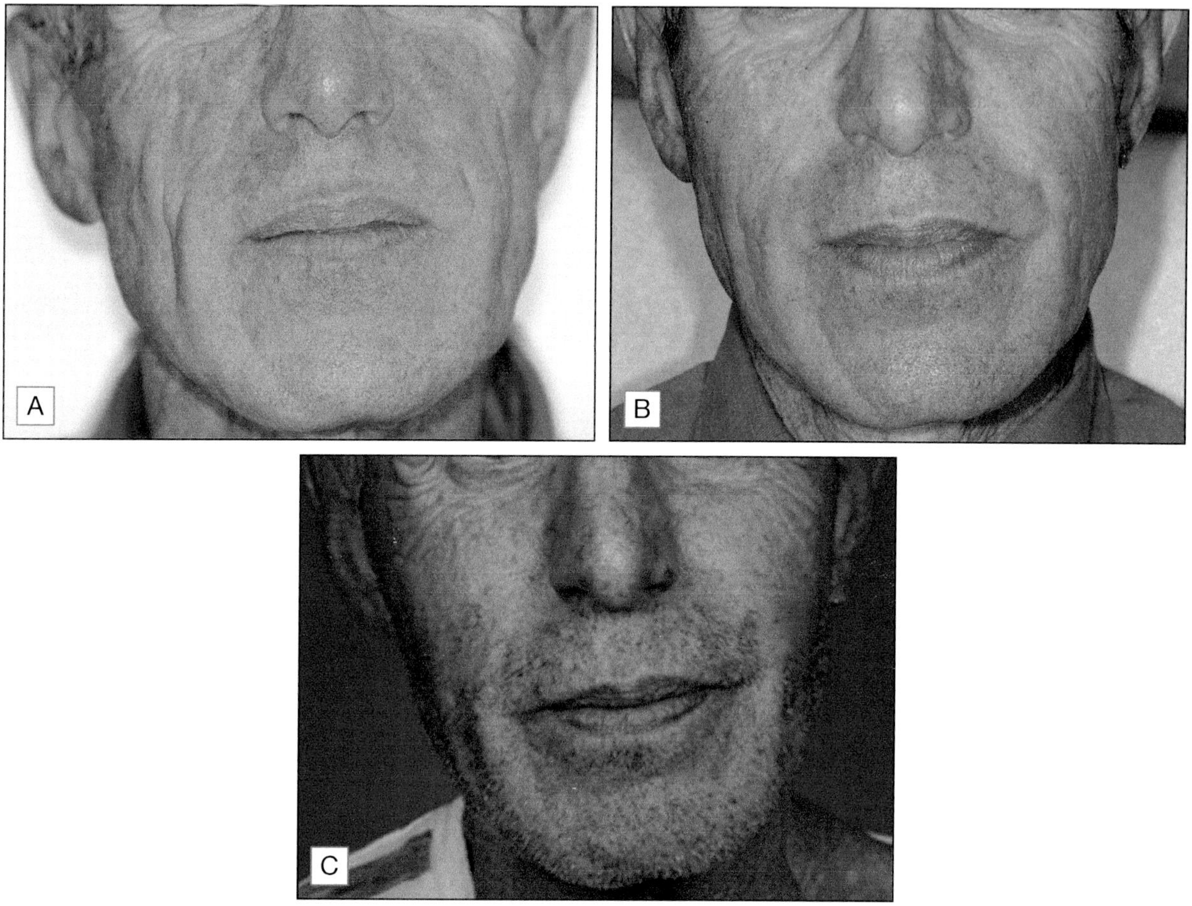

Fig. 14.2 (A) Human immunodeficiency virus (HIV) facial lipoatrophy after Gore-tex thread implants. Note the uneven facial contour. (B) After a series of monthly injections with Silikon-1000 to restore volume and even contour. (C) Ten-year follow-up.

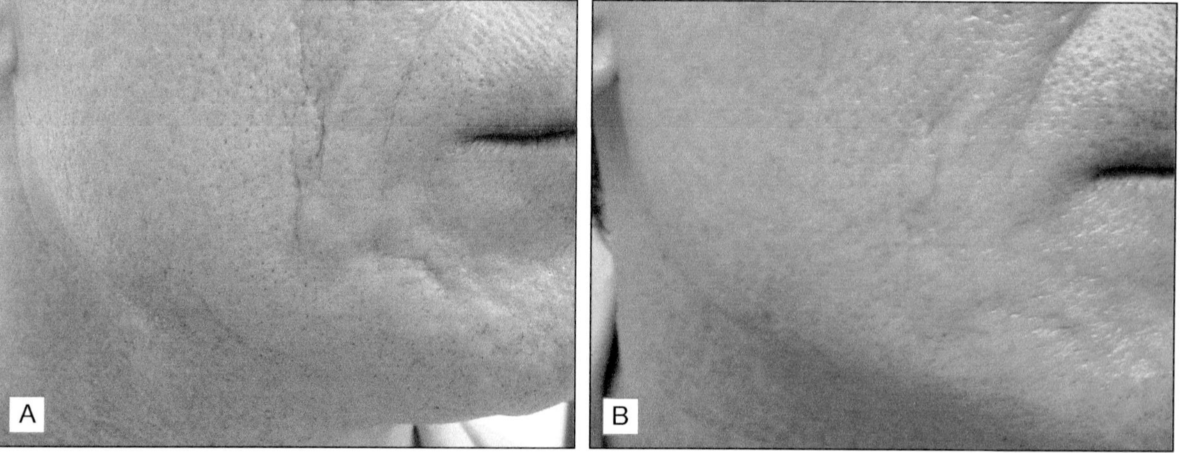

Fig. 14.3 (A) Acne scarring. (B) After a series of injections with Silikon-1000.

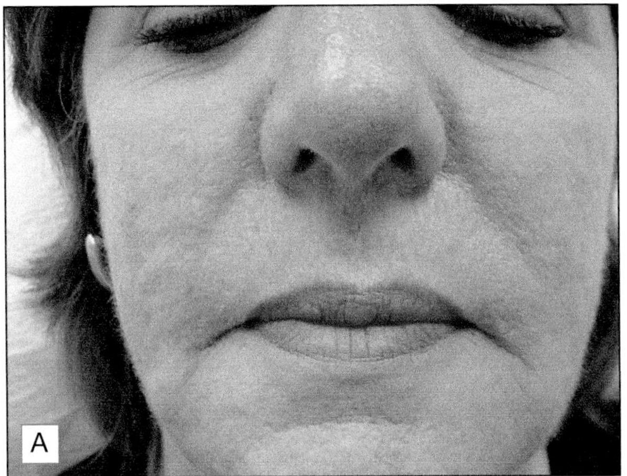

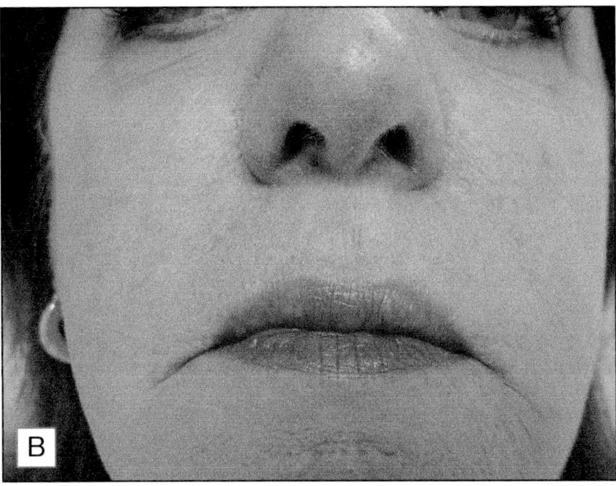

Fig. 14.4 (A) Acne scarring before treatment. (B) Improved appearance of acne scarring after a series of injections with Silikon-1000.

HPLIS were required for each stage of severity on the James/Carruthers lipoatrophy severity rating scale. No initial adverse events were noted. In this pilot trial, it was demonstrated that highly purified 1000 cs silicone oil is a safe and effective treatment option for HIV FLA.

Jones reported in 2010 on safety outcomes in 135 patients with 5-year and beyond follow-up after treatment with HPLIS for HIV FLA. At 5-year follow-up, 4 of the 135 patients experienced a palpable subcutaneous nodule or firmness at the injection site. All events responded completely to intralesional triamcinolone and oral minocycline, and none were considered serious. In 2016, Black and Jones presented a report on the safety outcomes in 113 patients with 10-year and beyond follow-up after treatment with HPLIS for HIV FLA. In 2019, an update was presented including the 2016 data in addition to the experience of two other practices, with a total of 164 patients with 10-year and beyond follow-up. Of the 164 patients, 10 experienced mild and treatable adverse events resulting from excessive fibroplasia manifesting as mild subcutaneous firmness or overcorrection. Two cases of severe adverse events were noted, manifesting as acute facial edema without warmth or tenderness. The specific histories of each patient support a bacterial and/or immunologic basis for such reactions. All adverse events were treatable. Jones currently prefers to treat these adverse events of late-appearing lumps and firmness, representing granulomatous reactions, with intralesional subcutaneous injections of injectable liquid 50 mg/mL 5-fluorouracil (5-FU), admixed with 40 mg/mL triamcinolone. Usually 0.1 mL of 40 mg/mL triamcinolone is added to 1 mL of 50 mg/mL 5-FU. This is injected monthly into the deep subcutis where the lump resides, until satisfactory improvement is achieved. Intradermal injection should be avoided to prevent dermal and epidermal injury or atrophy.

Using the microdroplet, multiple-injection technique, Barnett and Barnett have had success with injections of LIS for acne scars lasting over a 10-, 15-, and 30-year follow-up period (as reported by Jones in 2010). A phone follow-up in 2021 reveals no persistent lumps in the Barnett series. One of the authors (HJB) has duplicated their technique and success in a retrospective examination of 103 patients using the microdroplet techniques for depressed scars over 11 years with similar success, especially in difficult-to-treat-by-resurfacing patients of color. No persistent lumps have been seen. Temporary swelling of the scars after microneedling in one patient months after silicone treatment has been noted but resolved within a week and may have been due to the microneedling. This has not been noted in the Barnett series despite many of their cases that have been microneedled after LIS. The use of much smaller quantities of LIS with strict microdroplet technique for the treatment of acne scarring seems to produce much less occurrence of delayed lumps and reactions.

MATERIALS

The most appropriate HPLIS for off-label soft tissue augmentation is Silikon-1000 (Alcon, Fort Worth, TX) (Fig. 14.5); 5000 cs Adatosil (Bausch & Lomb, Rochester,

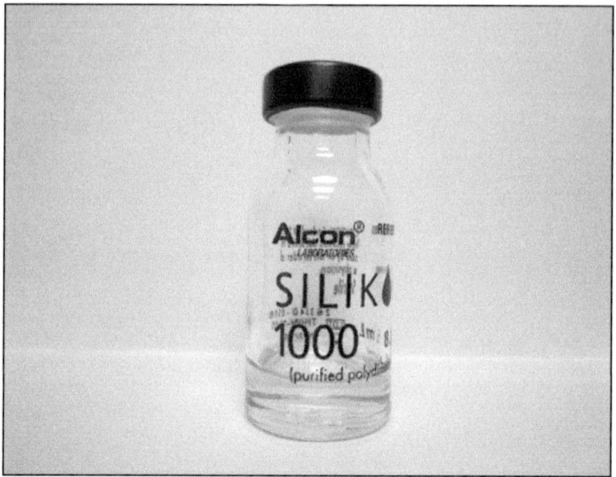

Fig. 14.5 Silikon-1000, which is specifically US Food and Drug Administration approved for ophthalmic use but may be legally used off-label for skin augmentation.

NY) may also be used off-label but is too viscous to inject through small-gauge needles. Using a 16-gauge Nokor needle, 0.5 mL of LIS is drawn into a 1-mL Becton Dickinson (BD) Luer-Lock syringe (Fig. 14.6), using sterile technique. As molecules from the rubber stopper of the syringe could theoretically contaminate the HPLIS after a long exposure period, it should be drawn into the injecting syringe immediately prior to treatment and should never be stored in the syringe. HPLIS is most easily injected through a 27-gauge 0.5-inch (6 mm) Kendall Monoject aluminum-hubbed needle. Plastic-hubbed needles tend to pop off with the higher injection pressures needed for injection through smaller-gauge needles. To increase injector comfort, 0.5-inch inner diameter rubber electrical bushings purchased from a hardware store may be autoclaved and placed over the barrel of the syringe to cushion the physician's second and third fingers during injection.

> **PEARL 1** Of the two FDA-approved liquid silicones, Adatosil-5000 and Silikon-1000, Silikon-1000 is more suitable for injection through small-gauge needles, and hence for skin augmentation, due to its lower viscosity.

> **PEARL 2** An autoclaved 0.5-inch internal diameter rubber electrical bushing purchased from a local hardware store may be placed over the barrel of the syringe to cushion the physician's second and third fingers during injection.

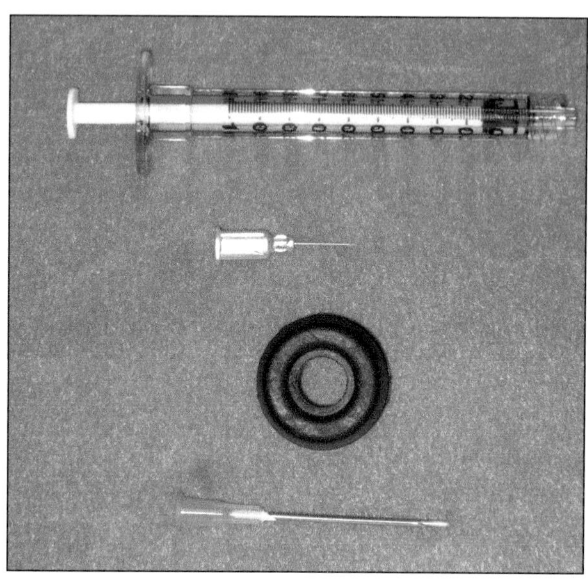

Fig. 14.6 Instrumentation. From top to bottom, 1-mL Becton Dickinson syringe, 27-gauge ½-inch needle, autoclaved electrical bushing, 16-gauge needle.

PATIENT PREPARATION

As with all fillers, patients should avoid blood thinners, such as aspirin, nonsteroidal anti-inflammatory preparations, and anticoagulants for 7 to 10 days prior to injection. It is mandatory to discuss with the patient the risks, benefits, and alternative treatments to HPLIS and document this prior to injection. Patients must understand that HPLIS is a permanent filler and is being used off-label and that late-appearing lumps and firmness may appear years after. Written informed consent must be obtained.

Furthermore, high-quality pretreatment photographs should be taken. Makeup is removed, and the skin is washed with an antibacterial cleanser and prepared with a povidone–iodine antiseptic or other surgical preparatory solution. Areas to be injected are outlined under good lighting, with the patient in a sitting position, using a fine-tip marking pen. Target areas for volume restoration should be marked in both the smiling and resting positions, as these often change remarkably with facial activity. When treating HIV facial lipoatrophy, midmalar depressions often become slightly elevated on smiling, and overcorrection of this area may result in a "chipmunk" appearance.

PEARL 3 High-quality, three-view two-dimensional or three-dimensional pretreatment photographs are mandatory and serve to document preexisting baseline defects and features.

PEARL 4 Areas to be treated should be carefully marked pretreatment using a fine-tipped marking pen.

PEARL 5 When treating HIV facial lipoatrophy, midmalar depressions may become elevated upon smiling. Overcorrection of this area may cause a "chipmunk" appearance when the patient smiles.

PEARL 6 A topical anesthetic, such as lidocaine or other topical amide mixture, is placed on the treatment area and wiped off after 30 minutes prior to injection with clean gauze.

INJECTION TECHNIQUE

Although temporary fillers may be injected with varied techniques, HPLIS should be injected only by the microdroplet technique originally described in 2000 by Orentreich. Other injection techniques risk undesirable consequences, including pooling or beading of silicone macrodroplets in the injection tract and possible migration via escape from the anchoring fibroplastic capsules. A microdroplet is defined as 0.005 to 0.01 mL of product, an amount that possesses a very large surface area-to-volume ratio. A larger surface area-to-volume ratio effectively allows the microdroplet to be anchored into place by the ensuing fibroplasia around the periphery. With larger macrodroplets, defined as greater than 0.01 mL, encapsulation may not be sufficient to prevent product migration. A given volume of HPLIS dispersed into many microdroplets provides for a greater total surface area than would be provided by fewer, larger droplets. Maximizing the total surface area of injected product effectively maximizes the degree of augmentation.

Injections are made into the immediate subdermal plane or deeper (Video 14.1). Often, as the needle enters the subdermal plane, there is a slight give in the tissue resistance to the needle. Intradermal injection should be diligently avoided, as it may result in dermal erythema and ridging. Attention should be given to make sure that the needle is in the subdermal plane prior to depressing the plunger. Furthermore, the injector's thumb should be removed from the plunger prior to removing the needle. Injections should be placed at 2- to 5-mm intervals along the skin surface at the optimal angle for penetration and deposition into the subdermal plane. The optimal angle varies with the intended depth of LIS placement. For areas where deeper placement is desired, a more oblique (approaching perpendicular to the skin surface) angle of insertion is best, whereas a more acute (approaching parallel to the skin surface) angle of insertion works best for more superficial deposition.

As a rule, multiple passes over the same treatment area in a single session should be avoided, although experienced injectors may sometimes make a second pass at a different subcutaneous level and use a tunneling technique to inject microdroplets in different subdermal areas. Importantly, greater correction should be accomplished over a longer period of time rather than with a larger per-session volume. Per-session treatment volumes should be limited to 0.5 mL for smaller surface areas, such as the nasolabial fold, and no more than 2.0 mL for larger surface areas, such as facial lipoatrophy. Such per-session volumes allow approximately 100 to 200 individual microdroplet deposits at 2- to 5-mm intervals, allowing a large treatment area to be covered in a single session if necessary.

Injection sessions should be spaced at least 1 month or more apart to allow for a limited fibrous tissue reaction to occur around each silicone microdroplet. Overcorrection should be avoided. As optimal correction approaches, treatment intervals should be extended to allow complete deposition of fibrous tissue prior to the next injection.

SIDE EFFECTS AND MANAGING COMPLICATIONS

The immediate injection-related side effects commonly seen with all fillers also occur with HPLIS. Needle-associated pain is usually well controlled with pretreatment topical lidocaine anesthetics. Pretreatment with oral analgesics (e.g., 0.5 mg alprazolam and two tablets of hydrocodone/acetaminophen 5/300 mg) 1 hour prior to treatment may occasionally be necessary in the pain-intolerant patient. Mild postinjection edema and erythema are common and resolve within a few days.

The transient edema may even be representative of what optimal correction may look like after several treatments. Purpura, when it rarely occurs, usually resolves within a few days and may be treated with a pulsed dye laser to hasten resolution.

When injected with the appropriate technique, LIS is remarkably similar in texture and sensation to natural soft tissue. However, when larger cumulative volumes are injected, as in HIV FLA, the treated area may occasionally feel slightly rubbery and firmer than natural soft tissue. Migration of injected liquid silicone is an often-mentioned and undesired adverse event. Using small volumes over multiple treatment sessions with the microdroplet technique avoids this problem because microdroplets of silicone are anchored to the surrounding soft tissue by fibroplasia. However, LIS may track along tissue planes in the path of least resistance when injected in large boluses all at once.

Skin dyschromia is a rare side effect of LIS, occurring most often when too much liquid silicone is inadvertently injected into the dermis. When the inflammatory response to LIS extends into the dermis, then postinflammatory erythema, postinflammatory hyperpigmentation, and telangiectasia may occur. Dermal ridging often occurs in conjunction with the dyschromia. Erythema and telangiectasia may be treated with a pulsed dye laser or intense pulsed light device. Hyperpigmentation may be treated with hydroquinone and sun protection. Dermal ridging may improve with intralesional steroid injection, but the response is often incomplete and the problem persistent.

A more concerning potential adverse event to LIS is granulomatous reactions presenting as a palpable subcutaneous nodule or firmness, often rocky hard, presenting many years or even decades after treatment Such reactions were described in 2009 by Jones with liquid silicone, as well as a variety of other permanent or longer-lasting fillers, such as polymethylmethacrylate and polylactic acid. They are thought to be immune mediated, and most often granulomatous. It has been postulated that granulomatous reactions may be a result of infection at a distant site because granulomatous reactions to liquid silicone have been noted to appear with the development of acute bacterial dental abscesses or sinusitis and to resolve upon treatment of the infection. Another theory, proposed by Christensen, is that bacterial biofilm formation around the LIS microdroplet may create a low-grade, chronic infection resulting in an inflammatory host response. Biofilms may occur if bacterial organisms are introduced upon filler injection, or seed the filler later during bacteremic episodes. Once present, they may remain dormant for months or years on foreign body surfaces, such as injected liquid silicone. Biofilms may serve as a target of a delayed immune response by the patient when organisms convert back to a planktonic state, explaining the potential for granuloma formation years after injection. Should granulomatous reactions develop, they may be treated with high concentrations of intralesional triamcinolone (20 to 40 mg/mL) at 2- to 4-week intervals. It should be noted that HIV infection or ritonavir (Norvir) might predispose individuals to adrenal suppression with higher doses of cortisone. In these cases, the addition of injectable 5-FU, providing known antifibrotic (antimitotic) and antimicrobial effects described by Beer and Avelar, may be beneficial. Based on the biofilm hypothesis, institution of a full-dose, broad-spectrum antibiotic, such as minocycline, once or twice daily should also occur. Isotretinoin and etanercept have also been used successfully to treat LIS granulomas, in studies by Desai et al., Lloret et al., and Pasternack et al. However, granulomas that fail to resolve may ultimately require surgical removal. Given the presence of such possible undesirable episodes, it is advised that HPLIS be used in circumstances and disease states in which the benefits outweigh the risk of adverse events.

> **PEARL 7** HIV infection or ritonavir (Norvir) may predispose individuals to develop adrenal suppression when higher doses of cortisone are used. In cases where higher doses may be needed to treat rare granulomatous reactions, injectable 5-FU may be useful.

CONCLUSION

The longevity of HPLIS and the relatively low cost provided a benefit that has given satisfaction to both the physicians and patients. HPLIS is a safe, effective filler when appropriately used by experienced injectors using the microdroplet technique. Currently, its greatest application is for the permanent correction of HIV FLA, although it is effective for the correction of a variety of facial atrophies, acne scarring, and deformities. Injectable liquid silicone has generated controversy in decades past. However, modern, highly purified silicone oils studied in controlled clinical settings have so far been demonstrated to be safe agents that warrant distinction. Physicians must be able to identify and treat complications, both mild and severe, that may be more difficult to treat, owing to the permanent nature of the product. For this reason, physicians must use proper injection method and inject only in appropriate patients who have had full disclosure as to the off-label nature of its use and adequate informed consent. Continued studies are ongoing to further examine both long-term safety and efficacy.

POSTSCRIPT At the time of this writing, oral angiotensin-converting enzyme inhibitors for the treatment of delayed inflammatory reactions to dermal hyaluronic acid fillers following COVID-19 vaccination as a model for inhibition of angiotensin II-induced cutaneous inflammation have been successfully reported. It is possible that lisinopril may be a viable treatment for delayed silicone reactions as well and may warrant further study (Munavalli et al., 2021).

FURTHER READING

Balkin, S. W. (2005). Injectable silicone and the foot: a 41-year clinical and histologic history. *Dermatol Surg., 31*(11 pt 2), 1555–1559.

Barnett, J. G., & Barnett, C. R. (2005). Treatment of acne scars with liquid silicone injections: 30-year perspective. *Dermatol Surg., 31*(11 pt 2), 1542–1549.

Baselga, E., & Pujol, R. (1994). Indurated plaques and persistent ulcers in an HIV-1 seropositive man. *Arch Dermatol., 130*(6), 785–789.

Beer, K., & Avelar, R. (2014). Relationship between delayed reactions to dermal fillers and biofilm: facts and considerations. *Dermatol Surg, 11*, 1175–1179.

Benedetto, A. V., & Lewis, A. T. (2003). Injecting 1000 centistoke liquid silicone with ease and precision. *Dermatol Surg., 29*(3), 211–214.

Black, J. M., & Jones, D. H. (2016). A report of 113 patients with 10-year and beyond follow up after treatment with highly purified liquid injectable silicone for HIV associated facial lipoatrophy. In *Poster abstract. American Society for Dermatologic Surgery Annual Meeting*. New Orleans, LA.

Chen, F., Carruthers, A., Humphrey, S., & Carruthers, J. (2013). HIV-associated lipoatrophy treated with injectable silicone oil: a pilot study. *Dermatol Surg., 69*(3), 431–437.

Christensen, L. (2007). Normal and pathologic tissue reactions to soft tissue gel fillers. *Dermatol Surg., 33*, s168–s175.

Delage, C., Shane, J. J., & Johnson, F. B. (1973). Mammary silicone granuloma: migration of silicone fluid to abdominal wall and inguinal region. *Arch Dermatol., 108*(1), 105–107.

Desai, A. M., Browning, J., & Rosen, T. (2006). Etanercept therapy for silicone granuloma. *J Drugs Dermatol., 5*(9), 894–896.

Diamond, B., Hulka, B., Kerkvliet, N., et al. (1998). *Summary of report of National Science Panel: silicone breast implants in relation to connective tissue diseases and immunologic dysfunction.* http://www.fjc.gov/BREIMLIT/SCIENCE/summary.htm. (Accessed 31 January 2009).

Duffy, D. M. (1998). Tissue injectable liquid silicone: new perspectives. In A. W. Klein (Ed.), *Augmentation in Clinical Practice: Procedures and Techniques* (pp. 237–263). New York: Marcel Dekker.

Duffy, D. M. (2002). The silicone conundrum: a battle of anecdotes. *Dermatol Surg., 28*, 590.

Duffy, D. M. (2005). Liquid silicone for soft tissue augmentation. *Dermatol Surg., 31*(11 pt 2), 1530–1541.

Duffy, D. M. (2006). Liquid silicone for soft tissue augmentation: histological, clinical, and molecular perspectives. In A. Klein (Ed.), *Tissue Augmentation in Clinical Practice* (2nd ed., pp. 141–237). New York: Taylor & Francis.

Fulton, J. E., Jr., Porumb, S., Caruso, J. C., et al. (2005). Lip augmentation with liquid silicone. *Dermatol Surg., 31*(11 pt 2), 1577–1586.

Hausauer, A. K., & Jones, D. H. (2018). Long-term correction of iatrogenic facial lipoatrophy with volumizing hyaluronic acid filler. *Dermatol Surg.*, S60–S62.

Hevia, O. (2009). Six-year experience using 1,000-centistoke silicone oil in 916 patients for soft-tissue augmentation in a private practice setting. *Dermatol Surg., 35*, 1646–1652.

Jones, D. (2005). HIV facial lipoatrophy: causes and treatment options. *Dermatol Surg., 31*(11 pt 2), 1519–1529.

Jones, D. (2009). Semi-permanent and permanent injectable fillers. *Dermatol Clin., 27*(4), 433–444.

Jones, D. (2010). A report of 135 patients with 5 year and beyond follow up after treatment with highly purified liquid injectable silicone (LIS) for HIV associated facial lipoatrophy (HIV FLA). In *American Society for Dermatologic Surgery Annual Meeting*. Chicago, IL.

Jones, D. H. (2014). Treatment of delayed reactions to dermal fillers. *Dermatol Surg., 40*(11), 1180.

Jones, D. H. (2002). Injectable silicone for facial lipoatrophy. *Cosmet Dermatol., 15*, 13–15.

Jones, D. H., Carruthers, A., Brody, H. J., et al. (2019). Ten-year and beyond follow-up after treatment with highly purified liquid-injectable silicone for HIV-associated facial lipoatrophy: a report of 164 patients. *Dermatol Surg., 45*, 941–948.

Jones, D. H., Carruthers, A., Orentreich, D., et al. (2004). Highly purified 1000-cSt silicone oil for treatment of human immunodeficiency virus-associated facial lipoatrophy: an open pilot trial. *Dermatol Surg., 30*, 1279–1286.

Lloret, P., Espana, A., Leache, A., et al. (2005). Successful treatment of granulomatous reactions secondary to injection of esthetic implants. *Dermatol Surg.*, *31*(4), 486–490.

Munavalli, G. G., Knutsen-Larson, S., Lupo, M. P., & Geronemus, R. G. (2021). Oral angiotensin converting enzyme inhibitors for the treatment of delayed inflammatory reaction of dermal hyaluronic acid fillers following COVID-19 vaccination—a model for inhibition of angiotensin II- induced cutaneous inflammation. *JAAD Case Rep*, *10*, 63–68.

Orentreich, D. S. (2000). Liquid injectable silicone: techniques for soft tissue augmentation. *Clin Plast Surg.*, *27*, 595–612.

Orentreich, D., & Leone, A. S. (2004). A case of HIV-associated facial lipoatrophy treated with 1000-cs liquid injectable silicone. *Dermatol Surg.*, *30*, 548–551.

Orentreich, D. S., & Jones, D. H. (2006). Liquid injectable silicone. In J. Carruthers, & A. Carruthers (Eds.), *Soft Tissue Augmentation* (pp. 77–91). New York: Elsevier.

Parel, J. M. (1989). Silicone oils: physiochemical properties. In B. M. Glaser, & R. G. Michels (Eds.), *3. Retina* (pp. 261–277). St Louis: Mosby.

Pasternack, F. R., Fox, L. P., & Engler, D. E. (2005). Silicone granulomas treated with etanercept. *Arch Dermatol.*, *141*(1), 13–15.

Price, E. A., Schueler, H., & Perper, J. A. (2006). Massive systemic silicone embolism: a case report and review of literature. *Am J Forensic Med Pathol.*, *27*(2), 97–102.

Rapaport, M. J., Vinnik, C., & Zarem, H. (1996). Injectable silicone: cause of facial nodules, cellulitis, ulceration, and migration. *Aesthetic Plast Surg.*, *20*, 267–276.

Rapaport, M. R. (2002). Silicone injections revisited. *Dermatol Surg.*, *28*, 594–595.

Selmanowitz, V. J., & Orentreich, N. (1977). Medical grade fluid silicone: a monographic review. *J Dermatol Surg Oncol.*, *3*, 597–611.

Spanoudis, S., & Koski, G. (2009). *Sci polymers*. http://www.plasnet.com.au/index.php?option=com_content&view=article&id=89:polymer-faq&catid=118:FAQ&Itemid=258. (Accessed 31 January 2009).

Turekian, K. K., & Wedepohl, K. H. (1961). Distribution of the elements in some major units of the earth's crust. *Bull Geol Soc Am.*, *72*(2), 175–192.

Wallace, W. D., Balkin, S. W., Kaplan, L., et al. (2004). The histological host response of liquid silicone injections for prevention of pressure-related ulcers of the foot: a 38-year study. *J Am Podiatr Med Assoc.*, *94*, 550–557.

15

Bellafill

Heidi B. Prather, Kachiu C. Lee, Neil S. Sadick, and Annie Chiu

SUMMARY AND KEY FEATURES

- Bellafill is currently the only US Food and Drug Administration (FDA)-approved long-term filler indicated for the correction of the nasolabial folds and atrophic acne scars.
- Bellafill is composed of smooth, round, and uniform microspheres (30–50 μm in diameter) of nonresorbable polymethylmethacrylate (PMMA).
- The PMMA microspheres of Bellafill are suspended in a water-based bovine collagen gel with lidocaine
- Bovine collagen is enzymatically cleaved at the ends to reduce immunogenicity.
- Type I and type III collagen production from PMMA microsphere stimulation results in a durable outcome, studied for up to 5 years with a favorable safety profile.
- Mindful patient selection, paired with skillful injection technique, makes Bellafill a desirable tool for optimizing long-term aesthetic outcomes.

INTRODUCTION

Soft tissue fillers have become one of the most popular minimally invasive aesthetic procedures in the past several decades. Most available fillers are reabsorbed in entirety to promote safety at the expense of durability. Polymethylmethacrylate (PMMA) microspheres in a water-based collagen gel suspension, currently branded as Bellafill, is the only US Food and Drug Administration (FDA)-approved long-term filler for correction of nasolabial folds and atrophic acne scars. Prior to its use in aesthetics, PMMA has long been used in medicine, particularly in the fields of orthopedics and dentistry. Early formulations of PMMA had an unfavorable safety profile due to its allergic reactivity. PMMA formulations have since undergone considerable development and refinements to meet current clinical and safety standards (Fig. 15.1). The first-generation product, called Arteplast (Arteplast, George Lemperle), was developed in the 1980s in Europe. This formulation consisted of small, rough PMMA particles of variable diameters suspended in gelatin, which allowed the microspheres to clump together and led to macrophage infiltration, particle phagocytosis, and subsequent inflammation. The second-generation product also developed in Europe, Artecoll (Artecoll, Rofil Medical), replaced gelatin with bovine collagen, which created a more consistent suspension of microspheres that were more refined but still variable in size with some rough surfaces. The addition of a wet sieving process eliminated some electrostatic charges to help minimize clumping. Bellafill, the third and latest generation of PMMA, previously called Artefill (Artefill, Artes Medical), is the result of 25 years of continuous scientific development to improve the safety and efficacy profile of PMMA. In Bellafill, the microspheres are small, consistent, and smooth. Seven wet sieving filters and an ultrasound bath remove negatively charged particles to eliminate clumping and create a uniform PMMA injectable filler safe for dermal injection.

Generation 1
Introduced in 1989

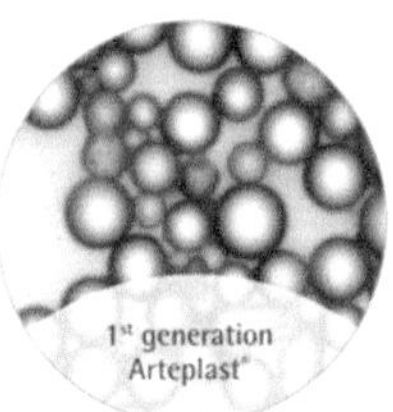

- High-bloom gelatin suspension
- Dry sieving process
- Non-uniform size of microspheres and rough surface
- Small microspheres (0.5–20 microns) may be phagocytosed by skin cells

Generation 2
Introduced in 1994*

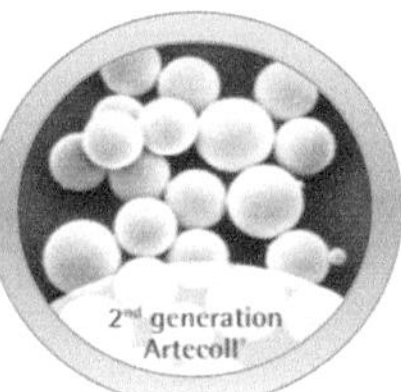

- Bovine collagen suspension
- Single wet sieving process introduced to eliminate negative charges on microspheres to minimize clumping
- More evenly sized microspheres but some less than 20 microns still present

Generation 3
Introduced in 2007

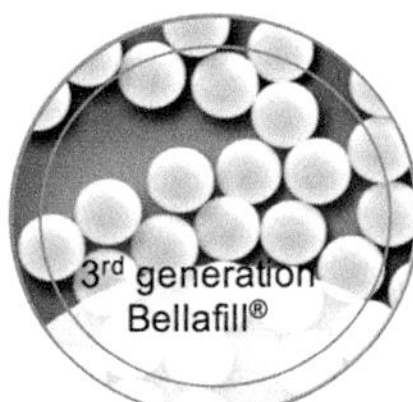

- Bovine collagen from a U.S. closed herd and U.S. manufacturing plant
- Additional wet sieving steps limit microsphere size to 30–50 microns and further reduce clumping
- PMMA particles in this range are not ingested by cells tested, nor do they stimulate TNFα production
- Smoother beads

Fig. 15.1 Overview of three generations of PMMA. *PMMA,* Polymethylmethacrylate; *TNFα*, tumor necrosis factor α.

PRODUCT OVERVIEW AND MECHANISM OF ACTION

Bellafill (previously branded as Artefill) is a nonbiodegradable injectable filler composed of 30 to 50 µm smooth, round PMMA microspheres (20% by volume) suspended in a water-based gel with bovine collagen and lidocaine. Bellafill has both an immediate and delayed mechanism of action (Fig. 15.2). The collagen containing water-based gel that constitutes 80% of the syringe volume provides an immediate lift and volumizing effect and contains 3.5% bovine collagen gel and 0.3% lidocaine. Over time, the collagen gel is reabsorbed, leaving the PMMA microspheres in the remaining 20% of the syringe to act as a matrix to stimulate collagen production. Histologic analysis has shown that within days of injection, monocytes infiltrate the injection sites, differentiate into fibroblasts, and produce a fibrous capsule around the microspheres. Collagen fibers can be detected as early as 3 weeks posttreatment, as dermal remodeling and angiogenesis progress. Over the next weeks to months, collagen fibers will continue to increase in density and volume; and after 4 months, dermal remodeling is complete.

TECHNICAL CONSIDERATIONS

Each Bellafill kit contains 5 × 0.85 mL syringes supplied with 10 × 26 G needles. Bellafill is made with lidocaine for injection comfort. To maximize comfort, topical local anesthetics can be applied to the treatment area prior to the procedure based on office protocols for injection but is not required. Bellafill product shelf life is 12 months and should be kept refrigerated at 3° C to 8° C. To decrease product viscosity and injector fatigue, the product should be allowed to warm to room temperature prior to injection. The product must be discarded if phase separation between the collagen and microspheres occurs.

Although the bovine collagen used in Bellafill is cleaved at the ends to minimize allergic reactions, it is still

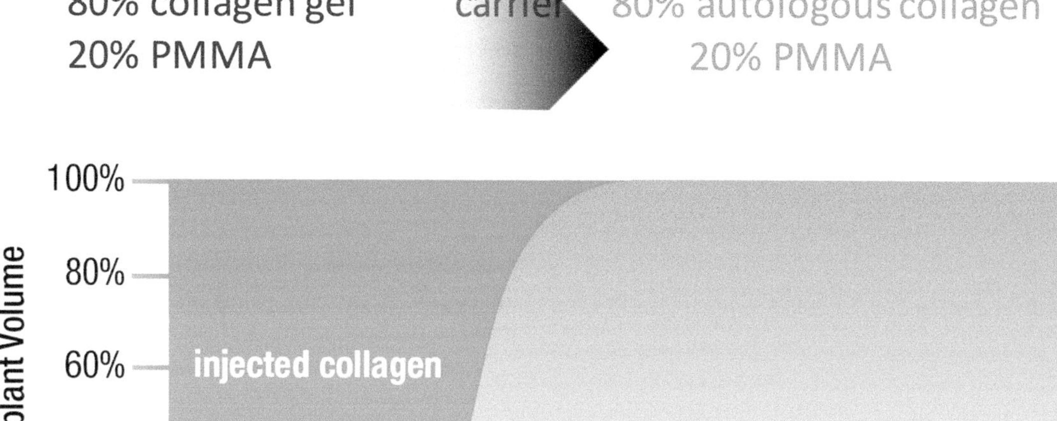

Fig. 15.2 Bellafill mechanism of action. *PMMA,* Polymethylmethacrylate.

recommended to allergy test 4 weeks prior to treatment using the intradermal collagen test kit from Bellafill to minimize any risk of hypersensitivity, especially in the setting of connective tissue disease, history of atopy or allergies and an existing allergy to beef. This recommendation is based on Artecoll data that are manufactured with a complete bovine collagen protein. Currently, correction of acne scars and nasolabial folds are the only FDA-approved clinical indications for Bellafill (Videos 15.1 and 15.2 in the online version at https://doi.org/10.1016/B978-0-323-83075-1.00015-8). Because of the durability and high G', injection into areas of thin skin, such as the lips or periocular "tear troughs," should be avoided.

Acne Scar Injection Technique

Bellafill is indicated for atrophic and distensible rolling acne scars. These scars are identified by their smooth borders and ability to disappear when the skin is stretched. Nondistensible scars indicate that subdermal tethers or adhesions are present and may prevent full correction without subcision, such as boxcar or ice pick scars (Fig. 15.3). Thorough skin preparation is paramount to minimize side effects with long-term fillers. Ideally, patients come in without makeup or sunscreen.

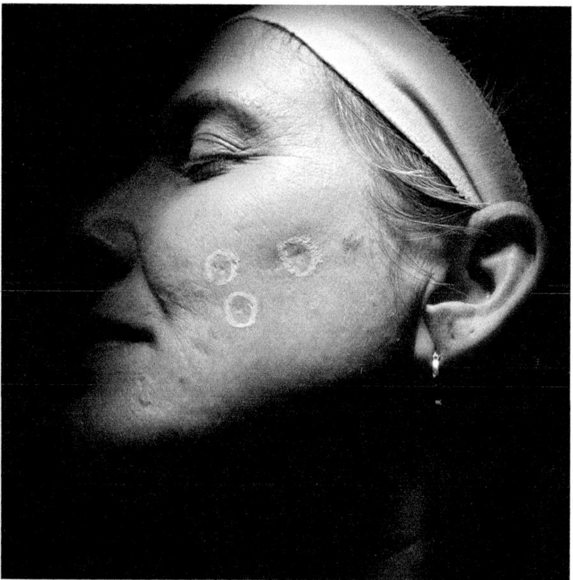

Fig. 15.3 Acne scar types: boxcar, ice pick, and rolling scars are illustrated from left to right.

Cleansing with soap and water should be followed with a 70% isopropyl alcohol wipe to ensure no residue of makeup or sunscreen remains. The authors recommend

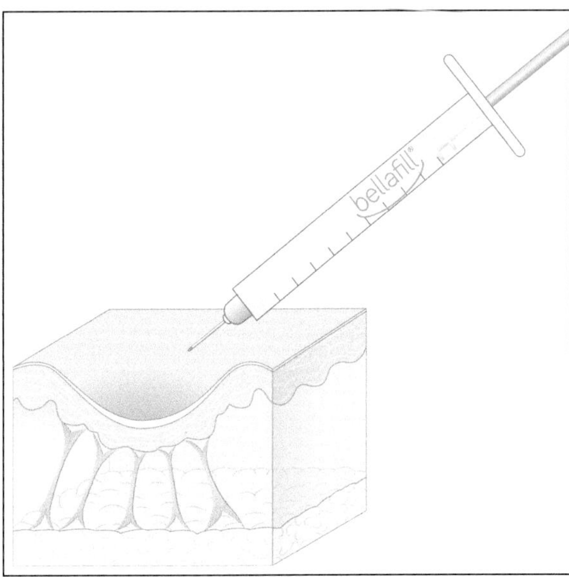

Fig. 15.4 Injection technique for acne scars.

an additional secondary step to further create an antiseptic field with either chlorhexidine or hypochlorous acid (Video 15.3 in the online version at https://doi.org/10.1016/B978-0-323-83075-1.00015-8). Chlorhexadine should be rinsed from the skin after treatment is complete due to skin irritation and care taken to avoid the eyes and ears which may result in keratitis and otitis. Mark appropriate scars and stretch the skin surrounding the scar with your index and thumb fingers to anchor the skin during injection. Insert the needle with the bevel up at a 30- to 40-degree angle relative to the surface of the skin just outside the scar border and advance the needle beneath the scar parallel to the surface in the dermal plane, moving forward and backward, creating a small potential space within the scar by microsubcision. Once released, simultaneously release microdroplets of Bellafill with continuous microsubcision until 100% scar correction is achieved (Fig. 15.4 and Video 15.4 in the online version at https://doi.org/10.1016/B978-0-323-83075-1.00015-8). A variety of injection techniques may be used to fill in the area underneath the scar, such as serial puncture or linear threading. Avoidance of overcorrection is recommended and when performing subsequent treatments, apply Bellafill above the previous filler implant to build a scaffold to support the tissue deficit (Figs. 15.5–15.7).

Nasolabial Fold Injection Technique

Ideal candidates for Bellafill treatment in the nasolabial folds are patients with moderate to severe volume loss without skin laxity. Patients with preserved skin elasticity and thickness are desirable to avoid visible or palpable deposits of Bellafill that may be more common in extremely thin or loose skin. Care should be taken to avoid lateral or superficial placement of Bellafill, which can stay viscous for the first few days after injection and potentially migrate with facial movement. Linear threading can be performed using the 26G needle supplied with the product, starting at the base of the Nasolabial folds and using retrograde deposits into the deep dermis while tenting the skin (Videos 15.5 and 15.6 in the online version at https://doi.org/10.1016/B978-0-323-83075-1.00015-8). Slow and deliberate injection technique is essential to avoid accidental cannulation of the angular artery that courses beneath the Nasolabial fold. Negative aspiration may not accurately represent vascular penetration due to the viscosity of the product (Fig. 15.8).

OFF-LABEL USE OF POLYMETHYLMETHACRYLATE

Given PMMA's 5-year indication in the nasolabial folds, the long-lasting benefits of PMMA has made it a consideration for other areas of off-label use, including the temporal fossa (with injections on bone) resistant to other types of fillers, nonsurgical rhinoplasty, and the dorsal hands. Use of PMMA in the temples can be clinically considered alone or in combination with other fillers in patients with significant volume loss in the temporal fossa. For these patients, often other fillers including PLLA, hyaluronic acid (HA), and calcium hydroxylapatite (CaHA) yield an unsatisfactory duration, especially in patients who are highly athletic. A 12-month retrospective study of PMMA for volume repletion in the dorsal hands reported that 92% of patients still had some degree of improvement at 12 months. The use of PMMA for nonsurgical filler rhinoplasty was shown also to be safe and effective in a small case series as patients often desire these corrections to be long term. The authors always suggest high experience prior to use in this area, as PMMA is not reversible, and intra-arterial embolism can lead to catastrophic blindness and tissue necrosis. When used off-label in high-risk areas, always consider multiple sessions of smaller volumes, injections with cautious force, and injecting only upon

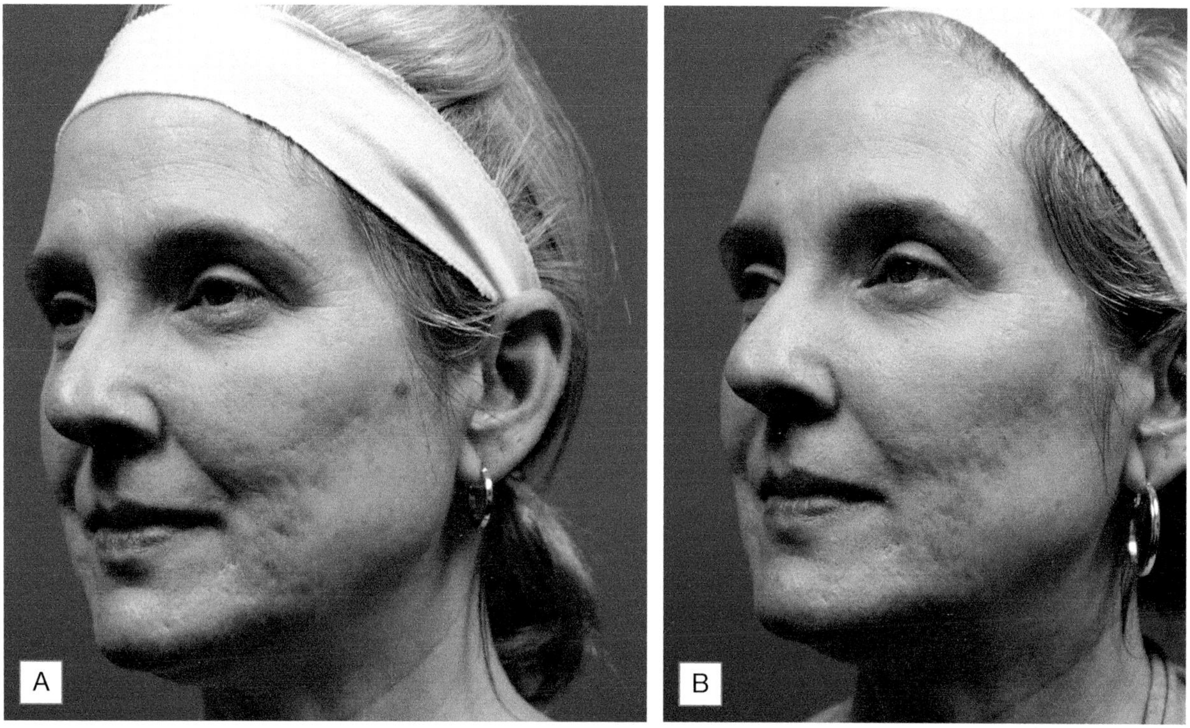

Fig. 15.5 Fifty-year-old patient before (A) and 1 month after (B) treatment with Bellafill 0.8 cc to atrophic rolling disensible scars on the cheeks and 0.8 cc to her nasal labial folds.

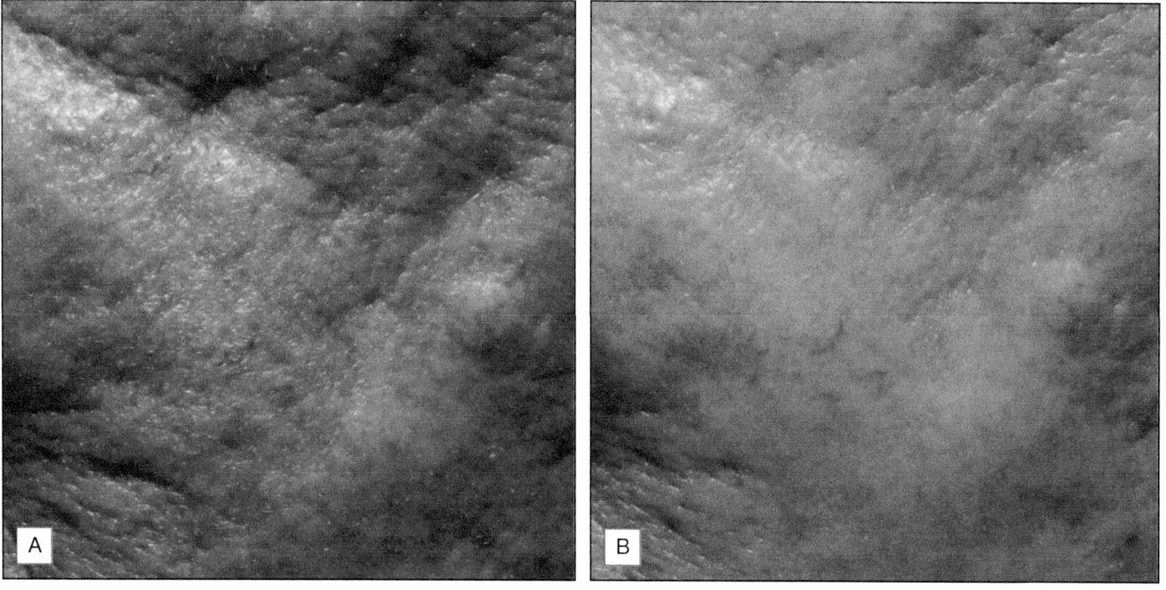

Fig. 15.6 A 35-year-old patient before (A) and 12 months after (B) two treatments of Bellafill for acne.

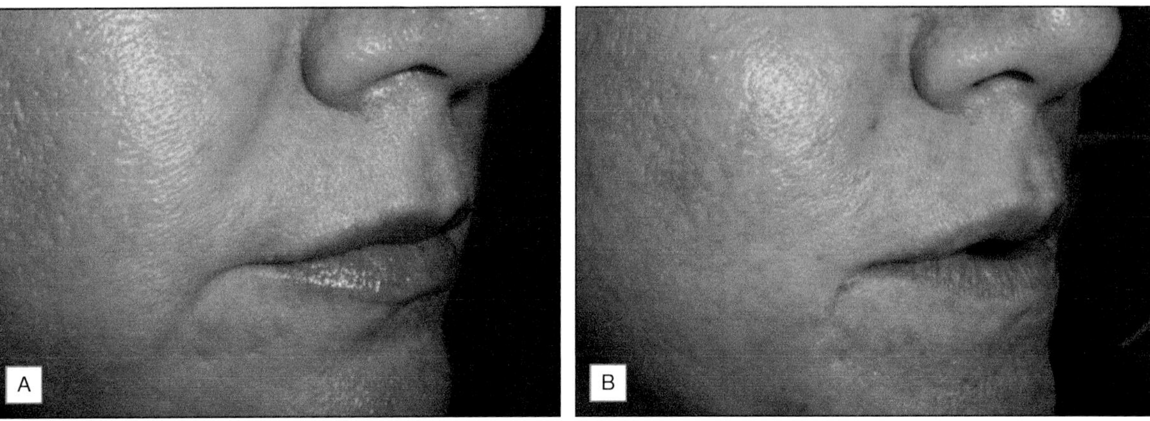

Fig. 15.7 A 50-year-old patient before (A) and after (B) 3 years of four treatments of Bellafill for acne.

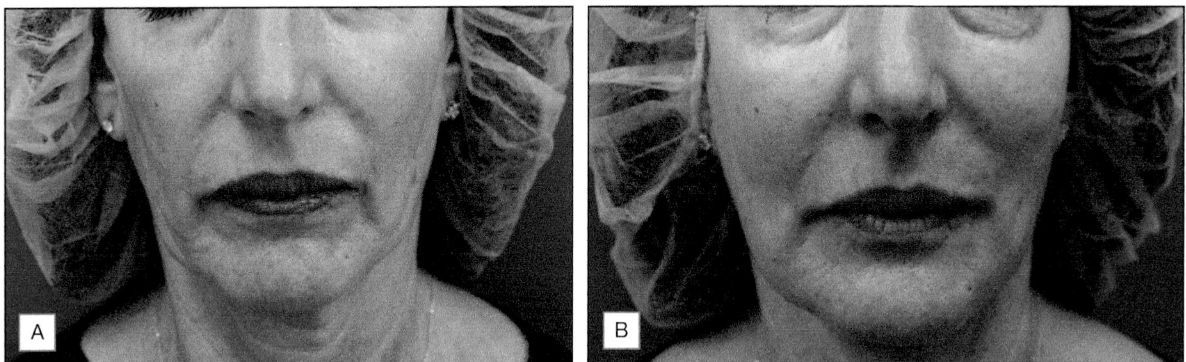

Fig. 15.8 A 65-year-old patient before (A) and 12 months after (B) two treatments of Bellafill for panfacial volumization.

retrograde withdrawal. Lastly, studies show PMMA filler treated areas can undergo combination therapy with laser, light, or ultrasound without any histological changes in the PMMA microspheres (Video 15.7 in the online version at https://doi.org/10.1016/B978-0-323-83075-1.00015-8).

PIVOTAL CLINICAL STUDIES

The efficacy and safety of Bellafill have only been demonstrated in the two pivotal clinical studies conducted for Bellafill FDA approval in the treatment of acne scars and nasolabial folds, respectively. In addition, off-label usage of Bellafill has also been investigated in prospective clinical trials.

The Bellafill US Acne Scar pivotal study was a prospective, randomized, placebo-controlled, double-blinded, multicenter (10 centers) clinical trial of 147 subjects older than 18 years who desired correction of moderate to severe, atrophic, distensible facial acne scarring. The primary effectiveness end point was the success rate at 6 months, based on the blinded evaluating investigator's (EI's) assessment using the validated 4-point Acne Scar Rating Scale (ASRS), with success defined as at least a 2-point improvement on the ASRS for at least 50% of treated scars. The average initial injection volume of Bellafill in randomized subjects was 0.11 mL per scar, and the average initial volume injected per subject was 0.93 mL. Touch-ups were conducted as needed at follow-up visits at weeks 2, 4, 6, and 8 and months 3, 6, 9, and 12. Results from the study showed that the primary effectiveness end point was achieved, with 64.4% responders in the Bellafill group and 32.6% responders in the control group (P = .0005) at 6 months. Subject satisfaction was assessed using the 6-point Subject's Assessment of Scar Correction (SASC) scale. More than 83% of Bellafill subjects judged themselves to be at least somewhat to very satisfied with the appearance of their treated scars at all time points. There were no treatment-related severe adverse effects. Unblinded evaluation out to 12 months confirmed a consistent level of effectiveness. Based on these results, acne scar treatment with Bellafill was shown to occur relatively quickly, was sustained, and was effective in all races, genders, and adults of all ages.

A large-scale 5-year postapproval study of Bellafill was required by the FDA to obtain full approval for the use of Bellafill for nasolabial folds with the aim of documenting the incidence of granuloma formation and satisfaction of long-term treatment. Thus, a prospective, multicenter, open-label postapproval study was conducted at 23 centers across the United States, and 1008 subjects were enrolled. Compliance with follow-up was outstanding, with an 87% completion rate (871/1008) at 5 years. Subjects received treatment with Bellafill in the nasolabial folds, and safety follow-up visits were conducted at 3 months and 60 months. Results of the study demonstrated an overall granuloma incidence rate of 1.7%, the majority of which were mild to moderate in severity. This 5-year study that represents the largest and longest follow-up study of a US-approved dermal filler product to date substantiated the safety and efficacy of Bellafill for use in nasolabial folds.

A 12-month, single-center, prospective study treated 23 subjects with Bellafill for midface volume restoration. Using the Midface Volume Deficit Scale and subject and physician improvement grading scales, investigators noted significant improvement at 12 months. Side effects were limited to swelling, bruising, tenderness, and pain with redness. Bellafill has also been evaluated for volume loss in the dorsal hands. A 12-month, single-center, prospective study evaluated the results of PMMA injections for correction of volume loss of the hands using the Merz 5-point Hand Grading Scale. All patients noted at least a 1-point improvement at 12 months postinjection with minimal adverse events (pinpoint bleeding, mild erythema, swelling). The mean Merz Hand Grading Scale score at baseline was 3.27 and 3.33 for the right and left hands, respectively. At 12 months postinjection, the mean Merz Hand Grading Scale scores were 1.5 for both the left and right hands.

Other notable studies using third-generation PMMA, branded as Artefill, include a single-center, open-label, pilot study of 14 qualified subjects treated for atrophic acne scars. Investigator ratings after 8 months postprocedure indicated that 96% of the atrophic acne scars showed some degree of improvement, with the majority of patients reporting a moderate correction. No adverse events or side effects were noted. In another prospective, multisite, open-label study including 24 patients with age-related lipoatrophy, Artefill was injected in the supraperiosteal layer of the malar region, at a maximum volume of 6 mL (3 mL/side). Touch-up injections were performed at weeks 4 and 6, up to a maximum total volume of 8.8 mL. Based on both the patient- and physician-rated evaluation, 95.8% of study participants were reported as being "improved" or "very much improved." The change in malar lipoatrophy grade was significantly improved from baseline to 1 year by 0.96 ± 0.98 ($P < .0003$). Patients also reported high levels of satisfaction, with 87.5% being "satisfied" or "very satisfied." There were no reported adverse safety events in the study.

COMPLICATIONS AND MANAGEMENT

As with any foreign material injected into the body, there is risk of complications, such as irregularity, incomplete correction, pain, bruising, swelling, infection, granuloma formation, and allergic response. However, Bellafill has been demonstrated to have a desirable safety profile. Injector skill is key to minimizing potential complications.

- In the case of potential technique-dependent adversities, such as uneven filler distribution that appears in the form of a string of pearls, a second implantation into the gaps may alleviate the problem.
- Deep placement of the filler in the subcutaneous fat, together with muscle movements, may result in inadequate treatment, in which case a successive implant is required.
- On the other hand, superficial treatment may lead to itching and erythema that can be treated with corticosteroid cream or intradermal corticosteroid injections. Irregularities or filler nodules that are palpable due to superficial injection can be removed by dermabrasion or shaving.
- Filler dislodgement or migration may be treated with intralesional corticosteroid injections or, if palpable intraorally, excision. Excision should be performed

thoroughly and completely because residual Bellafill may potentially cause secondary hypertrophic scarring, especially in patients prone to keloid formation (Asian and African American ethnicity).

- Patients with thin skin overlying the implant may experience visible dilated capillaries that can be treated and resolved by laser or intense pulsed-light (IPL) therapy.
- Granulomas are the most serious potential complications that occur with soft-tissue fillers, and the concern was more pronounced in the case of Bellafill due to the earlier product formulations and the filler being nonreabsorbable. The etiology of granulomas in dermal implants is multifactorial and potential factors include an excessive immunologic response, bacterial seeding of the implant acquired around the time of implantation, late contamination of the implant site with organisms presumptively spread hematogenously, and biofilms produced by seeded microorganisms. The safety results from the 5-year study of Bellafill demonstrated that the overall granuloma rate was only 1.7%, with all confirmed cases being mild to moderate and where treatment included intralesional corticosteroid injections with and without 5-fluorouracil. Granuloma treatment is difficult, and the most common treatment is with intralesional corticosteroid (Kenalog) injections. A 1:1 mixture of lidocaine and triamcinolone = fluorprednisolone ([Kenalog or Volon-A] up to 20 mg/mL or betamethasone [Diprosone] up to 5 mg/mL) can be injected safely through a 1-mL syringe with a Luer-Lock and a 30-gauge needle, using a lower concentration when more superficial to avoid delayed atrophy. The steroid must be injected strictly into the nodule while guiding the needle tip back and forth.

CONCLUSION

Bellafill, the latest generation of PMMA microspheres with collagen, has proven an important addition to the armamentarium of soft tissue fillers available for aesthetic correction. Based on 5-year data supporting its safety and efficacy, Bellafill is currently FDA approved for long-term correction of moderate to severe nasolabial folds and atrophic acne scars. In the author's collaborative experience, off-label use of Bellafill for panfacial augmentation and other off-label uses has favorable outcomes, especially in older patients who seek a longer-acting treatment, who need considerable structural facial support or have been poor responders to other fillers (Fig. 15.8). Bellafill may also serve as an adjunct to combination treatments with energy-based devices. Ultimately, it is the practitioner's responsibility to engage in judicious training of anatomic knowledge, injection technique, and current treatment protocols to capitalize the benefits and minimize patient risk when using a long-term filler such as Bellafill. When advising our patients for aesthetic rejuvenation and acne scar correction, it is important to keep in mind the value that Bellafill can add for patient outcomes when used appropriately.

FURTHER READING

Bagal, A., Dahiya, R., Tsai, V., & Adamson, P. A. (2007). Clinical experience with polymethylmethacrylate microspheres (Artecoll) for soft-tissue augmentation: a retrospective review. *Arch Facial Plast Surg.*, *9*(4), 275–280.

Broder, K. W., & Cohen, S. R. (2006). ArteFill: a permanent skin filler. *Expert Rev Med Devices.*, *3*(3), 281–289.

Cohen, S., Dover, J., Monheit, G., et al. (2015). Five-year safety and satisfaction study of PMMA-collagen in the correction of nasolabial folds. *Dermatol Surg.*, *41*(suppl 1), s302–s313.

Conejo-Mir, J. S., Sanz Guirado, S., & Angel, Munoz M. (2006). Adverse granulomatous reaction to Artecoll treated by intralesional 5-fluorouracil and triamcinolone injections. *Dermatol Surg.*, *32*(8), 1079–1081. discussion 1082.

Epstein, R. E., & Spencer, J. M. (2010). Correction of atrophic scars with artefill: an open-label pilot study. *J Drugs Dermatol.*, *9*(9), 1062–1064.

Haneke, E. (2004). Polymethyl methacrylate microspheres in collagen. *Semin Cutan Med Surg.*, *23*(4), 227–232.

Honma, T., & Hamasaki, T. (1996). Ultrastructure of multinucleated giant cell apoptosis in foreign-body granuloma. *Virchows Arch.*, *428*(3), 165–176.

Jones, D. H., Fitzgerald, R., Cox, S. E., et al. (2021). Preventing and treating adverse events of injectable fillers: evidence-based recommendations from the American Society for Dermatologic Surgery Multidisciplinary Task Force. *Dermatol Surg.*, *47*(2), 214–226.

Joseph, J. H., Eaton, L. L., & Cohen, S. R. (2015). Current concepts in the use of Bellafill. *Plast Reconstr Surg.*, *136*(5 suppl), 171s–179s.

Kadouch, J. A., Kadouch, D. J., Fortuin, S., van Rozelaar, L., Karim, R. B., & Hoekzema, R. (2013). Delayed-onset complications of facial soft tissue augmentation with permanent fillers in 85 patients. *Dermatol Surg.*, *39*(10), 1474–1485.

Karnik, J., Baumann, L., Bruce, S., et al. (2014). A double-blind, randomized, multicenter, controlled trial of suspended polymethylmethacrylate microspheres for the correction of atrophic facial acne scars. *J Am Acad Dermatol., 71*(1), 77–83.

Katz, B., Lehman, A., Misev, V., Vachon, G., & Saeed, S. (2021). A 12-month study to evaluate safety and efficacy of polymethylmethacrylate-collagen gel for correction of midface volume loss using a blunt cannula as measured by 3-D imaging. *Dermatol Surg., 47*(3), 365–369.

Lee, S. C., Kim, J. B., Chin, B. R., Kim, J. W., & Kwon, T. G. (2013). Inflammatory granuloma caused by injectable soft tissue filler (Artecoll). *J Korean Assoc Oral Maxillofac Surg., 39*(4), 193–196.

Lemperle, G., de Fazio, S., & Nicolau, P. (2006). ArteFill: a third-generation permanent dermal filler and tissue stimulator. *Clin Plast Surg., 33*(4), 551–565.

Lemperle, G., Sadick, N. S., Knapp, T. R., & Lemperle, S. M. (2010). ArteFill permanent injectable for soft tissue augmentation: II. Indications and applications. *Aesthetic Plast Surg., 34*(3), 273–286.

Lemperle, G., & Gauthier-Hazan, N. (2009). Foreign body granulomas after all injectable dermal fillers: part 2. Treatment options. *Plast Reconstr Surg., 123*(6), 1864–1873.

Lemperle, G., Rullan, P. P., & Gauthier-Hazan, N. (2006). Avoiding and treating dermal filler complications. *Plast Reconstr Surg., 118*(3 suppl), 92s–107s.

Mills, D. C., Camp, S., Mosser, S., Sayeg, A., Hurwitz, D., & Ronel, D. (2013). Malar augmentation with a polymethylmethacrylate-enhanced filler: assessment of a 12-month open-label pilot study. *Aesthet Surg J., 33*(3), 421–430.

Park, T. H., Seo, S. W., Kim, J. K., & Chang, C. H. (2012). Clinical experience with polymethylmethacrylate microsphere filler complications. *Aesthetic Plast Surg., 36*(2), 421–426.

Sadick, N. (2010). The manufacturer of the FDA approved non-resorbable aesthetic dermal filler Artefill. *J Drugs Dermatol., 9*(7), 751. author reply 751.

Smith, K. C., & Melnychuk, M. (2005). Five percent lidocaine cream applied simultaneously to the skin and mucosa of the lips creates excellent anesthesia for filler injections. *Dermatol Surg., 31*(11 pt 2), 1635–1637.

Solomon, P., Sklar, M., & Zener, R. (2012). Facial soft tissue augmentation with Artecoll(®): a review of eight years of clinical experience in 153 patients. *Can J Plast Surg., 20*(1), 28–32.

Yeh, L. C., & Goldberg, D. J. (2020). Twelve-month prospective study of polymethylmethacrylate/collagen dermal filler for volume loss of the dorsal of hands. *J Cosmet Dermatol., 19*(9), 2259–2266.

16

Forehead Reflation

Kavita Mariwalla and Marguerite Germain

SUMMARY AND KEY FEATURES

- Rejuvenation of the upper face relies on toxins, but for some patients with etched-in lines, true correction requires replacement of volume in the forehead concavity and filling of lines at the superficial dermal level. Although multiple fillers are available to correct the upper third of the face, we recommend calcium hydroxylapatite for deep volumization and hyaluronic acid fillers for fine lines specifically.
- Forehead correction is achieved by placing a bolus of material into the inferior frontal eminence. Fine-line correction is achieved by placing hyaluronic acid fillers directly into the lines themselves, although occasionally, a bolus to add support to the forehead concavity can be done simultaneously.
- Knowledge of forehead anatomy, especially of the arterial supply, is essential to safe and effective forehead filling.
- Postoperative edema is a common side effect that resolves spontaneously by 72 hours.
- Relative ptosis of the eyebrows is also a temporary side effect and is a result of lidocaine and edema, typically resolving within 24 hours.

INTRODUCTION

Although fillers are typically used for restoring volume loss to create a youthful appearance, an additional role of fillers is often overlooked—facial recontouring. The recontouring process not only corrects for defects but also aims to restore facial proportion that may or may not have been present naturally in the patient who presents for correction. As the use of toxin occurs consistently over years to decades in many patients, muscular atrophy also presents more commonly in our patients than it did in the past.

One of the prime areas amenable to restructuring through fillers is the forehead area. With time, the upper third of the face elongates as the hairline moves upward and the brow moves downward. Both intrinsic and extrinsic factors play a role. Gender, age, family history, and styling practices can influence hairline position, while gravity, smoking, and sun exposure can cause keratinocytic dysplasia, which manifests as coarse wrinkles and a rough skin surface.

Initially, changes associated with aging, such as rhytides, can be corrected through neurotoxin use. Over time, skin laxity and relative muscle atrophy create temporal wasting and some brow ptosis, leading to decreased efficacy of neurotoxin for this area. Even in patients who are neurotoxin naïve, brow descent can occur through repetitive contractions of forehead depressor muscles and loss of elastic fibers. Although many physicians focus on brow elevation, it is important to consider complementary filler placement in the forehead to optimize a younger appearance. (Coincidentally, brow elevation is on occasion noted in patients treated for forehead recontouring.)

In this chapter, we review a simple technique to replenish volume loss in the forehead, improve skin laxity, and reposition facial structures to correct for descent using calcium hydroxylapatite (CaHA; Radiesse or Radiesse Plus [Merz Aesthetics, Raleigh, NC]) and hyaluronic acid (HA) fillers. Although we primarily use CaHA and HA, autologous fat and poly-L-lactic acid (PLLA; Sculptra [Galderma Laboratories LP, Forth Worth, TX]) are also options and will be reviewed briefly.

PATIENT EVALUATION

Changes in the forehead region in terms of texture are typically sun related, whereas age-related changes cause volume loss, descent of brow position, and muscle atrophy, along with a seeming permanence of horizontal lines. For horizontal lines that are etched into the skin surface, it is important to use neurotoxin first to assess the degree of amelioration through that route, and evaluation for fillers in this region should only occur after the full effect of the neurotoxins has taken place. Questions regarding malignancy, human immunodeficiency virus (HIV) status, diabetes, and thyroid dysfunction should be asked because these are all medical conditions that can contribute to lipoatrophy. In addition, it is important to be aware if the patient is allergic to lidocaine or if he or she has had an adverse reaction to fillers in the past. This is especially important when using PLLA, which can cause granulomas. Informed consent should always be obtained in addition to preoperative photographs. Baseline facial asymmetry is also important to assess. Prior to injection, these authors recommend prepping the skin with alcohol or with chlorhexidine gluconate. Because additional diluted anesthetic is added to the product (CaHA is now available with lidocaine added to it), it is not necessary to anesthetize the patient topically prior to the procedure.

PATIENT CONSENT

As with any cosmetic procedure, informed consent is a must. In addition to the usual side effects of filler use, including bruising and edema, it is important to discuss the risk of nodule formation. In the forehead, incorrect placement of filler is unforgiving as this area of the face is mobile and even small nodules become very apparent depending on the lighting the patient is in. Filler migration should be discussed with patients as well as the possibility of vascular event. As will be discussed in the anatomy section, while intravascular injection is only sporadically reported in the literature, it can occur and can lead to skin necrosis. It is important to discuss this with patients and to include signs and symptoms in postfiller care so that patients know when to seek immediate medical attention. It is also imperative that staff receiving patient calls be aware of reports of bruising in this area which could be a sign of something more serious and may need physician evaluation.

A SPECIFIC NOTE ON PATIENT PREPARATION

With the more frequent use of different types of anticoagulant therapies, it is important to discuss the extent of bruising that can occur with forehead reflation as multiple entry points occur whether by needle or cannula. The direct oral anticoagulants—apixaban, dabigatran, rivaroxaban, and edoxaban—anecdotally have a greater chance of significant bleeding as compared to a single antiplatelet agent; however, oozing is easier to control on these agents. Although there is variability from medication to medication, it is important to alert patients to the significant bruising risk. That being said, it is not advised to have patients stop anticoagulant therapy for filler in this area. Added bleeding risk factors such as alcohol use and supplement use (e.g., St. John's Wort, Garlic) are discouraged for 72 h and 2 weeks prior to planned injection, respectively.

> **PEARL 1** Prior to injection in the forehead, three preoperative photographs should be taken at the following angles: full face, face at a 45-degree angle looking to the right, and face at a 45-degree angle looking to the left.

ANATOMY

Forehead

The skin of the forehead is typically thick compared with other areas on the face, is richly vascularized, and is abundant in sebaceous and sweat glands. Although the forehead appears to be a convex structure, there is a concavity that becomes more prominent with age in the suprabrow region. It is located between the frontal eminence of the forehead and the supraciliary arches. The superciliary ridges are prominences of the frontal bone above the orbital margins that meet in the midline in the glabella and are typically more visible in men.

The forehead constitutes the upper third of the face and is superiorly bordered by the hairline and inferiorly by the glabella and the eyebrows. For multiple reasons, the hairline is not a reliable landmark among individuals, and depending on the hairline, rhytids can extend almost into the lower hairline area. Remember that the frontal branch of the facial nerve passes through the temple and forehead, placing this nerve at risk of injury during filler use. For this reason, fanning is not encouraged because it can cause nerve injury. The frontal branch of the facial nerve supplies motor innervation to the muscles of facial expression of the eyebrows and forehead. The usual trajectory of the nerve is from a point 5 mm below the tragus to a point 15 mm above the lateral extremity of the brow. The most common method of finding this "danger zone" is to draw a line from the ear lobe to the lateral eyebrow and then from the tragus to the superior-most forehead rhytid. The result will be a zone that corresponds to the usual trajectory path of the frontal branch. Transection with a needle in this area can result in brow ptosis.

Injury to the supraorbital nerve is of concern when treating the forehead. The nerve exits the supraorbital notch, which lies along the orbital rim medially. Although we often teach palpation along the superior orbital rim to find this notch, notches are present bilaterally in only 49% of skulls. A compression injury to the nerve can be avoided by injecting laterally and at least 1 cm lateral to the supraorbital foramen. Adjacent to the supraorbital nerve is the supraorbital artery. Retrograde injection can decrease the risk of vascular embolization, as can the use of blunt-tipped cannulas, however the gauge of the cannula should be kept in mind as cannulas can still present a risk of vascular perforation (see Pearl 3).

The tissue layers of the forehead are as follows: skin, subcutaneous fat, galea aponeurotica, loose areolar tissue, and periosteum. In the region of the eyebrow, galea gives way to the muscles of facial expression. The preferred injection plane is posterior to the frontalis muscle. Transverse fibrous septa from the frontalis muscle to the dermis in the forehead are partially responsible for the deep, horizontal forehead creases. The subcutaneous prefrontalis muscle level has been used for PLLA injections. More cohesive fillers, such as CaHA, may not spread as easily and may require multiple injections, thus causing more tissue trauma. Cases of blindness have been reported when injecting near the glabella, making it critical to understand the anatomy of this area before injecting. For this reason, we often use HA fillers in patients with noticeable atrophy due to its pliability and ability to be dissolved.

Vascular supply is not as straightforward as it is often taught in medical school. Cadaveric dissection by Cong et al. has shown that there is variability in the topographic route of the supratrochlear artery and the supraorbital artery. In a type 1a schema, the layer superficial to the frontalis is supplied medially by the superficial branch of the supraorbital artery while the deep branch of the supratrochlear artery and the deep branch of the supraorbital artery are distributed deep to the frontalis. In type 1b, the layer superficial to the frontalis is supplied by the superficial branch of the supraorbital artery in addition to the central artery or the paracentral artery and the layer deep to the frontalis is same as that in type 1a. In a type II distribution, the layer superficial to the frontalis is supplied similarly to type 1a but only the deep branch of the supraorbital artery supplies the layer deep to the frontalis. It is important to recognize these variants as classically the supraorbital artery is described as passing through the supraorbital foramen and then dividing into a superficial and deep branch, which anastomose with the frontal, anterior branch of the temporal and the artery of the opposite side. Our anatomic understanding from cadaveric dissections has also evolved to recognize that fine perforations also supply the skin at the upper eyebrow area. One of the safest entry points, therefore, in the forehead for augmentation is lateral to the vertical plane of the supraorbital foramen to avoid vascular injury.

PEARL 2 Injections into the creases of the forehead are placed relatively superficially and are therefore painful. Topical numbing preparations often cause hyperemia and, combined with an already rich vascular bed, filler injections at this level can result in extensive bruising. To avoid this, we recommend numbing in sections using ice packs rather than topical numbing agents. It is also important to change the needle every five to six injection points.

PEARL 3 Blunt-tipped cannulas have become increasingly popular over the past several years, although we caution readers about reliance on the term "blunt-tipped." At 27 gauge, a blunt-tipped cannula can still pop an inflated balloon; it should still be considered a sharp instrument. If using a cannula, we recommend a 25 gauge, although some advocate for nothing smaller than a 22 gauge in this area. Although cannula use can minimize bruising, an insertion point must be created that is larger than a needle mark in all instances. We caution reliance on a cannula to prevent intravessel injection or to minimize risk of injection in the temple or forehead due to the complex anatomy in the area at baseline.

SELECTING THE RIGHT FILLER

There are many fillers to choose from when rejuvenating the upper third of the face. Autologous fat transfer can provide long-lasting results, although multiple treatment sessions are required and significant swelling and edema are postoperative consequences. Autologous fat is also less amenable in patients with HIV-associated lipoatrophy because the fat cells are more difficult to harvest and the fat graft tends to be less successful.

PLLA is another choice for filling, but again multiple treatment sessions spaced 4 to 6 weeks apart are required for optimal results. In these authors' experience the ideal dilution for PLLA is 8 mL of sterile water and 1 mL of 1% or 2% lidocaine. The product can be premixed days in advance, despite package instructions to mix 2 hours prior to injection with the final 1 mL of lidocaine added just prior to patient injection. Injection with 1 ¼-inch (35 mm), 25-gauge needles attached to 3-mL syringes allows for even injecting and controlled dispersion of the product. It is critical that the patient massage the area postprocedure using the "rule of fives" (5 times a day for 5 days for 5 minutes each time).

HA fillers are viable in this area and due to their ease of dissolution, recommended for filling in the forehead, especially for etched in lines. For concavity filling, the more viscous products, such as Restylane Lyft (Galderma Laboratories LP, Fort Worth, TX), Juvéderm Ultra Plus (Allergan, Irvine, CA), RHA 3 (Revance, Irvine, CA) are preferable, whereas for individual creases, Restylane Silk (Galderma Laboratories LP, Fort Worth, TX), Belotero Balance (Merz Aesthetics, Raleigh, NC) or RHA 2 or Redensity (Revance, Irvine, CA) are optimal. Some practitioners "thin" Juvéderm Ultra (Allergan, Irvine, CA) or Restylane (Galderma Laboratories LP, Fort Worth, TX) by adding 0.5 mL of lidocaine to a 1-mL syringe and injecting this into the mid-dermis in a small depot fashion along the horizontal forehead creases. Placement of these products can occur high in the dermis without Tyndall effect, making it an ideal choice for softening of lines in patients who have become toxin-immune or who require frontalis action to raise the brow and thus cannot tolerate toxin injection (especially the lateral frontalis). Placement of Restylane Silk, Belotero Balance, or RHA 2 directly into the lines will still allow for muscle movement, although it will create a relative softening. Some practitioners will use a tumescent saline technique to create a plane for a cannula to pass easily for forehead augmentation; however, it is the opinion of these authors that the tumescent technique leads to excessive edema and creates difficulty in assessing final results for etched lines.

The HA family of fillers is ideal when a reversible correction is desired. Adding 0.5 mL of 1% lidocaine per HA syringe and injecting the retrofrontalis muscle facilitates an even correction.

Again, assessments of the degree of frontal atrophy and skin thickness are necessary before choosing which product is best. For HA fillers, the duration of action is typically 4 to 6 months.

In our clinical practices, we use both HA and CaHA for these specific applications. The CaHA, especially mixed with lidocaine, lends itself to reliable placement without migration and provides longevity, whereas the HAs have a unique role in the correction of deep, etched in lines. Injection with CaHA and HA is described in detail in the following sections.

MATERIALS, INJECTION SITES, AND INJECTION TECHNIQUES

Materials

CaHA is a filler with relatively high viscosity. Alterations in the viscosity can be implemented without compromising long-term efficacy. Consequently, prior to administration of CaHA into the forehead, the product should be homogeneously mixed with lidocaine. In our clinical practice, the 1.5-mL syringe of CaHA is combined with 1.0 mL of 1% lidocaine/normal saline diluent mixture for the forehead. If using CaHA that already

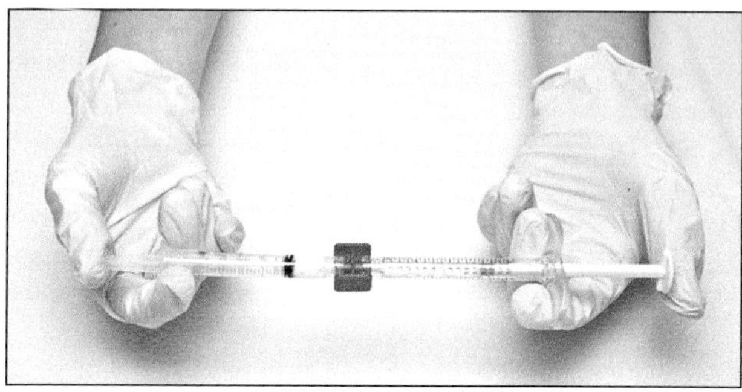

Fig. 16.1 A Luer-Lock connector is used to mix the 1.5-mL calcium hydroxylapatite syringe with the 3.0-mL syringe containing either lidocaine or lidocaine/normal saline diluent. (Courtesy of Merz North America, Inc., Raleigh, NC.)

contains 2% lidocaine, then constitute with 1.0 mL of normal saline diluent only. This mixing enhances the ease of distributing the product throughout the treatment area. It is known that this hyperdilute CaHA technique can stimulate neocollagenesis, which is another reason we prefer to use this product in the forehead.

An ordinary 3.0-mL syringe containing the diluent can be connected to the 1.5-mL syringe, using a female-to-female Luer-Lock adapter (Fig. 16.1). Typically, 10 to 15 passes of the CaHA and the diluent back and forth from syringe to syringe are sufficient for homogeneous distribution of both diluent and dermal filler. When using an HA, addition of diluent is typically not needed unless filling lines specifically—in this case, if a more viscous product is used (other than Restylane Silk or Belotero Balance), 0.5 mL of 1% lidocaine should be similarly added to the syringe. Voluma, Restylane Lyft, and Juvéderm Ultra Plus are not recommended for this area.

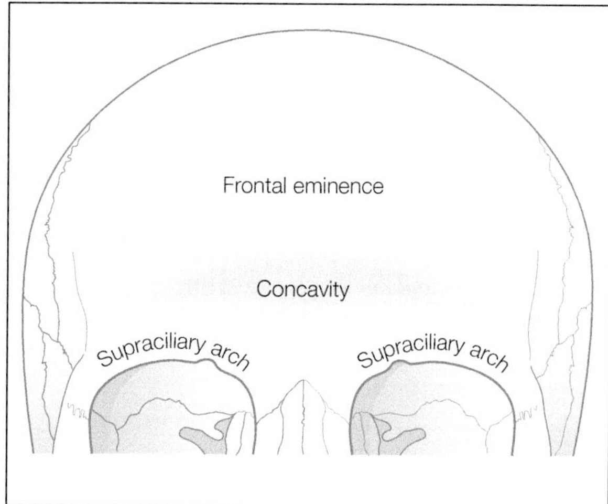

Fig. 16.2 The suprabrow concavity extends inferiorly to the frontal bone supraciliary ridge and superiorly to the frontal eminence.

Injection Site for the Forehead

The target in the suprabrow area is the suprabrow concavity. Specifically, this area extends inferiorly to the frontal bone supraciliary ridge and superiorly to the frontal eminence, approximately 3 cm away from the supraciliary arches. Laterally, the space to be injected is marked by extension into the temporal compartment below the temporal cheek fat (Fig. 16.2). The floor of the target injection area is the frontal supraperiosteum, and the ceiling is the frontalis muscle. Bone touch is an important safety check to make sure that the needle or cannular insertion point is deep to the frontalis.

When addressing the medial aspects of the area, injections should extend lateral to the projection of the supraorbital nerve. This projection is located more than 1 cm from the supraorbital notch or foramen. Injections should be executed at the subcutaneous level, with dermal filler placed at the supraperiosteal level behind the galeal fat pad (Fig. 16.3).

Safe zones for cannula entry should be considered with regard to the length of the cannula itself. The recommended entry point should be lateral to the vertical plane of the supraorbital foramen to avoid vascular injury and like needle use, employ the technique of bone touch to ensure that one is deep to the frontalis. The cannula should be guided along the superperiosteal layer until it reaches the medial area of the forehead. Once that area is reached, filler should be released.

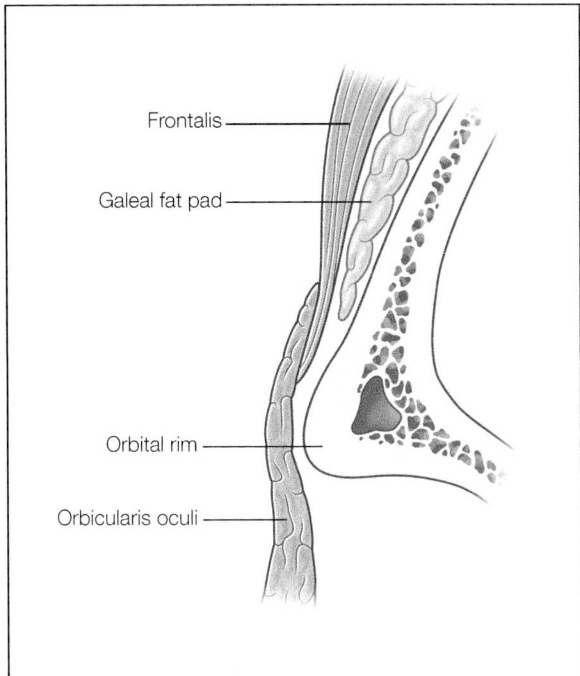

Fig. 16.3 Injections should be executed at the subcutaneous level when trying to ameliorate etched in lines or lines in patients in whom neuromodulators are not effective.

When correcting superficial lines that cannot be corrected with neurotoxin alone, place the needle of the HA filler (30 gauge) into the line itself in the dermal place with bevel up. Inject using a retrograde, threading technique, and massage the area immediately afterward. Keep in mind that overcorrection is not necessary with HA fillers and that swelling is common and should be expected for 24 to 48 hours after filler placement (Video 16.1).

> **PEARL 4** Patients taking blood thinners are susceptible to bruising. When reflating the forehead, bruising can be expected, and in patients on some of the newer blood-thinning agents that do not require routine blood monitoring, the bleeding risk is significant and can leave hemosiderin deposition, especially at the temples. For this reason, patients on blood thinners other than aspirin are asked to have an international normalized ratio (INR) check the day prior to the cosmetic appointment. For those on blood thinners that do not require monitoring, we extensively discuss the risk of bleeding and bruising. We have found the most bleeding from skin procedures occurs in patients on a combination of clopidogrel and aspirin or on prasugrel. Other thinners that cause extensive bruising are the direct oral anticoagulants.

Injection Technique for Forehead Recontouring

A 27-gauge, 1 ¼-inch (35-mm) needle is used to introduce the CaHA–lidocaine solution into the forehead. A threading bolus is used to place the product in the inferior frontal eminence (Fig. 16.4). The amount of product varies with each patient, but the stated objective is reconstitution of the suprabrow arch. When sufficient product has been deposited using retrograde injection for introduction of the bolus, the area is then massaged so that the product is evenly distributed throughout the borders described in the previous section. Volumes may range from 1.5 mL to 3.0 mL of CaHA, in addition to the volumes of diluent necessary for mixing.

In some cases, a brow lift has also been a fortunate consequence of forehead recontouring. This has occurred without any placement of product directly behind the brow. However, even in the absence of a brow lift, the filler placement of the patients in a "horseshoe" pattern has resulted in cosmetic benefits, including projection of the lateral eyebrow and reduction of transitions between the suprabrow, temporal, and cheek regions.

When filling individual lines, use a 30-gauge, ½-inch needle attached to the HA syringe. Be prepared to replace the needle frequently because 30-gauge needles can burr quickly after multiple injections into thick forehead skin. Inject in a retrograde motion with the bevel of the needle pointed up. Do not inject with the patient lying down because this will give a false sense

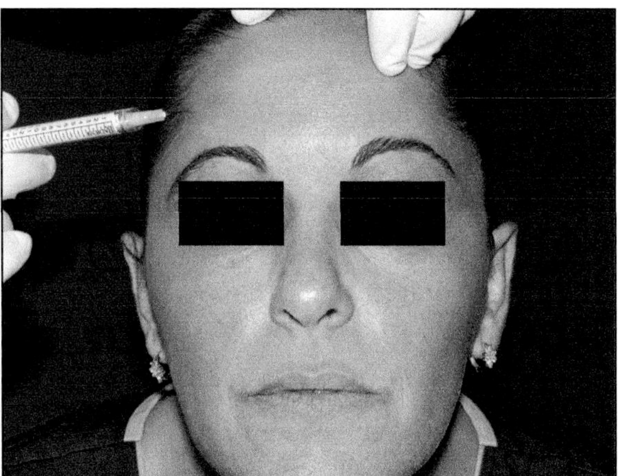

Fig. 16.4 A threading bolus is used to place calcium hydroxylapatite in the inferior frontal eminence. (Reproduced from Busso M. Forehead contouring with calcium hydroxylapatite. *Dermatol Surg*. 2010;36(s3):s1910–s1913.)

of improvement. For comfort, the patient should be at a 45-degree angle because patients who are sitting upright can sometimes develop vasovagal syncope due to the number of injections placed into individual lines. When using a low-viscosity filler, one may see extrusion of small amounts of filler through pores depending on the superficial plane one is injecting in.

> **PEARL 5** Using a bolus technique is preferable to fanning in the forehead region. A 1¼-inch (35 mm) needle facilitates placement.

Note: After injection, the treated area will likely become edematous. This condition is self-limiting and will resolve in as little as 24 hours in some cases but as long as 10 days in others. An initial temporary brow droop, as opposed to brow lift, is the likely consequence of the diffusion of the lidocaine in the injected solution. The droop is quite short lived, resolving within several hours.

SAFETY CONSIDERATIONS AND ADVERSE EVENTS

The anatomy of the forehead can pose a challenge to experienced and inexperienced physicians alike. The superficial temporal artery and the frontal branch of the facial nerve, both closely associated with the superficial temporal fascia, are to be avoided. Tenting the forehead may be difficult because of relatively low skin laxity, but tenting the temporal area can separate the subcutaneous layer from the fascia and help to identify the area where the filler is to be injected. Retrograde injection and the use of blunt cannulas can decrease vascular complications, although reliance on a cannula itself is not advised to avoid this complication.

Even with the most careful injection technique into the forehead, edema is likely. This edema is short lived and usually resolves without any need for ice, cool presses, or analgesic at home. However, our patients are always instructed to contact us when edema lasts beyond 72 hours. Delayed bruising is also possible with ecchymosis, appearing up to 48 hours after injection. To avoid excessive or long-lasting edema, upper face recontouring can be staged, limiting the total volume of CaHA to 1.5 mL per visit. Short-lived brow ptosis has also been observed in some patients, lasting only a few hours postinjection of filler.

CONCLUSIONS

As the 21st century opened, aesthetic physicians were accustomed to seeing the application of dermal fillers as an endeavor that involved chasing lines and wrinkles. Indeed, even the indications for CaHA and other fillers address remediation of fine lines and wrinkles. However, within 10 years, a sea change has occurred in the profession of dermatology in its approach to the use of fillers. Dermatologists now see fillers as tools to volumize the midface and lower face. We believe that the upper face can also profit from volumizing, in particular by restoring the original contours of the forehead and softening creases that are resistant to neurotoxin use alone. Although PLLA and perhaps even fat transfer may have utility in upper face recontouring, at present, we have found that CaHA and HAs offer us the best treatment option for the forehead and temples.

CASE STUDY 1

Sara is a 55-year-old female patient who consulted us to learn about nonsurgical options for facial rejuvenation. On examination, it was established that periorbital volume reconstitution should be part of the antiaging regimen. CaHA was injected at the retrofrontalis level. Soon after the injection was started, a treelike blanching with the base at the orbital rim was observed, most likely caused by vascular occlusion or compression of a supraorbital artery branch. Subsequent steps included immediate cessation of injection of filler and commencement of vigorous massage. No further changes were observed in subsequent days. Had an HA filler been injected, a hyaluronidase would have been administrated.

It is important to watch for any skin color changes while injecting any filler. Injecting lateral to the supraorbital vessels with a blunt cannula, in small amounts, diluted with anesthetic, will help to avoid this complication.

FURTHER READING

Busso, M. (2009). Vectoring approach to midfacial contouring using calcium hydroxylapatite and hyaluronic acid. *Cosmet Dermatol.*, *22*(10), 522–528.

Busso, M. (2010). Commentary on extrinsic addition of lidocaine to calcium hydroxylapatite. *Dermatol Surg.*, *36*(11), 1795.

Cong, L. Y., Phothong, W., Lee, S. H., et al. (2017). Topographic analysis of the supratrochlear artery and the supraorbital artery: implication for improving the safety of forehead augmentation. *Plast Reconstr Surg.*, *139*(3), 620e–627e.

Jones, D. (2009). Semi-permanent and permanent injectable fillers. *Dermatol Clin.*, *27*(4), 433–444.

Knize, D. M. (1996). An anatomically based study of the mechanism of eyebrow ptosis. *Plast Reconstr Surg.*, *97*(7), 1321–1333.

Knize, D. M. (2009). Anatomic concepts for brow lift procedures. *Plast Reconstr Surg.*, *124*(6), 2118–2126.

Le Louarn, C., Buthiau, D., & Buis, J. (2007). The face recurve concept: medical and surgical applications. *Aesthet Plast Surg.*, *31*(3), 219–231. discussion 232.

Rohrich, R. J., & Pessa, J. E. (2007). The fat compartments of the face: anatomy and clinical implications for cosmetic surgery. *Plast Reconstr Surg.*, *119*(7), 2219–2227.

Sundaram, H., Voigts, R., Beer, K., & Meland, M. (2010). Comparison of the rheological properties of viscosity and elasticity in two categories of soft tissue fillers: calcium hydroxylapatite and hyaluronic acid. *Dermatol Surg.*, *36*(S3), 1859–1865.

Sullivan, P. K., Salomon, J. A., Woo, A. S., & Freeman, M. B. (2006). The importance of the retaining ligamentous attachments of the forehead for selective eyebrow reshaping and forehead rejuvenation. *Plast Reconstr Surg.*, *117*(1), 95–104.

17

Soft Tissue Augmentation of the Temple

Adele Haimovic, Diane K. Murphy, and Derek Jones

SUMMARY AND KEY FEATURES

- Lipoatrophy of the temporal region can result from the aging process, low body fat, certain genetic disorders, treatment with antiretroviral therapy, or physical trauma.
- Effective augmentation of the temporal region with soft tissue fillers can produce gratifying results for both the patient and the physician.
- Administration of hyaluronic acid fillers to augment the temple has gained significant popularity because of their ease of use and predictable treatment outcomes.
- To decrease the risk of severe complications associated with vascular occlusion, precise knowledge of temporal anatomy and injection technique is essential to achieve safe and effective temple augmentation.

INTRODUCTION

The appearance of soft tissue fullness in the face results from the multifaceted interplay of all facial tissues, including bone, fat, muscle, and skin. Age-related lipoatrophy, the slow, symmetrical loss of subdermal adipose tissue, can result in loss of fullness in many facial areas, although lipoatrophy can also result from low body fat, certain genetic disorders, treatment with antiretroviral therapy, or physical trauma at any age. Disease-related lipoatrophy is often more rapid and asymmetric and may be associated with psychological issues (e.g., body image distortions, social anxiety/withdrawal).

One of the earliest and frequently unaddressed signs of aging is lipoatrophy of the temples (i.e., temple hollowing). With age, the temporal bone progressively becomes more concave, and the overlying temporalis muscle reduces in volume. Deflation of the temple causes the tail of the eyebrow to appear shorter, results in the loss of smooth arcs of light around the temporal orbit, and emphasizes the lateral orbital rim. Importantly, hollow temples may also be a hallmark of thin individuals and not related to aging. Regardless, individuals with substantial soft tissue loss, especially thinner patients, can have a hollowed, gaunt appearance and lose the temporal fullness that is associated with youth. Successful treatment and correction of the temporal region can produce satisfying results for both the patient and the physician.

> **PEARL 1** The temporal fossa is a large, concave area located on the lateral surface of the skull that extends almost to the end of the parietal bone and is bordered by the temporal fusion line, zygomatic arch, and anterior hairline. The anterior region near the temporal fusion line is the focus of cosmetic augmentation procedures.

AESTHETIC PROCEDURES USED FOR TEMPLE AUGMENTATION

Numerous aesthetic techniques have been used to volumize or augment hollowed temples, including surgical implants, autologous fat transfer, or soft tissue filler injections. Implants present challenges such as incorrect size or placement location, and migration or extrusion are possible outcomes. Limitations of autologous fat transfer include nonstandardization of fat harvesting and fat processing techniques, unpredictability of fat graft retention, and potential for fat necrosis, hematoma, seroma, nerve injury, and blindness. Poly-L-lactic acid (Sculptra, Galderma) is a biostimulatory injectable that can deliver natural-appearing temple augmentation for up to 2 years. However, numerous injections are required over several months to achieve the desired effect, and the effectiveness is dependent on the amount of fibroplasia the patient develops around the poly-L-lactic acid microparticles. Treatment may be unpredictable and, in some cases, result in nodule formation. Calcium hydroxylapatite (Radiesse, Merz Aesthetics) provides volume correction for 10 to 14 months and has an immediate effect due to the aqueous vehicle. It is important to note that, unlike hyaluronic acid (HA), both poly-L-lactic acid and calcium hydroxylapatite are generally not dissolvable if there are any complications or unsatisfactory aesthetic results.

Use of HA fillers for temple augmentation has substantially increased in popularity due to their ease of use, consistent, predictable outcomes, and physician and patient satisfaction. The immediate aesthetic effects of HA fillers can last up to 1 year or longer; however, these agents have the unique quality of being reversible (i.e., dissolvable) with hyaluronidase if vascular occlusion, nodule formation, or overcorrection occur. As shown in Fig. 17.1, temple augmentation can create a less concave appearance, provide an upward lift of the face and brow, and result in considerable enhancement of the upper face. Based on these outcomes, temple augmentation with HA fillers may be part of a comprehensive approach to facial aesthetic treatment.

SCALES TO ASSESS TEMPLE HOLLOWS

Standardized, graded scales are critical to provide objective assessments of the severity of temple hollowing before and after treatment. There are currently two validated photonumeric scales for physician assessment of temple volume deficit assessing temple appearance. The Allergan Temple Hollowing Scale is a 5-point scale (Fig. 17.2), which demonstrated almost perfect interrater and intrarater agreement, suggesting the substantial reliability of numerous assessments for the same individual across different raters and at different time points for the same rater. The scale also showed sufficient sensitivity to determine that a one-grade change represents a clinically significant improvement in temple volume deficit. Scale components include an assessment area diagram, verbal descriptors, morphed images, and real-world patient images representing both genders and several skin types. The Galderma Temple Volume Deficit Scale is a 4-point scale with verbal descriptors, morphed images, and real-world patient images, and it had substantial interrater and intrarater agreement. Because both scales were validated in live subjects and included both morphed and unaltered images, the scales can be applied in day-to-day clinical practice and in clinical trials of individuals seeking temple augmentation.

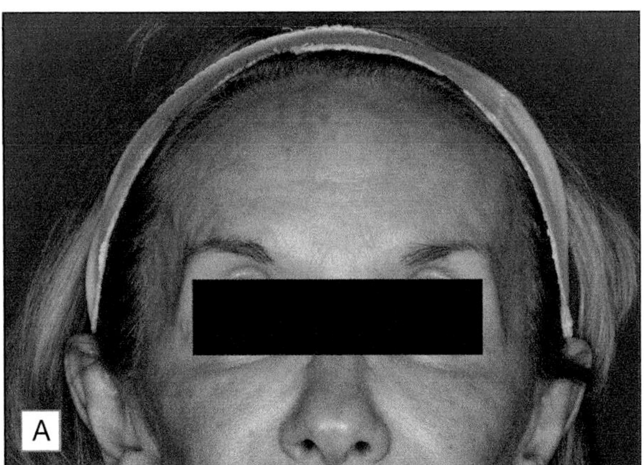

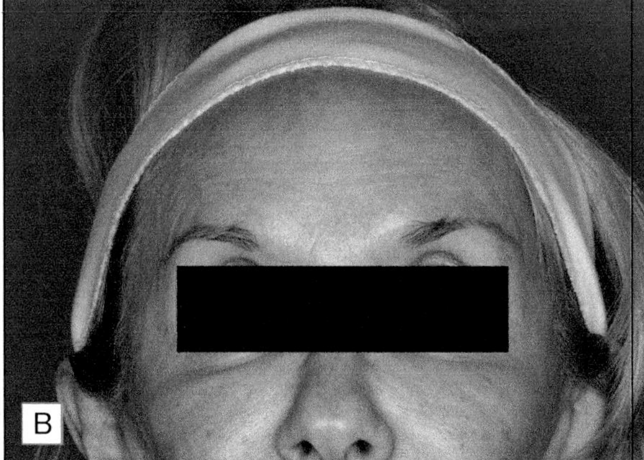

Fig. 17.1 Patient before (A) and after (B) Juvéderm Voluma XC treatment for temple hollows (2 mL injected per temple). (Photographs courtesy of Derek Jones.)

Allergan Temple Hollowing Scale

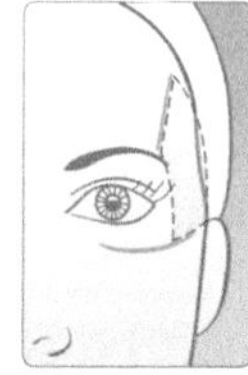

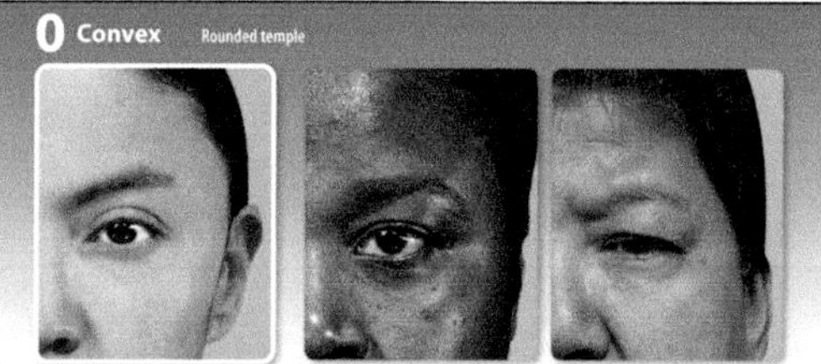

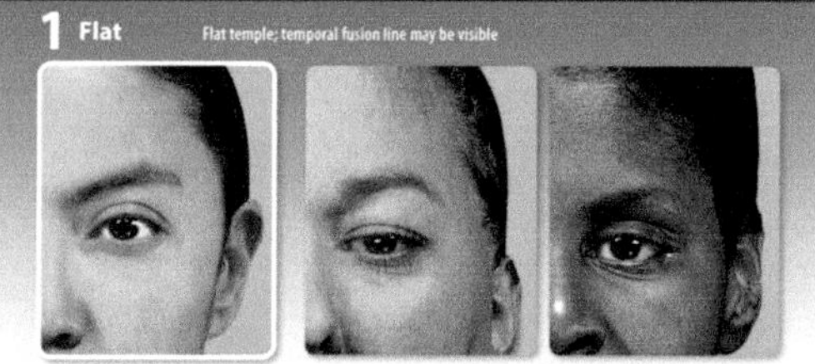

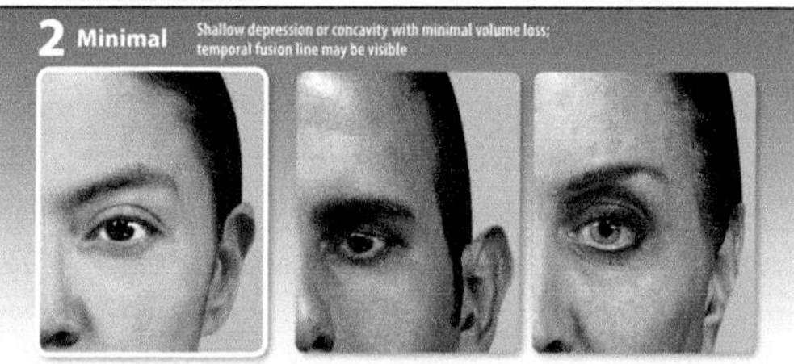

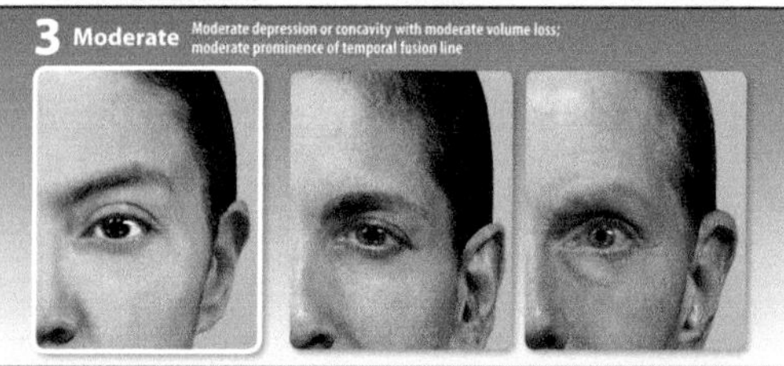

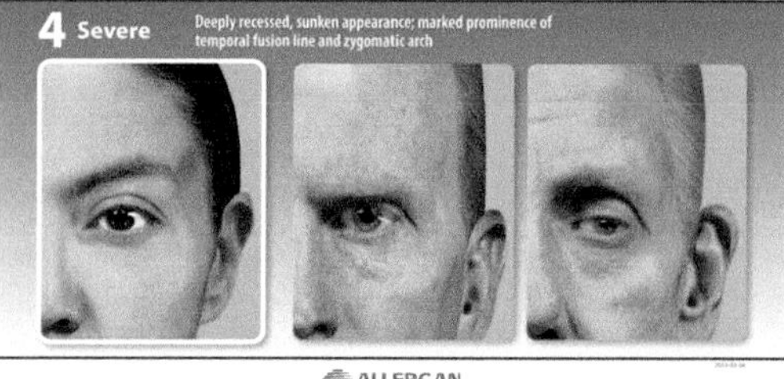

ALLERGAN

Fig. 17.2 The Allergan Temple Hollowing Scale. The extent of temple volume deficit (within area of diagram shown in upper right corner) is assigned a grade of 0 (convex) to 4 (severe). (Reproduced with permission from Carruthers J, Jones D, Hardas B, et al. Development and validation of a photonumeric scale for evaluation of volume deficit of the temple. *Dermatol Surg*. 2016;42(suppl 1):S203–S210.)

INJECTION TECHNIQUE FOR PLACEMENT OF HYALURONIC ACID FILLERS IN THE TEMPLE

Exceptional knowledge of temporal anatomy is critical to safely achieving optimal temple augmentation, and it should be performed only by advanced injectors. The complexity of the network of blood vessels in the temporal region increases the risk of vascular compromise and severe complications. Thus, it is paramount to know the exact location of these specific vascular structures to avoid injury to the patient. Branches of the superficial temporal artery reside in the superficial plane of the temporal fossa and have important communications with the vessels leading to the ophthalmic and retinal vessels. Furthermore, the location of the middle temporal vein (MTV) deep to the superficial layer of the deep temporal fascia presents challenges in avoiding this vein during injection, particularly since its maximal diameter can range from 0.5 to 9.1 mm (average 5.1 mm) and its length can range from 10 to 60 mm (average 24 mm). Likewise, the medial zygomaticotemporal vein (MZTV) is located within the same anatomic area and may also be prone to injection-related vascular damage. Based on anatomic knowledge of the temporal fossa area as well as clinical experience, it has been determined that the safest temple injections are deep to the temporalis muscle on the periosteum using a needle and avoiding the superficial and deep temporal arteries. Safe injection also depends on the type of filler being used. The physician should consider specific attributes of the product because formulations with higher viscosity or elasticity can resist any downward pull of the mid or lower face.

Prior to initiating the injection, the temporal region should be thoroughly cleaned with alcohol and chlorhexidine to prevent infection and formation of biofilm. An HA filler can be injected using a 27- or 30-gauge, half-inch needle, and the injection should be initiated within the safe treatment window, which includes three facial landmarks that serve as safety boundaries. The temporal fusion line represents the superomedial boundary beginning at the tail of the eyebrow; all injections should be placed posterior and lateral to this point. All injections should occur 1.5 cm above the zygomatic arch to avoid contact with the MTV and should be placed anterior to the facial hairline to avoid the deep temporal artery (Video 17.1).

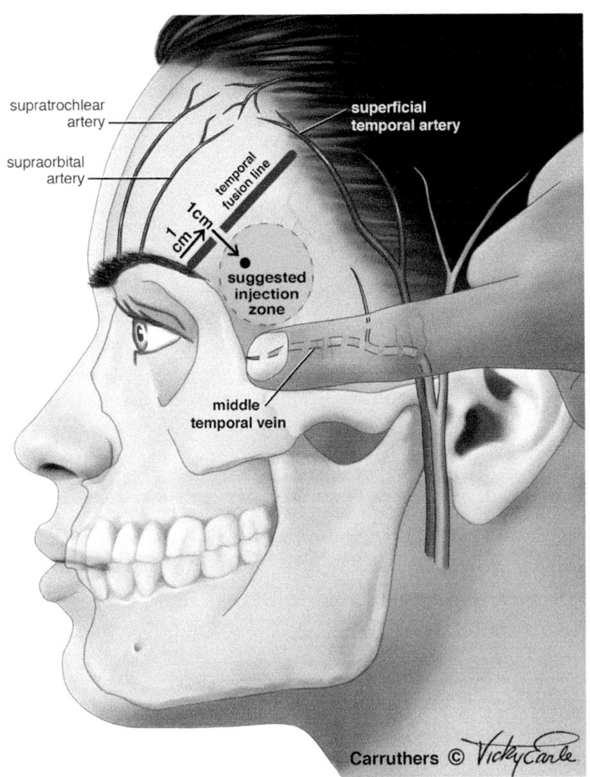

Fig. 17.3 Suggested safe injection zone for the temple lies between the superolateral bony orbital margin, approximately 1 cm inferior to the temporal fusion line and over 1 finger breadth above the superior border of the zygoma in order to avoid the middle temporal vein. (Reproduced with permission from Carruthers J, Humphrey S, Beleznay K, Carruthers A. Suggested injection zone for soft tissue fillers in the temple? *Dermatol Surg*. 2017;43(5):756–757.)

Recent evidence-based recommendations from the American Society for Dermatologic Surgery are for injections via needle on the periosteum deep to the superficial temple vessels. The suggested safe zone to avoid the MTV is 1 cm up from the superior orbital rim, 1 cm lateral to the temporal fusion line, and more than 2.5 cm above the zygomatic arch (Fig 17.3).

To successfully place the filler on the periosteum, the injector should insert the needle perpendicular to the skin and guide it deep until the needle makes contact with bone. Maintaining the needle tip in contact with bone is paramount to avoid intravascular injection. The injector should then aspirate the syringe for several seconds; this will help to confirm that the needle was not placed intravascularly, although this is not always foolproof, especially with small-bore needles. A slow, steady injection of 0.5 to 1.0 mL of HA filler is recommended for each treatment per temple, using bolus technique on bone. Larger volume, up to 2 mL per each temple, may be injected for more severe concavities. The injector may choose to place a finger posteriorly to ease the flow of product into the temple and prevent diffusion to the hairline and massage the temporal area to ensure even distribution of product and achieve smooth, optimal contour (Video 17.1). Injecting deep on bone too far posteriorly or inferiorly within the fossa is not recommended, as the deep temporal artery may reside in these locations.

For patients with mild volume loss in the anterior temple, a blunt cannula (25 gauge or larger) can be used for superficial filling with a low G' filler in the subdermal plane. This is a riskier, more advanced method as the temporal arteries reside in this more superficial plane. The contours of the cannula should be visible if you are in the correct plane, and the injector should slowly and steadily fan the cannula throughout the temporal region using a retrograde injection technique and massage the area to ensure even distribution of the filler. Less than 0.7 mL of HA product is often required to achieve desired results.

PEARL 2 Thorough knowledge of temporal anatomy and appropriate injection technique are critical to achieving optimal temple augmentation. The recommended technique is to inject volumizing HA filler deep to the temporalis muscle into the space directly on the periosteum, within the safe zone described in Fig. 17.3.

AVOIDING AND TREATING COMPLICATIONS OF INJECTING HYALURONIC ACID FILLERS

Potential complications associated with injection of HA fillers can be minimized or prevented with sufficient knowledge of the product and the injection technique. The most common adverse events associated with filler placement in the temples are often mild and transient and include lower eyelid bruising, prominence of superficial blood vessels, headache, injection site pain, and soreness or tenderness that worsens with chewing or eating. One study of temple augmentation with

Juvéderm Voluma XC (Allergan Aesthetics) found that 40% of the 30 subjects had self-limited mild to moderate jaw pain during mastication. This is because the temporalis muscle connects to the temporomandibular joint, and the pressure from the injections beneath the muscle can result in tension and transient pain in the joint. To avoid pain while chewing or eating, patients should be instructed to eat soft foods until the pain resolves. The relatively mild adverse events of bruising and pain may be minimized by having patients avoid any medications that may increase the risk of bruising (aspirin, nonsteroidal antiinflammatory agents, fish oil, garlic, gingko) for 7 to 10 days prior to the procedure. If prominent bleeding occurs upon needle withdrawal following injection, direct pressure should be applied to the injection site. Ice, pressure, and corticosteroids can be recommended for acute, intense swelling at the injection site, which is rare.

Severe complications associated with soft tissue temple augmentation, using either biostimulatory agents or HA fillers, may occur through accidental direct intravascular injection. Although rare, these complications can include skin ischemia distant from the injection site, severe skin pain, visual acuity changes, ocular pain, or permanent blindness. Occlusion of the MTV during HA filler placement may lead to stroke and central nervous system damage in that this vein is connected to the cavernous sinus, potentially leading to cavernous sinus embolization. The MZTV may also play a role in ocular complications given that this vein drains into the MTV. Avoiding vascular compromise and occlusion is therefore critical, and the risk is substantially reduced with injection of the HA filler in the preperiosteal space. In addition, aspiration must be performed prior to injection, and it is absolutely required that the filler is placed slowly without force. If the needle becomes clogged, it should be removed and replaced before reinitiating the injection. If signs or symptoms of vascular occlusion become apparent, including skin changes, severe pain, change in vision, or ocular pain, the needle should be removed immediately. Hyaluronidase should be liberally injected to dissolve any product responsible for the vascular occlusion. Other potentially beneficial treatments for vascular compromise with visual changes include ocular massage, breathing into a paper bag, aspirin, sildenafil, topical timolol, oral acetazolamide, among others. Evidence-based recommendations for treating vascular occlusion, including blindness and visual adverse events, have recently been published by the American Society for Dermatologic Surgery Task Force for prevention and treatment of adverse events from injectable fillers.

PEARL 3 Complications can be minimized by knowing the location of vascular structures to avoid injury to the patient. The safest injection site is on periosteum, 1 cm superior and 1 cm lateral to the temporal fusion line.

CONCLUSIONS

Hollowing of the temples can be successfully corrected using HA fillers. However, the complex anatomy of the temporal region increases the risk of potentially severe adverse effects and should not be overlooked. Safe, effective injections of HA fillers to the temple can be achieved with superior knowledge of temporal anatomy and through use of appropriate injection techniques.

FURTHER READING

Baumann, L. S., Weisberg, E. M., Mayans, M., & Arcuri, E. (2019). Open label study evaluating efficacy, safety, and effects on perception of age after injectable 20 mg/ml hyaluronic acid gel for volumization of facial temples. *J Drugs Dermatol.*, *18*(1), 67–74.

Beleznay, K., Carruthers, J. D. A., Humphrey, S., Carruthers, A., & Jones, D. (2019). Update on avoiding and treating blindness from fillers: a recent review of the world literature. *Aesthet Surg J.*, *39*(6), 662–674.

Breithaupt, A. D., Jones, D. H., Braz, A., Narins, R., & Weinkle, S. (2015). Anatomical basis for safe and effective volumization of the temple. *Dermatol Surg.*, *41*(suppl 1), s278–s283.

Carruthers, J., Humphrey, S., Beleznay, K., & Carruthers, A. (2017). Suggested injection zone for soft tissue fillers in the temple? *Dermatol Surg.*, *43*(5), 756–757.

Carruthers, J., Jones, D., Hardas, B., et al. (2016). Development and validation of a photonumeric scale for evaluation of volume deficit of the temple. *Dermatol Surg.*, *42*(suppl 1), S203–S210.

Cotofana, S., Gaete, A., Hernandez, C. A., et al. (2020). The six different injection techniques for the temple relevant for soft tissue filler augmentation procedures—clinical anatomy and danger zones. *J Cosmet Dermatol.*, *19*(7), 1570–1579.

Gause, T. M., 2nd, Kling, R. E., Sivak, W. N., Marra, K. G., Rubin, J. P., & Kokai, L. E. (2014). Particle size in fat graft retention: a review on the impact of harvesting technique in lipofilling surgical outcomes. *Adipocyte.*, *3*(4), 273–279.

Jones, D. H., Fitzgerald, R., Cox, S. E., et al. (2021). Preventing and treating adverse events of injectable fillers: evidence-based recommendations from the American Society for Dermatologic Surgery Multidisciplinary Task Force. *Dermatol Surg.*, *47*(2), 214–226.

Jung, W., Youn, K. H., Won, S. Y., Park, J. T., Hu, K. S., & Kim, H. J. (2014). Clinical implications of the middle temporal vein with regard to temporal fossa augmentation. *Dermatol Surg.*, *40*(6), 618–623.

Kapoor, K. M., Bertossi, D., Li, C. Q., Saputra, D. I., Heydenrych, I., & Yavuzer, R. (2020). A systematic literature review of the middle temporal vein anatomy: 'venous danger zone' in temporal fossa for filler injections. *Aesthetic Plast Surg.*, *44*(5), 1803–1810.

Lambros, V. (2011). A technique for filling the temples with highly diluted hyaluronic acid: the "dilution solution". *Aesthet Surg J.*, *31*(1), 89–94.

Moradi, A., Lin, X., Allen, S., Fagien, S., Norberg, M., & Smith, S. (2020). Validation of photonumeric assessment scales for temple volume deficit, infraorbital hollows, and chin retrusion. *Dermatol Surg.*, *46*(9), 1148–1154.

Moradi, A., Shirazi, A., & Perez, V. (2011). A guide to temporal fossa augmentation with small gel particle hyaluronic acid dermal filler. *J Drugs Dermatol.*, *10*(6), 673–676.

Othman, S., Cohn, J. E., Burdett, J., Daggumati, S., & Bloom, J. D. (2020). Temporal augmentation: a systematic review. *Facial Plast Surg.*, *36*(3), 217–225.

Rose, A. E., & Day, D. (2013). Esthetic rejuvenation of the temple. *Clin Plast Surg.*, *40*(1), 77–89.

Sykes, J. M., Cotofana, S., Trevidic, P., et al. (2015). Upper face: clinical anatomy and regional approaches with injectable fillers. *Plast Reconstr Surg.*, *136*(5 suppl), 204s–218s.

Szczerkowska-Dobosz, A., Olszewska, B., Lemanska, M., Purzycka-Bohdan, D., & Nowicki, R. (2015). Acquired facial lipoatrophy: pathogenesis and therapeutic options. *Postepy Dermatol Alergol.*, *32*(2), 127–133.

Wollina, U., & Goldman, A. (2020). Facial vascular danger zones for filler injections. *Dermatol Ther.*, *33*(6), e14285.

Yang, H. M., Jung, W., Won, S. Y., Youn, K. H., Hu, K. S., & Kim, H. J. (2015). Anatomical study of medial zygomaticotemporal vein and its clinical implication regarding the injectable treatments. *Surg Radiol Anat.*, *37*(2), 175–180.

18

Three-Dimensional Reflation of the Glabella and Adjacent Forehead

Sara Hogan, Jean Carruthers, and Alastair Carruthers

SUMMARY AND KEY FEATURES

- Soft tissue fillers are employed to restore lost frontal volume and lift the brow.
- The forehead is a high-risk location for complications from soft tissue filler injection. A detailed knowledge of the underlying neurovascular anatomy is essential to effective and safe treatment.
- Informed consent must include discussion of the potential for both superficial and deep vascular occlusion and its management.

INTRODUCTION

The arc of the forehead denotes youth and has been considered a sign of beauty since the Middle Ages. This contour is created by both forehead skin thickness and subcutaneous volume. Age brings about deflation and descent of soft tissue. This process begins earlier in women (i.e., 25 years) than in men (i.e., 45 years). Similar changes also affect the brow, glabella, and orbit, particularly the lateral orbicularis oculi. The result is flattened brows, furrowed glabellar and forehead skin, hooded upper eyelids, and a tired or discouraged expression (Fig. 18.1). Both women and men wish to eliminate this disempowered appearance. As such, the forehead and brow are an important focus of facial aging.

Botulinum toxin A (BoNT-A) alone may not be enough for the treatment of the aging forehead, especially in settings where treatment of the frontalis muscle results in further flattening and descent of the brow. Such brow ptosis produces a flat, uncaring, and rather wooden lack of forehead expression. The addition of intradermal hyaluronic acid (HA) fillers to BoNT-A to support glabella lines has been, for many years, typically successful. But this combination does not fully address age-related changes to forehead contour. An acceptable alternative, detailed in this chapter, is the deeper injection of soft tissue filler to restore forehead shape and a relaxed, open expression.

FAT COMPARTMENT ANATOMY

Our understanding of the fat compartments of the forehead was recently improved through anatomic dissection studies and computed tomography imaging. We now know that there exist three superficial fat compartments subcutaneously and three deep fat compartments deep to the frontalis and superficial to the periosteum. The central superficial fat compartment is continuous with the glabella, contains the prominent central frontal vein often noted clinically, and is bordered on both sides with the supraorbital neurovascular bundles. The two lateral superficial fat compartments contain smaller blood vessels and laterally abut temporal ligament adhesions. The central deep fat compartment is flanked on both sides by the supratrochlear neurovascular bundles. Soft tissue filler volumization is best achieved by injection within the forehead fat compartments boundaries, which are defined by fibrous ligament adhesions.

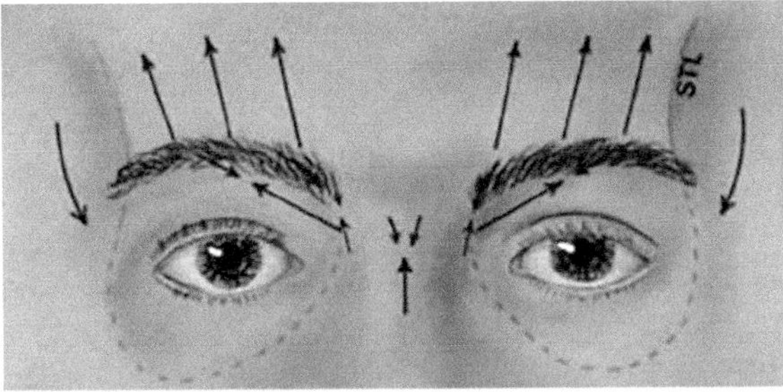

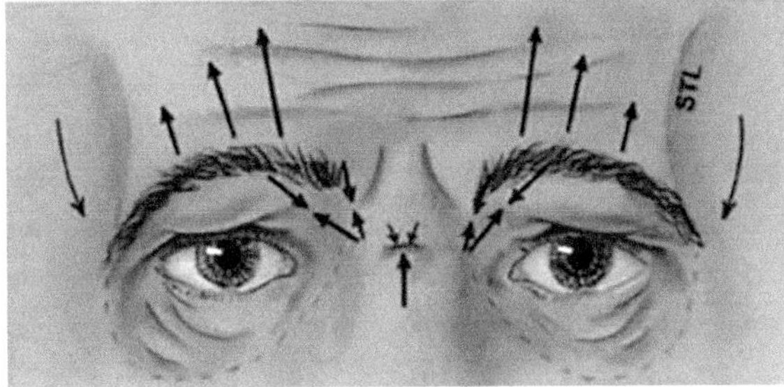

Fig. 18.1 The aging glabella and forehead.

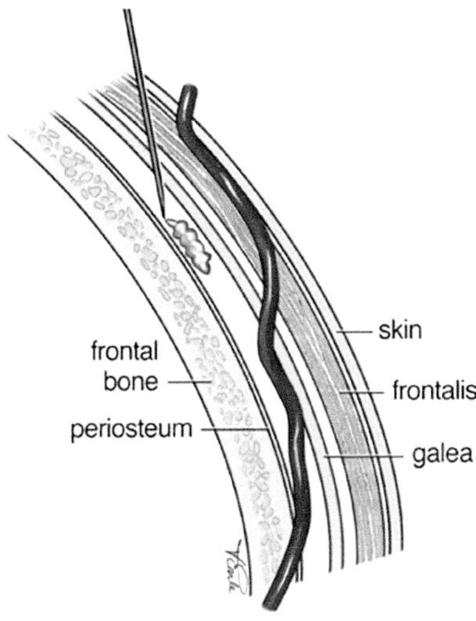

Fig. 18.2 Soft tissue filler injection plane for forehead volumization.

VASCULAR ANATOMY

The vascular anatomy of the forehead is complex and varies not only between individuals but also between halves of the face. The supratrochlear, supraorbital, and dorsal nasal arteries, all distal branches of the ophthalmic artery, provide vascular supply to the forehead.

The glabella is the nexus of the angular, formed from the terminal branch of the facial artery, and dorsal nasal vascular networks. The dorsal nasal artery originates from the orbital septum and can branch off to the central forehead artery, which anastomoses with the contralateral forehead central artery in the bottom third of the forehead. The supratrochlear arteries are found 18 to 22 mm lateral to the midline of the glabella and can communicate with the angular artery at the medial orbital rim. The supraorbital arteries exist the orbit at the supraorbital foramen approximately 1 cm lateral to the supratrochlear vessels and often anastomose with the superficial temporal arteries at the lateral orbital rim. The lateral superficial temporal arcades are often easily visible through forehead skin. The supratrochlear and supraorbital arteries are the two vessels most responsible for complications secondary to soft tissue volumization.

Inadvertent soft tissue filler delivery into one of these arteries, with an appropriate amount of pressure, can travel *retrograde* into the ophthalmic circulation. The clinical consequence can be skin necrosis, vision changes, or even blindness. Cerebral infarcts, intracranial hemorrhage, and superior sagittal sinus thrombosis have also been reported.

Given the many variation in vascular branching patterns, it is helpful to understand that there is a relatively vasculature-free zone between the periosteum and the galea. This is known as the forehead glide plane (Fig. 18.2).

EVALUATION

Forehead aging is due to numerous factors, all of which should be considered during patient evaluation. The patient should be evaluated while sitting upright. The position of frontal hairline and density of hair may influence forehead boundaries and arc and should be considered when planning volumization. Forehead height, shape, curvature (e.g., concave vs. convex), and horizontal rhytid number and depth should all be noted. Eyebrow height, shape, and movement should be evaluated to approximate the "true" brow position. The patient should be asked to open and close their eyes and raise their eyebrows to determine frontalis muscle force. Holding the brow in position with a finger while the patient opens their eyes also allows for assessment of between the eyebrow and the eyelid.

Patients should be asked about history of facial surgical procedures (e.g., brow lift, rhinoplasty), as this may increase risk of vascular complication given the possible development of collateral vessels. Patient expectations should be established prior to treatment. Full correction may not be achieved in a single treatment. The patient should be photographed from frontal, 45-degree, and 90-degree views at baseline to capture forehead height and curvature. The patient should be photographed before and after the injection session. Expected side effects include edema, bruising, and focal areas of tenderness or induration. Contour irregularity is a significant consideration that should be discussed with the patient. Full informed consent should also include the discussion of the rare possibility of iatrogenic filler-induced blindness, as well as management should this occur.

INJECTION TECHNIQUES

While different soft tissue fillers may be used to volumize the forehead, the authors prefer to use an HA filler. This is in part due to increased risk of delayed filler migration and granuloma formation seen with other soft tissue fillers.

Prior to injection, the authors mark the vessels to be avoided on the midforehead—supratrochlear and supraorbital vessels. As it is mostly avascular, soft tissue fillers are injected into the subgaleal, preperiosteal, or forehead glide plane (Fig. 18.2). Each 0.5 mL of a 1-ml syringe of HA filler may be diluted with 0.1 mL of 2% lidocaine with epinephrine 1:100,000 mixed with 20 back and forth movements through a double Luer-Lock syringe. An additional 0.4 mL of preserved saline is then added to each 0.5-mL syringe to bring the total volume in each syringe to 1 mL. This is also mixed with 20 back-and-forth movements using the double Luer-Lock.

There are two approaches employed, depending on the patient's anatomy and aesthetic goals.

The first technique involves deposition of a bolus of dilute HA filler in the glabella between the supratrochlear vascular arcades (Fig. 18.3). After injection below the dermis, the syringe plunger is withdrawn to see if any blood regurgitates into the needle hub. Then boluses are placed with slow and gentle anterograde injection and radially fanning technique (Video 18.1). These can be then massaged gently to distribute filler without further needling injections. In the second technique, boluses are injected inferior to the frontal hairline between the supratrochlear, supraorbital, and superficial temporal artery pathways (Fig. 18.4). At this location, the arteries are located superficially in the subcutaneous layer after coursing superiorly from their deep origins near the orbit. The boluses are then massaged into the appropriate concavity (Video 18.2 or 'Reinflation of Forehead'). Ice can be applied immediately following the procedure to reduce transient swelling and redness. It is important to explain to the subjects that for a period of 40 minutes to an hour, the lidocaine in the HA filler will affect the function of the frontalis and the brows may transiently drop.

These approaches may be performed at the same time as filler into intradermal glabellar folds, if needed. The result is softening of the glabellar folds, reflation of the forehead concavities, elevation of the glabella and the brows, and restoration of a relaxed open expression (Fig. 18.5). Importantly, some patients note softening of their horizontal frontalis rhytides without any drop of their brow or reduction in expressivity. Treatment results typically last for at least 10 to 12 months, and associated brow depressor treatment with BoNT-A is helpful in increasing longevity of response.

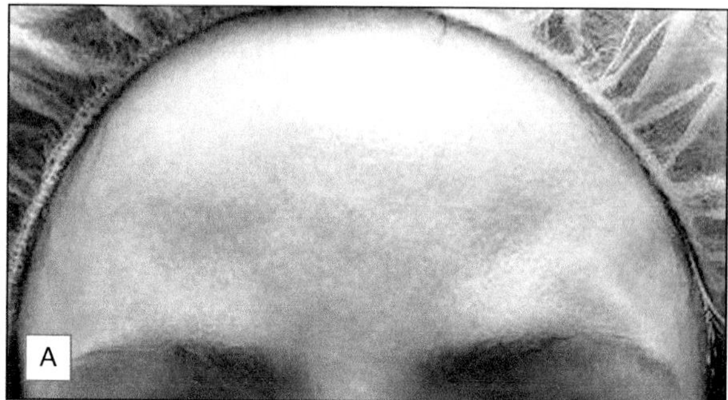

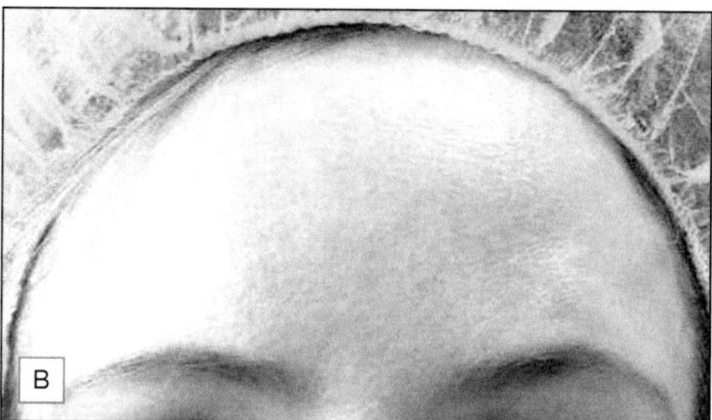

Fig. 18.3 Technique of anterograde subgaleal injection of diluted hyaluronic acid filler into the glide place between periosteum and galea. After the bolus of diluted filler is deposited, gentle upward digital massage distributed the product without further needle injections.

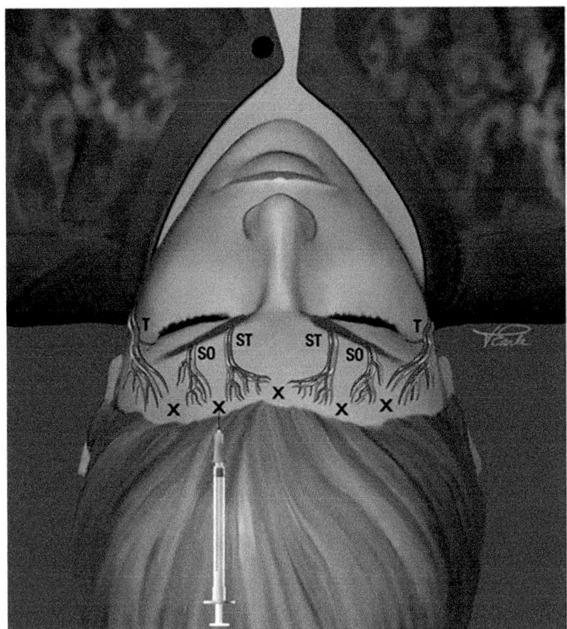

Fig. 18.4 Superior forehead subgaleal injection sites of for volumization. Key: SO = supraorbital; ST = supratrochlear, T = temporal. (From Carruthers JDA, Carruthers JA. Appreciation of the vascular anatomy of aesthetic. *Forehead Reflation Dermatol Surg.* 2018;44:S2–S4.)

CONCLUSION

Soft tissue fillers restore lost frontal volume, produce a lifting effect on the brow and less commonly, soften horizontal forehead rhytids. Three-dimensional filling has reinvented the rejuvenation of the upper face. The resulting brow elevation and continued frontalis action can give the subject back a rested and interested and positive expression, most helpful in all social interaction.

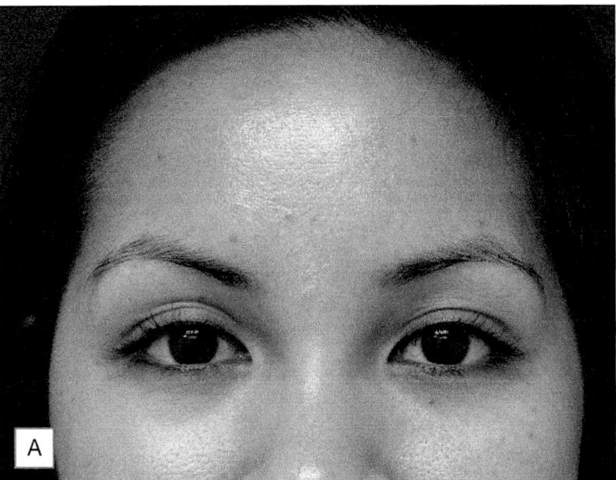

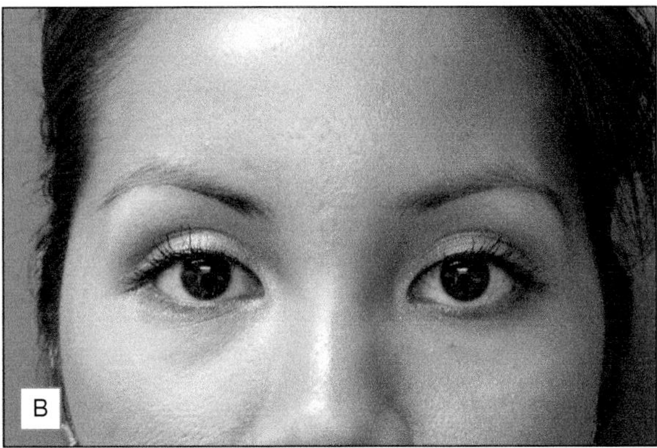

Fig. 18.5 (A) Before and (B) after three-dimensional reinflation of the forehead with injection of hyaluronic acid filler (Juvederm Voluma) to the midbrow.

FURTHER READING

Beleznay, K., Carruthers, J. D. A., & Humphrey, S. (2019). Update on avoiding and treating blindness from fillers: a recent review of the world literature. *Aesthet Surg J.*, *39*(6), 662–674.

Beleznay, K., Carruthers, J. D. A., Humphrey, S., & Jones, D. (2015). Avoiding and treating blindness from fillers: a review of the world literature. *Dermatol Surg.*, *41*, 1097–1117.

Carruthers, J., & Carruthers, A. (2015). Three-dimensional forehead reflation. *Dermatol Surg.*, *41*, S321–S324.

Carruthers, J., & Carruthers, A. (2003). A prospective, randomized, parallel group study analyzing the effect of BTX-A (Botox) and nonanimal sourced hyaluronic acid (NASHA, Restylane) in combination compared with NASHA (Restylane) alone in severe glabellar rhytides in adult female subjects: treatment of severe glabellar rhytides with a hyaluronic acid derivative compared with the derivative BTX-A. *Dermatol Surg.*, *29*, 802–809.

Carruthers, J. D. A., & Carruthers, J. A. (2010). Volumizing the glabella and forehead. *Dermatol Surg.*, *36*, 1905–1909.

Carruthers, J. D. A., & Carruthers, J. A. (2018). Appreciation of the vascular anatomy of aesthetic. *Forehead Reflation Dermatol Surg.*, *44*, S2–S4.

Carruthers, J. D. A., & Carruthers, J. A. (2018). Appreciation of the anatomy of aesthetic forehead reflation. *Dermatol Surg.*, *44*, S2–S4.

Carruthers, J. D. A., Fagien, S., Rohrich, R., Weinkle, S., & Carruthers, A. (2014). Blindness caused by cosmetic filler injection. *Plast Reconstr Surg.*, *134*(6), 1197–1201.

Coleman, S. R., & Grover, R. (2006). The anatomy of the aging face: volume loss and changes in 3-dimensional topography. *Aesthetic Surg J.*, *26*(suppl), S4–S9.

Cotofana, S., Mian, A., & Sykes, J. M. (2017). Update on the anatomy of the forehead compartments. *Plast Reconstr Surg.*, *139*, 864e.

Kleintjes, W. G. (2007). Forehead anatomy: arterial variations and venous link of the midline forehead flap. *J Plast Reconstr Aesthet Surg.*, *60*(6), 593–606.

Knize, D. M. (2009). Anatomic concepts for brow lift procedures. *Plast Reconst Surg.*, *124*(6), 2118–2126.

Langelier, N., Beleznay, K., & Woodward, J. (2016). Rejuvenation of the upper face and periocular region. *Dermatol Surg.*, *42*(suppl 2), S77–S82.

Paik, J. S., Wk, Cho, Park, G. S., et al. (2013). Eyelid-associated complications after autogenous fat injection for cosmetic forehead augmentation. *BMC Ophthalmol.*, *13*, 325.

Pao, S., Lin, S. M., & Chang, Y. H. (2016). Upper eyelid granuloma: a rare delayed-onset complication secondary to cosmetic filler injection on forehead. *Int Med Case Rep J.*, *9*, 155–157.

Park, Y. R., Choi, J. A., & La, Y. T. (2013). Periorbital lipogranuloma after cryopreserved autologous fat injection at forehead: unexpected complication of a popular cosmetic procedure. *Can J Ophthalmol.*, *48*, 6.

Prevot, M., Thomet, C., Cornette, T. B., et al. (2017). Forehead rejuvenation. *Ann Aesthet Plast Surg.*, *62*(5), 406–423.

Ramanadhan, S., & Rohrich, R. (2015). Newer understanding of specific anatomic targets in the aging face as applied to injectables: superficial and deep fat compartments—an evolving target for site-specific facial augmentation. *Plast Reconstr Surg.*, *136*, 49s–55s.

Richard, M. J., Morris, C., Deen, B. F., Gray, L., & Woodward, J. A. (2009). Analysis of the anatomic changes of the aging facial skeleton using computer-assisted tomography. *Ophthal Plast Reconstr Surg.*, *25*, 382–386.

Shaw, R. B., Jr., Katzel, E. B., Koltz, P. F., et al. (2011). Aging of the facial skeleton: aesthetic implications and rejuvenation strategies. *Plast Reconstr Surg.*, *127*(1), 374–383.

Sykes, J. M., Cotofana, S., & Trevidic, P. (2015). Upper face: clinical anatomy and regional approaches with injectable fillers. *Plast Reconstruct Surg.*, (November Supplement), 204S–218S.

Wong, C., & Medelson, B. (2015). Newer understanding of specific anatomic targets in the aging face as applied to injectables: aging changes in the craniofacial skeleton and facial ligaments. *Plast Reconstr Surg.*, *136*, 44s–48s.

Yao, B., Shen, F., Zhao, X., et al. (2019). Ophthalmic artery occlusion combined with superior sagittal sinus thrombosis caused by hyaluronic acid injection for facial soft tissue augmentation: a case report. *Medicine (Baltimore).*, *98*(36), e17048.

19

Volumetric Treatment of the Brows

Val Lambros

SUMMARY AND KEY FEATURES

- Orbits that are large, round, and hollow are associated with age, not youth.
- Young orbits are almond shaped, the bone is not visible, and there may be considerable fullness of the upper lid.
- The same configurations that are seen in younger patients may be perceived as looking old in older ones.
- Communication is difficult in the periorbital area. Many patients want the eye "lifted" or skin and fat removed because that is what they have been told is done. Moreover, some patients like the hollow and defined look because it may look more dramatic and makeup can be used more liberally.
- The author prefers using a trial of local anesthetic in the upper lid to demonstrate the visual effect of filling in the upper lids and brow. If the patient likes the look, the injection is performed immediately; there is no need to wait. Local anesthetic provides a vasoconstricted environment. There is no better way of communicating the visual effect of the brow fill.
- Putting in the local anesthetic and avoiding overfills and fluid blobs in the upper lid are difficult to do well and easily; some practice is involved. The area is massaged, and a few minutes should elapse to let the local anesthetic distribute before showing the patient.
- Underfill is better than overfill. This is not a method to fill in an abundance of skin, although the fill does inflate some skin. Nor is it a method to lift brows, although the brow can elevate in a few patients. Someone with full heavy lids is not a candidate for this procedure.
- The author favors hyaluronic acid (HA) products in the brow because they have more projection.
- One should expect at least 2 years' duration in this location with HA products.
- The injector should always be aware of the presence of the globe. Some upper orbits are very shallow, and the globe is immediately adjacent to the bone.

INTRODUCTION

Thinning, deflation, and loss of subcutaneous volume are characteristic of periorbital aging. Although by no means universal, and seen largely in people who have not gained facial weight, this pattern of aging has been known through the ages and is frequently used as a caricature of the aging process. The term "nursing home eyes" provides an instant visual image of the problem.

Traditional treatments around the upper lid have been largely surgical, mainly because until recently the only tools available were excisional. "Extra" skin and fat around the upper lid were removed; for many eyes, this proved to be an entirely satisfactory remedy. However, for some patients, the apparent extra skin was secondary to a volume loss in the upper lid and brow, and removing further tissue had the dual effect of making the orbit look more defined but rounder and more hollow. Both of these have traditionally been considered beneficial. The perceived advantage of this look is that the orbit looks larger and dramatic in the vertical dimension and leaves more room for makeup. It is also the traditional look of upper lid "rejuvenation" and familiar. However, these are also characteristics of the nursing home eye, and in some people the overall appearance of the eye is clearly older, smaller, and more tired. With the advent of tools to reestablish volume in the face, alternatives have become available, which the patient (and clinician) should be aware of before making treatment decisions in the periorbital area.

There is nothing new in these observations. Volume fillers were used exactly as they are now in the 1890s, well before facelift surgery was developed. Unfortunately, all that was available at the time was paraffin and petroleum jelly (Vaseline); the complication rate was high, and these treatments fell into disfavor, as described by Kolle and by Goldwyn.

THE "LOCAL PREVIEW"

Patients usually have their own predetermined ideas about what looks good. If one has a choice of filling an area or defining it by removing tissue, the different potential effects must somehow be communicated to the patient. In other words, an adequate consultation should be able to explain the aesthetic alternatives to the patient. We have found no way in words to describe how the effects of filling the brow will improve the patient's overall look; this is entirely a visual concept. It is like trying to describe a dress and assuming that the customer will like it without trying it on.

What has proven extremely useful is the "local preview," as (VL) have described (2009); 1 cc or two of 1/4% lidocaine with epinephrine is injected into the brow with the intention of visualizing the effect of filling the area and also to make it numb and vasoconstricted (Fig. 19.1). With the use of an ice cube for the initial injections, this is almost painless.

Filling the brow with local anesthetic in a realistic way is not easy but is good practice for the final injection. The tendency for inexperienced injectors is to place the needle superficially and make individual lumps of fluid. This is convincing of nothing. The correct plane is around the orbicularis muscle or deeper, and the needle must be withdrawn on injection, leaving a horizontal and even flow of local anesthetic. This is performed across the brow, trying to anticipate the final intended result. The area is massaged a little. After a few minutes the product has diffused enough to demonstrate the intended look.

We tell patients that what they see is approximately 80% accurate as to the final result. Most people, if correctly selected, like the look and say that it "opens their eyes." This is perceptually interesting because in reality the orbit is being narrowed. In addition to the demonstrative ability of the preview, the area is now vasoconstricted, making the possibility of an intravascular injection smaller. Strictly speaking, brow filling could be performed with topical anesthetic or none at all, but the communicative power of the preview is invaluable—patients determine whether they like the look before the clinician does anything definitive. The latter can also see whether he or she likes the effect. Because patients have seen the results of the injection and approved it before

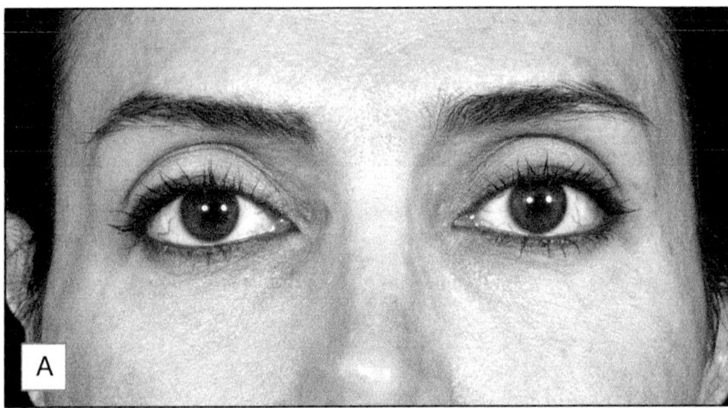

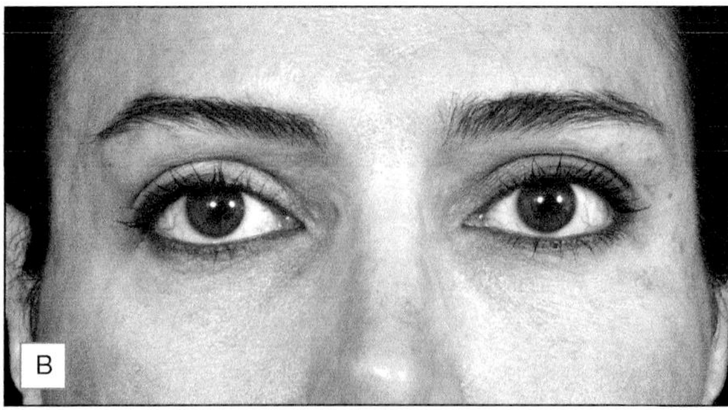

Fig. 19.1 The "local preview." It is difficult to communicate the visual effects of volume around the orbit without actually seeing it. An invaluable way of doing this is to inject the area with local anesthetic, which demonstrates the effect of fill and numbs and vasoconstricts the area at the same time. Patients approve or disapprove of the visual effect before any product is injected. It usually takes more fill—approximately 1/2 to 1 mL per side—than the actual product injection. The long-term result looks like the result at the end of the procedure and typically lasts 2 to 3 years. (A) Before and (B) after injection.

the product injection, no one in my experience has asked to have product removed. If they do not like the look of the preview, then nothing further is performed; no product has been injected, and other alternatives can be explored. Patients love the idea that they can see the results before a procedure is performed and embrace the concept enthusiastically.

> **PEARL 1** There is a population of patients who have anxious-looking eyes with level brows. These patients do not have a well-developed medial upper lid crease, or it is absent. Restoring this crease makes the eyes look much more normal and less anxiety projecting.

> **PEARL 2** There are patients with small excesses of lid skin that get used up by increasing the volume of the brow down to the orbital rim.

> **PEARL 3** The anterior orbital rim can be pushed forward in some eyes, hiding the upper lid crease and making the eye look less bulgy.

THE INJECTION

At the time of writing, hyaluronic acid (HA) products, calcium-based products, and poly-L-lactic acid are available. I use only HA fillers outside of the operating room, where I may use autologous fat. They are easy to use and can be removed with hyaluronidase if necessary. The duration of HA products in the brow and tear trough is 2 to 3 years, equal to or greater than other available products. To my mind there is no advantage to using products other than HAs in the periorbital region.

> **PEARL 4** The author does not favor using non-HA injectable fillers here. The duration of other products is greatly exaggerated and cannot be reversed. The author quotes patients' duration of 2 years but has seen HAs last up to 4 years in the periorbital area.

This is not an area for novice injectors. If the clinician has performed only lips and nasolabial folds and injects them with bolus injections and massage, the upper lid will be a source of disappointment and complications, some of them potentially catastrophic. Although not difficult for experienced injectors, technique in the upper lid is important. The goal is to create a pleasing shape across the brow, not just to fill a hollow. The depth of this injection should be around the level of the orbicularis muscle. There are very large immobile arteries at the periosteal level that one should avoid. Injection into the sulcus of the upper lid may result in ptosis, as described by Coleman. Keeping the plane of injection superficial to the bone also keeps the needle farther away from the globe, as mentioned further in the chapter.

I begin the injection at the conclusion of the local preview after the patient has approved the look. The area is now vasoconstricted and numb. The presence of the anesthetic in no way alters the ability to distribute the product evenly, which is performed partially visually and partially by feel. Although I cannot prove it, I believe that HAs distribute more evenly in a very wet environment.

As illustrated in Fig. 19.2, my preferred technique is to begin laterally and place three fanning longitudinal

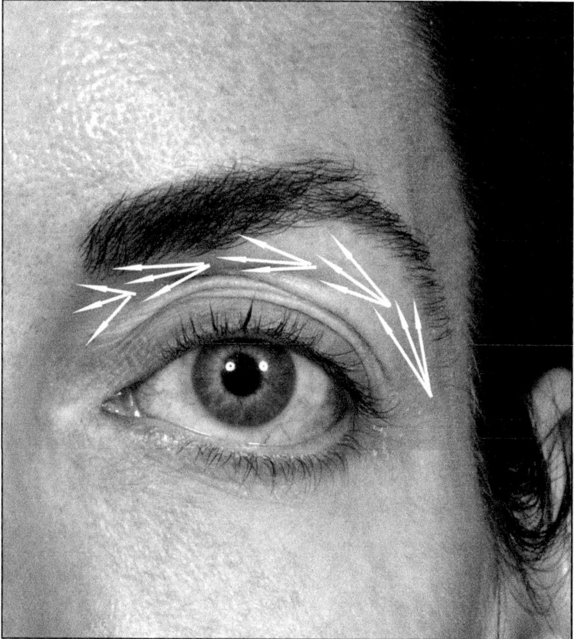

Fig. 19.2 Author's injection technique: after the area is numb and vasoconstricted, I use three passes from each injection site—high, medium, and low. The injection is repeated across the brow and repeated if necessary. The presence of local anesthetic in no way alters the ability of the injector to visualize the results.

fills with a 30-g 1/2-inch (6-mm) needle: high, middle, and low. The process is repeated across the brow. Tiny amounts are placed with each pass. If the thumb moves perceptibly, then the volume is excessive. A small needle like the 30-g 1/2-inch one is protective in avoiding overfills. Palpation is an excellent way to determine the evenness of the injection. Typically, the injection should not go inferior to the border of the orbital bone laterally and centrally. Unless one is confident of the intention and results, it is very easy to create irregularities or worse here. The expansion of the curve of the orbital bone suffices to improve the hollow of all but the most deep-set and hollow orbits. As one proceeds medially, the injection might need to drop inferior to the level of the bone somewhat. Usually, 1/2 mL per side is injected. For economic reasons, this seems a good place to start, and indeed most brows and the expressive qualities of the face are improvable by even this small amount, even if undercorrected. I am always amazed by the ability of such a small amount of filler to create as much difference as it does. With experience, it is obvious where the product needs to be placed.

PEARL 5 The author favors making small radial passes in the brow from lateral to medial, deep to the orbicularis muscle but superficial to the bone. Three passes—high, middle, and low—are usually sufficient to make the brow fill in an even manner. The injection point is then walked across the brow.

PEARL 6 A half milliliter of product per side creates a convincing but slightly undercorrected result. Patients can be made to look astonishingly odd by overdoing the injections.

The injection should not be overdone. More is not better. The patient is given an ice pack to use later in the day. Bruising is occasional. There is not much swelling, although there is some. Usual complications are minor and are usually related to irregularities that can be dissolved or added to. In general, the appearance at the end of the injection is the final result.

INTRAARTERIAL INJECTION

Injections are by and large innocuous and low risk. However, the specter of intraarterial injection is ever present although fortunately uncommon. For this to occur, the needle tip must be in an artery and a bolus of sufficient size injected to cause upstream flow, as blindness from a periocular injection, or distal embolization, as in a lip or nasal necrosis from injection into the nasolabial fold, as described by Coleman. These are excellent arguments for not doing bolus injections. We favor threading injections, always keeping the tip of the needle moving with small low-pressure flows and vasoconstriction. We believe that this complication is largely technical and avoidable.

Some orbits are flat superiorly, without an upper lid sulcus. In orbits like these, the globe is immediately adjacent to the orbital rim, and there is a distinct possibility of a direct needle injury. We have never seen this complication, but it is easy to see how it could happen. The clinician must focus on the position of the globe and needle tip. Keeping the tip of the needle away from the orbital bone will also keep it away from the globe. We are uncertain of the use of blunt cannulas here. Although they are blunt, they are also long and whippy and could easily track subcutaneously and wind up in unexpected places.

WHO IS A CANDIDATE FOR BROW VOLUME TREATMENTS?

Unlike the lip or nasolabial fold, one cannot rely on formula or dogma to treat the brow. Although some brows may have been fuller when younger, the look of the eye might be worse on restoring or amplifying the brow volume. There are configurations that lend themselves to this treatment and configurations that are made worse by adding volume. In general, except for some Asian eyelids, full upper lids are not made better by additional filling. Very hollow eyes are made only modestly better. As mentioned by Mancini et al., there is concern that injection into the actual sulcus may cause a space-occupying ptosis.

PEARL 7 This is not a technique that all eyes need. Experience will show which eyes improve.

Brows that have deflated evenly (Figs. 19.3 to 19.5) and brows in which the medial supraorbital crease peaks medially are excellent candidates. This latter group is interesting in that a medial peak of the

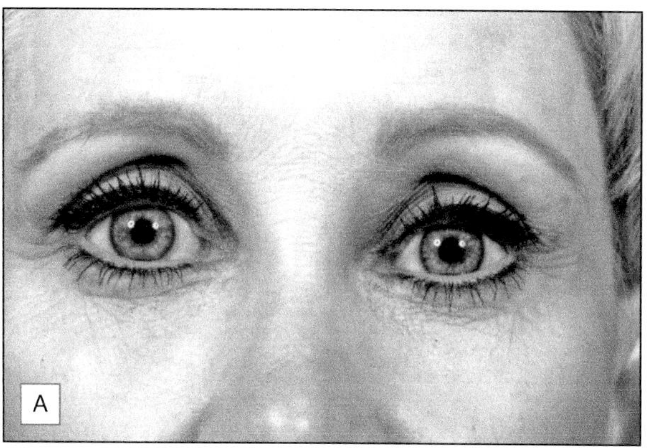

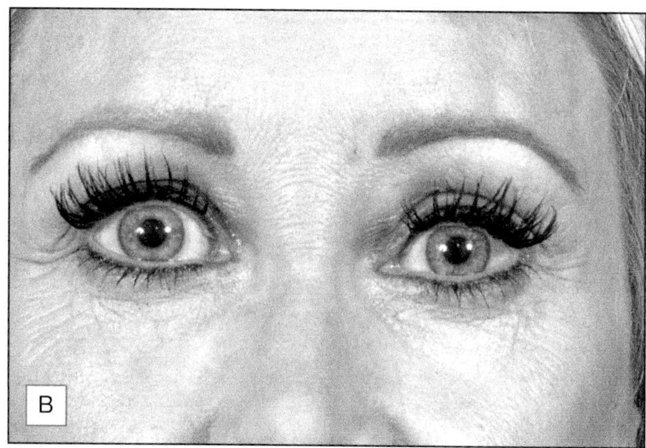

Fig. 19.3 (A) A 56-year-old patient seen in 2009, (B) for whom 1/2 mL Restylane was injected into each brow. The patient returned in 2016 reporting no further surgery or injections into her brows, although she has had lip fillers. This is the most longevity I have seen with hyaluronic acid fillers in this location. Like the temples and tear troughs, 2 years is usual and 4 years is common, but a 7-year duration is remarkable. The product could be palpated, as well as seen. Note the appearance of anxiety in the preinjection image, which is gone post injection. (Photo courtesy of V. Lambros, MD.)

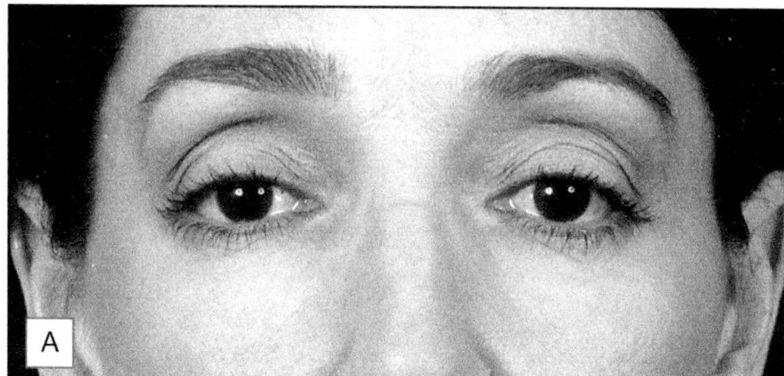

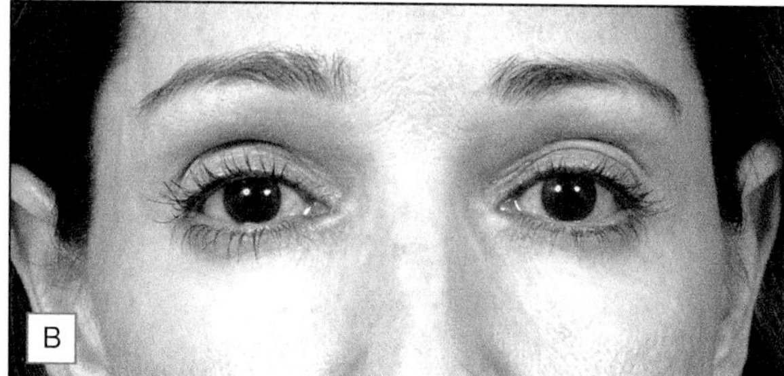

Fig. 19.4 (A) A 58-year-old patient with hollow superior orbit, (B) seen 3 years after brow injection 1 mL per side. The temples were also filled 6 months previously.

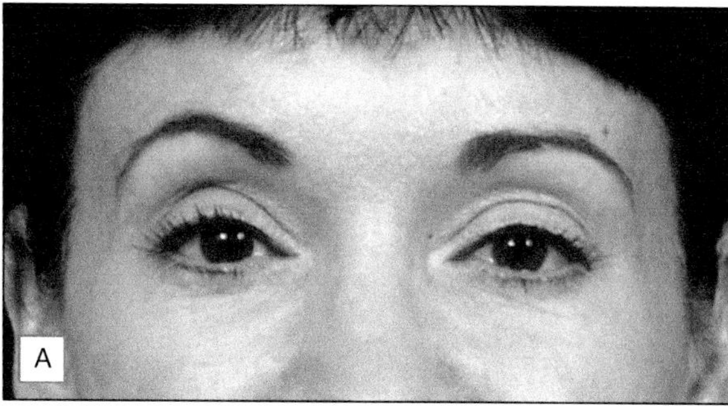

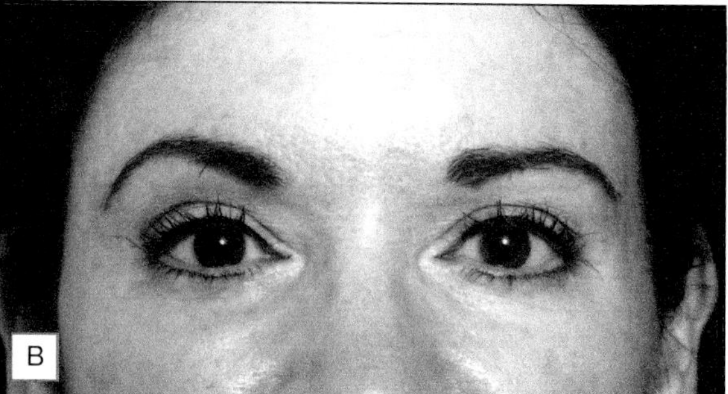

Fig. 19.5 (A) A 68-year-old patient with hollow brows, (B) 3 years after 1 mL hyaluronic acid filler was placed in each brow.

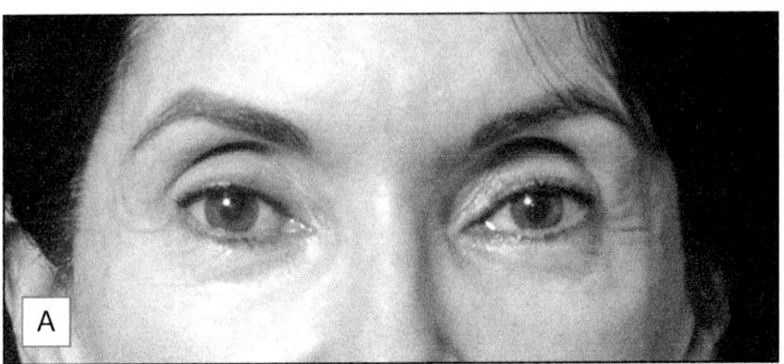

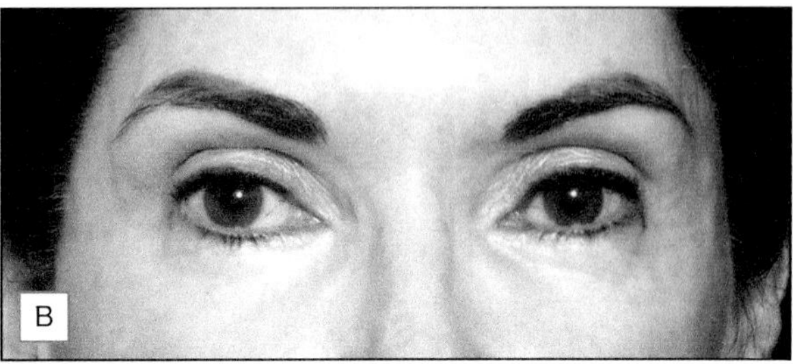

Fig. 19.6 (A) A 54-year-old patient with very hollow and anxious eyes, (B) seen here 3 years after 1 mL HA filler per side and 10 months after a fill of her temples 2 mL per side with diluted HA fillers.

supraorbital crease gives people a look of anxiety or worry. A very small amount of filler in this location alters the emotional projection of the face (Fig. 19.6). Although actual elevation of the brows of a millimeter or two is sometimes seen with injection, we believe that the impression of elevation is largely illusory, based on greater light reflection from the now-filled and rounder brow. In any event, trying to lift brows with volume may provide a slight elevation at the cost of an unnaturally overfilled eye.

The point with these treatments is not necessarily to make the orbit fuller; rather it is to make the periorbital area look better, and if one does not have at least a rudimentary appreciation for what looks good on the face, one will have limited success in treating the area.

FURTHER READING

Coleman, S. R. (2006). Hyaluronic acid fillers. *Plastic Reconstructive Surgery, 117*(2), 661–665.

Goldwyn, R. M. (1980). The paraffin story. *Plastic Reconstructive Surgery, 65*(4), 517–524.

Kolle, F. S. (1911). *Plastic and Cosmetic Surgery*. New York: Appleton.

Lambros, V. S. (2007). Observations on periorbital and midface aging. *Plastic Reconstructive Surgery, 120*(5), 1367–1376. discussion 1377.

Lambros, V. (2009). Volumizing the brows with HA fillers. *Aesthetic Surgery Journal, 29*, 177–179.

Mancini, R., Taban, M., Lowinger, A., et al. (2009). Use of hyaluronic acid gel in the management of paralytic lagophthalmos: the hyaluronic acid gel 'gold weight'. *Ophthalmic Plastic Reconstructive Surgery, 25*(1), 23–26.

20

Infraorbital Hollow and Nasojugal Fold

Femida Kherani and Allison Sutton

SUMMARY AND KEY FEATURES

- The infraorbital hollow (IOH) refers clinically to the curvilinear depression below the eyes and comprises the tear trough, nasojugal fold, and palpebromalar groove.
- With thin skin overlying bone and little to no subcutaneous fat in this region, the IOH can be an unforgiving region and challenging to treat with injectable agents.
- Periocular filler injections yield better outcomes in patients with thicker, smoother skin with a well-defined tear trough, minimal prolapsing lower eyelid fat, and minimal lower eyelid laxity.
- Hyaluronic acid (HA) is currently the injectable agent treatment of choice for IOHs and lower eyelid and periorbital enhancement.
- Meticulous injection with small volumes, reduced injection speed, supraperiosteal placement, and minimal number of injection sites may reduce complications.
- Some patients are not suited for fillers alone and require adjuvant therapy or surgery for periorbital rejuvenation.

INTRODUCTION

The eyes are the primary focal point of the face, playing important roles in conveying emotion and our perception of beauty. As the face ages, changes to the infraorbital region occur, negatively affecting our perception of beauty and potentially evoking emotions of sadness and fatigue. Consequently, periocular rejuvenation is a frequent patient request for aesthetic improvement.

The infraorbital hollow (IOH) refers to the curvilinear or U-shaped depression under the eyes from the nasal bone to the outer corner of the eye and comprises three core elements: the "tear trough" and "nasojugal fold" medially and the palpebromalar groove laterally (Fig. 20.1). The terms "tear trough" and "nasojugal fold" have historically been used interchangeably. The tear trough occurs mildly in all people across all ages and refers to the superior aspect of the nasojugal fold. A sign of early aging, the deepening of the tear trough leads to a true indentation at the junction of the thin eyelid skin above and thicker skin of the cheek below. Later, the midcheek may descend, accentuating a flat or hollow crescent below the eye and lengthening of the lower eyelid. The appearance of hollows and dark circles under the eye is the interplay of various factors. Genetics, habits and environmental exposures lead to dyschromias and pigmentation changes, soft tissue laxity, subcutaneous volume alterations, changes in bone, and redistribution of superficial fat; all of which contribute to shadowed contours and deepening folds. Periorbital volumetric shifting and loss is not an isolated event but part of a global shift in the contours of the aging face.

There is minimal fat below the lower eyelid. The orbicularis oculi muscle has direct bony attachments to the orbital rim, from the nasal bone to the medial limbus. Laterally, orbicularis-retaining ligaments connect

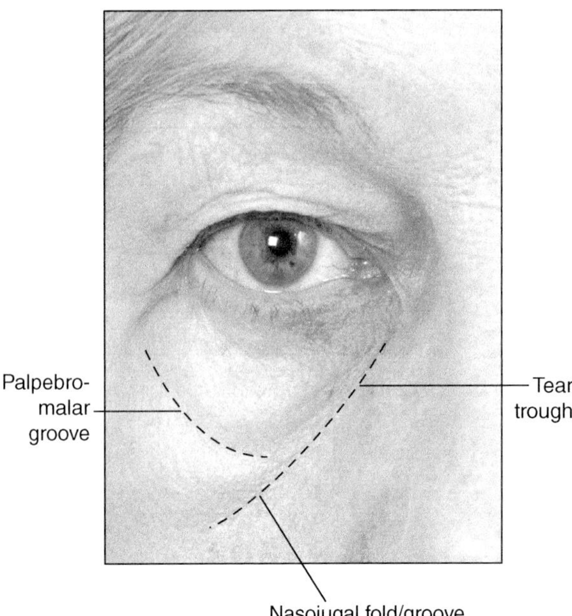

Fig. 20.1 Anatomy of the infraorbital hollow

the deep surface of the skin to bone. Retaining ligaments weaken, facial bones recede, and volume decreases in the deep fat pads, causing the cheek to descend and superficial fat to prolapse below the eye, all of which combine with genetically predisposed discolorations and bony changes to contribute to the perception of hollowed and sometimes baggy eyes, deep and shadowed tear troughs, and an aged, fatigued appearance refractory to cosmetic attempts at concealment.

Treatment of the periorbital area with injectable agents allows little room for error. Optimal outcomes require careful patient selection, discriminating choice of filling agent, and precise techniques to avoid complications.

CANDIDATES FOR AUGMENTATION OF THE INFRAORBITAL HOLLOW

Appropriate patient selection is critical and relies on careful medical and ophthalmic history and physical assessment. Poor candidates are unlikely to obtain optimal results, may not be satisfied with results, and are at higher risk of side effects such as visibility and irregularity (Table 20.1). Patients with diseases or metabolic conditions that predispose to lower eyelid irregularity, bleeding, and infection should be excluded. All

TABLE 20.1 Identifying Candidates for Augmentation of the Infraorbital Hollow

Best candidates	Poor candidates
Young patients with good skin elasticity	Elderly patients with poor skin elasticity
Thick smooth skin	Very thin skin
Good skin tone	Transparent or dyspigmented skin
Minimal laxity	Significant skin laxity
Mild to moderate tear troughs	Extremely deep tear troughs

anticoagulant medications and supplements should ideally be discontinued if medically appropriate. Some patients have genetically determined pigmentation that may appear like a tear trough but without an indentation that can be filled. Pigmented dark lower eyelid circles cannot be improved by fillers and can indeed be worsened by treatment. Older patients with thinner, crepelike, inelastic skin and individuals with preexisting malar edema—whether metabolic (thyroid disease) or otherwise (chronic sinus disease, prior surgery, etc.)—may not respond well and also have an increased risk for adverse events and dissatisfaction with results. It is prudent to identify the ideal candidate for periorbital fillers in consultation. Patients with orbital fat herniation and significant skin laxity would benefit first from lower lid blepharoplasty with possible midface lift or other adjuvant procedures. Injection works best in patients with thick and smooth skin with a well-defined tear trough or defined maxillary retrusion or hypoplasia (commonly noted in young Asian females), without excessive prolapsed eyelid fat or excess eyelid skin. Lower eyelids should be evaluated for orbicularis hypertrophy, eyelid laxity and prolapsed orbital fat (Table 20.2).

APPROPRIATE FILLING AGENTS

Thin skin directly overlying bone with ligamentous attachments allow any irregularity to be readily visible. Furthermore, the periocular treatment area is highly vascularized and maintains a high propensity for discoloration. The ideal filler is one with a low extrusion force or density to allow precise and delicate injection through lower-gauged needles or cannulas, and is reversible or, at the very least, biodegradable. Because

TABLE 20.2 **Anatomical Characteristics and Treatment Considerations**

Image	Diagnosis	Treatment considerations
	Pretarsal orbicularis oculi hypertrophy	Can be treated with neuromodulators
	Skin hyperpigmentation	May be due to various causes. If a tear trough depression and hyperpigmentation coexist, it is reasonable to treat with HA filler.
	Laxity/skin wrinkles	Best results for fillers are with skin that is firm and thick although HA fillers may improve this to a degree.
	Fat pad prolapse	HA filler may help but it is important to consider surgical correction
	Lower eyelid and/or malar edema	HA could aggravate this due to its hydrophilicity as well as possible compression of lymphatic structures

HA, Hyaluronic acid.

there is a tendency for anything injected into this area to form visible lumps, particularly on facial animation, permanent fillers should be considered only with great caution. In fact, the eye muscles are the most active muscles in the body and consequently, fillers placed in this dynamic area have to seamlessly integrate and withstand the muscle movements.

Hyaluronic acid (HA)—with its gel consistency, varying concentrations and the possibility of dilution, favorable flow characteristics, fewer side effects, and nonpermanence—has emerged as the treatment of choice by many aesthetic physicians for periocular rejuvenation. Lumps or irregularities can be avoided with careful and precise injection techniques and can also be easily reversed with hyaluronidase injection, which is an important consideration when injecting in delicate areas requiring the most precise placement of fillers. Surprisingly, HA fillers in the periorbital region yield better than expected longevity. Lambros (and others) has described the persistence of effect, often in excess of 1 year. Donath et al. used three-dimensional imaging in 20 patients treated in the tear trough with HA and found an average 85% maintenance of effect at the final follow-up visit (average 14.4 months); the patient with the longest duration retained 73% volume augmentation at 23 months without any touch-ups. In practice, it is not uncommon to see persistence of HA filler effect for many years after it was originally placed. Common side effects with HA fillers may include nodules, a bluish tint (the Tyndall effect), along with injection- related bruising and swelling (see Complications section later). Additionally, given the proximity to the infraorbital artery, infratrochlear artery, dorsal nasal artery, and angular artery, there is a risk of vascular occlusion and even rarer, injection related visual adverse events.

Calcium hydroxylapatite (CaHA) has yielded positive outcomes in other areas of the face, and Hevia has detailed successful outcomes in the infraorbital region using CaHA diluted by 10% to 30% with 2% lidocaine. However, CaHA has a history of palpable (and sometimes visible) nodules, particularly in the lips, and Goldman has reported a case of superficial nodularity after injection of CaHA in the IOH. Its major drawback remains the lack of reversibility. Despite its biodegradable nature, if an adverse event occurs, there is little to do but wait until the product has naturally resorbed.

AUGMENTATION TECHNIQUES

Techniques for augmentation under the eye vary. Replacing periorbital volume entails not only focusing on specific regions in the IOH requiring augmentation—the tear trough, the central and lateral aspect of the orbital rim, the palpebromalar groove—but also other areas that influence the appearance of the lower eye. A deflated medial cheek, for example, will look unnatural without concurrent augmentation, particularly with animation. Correction of the cheek will sometimes improve the appearance of the IOH, necessitating smaller volumes of filling agent to achieve optimal results. Hill et al. have demonstrated that treatment of the medial cheek alone does not significantly improve the tear trough deficit. Although a small sample size, their study showed that direct treatment of the tear trough with HA had a more profound improvement of the tear trough depth than isolated HA gel volume augmentation of the deep medial cheek. Ideally, periorbital volume augmentation should be performed in conjunction with rejuvenation of the midface and sometimes the entire face to preserve harmony and restore aesthetic proportions. Treatment of the lateral cheek may have a beneficial effect on the tear trough.

Skin Preparation, Anesthetic, and Syringes

Patients are ideally treated sitting in an upright position with the backrest reclined to approximately 80 degrees. Pretreatment photographs should be taken without makeup and with controlled lighting to illuminate the appearance of rhytides, tear trough deformity, and lower lid fat prolapse. Hair is tied back, makeup is removed, and the skin is thoroughly cleansed. Marking of the treatment area is done; the patient is asked to look upward to accentuate and delineate the borders of the tear trough, and areas of planned injection are marked using a marker, including adjacent areas requiring augmentation. The authors often mark the inferior orbital rim from medial to lateral canthus, noting that injections should not occur above this line as that would risk injecting into the retro-orbital space. The location of the infraorbital artery should also be marked and avoided during injections. The infraorbital foramen can be found by running a finger along the inferior orbital rim until a notch is felt. This is often in line with the medial limbus approximately 8 to 11 mm below the inferior orbital rim.

The choice of anesthetic depends on the patient's tolerance and the number of injection sites. Typically, a combination of topical anesthetic and the use of HA agents containing lidocaine provide optimal patient comfort. Direct infiltration or infraorbital nerve blocks are rarely necessary. Use of ice packs, "talkesthesia" and vibration are all helpful tools to distract and minimize pain.

Tools for injection range from 22- to 25-gauge blunt-tipped cannulas to 27- to 32-gauge needles, depending on injector preference, treatment area, and technique used. Larger-bore, blunt tipped cannulas may possibly decrease the risk of inadvertent intravascular injection; however, some injectors believe that needles allow more precise placement of filler material in the periorbital region.

> **PEARL 1** Anatomic areas of concern in the IOH include the infratrochlear artery, infraorbital artery, angular artery, and dorsal nasal artery.

General Techniques

The area is prepped with alcohol or chlorhexidine. Small amounts of filler, generally no more than 1 mL in total for both sides, are injected. Injections are performed under low pressure to minimize complications such as a "sausage roll" appearance under the eye. If 0.2 to 0.4 mL of HA does not lead to a noticeable improvement, it is possible—or even likely—the filler has been misplaced. The objective is to place a confluent deposit of filler material along the orbital rim, beneath the apparent "hollow" without complete volume filling of the agent and allowing the additional physical properties of these filling agents (including hydrophilicity) to augment the overlying soft tissues to reduce the appearance of the "trough" (Video 20.1).

Injections are deep in the suborbicularis oculi plane at or below the orbital rim at the supraperiosteal level except in the medial aspect where the orbicularis oculi attaches to bone and requires direct injection. Superficial injections in the periorbital region increase the risk of visibility and skin discoloration secondary to the Tyndall effect (see Complications section later), although some researchers, such as Hirmand et al., have described the occasional need for a very superficial subdermal injection using a 32-gauge needle for spot application over a 1- to 2-mm surface area to "lift" the overlying skin. The medial aspect of the tear trough extending to the mid pupillary line is the highest risk zone of injection given the vascular anatomy.

Use of the smallest possible gauge but longer needles (i.e., a 1-inch [12-mm] 30-gauge needle) and reducing the number of injection sites can minimize postinjection bruising caused by trauma to blood vessels as the needle passes through the skin and the underlying orbicularis oculi muscle. Attempting to use the fewest injection points possible will also help to decrease risks of bruising and swelling. When using multiple passes and layered techniques, it is best to withdraw the needle just enough to reposition it without exiting back through the muscle. Use of blunt tipped cannulas can also help to decrease the risk of bruising.

Augmentation of the Infraorbital Hollow

Preferred injection techniques include linear threading with anterograde or retrograde injection via a cannula or needle or serial depot injections at the supraperiosteal level with a needle perpendicular to the skin at the supraperiosteal level. The vertical supraperiosteal depot technique, pioneered by Sattler, involves the vertical deposition of small HA aliquots through a needle at the supraperiosteal level. Recently, Hussein described the Tick Technique for treating IOHs, which involves a three-point injection technique using back-filled BD syringes with 31 g 6-mm needles. He uses the same perpendicular approach with supraperiosteal depots at these three sites. The first injection point is at the junction between the inferolateral aspect of the tear trough and nasojugal groove at the midpupillary line. The second is the medial infraorbital area between the medial canthus and medial limbus. The third is the lateral infraorbital area 1 cm lateral to the lateral limbus at the lid-cheek junction. Small boluses of 0.1 to 0.2 mL are injected at each site, supraperiosteally followed by gentle molding and massage. Some may prefer to initiate their injections at the lateral aspect of the inferior orbital rim because this can stretch the skin and reduce the hollow over the medial tear trough. This would then potentially reduce the volume of product required medially which tends to be the least forgiving region to inject.

If a cannula is chosen, a commonly used entry point for cannula use is found by drawing a line from the nasojugal fold and extending it inferolaterally. Where this line intercepts with a line drawn inferiorly from the lateral canthus is an excellent entry site. The cannula should be inserted perpendicularly until it reaches periosteum and then angled toward the medial canthus, staying ideally in the supraperiosteal plane and beneath the orbicularis oculi muscle. The index finger of the nondominant hand can ensure the correct location of the cannula tip. Small aliquots of filler are deposited in a retrograde fashion either as linear threads or small boluses.

Choice of injection technique may be due to patient factors and physician preference. It is also possible to use both techniques in the same patient, for instance, using supraperiosteal needle depots on bone laterally and a cannula medially.

Extra caution must be taken in the medial portion of the IOH to avoid inadvertent injection of the infratrochlear, infraorbital, dorsal nasal, and angular arteries. Some advocate for a small depot of filler to be injected in this area and then to use digital manipulation to "push" the filling agent into the desired location (see Fig. 20.2A,B).

Posttreatment Management and Follow-up

After treatment, gentle pressure and the application of ice can minimize localized edema and erythema. The patient should be warned to expect swelling and bruising for up to 2 weeks; massage or manipulation of the area should be avoided until these effects subside. More specific aftercare procedures will vary according to clinical preferences but may include the avoidance of alcohol and exercise for up to 48 hours and the addition of *Arnica montana* tablets for 3 days.

> **PEARL 2** Taking *Arnica montana* tablets; using a careful, slow injection technique; using very small needles or a cannula; and applying ice may minimize bruising, although this remains a common side effect in the infraorbital area.

Follow-up within 2 to 4 weeks of treatment allows evaluation of response and contour or volume irregularities. Touch-up injections or hyaluronidase may be required. HA in the IOH can last for a year or more; regular follow-up visits and touch-ups before the filling agent has dissipated will maintain the aesthetic effect.

> **PEARL 3** Patients should be evaluated in animation throughout the procedure to identify and correct bulging or dimpling that can occur with motion.

COMPLICATIONS

Ecchymosis and edema are the most common injection-related side effects. Ecchymosis may last up to 10 days, while edema can last for up to 3 weeks or more depending on the causality. Edema may last longer in individuals treated simultaneously with neuromodulators in the orbicularis oculi at the same visit. Visible irregularities in patients with thin or lax skin can be massaged away over several weeks. Superficial injection increases the risk of lumps that are often difficult to resolve without

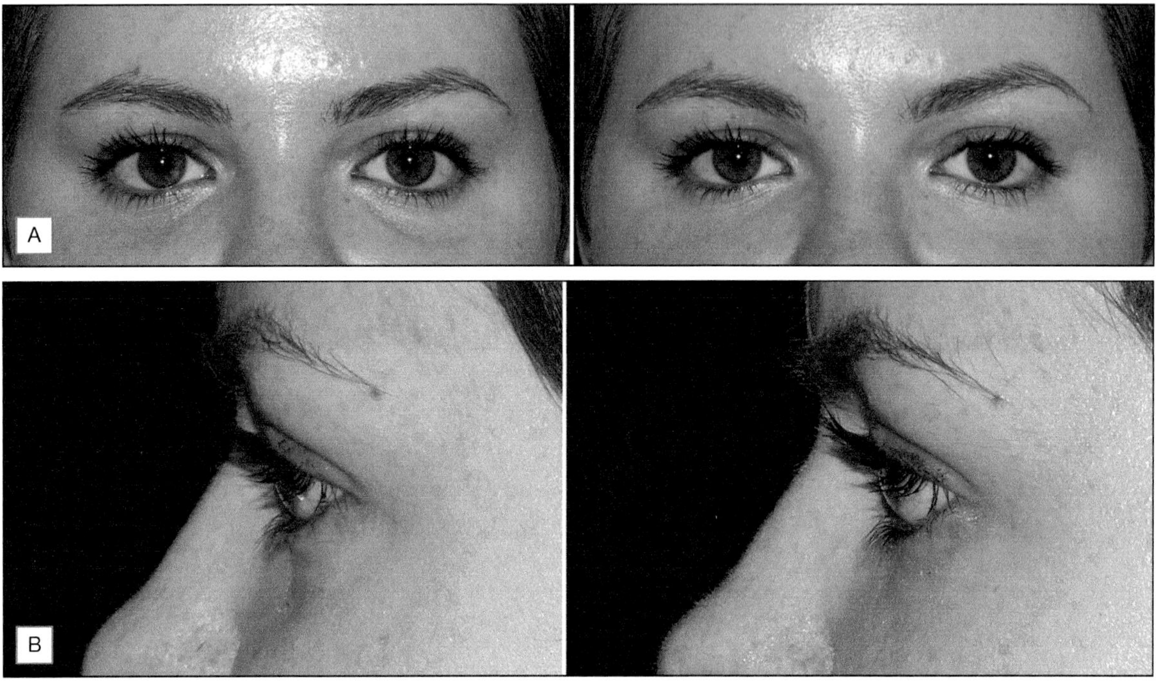

Fig. 20.2 (A) Patient before and after hyaluronic acid (HA) filler treatment from the frontal view. (B) Patient before and after HA filler treatment from the lateral view. (Courtesy of Dr. A. Sutton.)

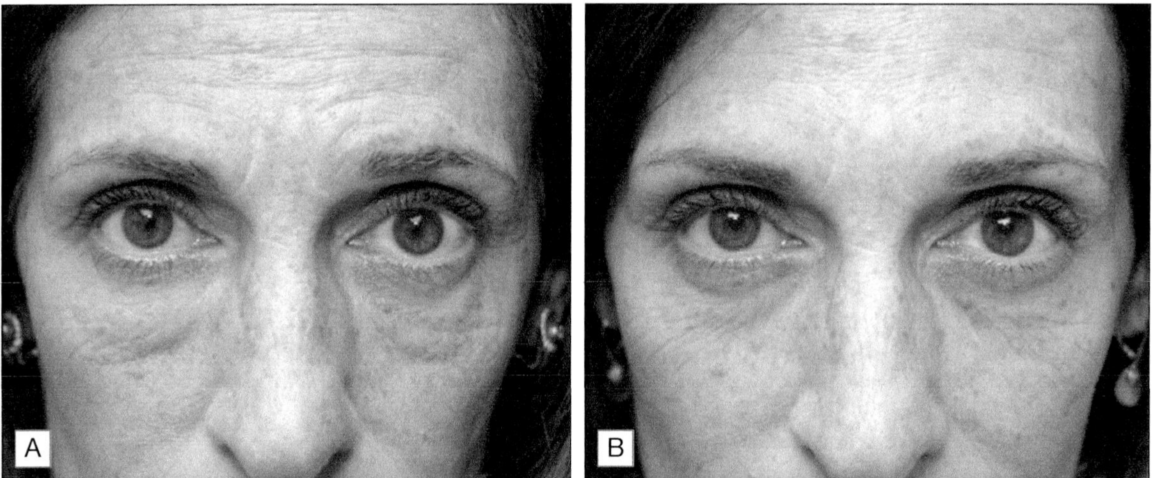

Fig. 20.3 (A) Edema in the lower lid following hyaluronic acid injection into the tear trough; (B) edema resolved after a "watchful waiting" approach.

injections of hyaluronidase to dissolve the implant (Fig. 20.3).

Injections placed too superficially can yield the appearance of a bluish-gray tint secondary to the Tyndall effect, in which the injected filler, readily visible under thin skin, causes preferential scattering of blue light (Fig. 20.4). Overcorrection may lead to unnatural bulges and festooning or a "baggy" eyelid. It is critical to address other areas of deficit; undercorrection of the lateral orbit or mid-face will make the appearance of an

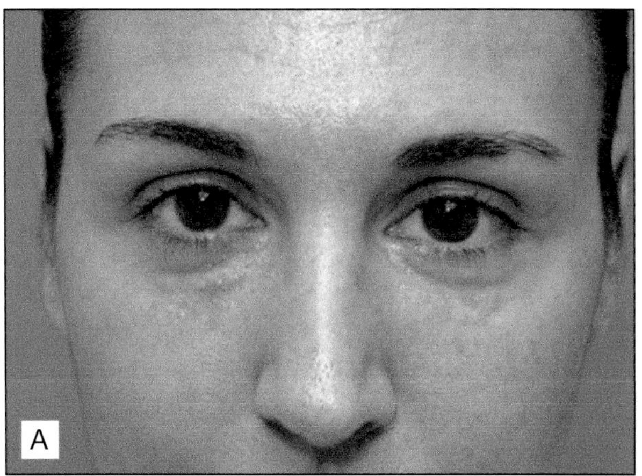

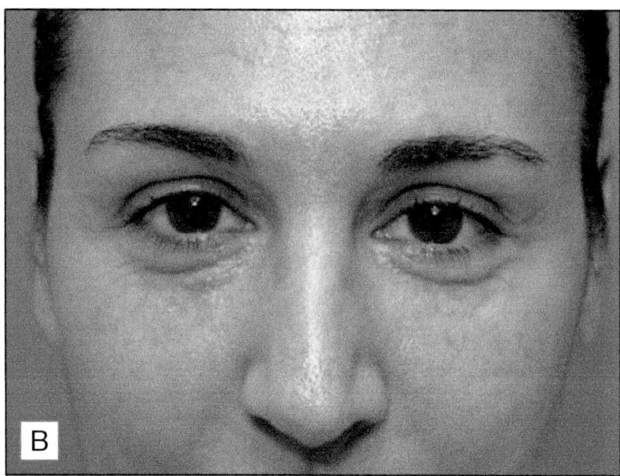

Fig. 20.4 Bluish-gray tint secondary to the Tyndall effect apparent (A) at rest and (B) when smiling.

augmented tear trough unappealing. Undercorrection or overcorrection can be assessed at follow-up and treated appropriately.

> **PEARL 4** Remember the adage, "Less is more."

More serious but rare complications in the IOH include occlusion of the vascular supply leading to skin necrosis, blindness, or stroke. The risk of intravascular injection can be decreased by particular attention to anatomy combined with careful injection techniques.

> **PEARL 5** Patients with eyelid edema from seasonal allergies or other causes may be poor tear trough injection candidates as injection in this area may lead to further edema.

ADJUNCTIVE THERAPY

Some patients are not suited to fillers alone and require adjuvant therapy for complete restoration of the IOH. Dark circles under the eye may be due to a number of variables; identifying the cause enables appropriate treatment. Hyperpigmentation of the skin may respond to α-hydroxy acid chemical peels and agents that reduce pigment formation, such as topical kojic acid or hydroquinone combined with topical retinoids. Dark circles due to excessive pigmentation have also been successfully treated with various pigment lasers (such as the Q-switched or picosecond Nd:YAG or alexandrite lasers). Skin laxity and tear trough deformity can be treated through ablative and nonablative resurfacing, although the side effects associated with the former—prolonged erythema, pigmentary changes, infections, or even scarring—have led clinicians and patients to less invasive, nonablative light-based therapies. Dark shadows under the eye caused by a hypertrophic pretarsal orbicularis oculi can be improved by injections of botulinum toxin and/or surgery. Finally, excess lower eyelid skin, eyelid laxity, or fat prolapse often requires surgical correction with fat removal or reposition (blepharoplasty).

CONCLUSIONS

The use of dermal fillers has become a common treatment to address hollowness of the periorbital region; however, it may be associated with significant complications. Best practice requires in-depth knowledge of regional anatomy, including the delicate and vascular nature of the surrounding tissues, careful patient selection, and precise injection techniques to produce optimal results and avoid serious complications.

FURTHER READING

Anido, J., Fernandez, J. M., Genol, I., Ribe, N., & Sevilla, G. P. (2021). Recommendations for the treatment of tear trough deformity with cross-linked hyaluronic acid filler. *J Cosmet Dermatol.*, *20*, 6–17.

Bagci, B. (2018). A new technique for the correction of tear trough deformity via filler injections. *Plast Reconstr Surg Glob Open.*, *6*, e1901.

Bellman, B. (2006). Complication following suspected intra-arterial injection of Restylane. *Aesthet Surg J., 26*, 304–305.

Bosniak, S., Sadick, N. S., Cantisano-Zilkha, M., Glavas, I. P., & Roy, D. (2008). The hyaluronic acid push technique for the nasojugal groove. *Dermatol Surg., 34*, 127–131.

Carruthers, J. D., & Carruthers, A. (2005). Facial sculpting and tissue augmentation. *Dermatol Surg., 31*(11 pt 2), 1604–1612.

Coleman, S. R. (2002). Avoidance of arterial occlusion from injection of soft tissue fillers. *Aesthet Surg J., 22*, 555.

Donath, A. S., Glasgold, R. A., Meier, J., & Glasgold, M. J. (2010). Quantitative evaluation of volume augmentation in the tear trough with a hyaluronic acid-based filler: a three-dimensional analysis. *Plast Reconstr Surg., 125*, 1515–1522.

Donofrio, L. M. (2003). Technique of periorbital lipoaugmentation. *Dermatol Surg., 29*, 92–98.

El-Garem, Y. F. (2015). Estimation of bony orbit depth for optimal selection of the injection technique to correct the tear trough and palpebromalar groove. *Dermatol Surg., 41*, 94–101.

Goldberg, R. A., & Fiaschetti, D. (2006). Filling the periorbital hollows with hyaluronic acid gel: initial experience with 244 injections. *Ophthal Plast Reconstr Surg., 22*, 335–343.

Goldman, M. P. (2010). Superficial nodularity of hydroxylapatite filler to fill the infraorbital hollow. *Dermatol Surg., 36*, 822–824.

Hevia, O. (2009). A retrospective review of calcium hydroxylapatite for correction of volume loss in the infraorbital region. *Dermatol Surg., 35*, 1487–1494.

Hill, R. H., 3rd, Czyz, C. N., Kandapalli, S., et al. (2015). Evolving minimally invasive techniques for tear trough enhancement. *Ophthal Plast Reconstr Surg., 31*, 306–309.

Hirmand, H. (2010). Anatomy and nonsurgical correction of the tear trough deformity. *Plast Reconstr Surg., 125*, 699–708.

Hirsch, R. J., Carruthers, J. D. A., & Carruthers, A. (2007). Infraorbital hollow treatment by dermal fillers. *Dermatol Surg., 33*, 1116–1119.

Hirsch, R. J., Cohen, J. L., & Carruthers, J. D. (2007). Successful management of an unusual presentation of impending necrosis following a hyaluronic acid injection embolus and proposed algorithm for management of hyaluronidase. *Dermatol Surg., 33*, 357–360.

Hirsch, R. J., Narurkar, V., & Carruthers, J. D. (2006). Management of injected hyaluronic acid induced Tyndall effects. *Lasers Surg Med., 38*, 202–204.

Hussein, S., Mangal, S., & Goodman, G. (2019). The Tick technique: a method to simplify and quantify treatment of the tear trough region. *J Cosmet Dermatol, 18*, 1642–1647.

Lambros, V. S. (2007). Hyaluronic acid injections for correction of the tear trough deformity. *Plast Reconstr Surg., 120*, 745–805.

Lambros, V. S. (2010). Discussion: quantitative evaluation of volume augmentation in the tear trough with a hyaluronic acid-based filler: a three-dimensional analysis. *Plast Reconstr Surg., 125*, 1523–1524.

(2003). Lowe NJ Arterial embolization caused by injection of hyaluronic acid (Restylane). *Br J Dermatol., 148*, 379.

Morley, A. M. S., & Malhotra, R. (2011). Use of hyaluronic acid filler for tear-trough rejuvenation as an alternative to lower eyelid surgery. *Ophthal Plast Reconstr Surg., 27*, 69–73.

Murthy, R., Roos, J., & Goldberg, R. A. (2019). Periocular hyaluronic acid fillers: applications, implications and complications. *Curr Opin Ophthalmol., 30*(5), 395–400.

Pessa, J. E., Desvigne, L. D., Lambros, V. S., Nimerick, J., Sugunan, B., & Zadoo, V. P. (1999). Changes in ocular globe-to-orbital rim position with age: implications for aesthetic blepharoplasty of the lower eyelids. *Aesthet Plast Surg., 23*, 337–342.

Roh, M. R., & Chung, K. Y. (2009). Infraorbital dark circles: definition, causes, and treatment options. *Dermatol Surg., 35*, 1163–1171.

Rohrich, R. J., Arbique, G. M., Wong, C., et al. (2009). The anatomy of suborbicularis fat: implications for periorbital rejuvenation. *Plast Reconstr Surg., 124*, 946–951.

Sadick, N. S., Bosniak, S. L., Cantisano-Zilkha, M., Glavas, I. P., & Roy, D. (2007). Definition of the tear trough and the tear trough rating scale. *J Cosmet Dermatol., 6*, 218–222.

Saylan, Z. (2003). Facial fillers and their complications. *Aesthet Surg J., 23*, 221–224.

Schanz, W., Schippert, W., Ultmer, A., Rassner, G., & Fierlbeck, G. (2002). Arterial embolization caused by injection of hyaluronic acid (Restylane). *Br J Dermatol., 146*, 928–929.

21

Midface

Ada Regina Trindade de Almeida, Luciana de Abreu, and André Vieira Braz

SUMMARY AND KEY FEATURES

- The midface is considered the region between the lower eyelid and the oral commissure.
- A full, wide, and naturally projected midface is related to youth and beauty.
- Similar to other facial areas, local aging encompasses bone, muscles, retaining ligaments, fat, and skin changes in a multifactorial process.
- Structure and contour evaluation of the different facial shapes can be an important tool used in facial assessment determining which facial areas will be prioritized in restoration and/or volumization.
- Biodegradable fillers and biostimulators are optimal choices for nonsurgical rejuvenation of the midface, due to their safety, effectiveness, reversibility and natural looking results.
- Knowledge of facial anatomy, including bone prominences, fat compartments, mimetic muscles, and risk areas, is crucial to achieve better results and to avoid complications.

INTRODUCTION

The midface is considered the area between the lower eyelid and the oral commissure.

A young and attractive face is characterized by a well-contoured and adequately covered zygomatic arch and a anteriorly projected cheek, with a smooth transition from and to the neighboring regions, e.g., no visible delimitation between the cheek and the lid, the nasolabial fold (NLF), and the jowls.

Due to anatomical, ultrasonographic, tomographic, and magnetic resonance imaging, the understanding of the midface aging process has evolved exponentially in the last decade. Similar to other facial areas, local aging encompass bone, muscles, retaining ligaments, fat and skin alterations in a multifactorial process. Individual genetics and/or anatomical features can influence how early or late the aging signs will be apparent.

Biodegradable hyaluronic acid (HA) fillers and biostimulators are optimal choices for nonsurgical rejuvenation of the midface, owing to their safety, effectiveness, reversibility, and natural-looking results.

ANATOMICAL CONSIDERATIONS

In the midface, the maxillary bone is more flattened in men, giving less anterior projection to the face, and the zygomatic prominence is more angled. In females, on the other hand, the zygomatic prominence is rounder, and the maxillary bone is more projected. For both genders, with aging, the orbital floor and the pyriform aperture enlarge inferiorly and laterally, facilitating the descent of the midface.

The facial subcutaneous fat tissue is compartmentalized by septal boundaries in superficial and deep portions, separated by the superficial muscle aponeurotic system (SMAS) and also by the muscles of facial expression. In the midface, the deep fat compartments are deep nasolabial or pyriform fat compartment (DNL), deep medial and deep lateral cheek fat portions (DMC and DLC), as well as two portions located under the orbicularis oculi muscle (medial and lateral suborbicularis oculi fat [SOOF]) (Fig. 21.1A). There are four superficial fat compartments: superficial nasolabial and the three malar portions: superficial medial cheek, superficial middle cheek, and superficial lateral cheek fat compartments (Fig. 21.1B). Volume replacement in the deep fat compartments results in structural support for midface rejuvenation.

Important retaining ligaments in the midface are the orbital retaining, the malar septum or zygomatic-cutaneous, and the MacGregor patch or zygomaticus.

A transverse facial septum attached to the underside of the zygomaticus major muscle was recently described, providing support for the deep medial and lateral cheek fat compartments. Contraction of the zygomaticus major muscle during smiling may "tense" this septum, promoting cranial shift of midfacial fat compartments, projecting the midface anteriorly.

The facial arteries run along the borders of the superficial fat compartments but are located deep to them. The facial artery is a main vessel that irrigates the midface directly or through derived branches, but several variations of its anatomic course have been described in recent papers.

Usually, it arises from the external carotid artery, crosses the lower border of the mandible anteriorly to the masseter muscle and then continues its way up laterally to the nose, sending some ramifications like the

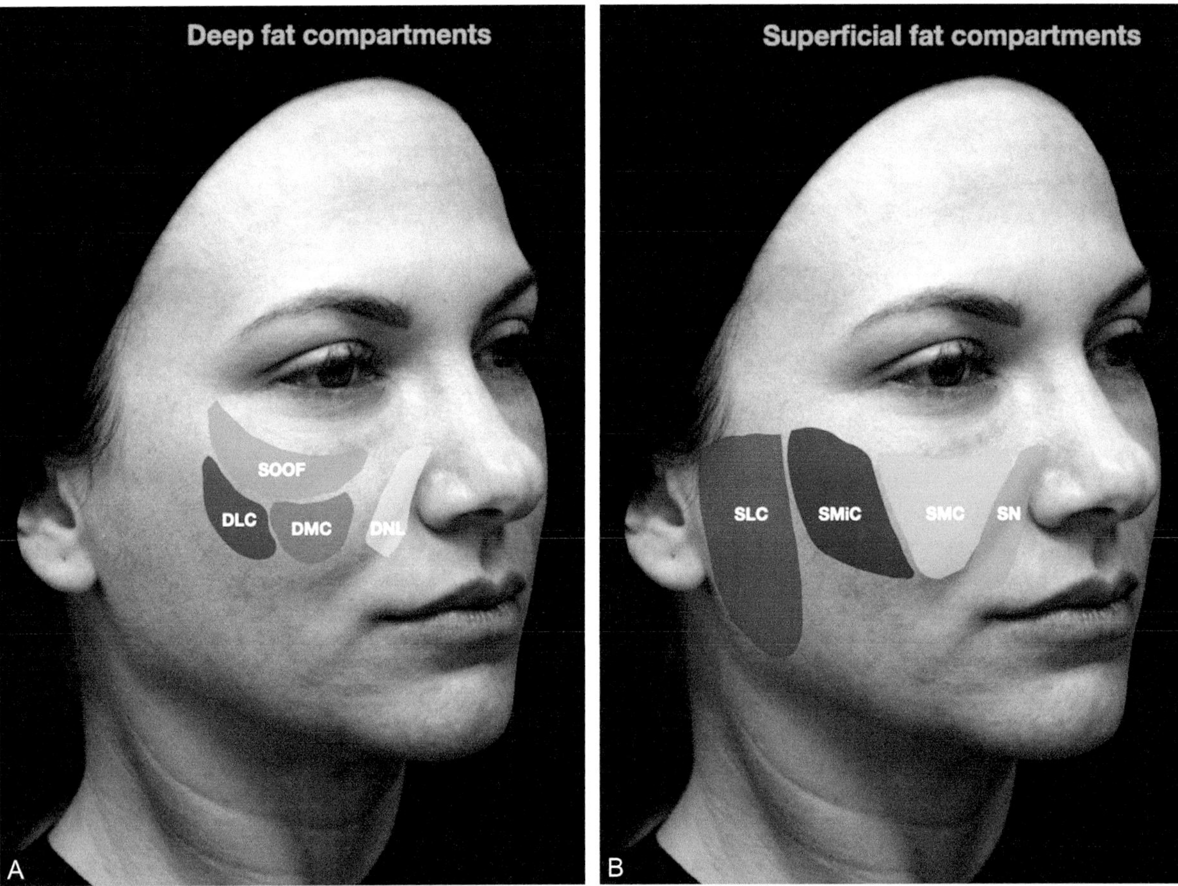

Fig. 21.1 (A) The deep fat compartments are deep nasolabial *(DNL)*, medial and lateral suborbicularis oculi fat *(SOOF)*, and deep medial and deep lateral cheek fat portions (*DMC* and *DLC*). (B) The superficial fat compartments are the superficial nasolabial *(SN)*, superficial medial cheek *(SMC)*, superficial middle cheek *(SMiC)*, and superficial lateral cheek *(SLC)*.

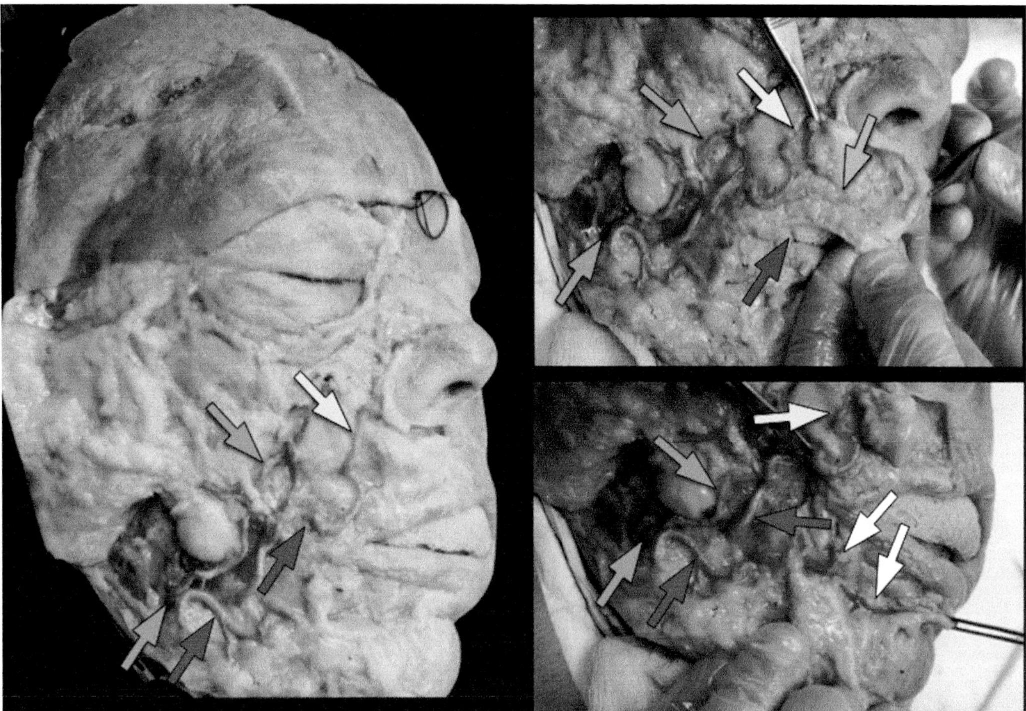

Fig. 21.2 Anatomic specimen illustrating the main vessels of the midface: facial artery *(red arrows)*, facial vein *(blue arrows)*, angular artery *(yellow arrows)*, superior labial artery *(gray arrow)*, and inferior labial artery *(white arrows)*.

lower and the upper lip and the lateral nasal branches. From the mouth corner to the NLF, the facial artery, now called as *angular artery*, runs in the subcutaneous plane, above facial muscles. From there it courses superiorly and may anastomose with the dorsal nasal, the infraorbital and transverse facial arteries, connecting external and internal carotid systems.

Because of its location and anastomosis to other vessels, the angular artery is the vessel most likely to be compromised after filler injections to the midcheek, NLF, and periorbital area (Fig. 21.2).

PEARL 1 The angular artery is the vessel most likely to be compromised after filler injections to the midcheek, NLF, and periorbital area.

The sensitive innervation of the midcheek is done by the maxillary branch of the trigeminal nerve, while the motor innervation is performed by the temporal and zygomatic branches of the facial nerve.

AESTHETIC GOALS

A full, wide, and naturally projected midface is related to youth and beauty. The ideal cheek contour follows the Ogee curve, an S-shaped curve formed by a concave arc going from the inferior lid, moving to a convex arc that includes the malar or cheek-bone prominence, and a gentle slide to the submalar (SM) hollow. Its restoration helps to obtain a natural looking rejuvenation of the midface.

Gender differences should be kept in mind when planning to address the midface with fillers in order to preserve or increase the angled male face or the more round/oblique female facial curves for natural looking results. For the female patient, the midface is stronger than the lower face, meaning that the bizygomatic distance is wider than the bigonial distance, while in men, these distances are almost the same and the lower face is stronger (Fig. 21.3A,B).

According to Remington and Swift, the female cheek is ovoid, with the apex angled and located high on the midface, below and lateral to lateral canthus. The male

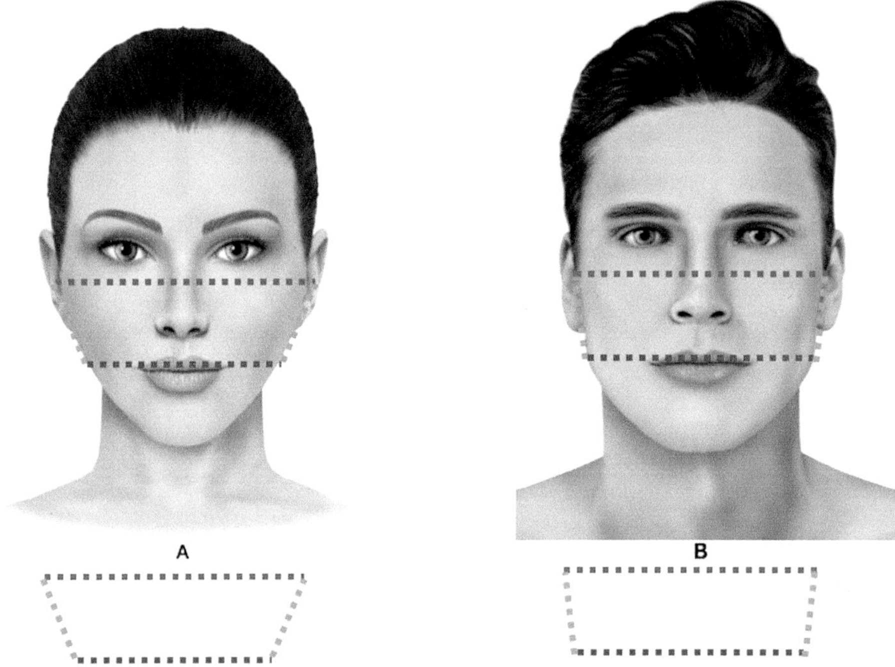

Fig. 21.3 Gender differences in midface. For the female patient (A), the midface is stronger than the lower face, meaning that the bizygomatic distance (horizontal blue dotted line) is wider than the bigonial distance (horizontal red dotted line), while in men (B), these distances are almost the same and the lower face is stronger (square shape).

cheek has a broader malar base, a more modest apex, located more inferomedially than the female cheek. But for all genders, in a young and attractive subject, the transition from the lid-cheek junction to the midface as well as from the cheek to the lower face has to be smooth and even, without any abrupt changes.

Based on four facial shapes (oval, heart, round, and angular), an innovative technique and facial approach for facial fillers placement, called AB face (Anatomy of Beauty) technique, was recently described by Braz and Cazerta (Fig. 21.4). It is a guideline to highlight the positive features of each facial shape, improving facial proportions and contours, restoring support and lifting the face, as well as contributing to delay the aging process. It also offers the possibility of reshaping a face into another facial format for individual beautification purposes.

It is divided into two steps: AB face structure and AB face refinement, including lower and midface approaches, but only the latter will be addressed in this chapter. In the first step (the AB face structure), the goal is to improve facial structure, restoring volume loss and improving contours and proportions of each facial shape. The aesthetic goal of the second step (AB refinement) is to treat the remaining sulcus and grooves, promoting a smooth transition and connection between the previously treated areas. The suggested anatomical areas for treatment are illustrated in Fig. 21.5.

TREATMENT AREAS

Before the procedure, all makeup is removed and the skin is cleaned with 4% chlorhexidine gluconate. Topical anesthetic creams may be applied to enhance patient comfort. Before and during the injection procedure, skin cleaning with 4% chlorhexidine gluconate is repeated several times.

Malar Area

Amazing results in facial rejuvenation can be achieved through volume restoration of the malar fat pad and SOOF compartments with fillers. Recent studies found that the SOOF compartments together have the highest surface volume coefficient (SVC), meaning that 95% of an injected product is translated into surface projection.

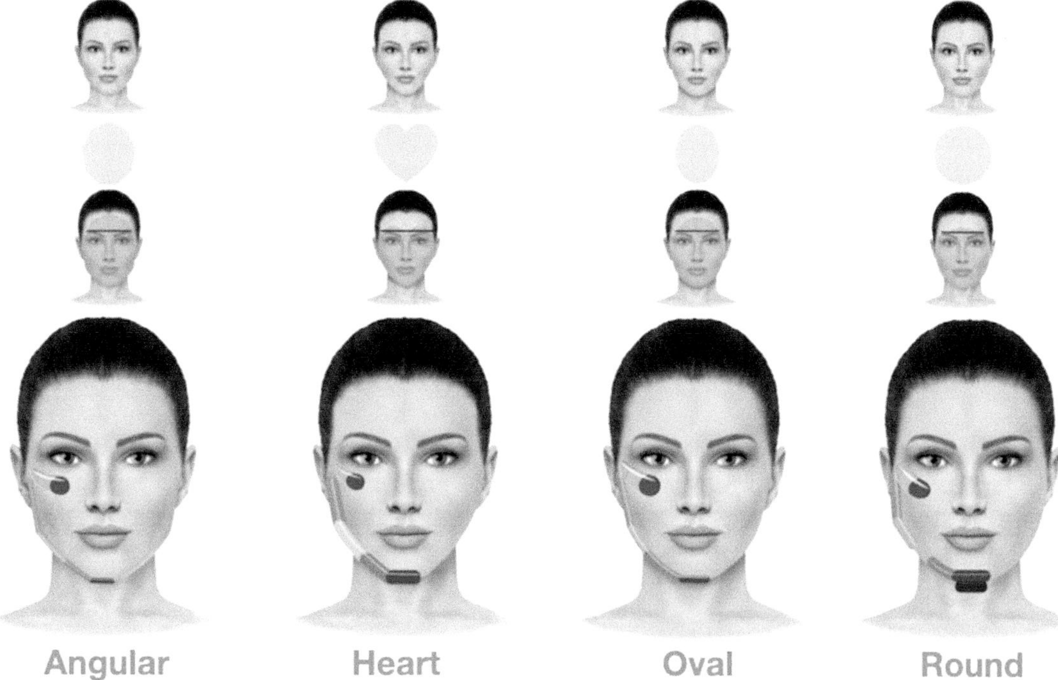

Fig. 21.4 The four facial shapes: angular, heart, oval, and round. On the bottom line are shown each facial shape with the respective areas (colored spherical and elliptical figures) suggested for treatment by the Anatomy of Beauty face structure technique. The treatment areas are very similar; however, the amount of filler used in each format changes according to the need of each one, and their strengths and weaknesses. For example, the priorities in the heart shape are in the lower face, whereas in the angular shape, the most important is to treat the midface.

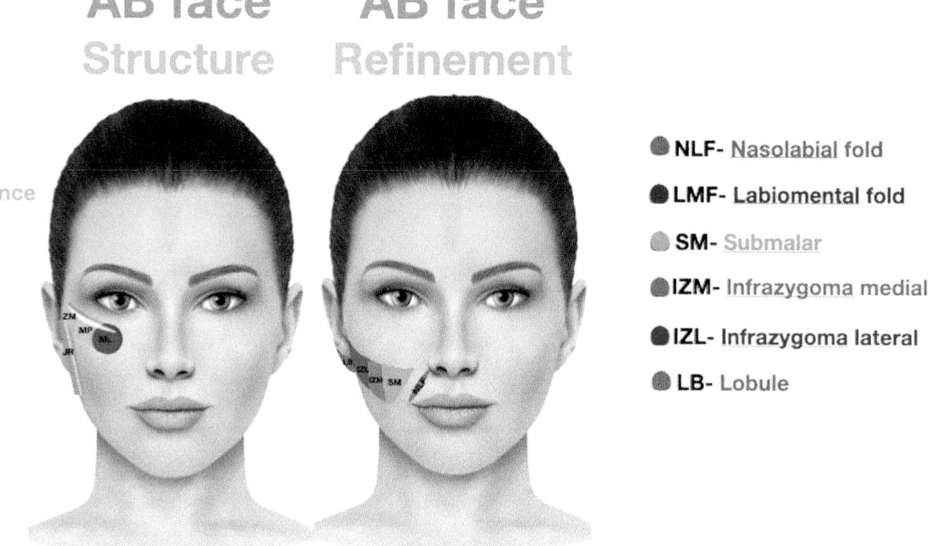

Fig. 21.5 Midface anatomical facial areas that can be treated with fillers in the Anatomy of Beauty face structure and refinement techniques, respectively. The use of 22–25-gauge cannulas is strongly recommended for these techniques.

The best area for volume restoration is identified by marking two lines: one linking the external corner of the eye to the labial commissure and another from the upper tragus to the superior part of the nasal ala. The intersection of these two lines sets up a point, referred as AB, that identifies the limit between the malar lateral or zygomatic eminence and the maxilla bone (malar area) (Fig. 21.6, *blue circle*). From there, a concave line is traced following the inferior limit of the tear trough, limited by the orbital rim (Fig. 21.6, *superior black line*). A second concave line is traced starting from point AB downward, following the posteroinferior border of the malar bone (Fig. 21.6, *lateral green line*). And finally, a convex line connecting the free corners of the two concave lines is traced, outlining the anterior limit of volume loss (Fig. 21.6, *anterior brown line*). The delimitated area corresponds deeply to the medial SOOF and superficially to the malar fat pad region, and its convexity is proportional to the area of volume loss (Video 21.1).

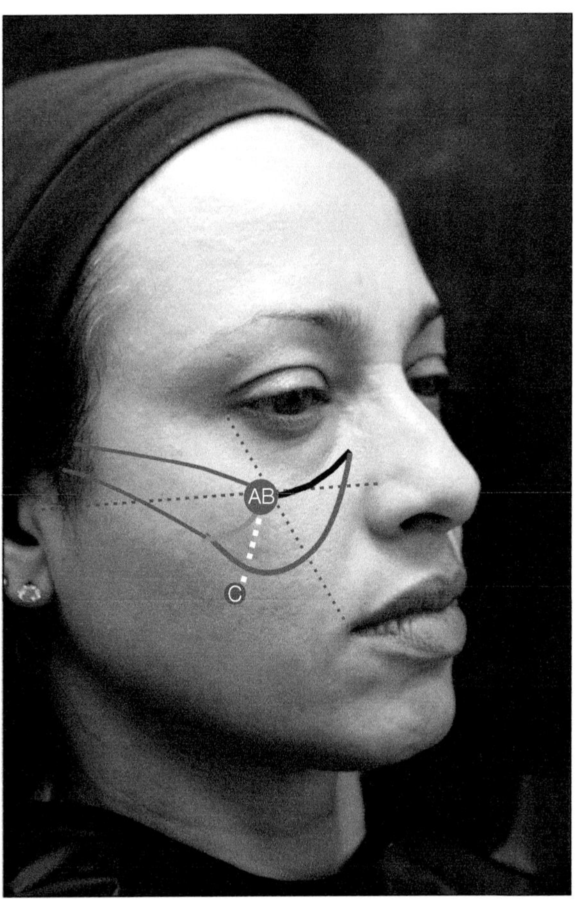

Fig. 21.6 Markings for malar and zygomatic areas augmentation.

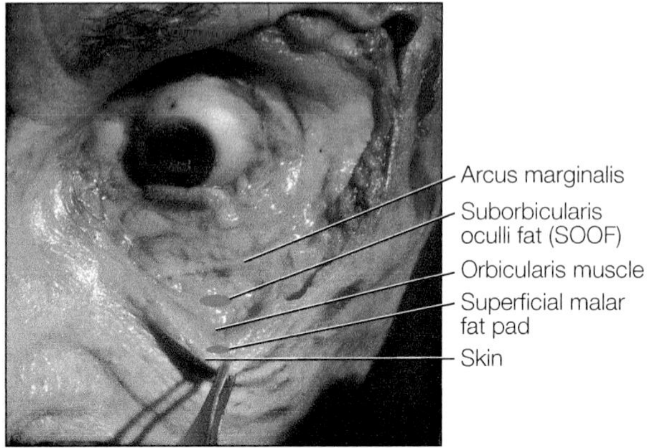

Fig. 21.7 Anatomic view of superficial (superficial malar fat pad) and deep (suborbicularis oculi fat) sites of injection for malar area.

Deep placement of small boluses of a high G' and lift capacity HA filler with lidocaine is the initial step to restore the structural support of the anterior cheek. To avoid the risk of inadvertent injection into infraorbital foramen, 22 to 25 G, 40-mm-long cannulas are preferred. The filler is deposited by retrograde injection tunnels, followed by gentle molding massage. It can also be delivered in the superficial fat compartments if needed to improve the natural projection (Fig. 21.7). The total amount injected varies according to the degree of volume depletion, ranging from 0.5 to 2 mL per side (Video 21.1).

Zygomatic Area

Although in a smaller degree than the fat pad reduction, the malar bone also retracts and loses volume with aging and needs treatment for a natural and rejuvenated look.

After palpation of the zygomatic bone, we draw two lines highlighting the superior and inferior margins of the zygomatic arch, beginning on the malar eminence (point AB). The filler is placed between the two lines, along the zygomatic arch, deep to the bone, until a point corresponding to the tail of the eyebrow (Fig. 21.8). When injecting in the supraperiosteal layer, using needles or cannulas, the filler will be placed between the bone and the lateral SOOF (Fig. 21.8). The filler placement in these lateral zygomatic cheek areas will promote a lifting effect of the midface and improvement in the lower-eyelid appearance (Fig. 21.9) (Video 21.2).

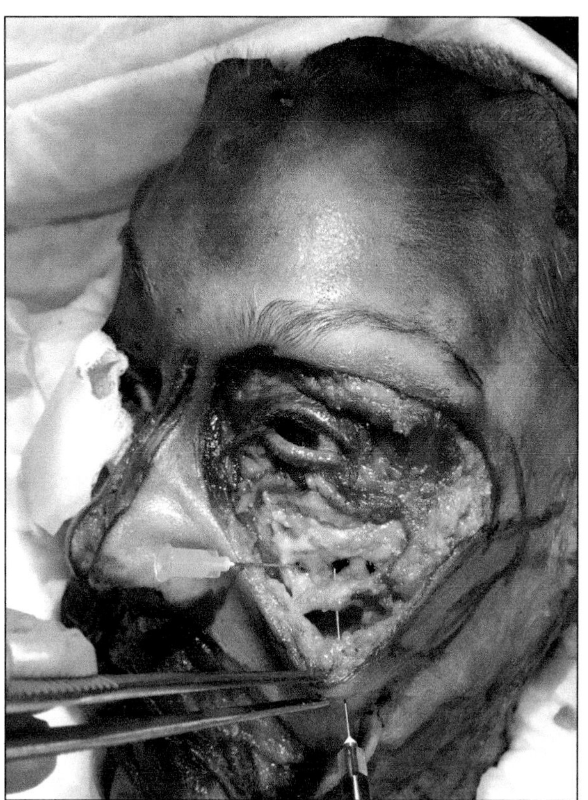

Fig. 21.8 Anatomic demonstration of filler deposits with needle *(green hub)* and cannula *(red hub)* along the zygomatic arch.

Submalar Region

Reflation of the SM region helps to efface and lift the lower part of the NLF and lower third of the face. The aesthetic goal is to keep the natural "shadow" to the midface, highlighting the cheek apex but maintaining the "Ogee curve." To allow a smooth transition from the upper cheek, the HA filler is placed in the superficial subcutaneous plane by retrograde fanning technique using 25 or 22 G cannulas. In some very hollowed subjects, like runners, deeper fat compartments also need to be treated to replace the volume loss.

To improve deep smile lines, one option is to inject lower G' HA filler using small-bore needles (27–31 G), in retrograde or anterograde linear threading, serial puncture, or fanning. Be careful not to overfill this area, or instead of the ideal oval shape, the result will be a round face with the appearance of being overweight (Fig. 21.10).

Another alternative is to inject diluted calcium hydroxyapatite (1:1, i.e., 1.5 mL of product plus 1.5 mL of diluent) using the fanning technique with 25 G cannulas in the subdermal level or parallel, serial retrograde linear threads with 27 G needles in the deep dermal plane.

After the procedure, gentle massage to the overlying skin as well as from the intraoral surface is applied to obtain an even distribution of the injected product.

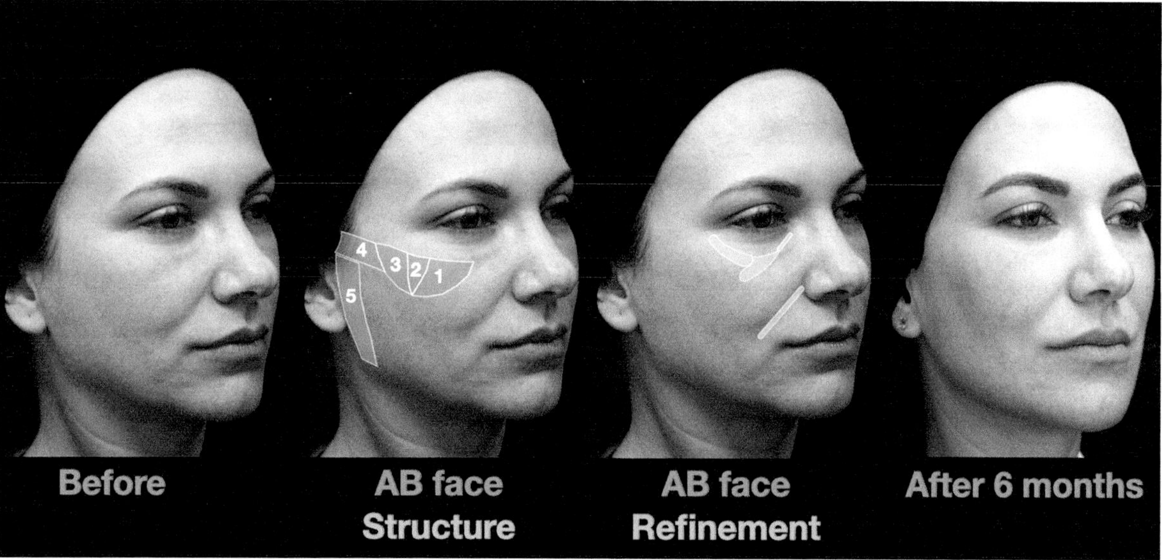

Fig. 21.9 Before and 6 months after midface augmentation with hyaluronic acid fillers using AB face structure and refinement techniques. Anatomical treated areas (AB face structure): malar lateral *(1)*, malar prominence *(2)*, medial zygoma *(3)*, lateral zygoma *(4)*, and jaw ramus *(5)*; and AB face refinement treated areas (in *yellow*): nasojugal groove, eyelid cheek junction, palpebral malar groove, and nasolabial fold.

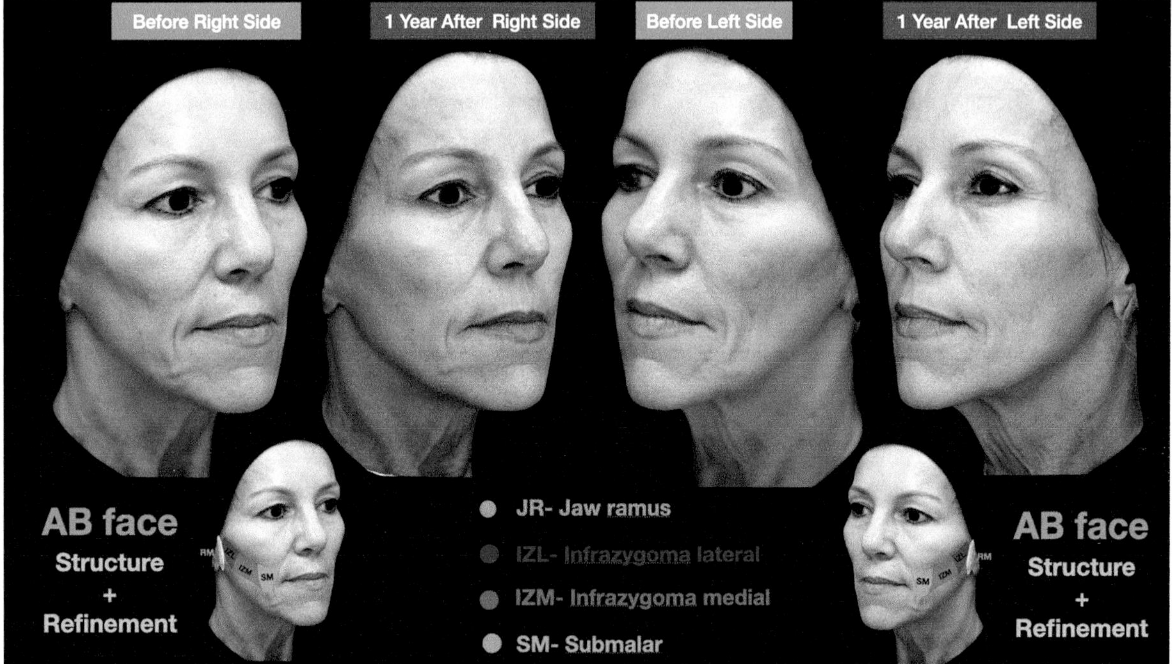

Fig. 21.10 Before and 1 year after midface augmentation with hyaluronic acid fillers using AB face structure and refinement techniques. Anatomical treated area (AB face structure): jaw ramus *(JR)*; and AB face refinement treated areas: submalar *(SM)*, infrazygoma medial *(IZM)*, infrazygoma lateral *(IZL)*.

> **PEARL 2** Reflation of the SM region also helps to efface and lift the lower third of the NLF.

Preauricular or Superficial Lateral Cheek Region or Jaw Ramus

This region gained relevance recently with the new concept of the line of ligaments—an imaginary line connecting the four major facial ligaments: temporal ligamentous adhesion (temple, upper face), lateral orbital thickening (periorbital, upper/middle face), zygomatic (zygomatic arch, middle face), and mandibular ligaments. This line separates a difference in soft tissue plane arrangement: medially, they are displayed obliquely to the skin surface, while laterally, they are arranged in parallel layers. Treatments of the lateral face, as the preauricular or lateral cheek region, will result mainly in lifting effects, whereas these treatments in the medial face will promote volumizing or projecting effects (Fig. 21.11).

Some relevant structures to remember here are the parotid gland and duct, the transverse artery and vein, all of them located below the SMAS, which is thicker in this region.

This area is considered the jaw ramus in the AB face structure and the infrazygoma lateral (IZL) in the AB face refinement technique. Between the IZL and SM areas, we describe the infrazygoma medial (IZM) (Fig. 21.10).

The correct plane of injection is subdermal, to address the superficial lateral fat compartment, using 22 to 25 G cannulas. Lower or high G' HA fillers, as well as diluted calcium hydroxyapatite, can be used to replace the depleted volume as needed.

The entry points can be in the medial cheek, in the mandibular angle, or even in the preauricular area, and sometimes, more than one may be necessary. The filler or the diluted calcium hydroxyapatite is deposited in small aliquots of 0.05 to 0.1 mL per line in retrograde injections in a fanning technique. Gentle massage would help to spread the product, ensuring an even surface at the end of the procedure, although some defects may be difficult to correct due to parotid fascia attachments.

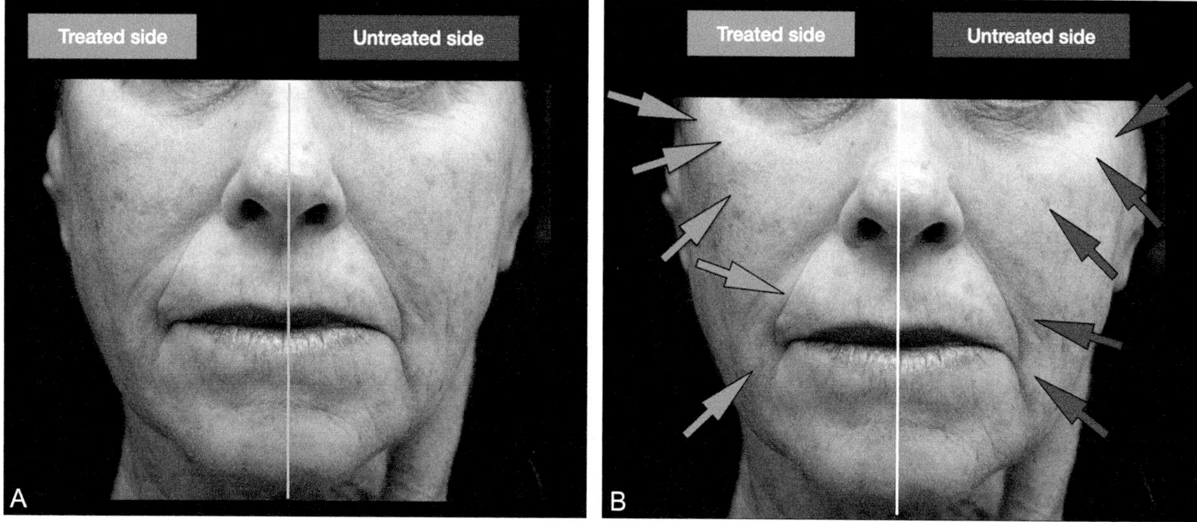

Fig. 21.11 Comparison of treated side (A—*blue arrows*) and untreated side (B—*red arrows*) after midcheek augmentation with hyaluronic acid fillers: improvement of eyelid cheek junction, nasolabial fold, and labiomental fold (blue arrows) resulting in lifting effects.

Correction of the preauricular region helps to finish the "frame" of the cheek, giving a natural-looking effect for the rejuvenation of the midface.

CONCLUSION

The midface projection and proportion impact our perception of youth and beauty. Aging of this region is manifested predominantly by volume loss, revealed by shadows. Biodegradable fillers are the best options for treatment because they are safe, reversible, with long-lasting results. Calcium hydroxyapatite is also safe and effective and can be used alone or associated to AH fillers. For all indications, proper training is crucial to promote natural-looking results and patient satisfaction and to avoid complications.

FURTHER READING

Avelar, L. E., Cardoso, M., Bordoni, L., & Avelar, L. (2017). Aging and sexual differences in the human skull. *Plast Reconstr Surg Glob Open.*, *5*, e1297.

Avelar, L. E., Cazerta, C., Avé, M., & Shitara, D. I. (2018). Dynamic changes of facial supporting cornerstones (pillars): considerations in aesthetic approach. *J Drugs Dermatol.*, *17*(4), 611–615.

Braz, A. V., & Sakuma, T. (2012). Midface rejuvenation: an innovative technique to restore cheek volume. *Dermatol Surg.*, *38*(1), 118–120.

Braz, A., & Eduardo, C. C. P. (2020). The facial shapes in planning the treatment with injectable fillers. *Indian J Plast Surg.*, *53*(2), 230–243.

Braz, A., & Eduardo, C. C. P. (2020). Reshaping the lower face using injectable fillers. *Indian J Plast Surg.*, *53*(2), 207–218.

Casabona, G., Bernadini, F., Skippen, B., et al. (2019). How to best utilize the line of ligaments and the surface volume coefficient in facial soft tissue filler injections. *J Cosmet Dermatol.*, *19*(2), 303–311.

Cotofana, S., & Lachman, N. (2019). Anatomy of the facial fat compartments and their relevance in aesthetic surgery. *J Deutsch Dermatol Ges.*, *17*(4), 399–413.

Cotofana, S., Gotkin, R., Frank, K., et al. (2019). The functional anatomy of the deep facial fat compartments: a detailed imaging-based investigation. *Plast Reconstr Surg.*, *143*, 53–63.

Cotofana, S., Gotkin, R., Frank, K., et al. (2020). Anatomy behind the facial overfilled syndrome: the transverse facial septum. *Dermatol Surg.*, *46*(8), e16–e22.

Cotofana, S., Koban, K., Konstantin, F., et al. (2019). The Surface-volume coefficient of the superficial and deep facial fat compartments: a cadaveric three-dimensional volumetric analysis. *Plast Reconstr Surg.*, *143*(6), 1605–1613.

Cotofana, S., Schenck, T., Trevidic, P., et al. (2015). Midface: clinical anatomy and regional approaches with injectable fillers. *Plast Reconstr Surg.*, *136*, 219S–234S.

Furukawa, M., Mathes, D. W., & Anzai, Y. (2013). Evaluation of the facial artery on computed tomographic angiography using 64-slice multidetector computed tomography: implications for facial reconstruction in plastic surgery. *Plast Reconstr Surg.*, *131*(3), 526–535.

Goldie, K., Peerts, W., Alghoul, M., et al. (2018). Global Consensus guidelines for the injection of diluted and hyperdiluted calcium hydroxyapatite for skin tightening. *Dermatol Surg.*, *44*(suppl 1), S32–S41.

Lam, S., Glasgold, R., & Glasgold, M. (2015). Analysis of facial aesthetics as applied to injectables. *Plast Reconstr Surg.*, *136*, 11S–21S.

Pilsl, U., Anderhuber, F., & Neugebauer, S. (2016). The facial artery—the main blood vessel for the anterior face? *Dermatol Surg.*, *42*, 203–208.

Ramanadhan, S., & Rohrich, R. (2015). Newer understanding of specific anatomic targets in the aging face as applied to injectables: superficial and deep fat compartments—an evolving target for site-specific facial augmentation. *Plast Reconstr Surg.*, *136*, 49S–55S.

Sadick, N., Dorizas, A., Krueguer, N., & Nassar, A. (2015). The facial adipose system: its role in facial aging and approaches to volume restoration. *Dermatol Surg.*, *41*, S333–S339.

Schaverien, M. V., Pessa, J. E., & Rohrich, R. J. (2009). Vascularized membranes determine the anatomical boundaries of the subcutaneous fat compartments. *Plast Reconstr Surg.*, *123*, 695–700.

Swift, A., & Remington, K. (2011). BeautiPHIcation! A global approach to facial beauty. *Clin Plast Surg.*, *38*, 347–377.

Trindade de Almeida, A., Figueiredo, V., et al. (2019). Consensus recommendations for the use of hyperdiluted calcium hydroxyapatite (Radiesse) as a face and body biostimulatory agent. *Plast Reconstr Surg Glob Open*. 7e2160.

Wang, W., Xie, Y., Hunag, R., et al. (2017). Facial contouring by targeted restoration of facial fat compartment volume: the midface. *Plast Reconstr Surg.*, *139*, 563.

Wong, C., & Medelson, B. (2015). Newer understanding of specific anatomic targets in the aging face as applied to injectables: aging changes in the craniofacial skeleton and facial ligaments. *Plast Reconstr Surg.*, *136*, 44S–48S.

22

The Anatomical Basis for Safe Injection Rhinoplasty

Woffles T.L. Wu and Steven Liew

INTRODUCTION

Injection rhinoplasty is not a new concept. Beauticians and unlicensed practitioners have been injecting paraffin, silicone oil, cooking oil, and other permanent "filler" materials into the nose for decades, especially in Asia, where the desire to augment the nose is high.[1] This has led to a slew of foreign body complications that included abnormal swelling, migration, granulomas, infection, and even cavernous sinus thrombosis. In time, many of these patients developed a similar dysmorphic facies with a bloated elephantine nose. Removal of the impregnated permanent material with a restoration to a normal nasal contour is extremely challenging.

Since the 1990s, fat and a variety of newer fillers have been used for injection rhinoplasty. The newer range of synthetic fillers started first with collagen (Zyplast), then progressed to a variety of cross- or non-cross-linked hyaluronic acid (HA) fillers, calcium hydroxyapatite, and other fillers containing different substances. These have typically been injected into the nose using sharp needles or blunt cannulae by physicians of all levels, having the perception that this is a simple, straightforward procedure. As a result it has become one of the most popular injectable techniques for correcting underprojected Asian noses or Caucasian noses, which may have irregularities or mild contour problems.

Injection rhinoplasty is a procedure that carries catastrophic albeit extremely rare complication. In fact, injection rhinoplasty, together with injections of the glabellar frown lines, temples, and forehead, is now considered to be the anatomical regions with the highest vascular risks, fraught with inherently disastrous potential complications that include skin necrosis, blindness, and strokes. In the last 10, years there have been countless cases of skin necrosis, over 200 cases of blindness have been reported in the literature, and more than 40 patients have suffered strokes. The true number of unreported cases could be much higher.

In all cases of blindness, the visual loss was permanent despite any remedial measures being implemented. Of these cases, approximately half were due to fat and the other half were due to a variety of synthetic injectable fillers. Surprisingly, over 75% of these complications were associated with the use of a cannula, indicating that its use may not be as safe as we once believed. It is therefore timely to review the anatomy of the nose and its immediate surroundings to understand why these complications occurred and how we can develop safe techniques for injection rhinoplasty.

THE ANATOMICAL BASIS FOR SAFE INJECTIONS

Understanding nasal anatomy allows us to formulate clear strategies when performing injection rhinoplasty. In 1990, Wu described the five soft tissue layers overlying the osseocartilaginous framework of the nose, namely, the skin envelope (thicker at the tip than over the dorsum or radix), the superficial fibrofatty areolar layer, the middle fibromuscular layer, the deep areolar layer, and the periosteum or perichondrium depending on whether it is at the bony vault or the cartilaginous portion of the nose (Fig. 22.1A,B).

The skin of the nasal tip is thick, firm, and difficult to inject into. The periosteum and perichondrium are both tightly affixed to the underlying osseocartilaginous framework and similarly difficult to inject into or beneath. This leaves a plane of least resistance sandwiched

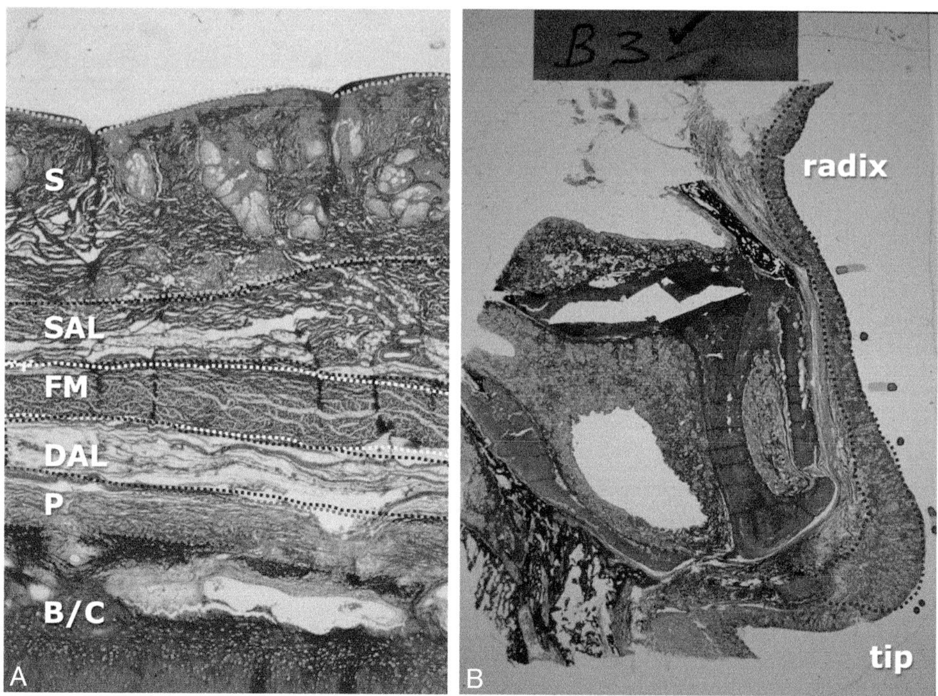

Fig. 22.1 (A) The five different soft tissue layers overlying the bony cartilaginous framework (*B/C*), namely: the overlying skin (*S*), superficial areolar layer (*SAL*), fibromuscular layer (*FM*), deep areolar layer (*DAL*), periosteum or perichondrium (*P*). (B) Sagittal section of the nose and septum showing the fibromuscular layer appearing as a continuous sheet sandwiched by the superficial and deep areolar layers. The thickness of the nasal skin increases from the radix to the tip.

between the outermost and innermost layers, made up of the fibromuscular layer, and the two loose areolar layers above and below it. The superficial and deep areolar layers represent two natural planes of dissection that allow the skin to be easily dissected off the fibromuscular layer (Fig. 22.2A) or the fibromuscular layer from the perichicondrial/periosteal layer (Fig. 22.2B). The vascular network of the nose lies on the surface of this fibromuscular layer, with very few vascular branches beneath it (Fig 22.3A,B). Over the alar lobules, all five layers are densely adherent to one another, while over the tip and dorsum, the skin is easily dissected free at the level of the superficial areolar (subcutaneous) layer.

The vascular supply of the nose is derived from both the internal and external carotid artery systems, which anastomose with each other at several points in the face (Fig. 22.4). This provides the anatomical basis for any filler material that is inadvertently injected into the facial artery, superficial temporal artery, or a nasal blood vessel to be propelled retrogradely into the orbit through these anastomotic channels and thereby occlude the ophthalmic artery, causing visual compromise, or even a stroke.

The main blood supply of the nose is derived from the columellar and alar branches of the facial artery (the external carotid system) as it winds its way upward to the medial corner of the eye to become the angular artery. These branches supply the lower two thirds of the nose. The upper third of the nose is also supplied by the dorsal nasal artery, which is a branch of the supratrochlear artery, which is itself a terminal branch of the ophthalmic artery (the internal carotid system). In a high percentage of cases, the angular artery may anastomose directly with the supratrochlear artery, thus providing a direct communication between the internal and external carotid artery systems.

In addition, the dorsal nasal, alar, and columellar arteries of each side of the nose enter into a dense vascular plexus that covers the tip and soft tissue lobule of the nose. In many anatomical specimens, the alar artery can

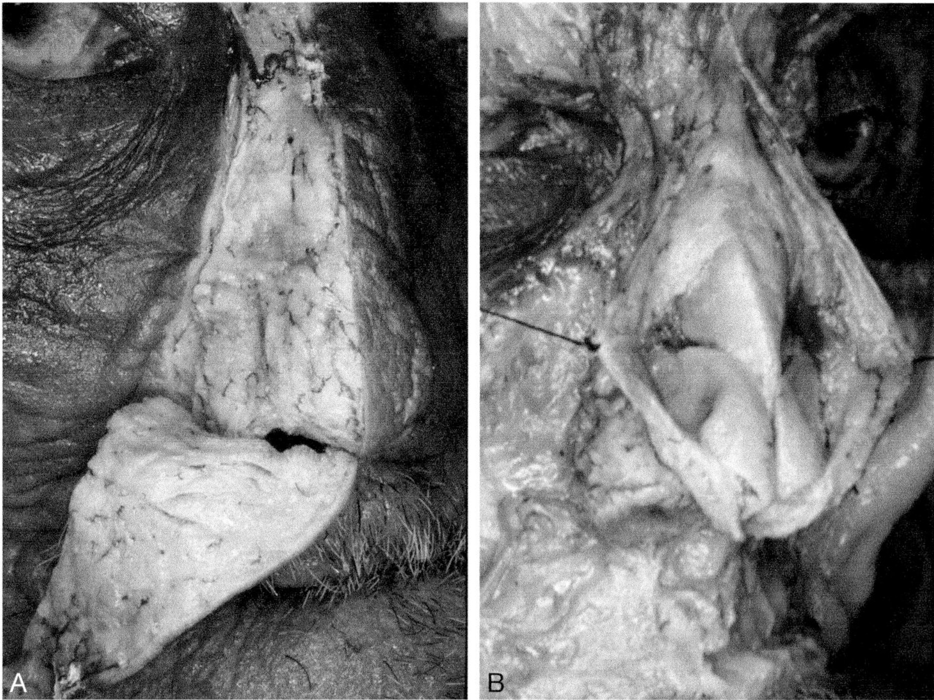

Fig. 22.2 (A, B) Anatomical dissection of the nose and its soft tissue layers. In (A), the skin envelope has already been dissected free at the level of the superficial areolar layer, exposing the vessels on top of the fibromuscular layer. In (B), the fibromuscular layer has been split in the midline and reflected at the level of the deep areolar layer, to show the underlying osseocartilaginous framework. No blood vessels lie beneath the fibromuscular layer. All major blood vessels lie on its superior surface. Therefore, the safest place to inject a filler in the nose is deep on the bone or periosteum itself or on the dorsal edge of the cartilaginous septum.

be seen communicating directly with the dorsal nasal artery. All the major blood vessels of the nose are paired symmetrically on either side of the nose with a resultant watershed running down the midline from the glabellar down to the anterior nasal spine (Fig. 22.3).

It would therefore appear that the safest way to deliver an injection of filler material to the nose is to stay in the midline and inject directly "on the bone" or dorsum of the cartilaginous septum, therefore avoiding any of the major blood vessels that mostly lie on the surface of the fibromuscular layer. For this reason, the use of a sharp 27 or 30 G needle for all injections on the nose may be safest as the needle tip can target the periosteal layer and bone most accurately and the droplet size can be kept small and well controlled. "On the bone" does not imply that the filler is actually subperiosteal and on the bone because that is a physical impossibility. But consciously touching the bony surface with the needle tip does ensure that the delivery of the filler droplet is as deep as possible and hopefully away from the major blood vessels. At the time of injection, the needle tip should remain in contact with the "bone."

Cannulae for nasal injection have traditionally been thought to be the safer alternative of delivering filler just like the rest of the face. However, this has proven not to be the case, with majority of reported vascular complication in the nose being associated with cannula usage. The cannulas have a tendency to enter into the first plane of least resistance, this being the superficial areolar tissue plane. With the cannula aims toward the deeper layer, it will glide in the middle plane of the superficial muscular aponeurotic system (SMAS), which unfortunately is where the major blood vessels are located. This may explain why most cases of blindness have been associated with the use of cannulae and not needles. Cannulae have been postulated to penetrate

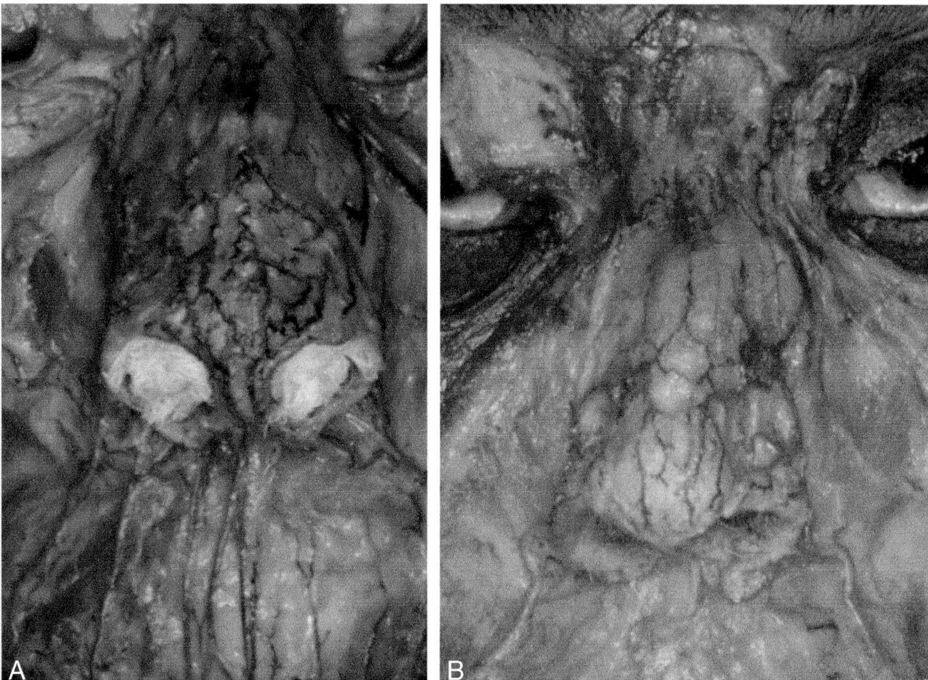

Fig. 22.3 (A, B) Over the nose, the arterial supply is from paired the alar, columellar (derived from the facial artery), and dorsal nasal (a branch of the ophthalmic artery) arteries on either side, with a vascular watershed in the midline. The midline of the nose is therefore an anatomically safe place for sharp-needle injections, which should endeavor to be delivered deep on the underlying bone or cartilage of the nose. In these separate specimens, the facial artery is seen coursing upward through the nasolabial region to the junction of the alar lobule with the lip, where it splits into a robust columellar artery, which runs in the nostril sill, and then along the columella to the tip of the nose and an alar artery, which curves around the alar groove and supplies the alar lobule (B). An attenuated tributary of the alar artery continues toward the medial canthus of the eye, where it anastomoses with the dorsal nasal artery, which in turn is a terminal branch of the ophthalmic artery (A). Note the paired columellar arteries running superficially along the columella to the tip of the nose, where they anastomose with the alar plexus, which unites branches from the columellar, alar, and dorsal nasal arteries.

the vessel at the fork of a bifurcation where it is most stationery. Larger-bore cannulae may be intuitively safer but may cause more discomfort and the entry point can leave a visible mark on the nose.

We are aware of an anecdotal case of blindness[29] following retrograde injections of a HA filler using a 21 G cannula inserted from the tip of the nose over the dorsum to the glabellar region. The surgeon noticed periorbital blanching, almost immediately after which the patient complained of blurring of vision. Despite emergency cannulation of the supraorbital and supratrochlear arteries and infiltration of hyaluronidase, the patient became blind in one eye. This an awful complication.

INDICATIONS

Injection rhinoplasty is indicated in patients who wish to have cosmetic enhancement of the nose without surgery. Younger patients are more concerned with correcting any perceived structural deficiencies and usually request significant changes to the shapes of their noses. Older patients on the other hand are more appreciative of the rejuvenative effects that result from volumizing the root and bridge of the nose or uplifting a drooping tip. Ethnic considerations play a significant role in the choice of fillers.

Asian noses tend to be broad and flat with a low dorsum, a fleshy bulbous tip, and widely spread alar lobules. The common indications for injection rhinoplasty for

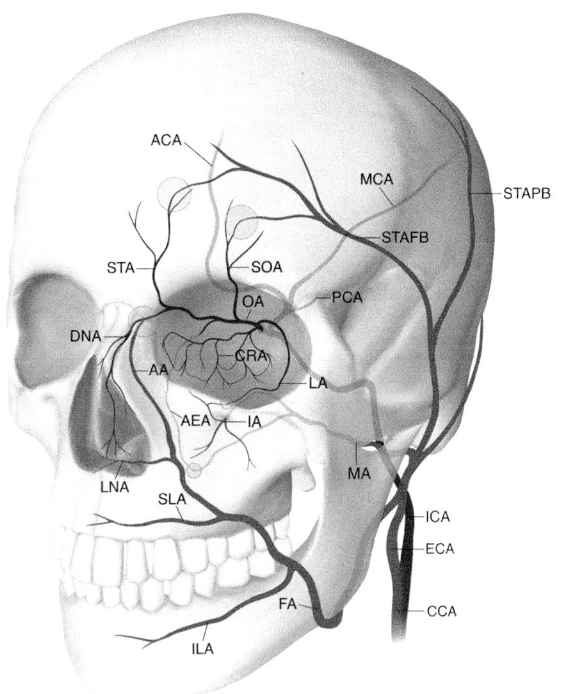

Fig. 22.4 Schematic diagram showing the extracranial branches of the ophthalmic artery and the anastamotic branches (*purple circle*) of the internal carotid artery (*blue*) and the external carotid artery (*red*). *AA*, angular art; *ACA*, anterior cerebral art; *AEA*, anterior ethmoidal art; *CCA*, common carotid art; *CRA*, central retinal art; *DNA*, dorsal nasal art; *ECA*, external carotid art; *FA*, facial art; *IA*, infraorbital art; *ICA*, internal carotid art; *ILA*, inf labial art; *LA*, lacrymal art; *LNA*, lateral nasal art; *MA*, maxillary art; *MCA*, middle cerebral art; *OA*, Ophthalmic art; *PCA*, posterior cerebral art; *SLA*, superior labial art; *SOA*, supraorbital art; *STA*, supratrochlear art; *STAFB*, superficial temporal artery frontal branch; *STAPB*, superficial temporal artery parietal branch. *Artwork created by R. Dong, reproduced with permission from the author.*

this group of patients are to increase the dorsal height, nasal tip projection, and elongation of the nasal tip with overall aim of increasing the three-dimensional definition of the nose as well as a "slimming effect" of the nasal shape. Such noses require fillers with a high cohesivity to resist the contracting forces of the tight, thick overlying skin envelope to elevate the bridge, project the tip of the nose anteriorly, or elongate the nose inferiorly. A small amount of filler placed lateral to the upper portion of the nasolabial fold can also displace the alar lobules medially, giving the impression of a narrower nasal base (Figs. 22.5A–D and 22.6A–F).

Caucasian noses usually have sufficient dorsal height, better projection, and definition of the tip due to the thinner skin envelope but may suffer from a dorsal hump, a narrow nasal bridge with an acute orbitonasal line, or a plunging tip. The common indication for this group is to correct some dorsal irregularities with a straighter dorsal and frontonasal profile, dorsal rotation of the nasal tip, and widening of the dorsal root of the nose. Fillers with a high cohesivity are desirable to provide structural support where it is needed, but fillers with a softer cohesivity can smoothen out surface or contour irregularities better. Patients with less-than-ideal results following surgical rhinoplasty can benefit from judicious and careful use of filler to smooth out any dorsal irregularities, camouflage some visible cartilage graft and correct excessive ski jump appearance (Fig. 22.7A–D). Plunging tips can be elevated by providing support at the anterior nasal spine and the columella. Treating any patients who had previous surgery or accident to the nose requires special skills and knowledge for it has an even higher risk of vascular complication than normal due to altered vascular anatomy and scar tissue. It is best reserved for those who operate in the area or those who have enough expertise in treating this area.

In the past, fillers were used only to augment the nasal dorsum, but today, with a variety of fillers having different degrees of cohesivity available, we are able to achieve better sculpting and shaping of the tip, columella, and base of the nose as well. The aesthetic considerations for injection rhinoplasty should be no different from performing a surgical augmentation rhinoplasty, with the fillers taking the place of either the implant or any cartilage grafts. In some cases, such as blending the dorsal aesthetic line with the medial end of the brow (the orbitonasal line), a filler can be more useful than an implant alone as it creates an aesthetically smoother and curved transition between the side of the nose and the medial end of the eyebrow. Implants on their own may actually aggravate the vertical glabellar furrows with a groove unesthetically breaking up the continuous orbitonasal line.

PAIN RELIEF

One of the authors (WW) routinely employs the following to provide anesthesia to the nose in anxious patients, prior to injection: a small amount (0.25 mL) of plain lidocaine 1% (without adrenaline) is administered to

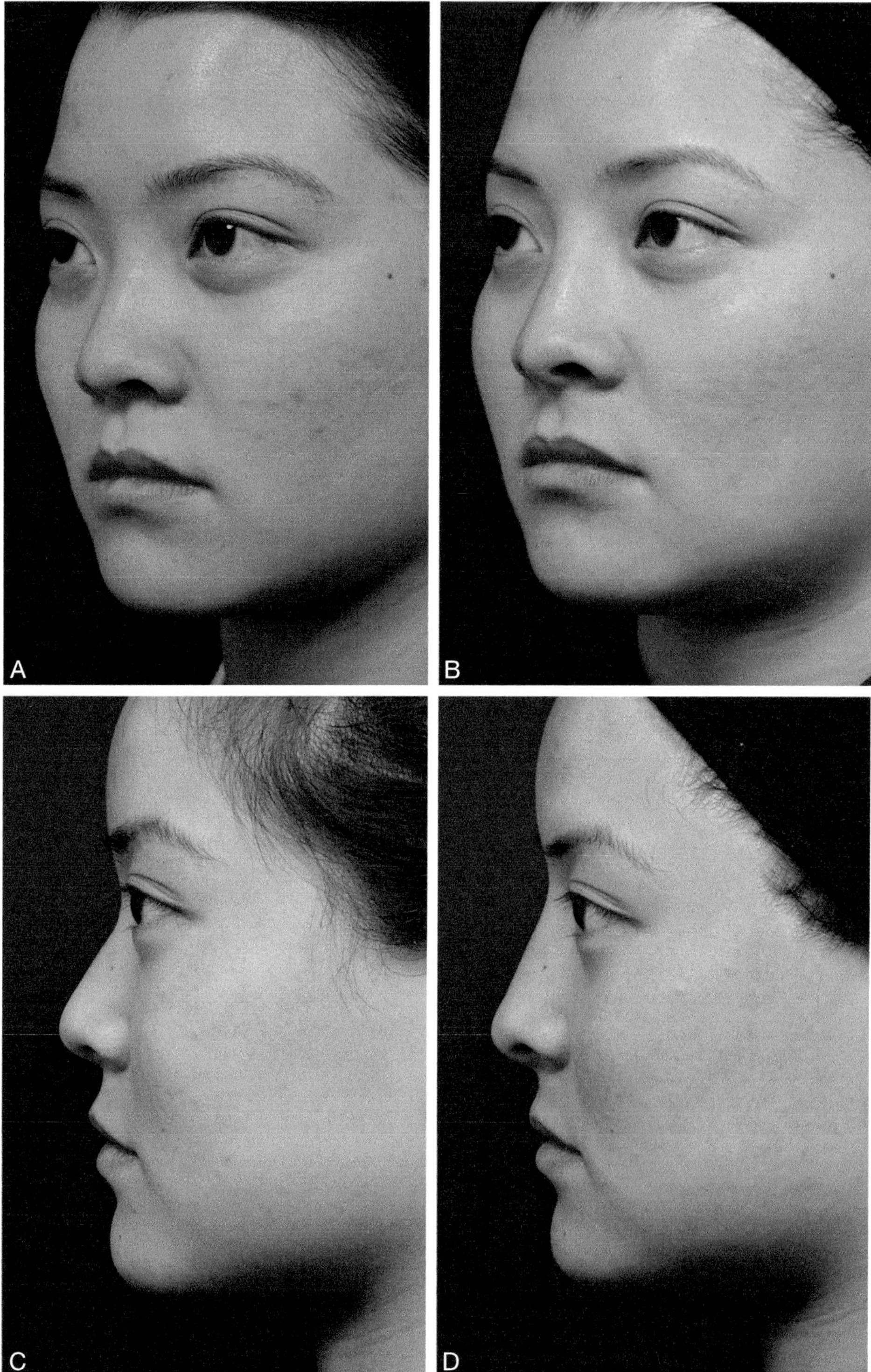

Fig. 22.5 (A–D) A young Asian female requested a higher nasal dorsum and more definition to her nose tip. A total of 1.5 mL of hyaluronic acid (HA) was used: 0.9 mL of the HA filler was placed at the nasal spine and columella to create a better projection of the nasal tip from the facial plane, whereas 0.6 mL of the same HA filler is placed on the nasal dorsum and nasal tip to create a higher nasal bridge, better definition of the nasal tip, and elongation of the nasal profile.

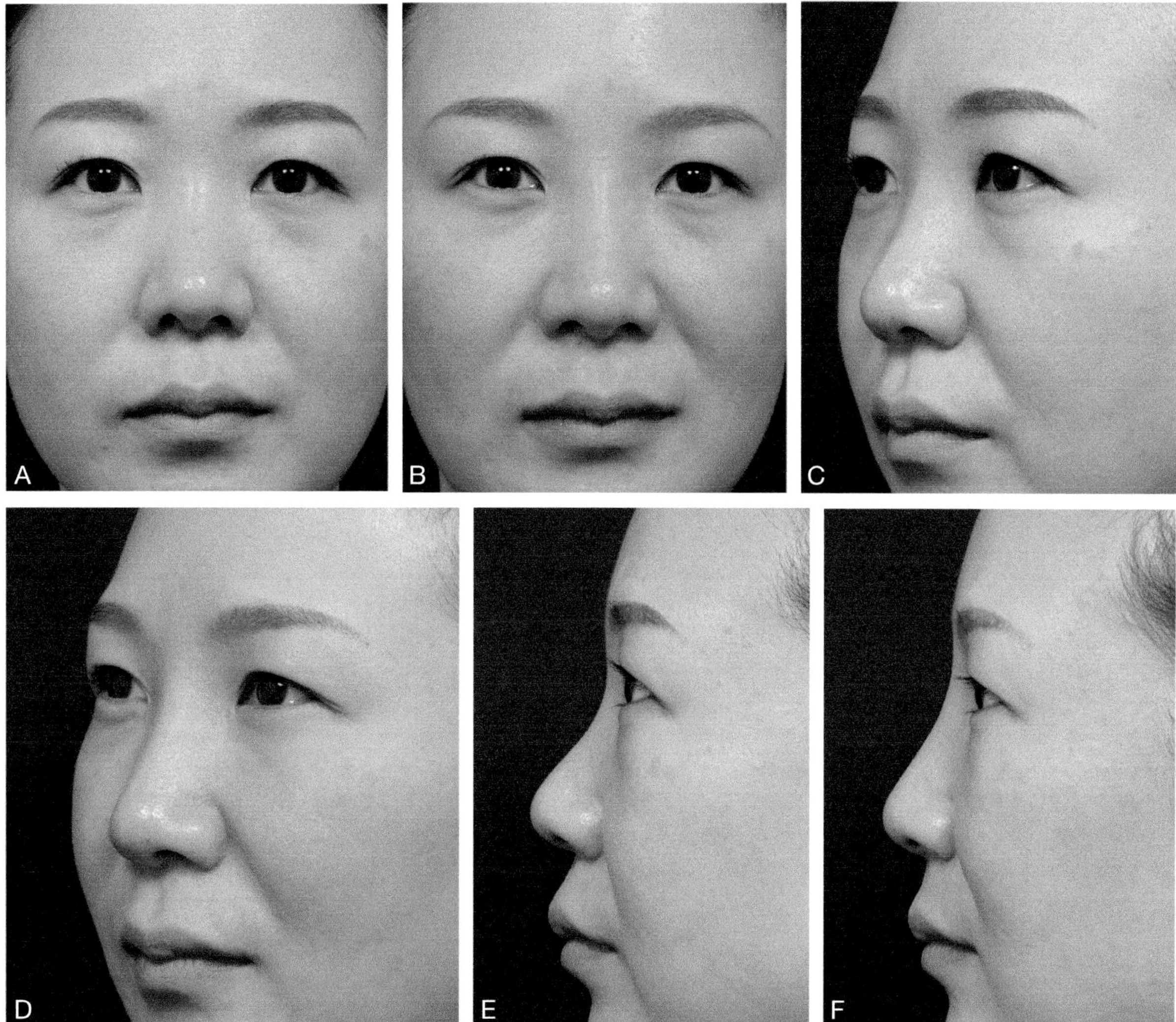

Fig. 22.6 (A–F) A young Asian female requested a more balanced and petite nasal appearance especially reducing the wide nasal lobules. A total of 1.6 mL of HA filler was used: 1.1 mL was placed on the nasal spine, columella, and ala base and 0.5 mL was used to augment the nasal dorsum and refine the nasal tip. The end result is a narrower nasal appearance with a more projected nasal tip, more acute columellar labial angle, and higher and defined nasal dorsum.

each of the supraorbital and infraorbital nerves, taking care not to allow the needle to enter into the foramina where the emerging blood vessels or nerves might be damaged. An additional bolus of 0.25 mL is also injected into the columellar-labial angle. With this combination, adequate anesthesia of the nose is achieved. Lidocaine with adrenaline should not be used as the blanching that inevitably happens due to vasoconstriction may mask a vascular obstruction.

INJECTION TECHNIQUE

Personal preference and the physician's own experience and familiarity with their tools will determine whether a cannula or a sharp needle will be used to deliver the fillers to the nose. Equally good results can be obtained using either technique. We prefer the sharp-needle technique using a half-inch 30 G or 27 G needle with the bevel facing downward for injecting the nose as it provides more "feel" and aids in a more accurate placement

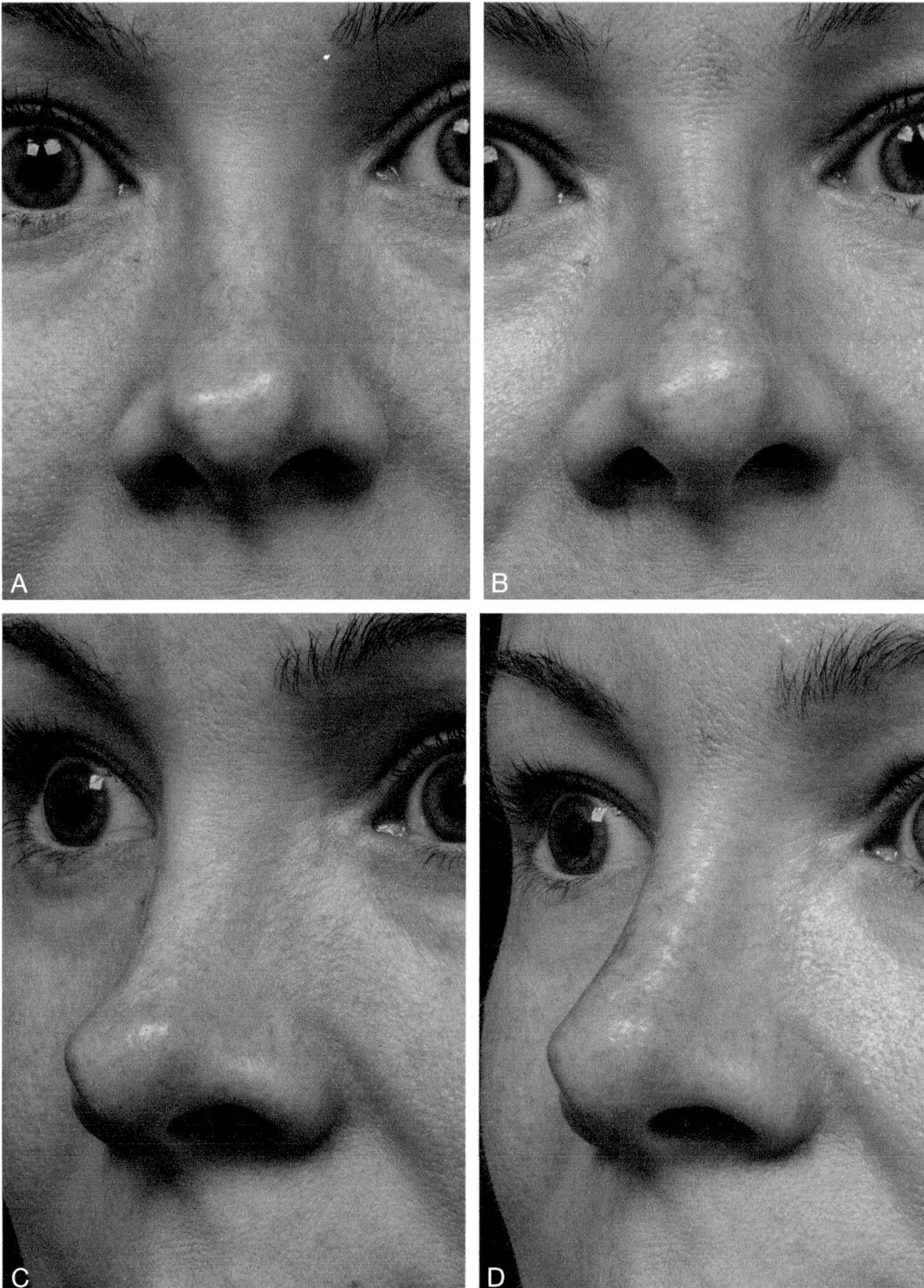

Fig. 22.7 (A–D) This patient requested a straighter nose, a straighter nasal profile to reduce dorsal irregularities, and ski-jump profile following surgery. She also disliked the visibility of her nasal tip cartilages. A total of 0.5 mL hyaluronic acid was in the form of multiple small aliquots on the bony and cartilage layer, along the dorsum and nasal tip. This was followed by gentle but thorough massage. The patient was kept in the office for a 30-minute observation period prior to discharge to ensure no vascular compromise. The result at 6 weeks showed a softer and straighter nose with a more pleasing nasal profile with good camouflage of the nasal tip cartilage. Vascular laser was offered to deal with her longstanding telangiectasia following her nasal surgery.

of the fillers in the desired layer of the nose, which in most situations should be directly onto the bone. The injection flow should be slow and steady. A 30 G needle slows down the flow of injection and reduces rapid delivery under high pressure. Slowing down the injection also creates greater awareness of the volumization process and the subtle changes in nasal shape that can be achieved. As long as the injection is deep on the bone and in the midline, problems of vascular occlusion can be minimized. One must always be mindful of the underlying vacular anatomy and minimize the risks of vascular compromise.

Level 1—the Six-Point Injection Technique

This is a simple, safe approach to augmenting the dorsum and tip of the nose as all the six injection points described are in the midline and injected deeply onto the bone or cartilage. A 27 or 30 G needle is used and introduced perpendicularly through the skin and soft tissue until the tip of the needle rests on the bone. The plunger is gently withdrawn to check for any backflow of blood. A bolus of filler is then slowly injected keeping the pressure steady as the needle continues to make contact with the bone or dorsum of the septal cartilage. Each bolus delivered is no larger than 0.1 to 0.2 mL. Careful attention must be paid to any sudden blanching or intense pain felt by the patient that might indicate a vascular occlusion requiring immediate treatment with hyaluronidase.

Point 1—this is the lowest point of the root of the nose usually at a level midway between the medial eyebrow and the medial canthus of the eye.

Point 2—this is halfway between point 1 and the dorsal hump or K-point of the nose.

Point 3—this point is just inferior to the projection of the dorsal hump and is injected onto the cartilaginous dorsum.

Point 4—this is at the supratip depression, also injected onto the dorsal edge of the cartilaginous septum.

Point 5—the needle is passed through the apex of the tip of the nose and inserted deeply toward the anterior nasal spine, traversing the columellar between the medial crura. Here, the injection starts deeply and continues as the needle is withdrawn retrogradely toward the tip, creating a column of filler that projects the tip forward or upward.

Point 6—this point is slightly above point 5, and here, a very small droplet of filler is injected intradermally or immediately subdermal to shape the tip and create an aesthetic nuance (Fig. 22.8A–F) (Video 22.1).

Level 2—the Eight-Point Injection Technique

This has two additional points (points 7 and 8) on either side of the midline and halfway between point 1 and the medial edge of the eyebrow. This widens the root of the nose and creates a more aesthetic orbitonasal line. The injection should be deep onto the bone to avoid injecting into a vessel. Injections anywhere other than subcutaneous or deep on the bone vascular compromise with necrosis of the supratrochlear territory are a potential risk. An example of a case receiving the eight-point injection technique is shown in Fig 22.9A,B.

Level 3—the 10-Point Injection Technique

Great care must be taken when performing this technique. Two further points, 9 and 10, are injected on either side of the alar lobule at the upper end of the nasolabial fold in order to narrow the apparent width of the nose. The filler is injected deeply as a bolus directly onto the bone by the side of the pyriform fossa, employing slow steady pressure (Fig. 22.9C). These injections may potentially occlude a branch of or even the facial artery itself if improperly delivered. As long as the needle touches the bone, there is less risk of any vascular compromise as there are no major blood vessels on the periosteum. It is when the injection is given too superficially in this region that the risk increases as the facial artery is, at this point, very superficial.

10 USEFUL TIPS FOR GOOD INJECTION OUTCOMES

1. Seat the patient upright, head stable, with good lighting.
2. HA fillers are safest.
3. Have hyaluronidase mixed and ready before you start injecting. Severe complications can occur very quickly.
4. Use a 27 or 30 G sharp needle for all injections as the needle tip can accurately make direct contact with the bone or the cartilage.
5. Once the needle tip contacts the bone or cartilage, do not move as the plunger is pressed
6. 30 G needles slow down the injection speed and help you focus on delivering the correct amount of filler.
7. Stay in the midline.

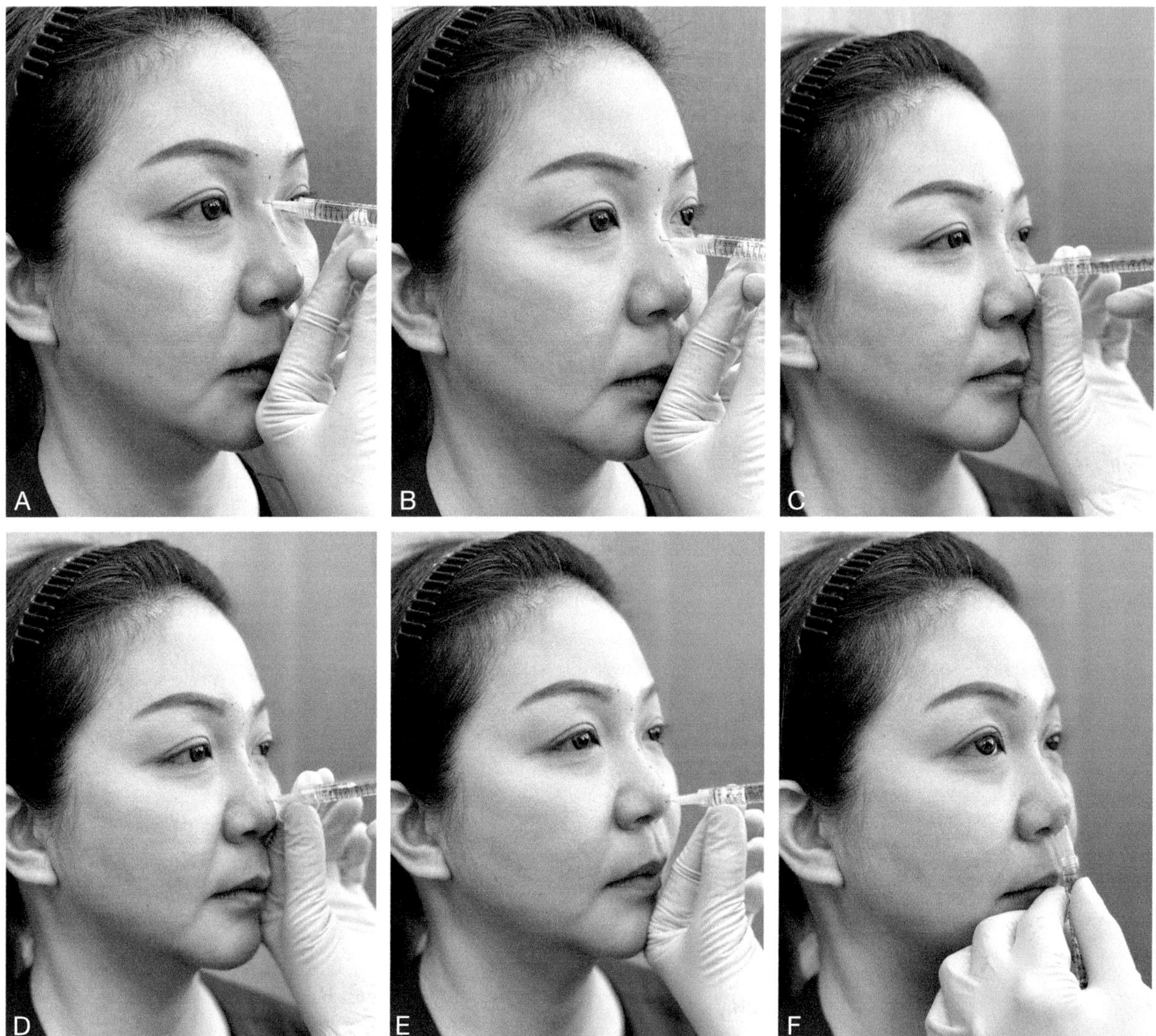

Fig. 22.8 (A–F) Six-point injection technique for nasal augmentation and contouring. The patient should be seated upright with the head rested comfortably on the back of the procedure chair. (A) Hyaluronic acid filler using a 27 or 30 G needle is aimed perpendicularly down to the bone of the nasal radix in the midline (point 1). A small bolus is delivered directly into the bone until the desired height of the nose is achieved. (B, C, D) The needle is removed and replaced at a point lower down from the previous injection to create a series of disconnected boluses that collectively create a slim aesthetic bridge (points 2, 3, and 4). (E) A columellar strut is created by retrogradely injecting a long column of filler from the anterior nasal spine to the tip (point 5). This linear injection should pass deeply between the medial crura and not on its surface as the columellar arteries run superficially just under the skin of the columellar. (F) For additional tip projection and refinement, a small amount of filler can be injected intradermally or immediately subdermal in the midline of the tip, thereby avoiding any major blood vessels.

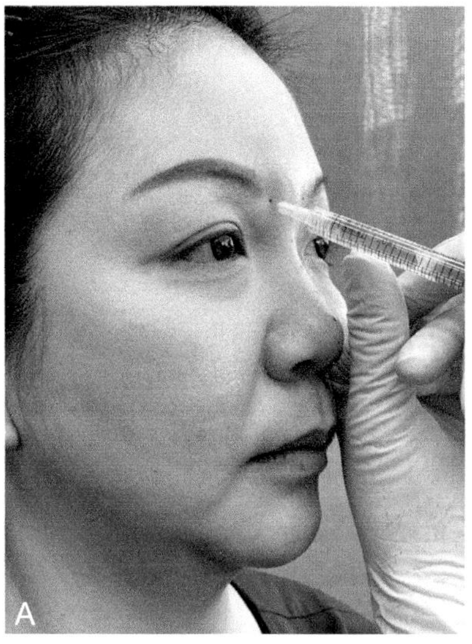

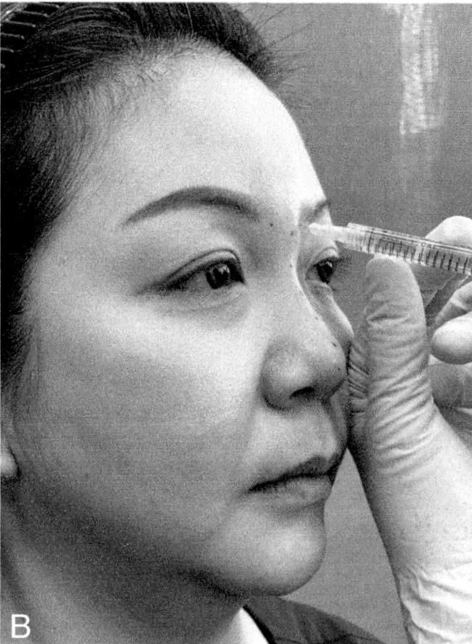

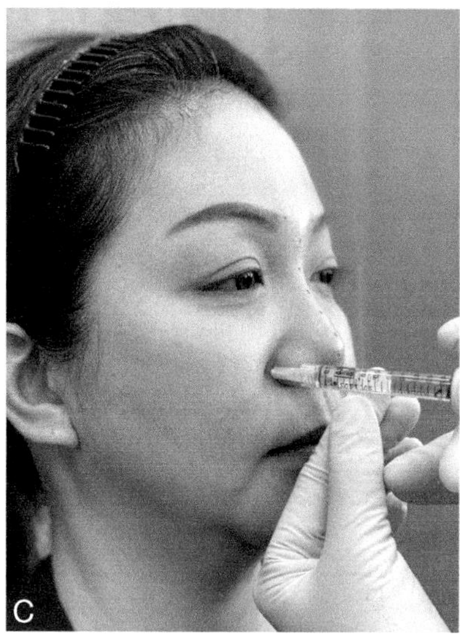

Fig. 22.9 (A, B) The nasal shape is completed by adding small boluses at either side of the radix (points 7 and 8) to create a smoothly curved naso-orbital aesthetic line or at points 9 and 10, deeply in each pyriform fossa (C).

8. Be aware of the underlying anatomical structures and stay away from bony foramina.
9. Be cautious of using a cannula as this tends to slip into the plane of least resistance which is where the vessels are. It is difficult to keep the cannula tip in contact with the bone of the nasal dorsum. If using a cannula, make sure the tip is moving all the time
10. Avoid a long, continuous line of filler along the nasal bridge as this gives an unaesthetic sausage-like appearance.

FURTHER READING

Beleznay, K., Carruthers, J. D. A., Humphrey, S., & Jones, D. (2015). Avoiding and treating blindness from fillers: A review of the world literature. *Dermatologic Surgery, 41*(10), 1097–1117.

Carruthers, J. D., Fagien, S., Rohrich, R. J., Weinkle, S., & Carruthers, A. (2014). Blindness caused by cosmetic filler injection: A review of cause and therapy. *Plastic and Reconstructive Surgery, 134*(6), 1197–1201.

Chatrath, V., Bannerjee, P. S., Goodman, G., & Rahman, E. (2019). Soft-tissue filler associated blindness: A systematic Rreview of case reports and case series. *Plastic and Reconstructive Surgery. Global Open, 7*(4), e2173.

De Lacerda, D. A., & Zancanaro, P. (2007). Filler rhinoplasty. *Dermatologic Surgery, 33*, S207–S212.

De Lorenzi, C. (2014). Complications of injectable fillers, part 2: Vascular complications. *Aesthetic Surgery Journal, 34*(4), 584–600.

Fukuta, K. (2016). Case report of blindness following injection rhinoplasty. Presentation ated at: 23rd Biennial Congress of ISAPS,; 23-27 Oct. 23–27, 2016.

He, M. S., Sheu, M. M., Huang, Z. L., Tsai, C. H., & Tsai, R. K. (2013). Sudden bilateral vision loss and brain infarction following cosmetic hyaluronic acid injection. *JAMA Ophthalmology, 131*, 1234–1235.

Humphrey, C. D., Arkins, J. P., & Dayan, S. H. (2009). Soft tissue fillers in the nose. *Aesthetic Surgery Journal, 29*(6), 477–484.

Jiang, X., Liu, D. L., & Chen, B. (2014). Middle temporal vein: A fatal hazard in injection cosmetic surgery for temple augmentation. *JAMA Facial Plastic Surgery, 16*(3), 227–229.

Kim, E. G., Eom, T. K., & Kang, S. J. (2014). Severe visual loss and cerebral infarction after injection of hyaluronic acid gel. *The Journal of Craniofacial Surgery, 25*(2), 684–686.

Kim, Y. J., Kim, S. S., Song, W. K., Lee, S. Y., & Yoon, J. S. (2011). Ocular ischemia with hypotony after injection of hyaluronic acid gel. *Ophthalmic Plastic and Reconstructive Surgery, 27*(6), 152–155.

Lazzeri, D., Agostini, T., Figus, M., Nardi, M., Pantaloni, M., & Lazzeri, S. (2012). Blindness following cosmetic injections of the face. *Plastic and Reconstructive Surgery, 129*(4), 995–1012.

Lazzeri, S., Figus, M., Nardi, M., Lazzeri, D., Agostini, T., & Zhang, Y. X. (2013). Iatrogenic retinal artery occlusion caused by cosmetic facial filler injections. *American Journal of Opthalmology*, *155*(2), 407–408.

Liew, S., Wu, W. T. L., Chan, H. H., Ho, W. W., Kim, H. J., Goodman, G. J., Peng, P. H., Rogers, J. D., et al. (2015). Consensus on changing trends, attitudes, and concepts of Asian beauty. *Aesthetic Plastic Surgery*, *40*(2), 193–201.

Liu, O. G., Chunming, L., Juanjuan, W., & Xiaoyan, X. (2014). Central retinal artery occlusion and cerebral inrfarction following forehead injection with a corticosteroid suspension for vitiligo. *Indian Journal of Dermatology, Venereology and Leprology*, *80*, 177–179.

Park, S. W., Woo, S. J., Park, K. H., Huh, J. W., Jung, C. L., & Kwon, O. K. (2012). Iatrogenic retinal artery occlusion caused by cosmetic facial filler injections. *American Journal of Opthalmology*, *154*(4), 653–662.

Piggot, J. R., & Yazdani, A. (2011). Hyaluronic acid used for the correction of nasal deviation in an 18 year old Middle Eastern man. *The Canadian Journal of Plastic Surgery*, *19*(4), 156–158.

Redaelli, A. (2008). Medical rhinoplasty with hyaluronic acid and botulinum toxin A: A very simple and quite effective technique. *Journal of Cosmetic Dermatology*, *7*, 210–220.

Samizadeh, S., & Wu, W. T. L. (2020). Ideals of facial beauty amongst the Chinese population: Results from a large national survey. *Aesthetic Plastic Surgery*, *42*(6), 1540–1550. https://doi.org/10.1007/s00266-018-1188-9.

Tansatit, T., Apinuntrum, P., & Phetudom, T. (2015). Temporal vein and the drainage vascular networks to assess the potential complications and the preventive maneuver during temporal augmentation using both anterograde and retrograde injections. *Aesthetic Plastic Surgery*, *39*(5), 791–799.

Wang, H. C. W., Yu, N. Z., Wang, X. J., et al. (2022). Cerebral embolism as a result of facial filler injections: A literature review. *Aesthetic Surgery Journal*, *42*(3). NP162–NP175.

Wu, W. T. L., Carlisle, I., Huang, P., et al. (2010). Novel administration technique for large particle stabilised hyaluronic acid-based gel of non-animal origin in facial tissue augmentation. *Aesthetic Plastic Surgery*, *34*(1), 88–95.

Wu, W. T. L., Liew, S., Chan, H. H., et al. (2015). Consensus on current injectable treatment strategies in the Asian face. *Aesthetic Plastic Surgery*, *40*(2), 202–214.

Wu Woffles, T. L. (2017). Aesthetic contouring of the upper and central third of the face with soft tissue fillers. In V. Tonnard (Ed.), *Centrofacial rejuvenation* (pp. 278–288). Publishers Thieme. chapter 10.

Wu, W. T. L. (2019). Injection rhinoplasty—aesthetic considerations and the anatomical basis for safe injection techniques. In D. Jones, & A. Swift (Eds.), *Injectable fillers: Facial contouring and shaping* (2nd ed., pp. 131–147). Wiley Publishing. chapter 7.

Woffles, T. L., & Wu, W. T. L. (2009). Periorbital rejuvenation with injectable fillers. In S. R. Cohen, & T. M. Born (Eds.), *Facial rejuvenation with fillers. techniques in aesthetic plastic surgery series* (pp. 93–105). Saunders. chapter 8.

Wu, W. T. L. (1992). The oriental nose: An anatomical basis for surgery. *Annals of the Academy of Medicine, Singapore*, *21*, 176–189.

Zhang, L., Feng, X., Shi, H. Y., Wu, W. T. L., & Wu, S. F. (2020). Blindness after facial filler injections: The role of extravascular hyaluronidase on intravascular hyaluronic acid embolism in the rabbit experimental model. *Aesthetic Surgery Journal*, *40*(3), 319–326.

Zhang, L., Feng, X., Shi, H. Y., Wu, W. T. L., & Wu, S. F. (2019). Clinical observation and the anatomical basis of blindness after facial hyaluronic acid injection. *Aesthetic Plastic Surgery*, *43*(4), 1054–1060.

23

Filler Injection of the Melolabial Folds and Marionette Lines

Britney N. Wilson, Andrew F. Alexis, and Kent Remington

SUMMARY AND KEY FEATURES

- Addressing the melolabial folds and marionette lines is a key issue in facial rejuvenation. Understanding the underlying anatomy of the perioral region, careful consideration of filler properties, and tailoring treatment to the patient's individual goals are key to achieving optimal outcomes.
- Discussion of the underlying factors that contribute to the development of melolabial folds and marionette lines.
- Expert recommendations for filler selection and optimal injection technique.

INTRODUCTION

Drooping and line formation near the corner of the mouth are among the most recognizable signs of facial aging. Addressing the melolabial folds and marionette lines is a key issue in facial rejuvenation. Best outcomes are achieved with an understanding of the underlying factors that lead to the development of these folds or lines—namely, the evolving anatomy of the aging lateral oral commissure, marionette zone (also referred as the labiomandibular or melomental folds), and prejowl sulcus. The loss of chin volume that occurs with aging results in the formation of a chasm into which the lateral oral commissure droops. This, combined with an increased prominence of the marionette zone that occurs with aging, results in the downward turn of the oral commissures. Together, these changes cause the individual to have an appearance of sadness. The underlying anatomy—specifically hyperreactivity of the platysma and depressor anguli oris (DAO)—are responsible for these unwanted signs of aging.

UNDERLYING ANATOMY AND KEY CONCEPTS

In-depth knowledge of midface anatomy is needed as the development of marionette lines can be linked to midface changes like the loss of midface elasticity and soft tissue volume. Buccal fat produces the appearance of youthfulness, but with age, it can move inferiorly. As we age, the marionette zone becomes even more conspicuous due to a loss of cheek support and inferior pull from jowl fat. Treating deeper prominent class III to IV melomental folds may require targeting of the initial midface changes through reflating and revolumizing buccal fat. This minimizes the pseudoptosis responsible for aggravating age-related changes of the marionette zone and melolabial folds.

Dynamic discord is an important concept to understand in the development of the melolabial folds and marionette lines. The muscles of facial expression overpower tissue resistance with time, creating the folds and lines characteristic of facial aging. While extrinsic factors such as sun exposure and cigarette smoking play a role, facial animation contributes the greatest influence on wrinkle formation in the perioral region. Idiosyncratic expressions, of which patients are generally unaware, lead to the development of lines and folds over time. This is more evident in the perioral (and periorbital) zones and at first, is only visible with animation but with time becomes visible even without animation. Constant activation of the downward-pulling DAO muscle is a key contributor to these lines and folds.

KEY CONSIDERATIONS AND PRACTICAL RECOMMENDATIONS FOR FILLER INJECTION

Hyaluronic acid (HA) fillers are key to rejuvenation of the perioral region, including the marionette and melolabial zones. They address what the current author (KR) refers to as the "7 dimensions (7 Ds)" of facial rejuvenation: (1) lines and wrinkles; (2) creases and folds; (3) reflation and facial contouring; (4) creating harmony, balance, and phi proportions; (5) balancing form and function through synergistic use of fillers and neuromodulators; (6) myomodulation of muscles of animation; and (7) neuro-myomodulation combining HA filler with a neuromodulator. A multimodal approach utilizing HA with a neuromodulator targets two key contributors to the aging melomental fold—mimetic muscle activity and volume loss. To compound the synergistic lifting and stabilizing of the lateral oral commissure, the marionette zone and the prejowl sulcus need to be shaped and lifted—with HA fillers and neuromodulator to the DAO muscle group. Injecting an HA with stretch and strength into and just above the DAO muscle may create some myomodulation effect with improved neuromuscular activity and connectivity. Injecting the DAO with a neuromodulator increases the persistence of HA by decreasing the mimetic muscle activity of this region. This may create a neuromyomodulation effect compounding the positive reversal of the DAO muscle on the lateral oral commissure. This impacts the positive result and improves the longevity of the outcome.

Choosing the right "personality" of the filler is important: it needs to be flexible and have some lift and bendability. The personality of a filler is influenced by factors like the concentration of HA, cohesivity, the degree of cross-linking, and gel hardness (G′). It is important that the HA filler has enough stretch and strength to be flexible with animation, which is a key contributor to patient satisfaction. HA fillers with a higher G' and low water uptake like Voluma (Allergan, Irvine, CA) provide tissue support and are suitable for deeper injections in regions like the prejowl sulcus and marionette regions where both support of overlying tissues and a change in volume are desired. Restoring the lateral oral commissure, marionette zone, and prejowl sulcus contributes to the restoration of a youthful lower face and should not be overlooked when reflating the deflated chin. Juvederm Volift, a more diluted gel that adds filler with a softer, less lifted appearance, can also be used in the marionette zone either alone or layered above Voluma. Others have reported that other fillers such as Perlane-L (Galderma Laboratories LP, Fort Worth, Tex.), with a high G' and lifting capacity, can also be utilized in this region.

The lateral oral commissure (LOC) zone is a "minefield of blood vessels." As such, one of the authors (KR) prefers the use of cannulas for HA fillers to reduce the risk of bruising, tissue damage, and posttreatment swelling. The Flying V technique developed by author KR can be a very rewarding technique for your patients and clinic. Starting at the angle of the jaw (see media for a complete narrated video demonstration of procedure, Video 23.1), a 25-G 50-mm cannula is directed in a horizontal flying V pattern aimed toward lateral oral commissure. Starting right above the red part of the upper lip using a twirling and spinning motion, the cannula is gently injected subcutaneously, aiming just above and medial to the lateral oral commisure (LOC) corner. The corner of the mouth is then lifted with the "smart hand" (i.e., hand opposite to the one being used for injection) while injecting to recreate the support of the LOC. The marionette zone is reflated and contoured with a "windshield wiper"-like effect and the product is injected anterogradely and retrogradely. This allows for the development of a zone of filler, rather than an unwanted band of filler. It is important to also inject the modiolus and the area under the DAO muscle. With the patient's mouth slightly open, injection of the modiolus can be achieved using the nondominant hand to hold the skin taut between the index finger positioned above the lip and the thumb positioned below the lip. This allows for the development of countertraction, which aids in the injection of filler.

In very animated patients, it may be necessary to inject under and on top of the muscle in addition to subcutaneously. In the current author's (KR's) experience, using the thenar eminence when injecting the plunger head allows for finer, better, and more precise cannula control. The amount of HA required for correction of the lateral oral commissure–marionette zone–prejowl sulcus depends on various factors including length, width, depth, associated volume loss, and presence or absence of a crease, with the average being 1.5 mL per session. After injection, molding and blending of the HA filler outside and inside the corner of the mouth with ultrasound gel are a useful technique.

A thorough understanding of the underlying anatomy of the perioral region of the face is essential. The inferior aspect of the melomental fold may house the mental nerve, artery, and vein. Being aware of these anatomical sites will help prevent patient discomfort and vascular compromise. When injecting this area, safety precautions should also be taken to avoid inadvertently weakening of the depressor labii inferioris (DLI), which can result in oral incompetence and/or lower lip asymmetry.[7]

CONCLUSIONS

The melolabial folds and marionette lines are defining features of the aging face. These changes are not only aesthetically displeasing but also have unwanted social implications. Ptosis of the oral commissures conveys an image of sadness or displeasure, and this has the propensity to influence how people are perceived by others.[13,15] These social implications can have economic consequences. Youthful appearances achieved through cosmetic surgery have been linked to workplace success, while an aged appearance has been cited as a barrier to employment time.

Fortunately, the advent of soft tissue fillers has revolutionized the ability to reduce signs of aging in this particular perioral location. HA fillers are a safe and minimally invasive technique that can significantly improve patient appearance and minimize signs of aging. They have the added benefit of simple titration and stepwise correction, making it easier to achieve the patient's desired appearance. Tailoring treatment to the individual's current appearance and youthful prior appearance alongside in-depth awareness of the perioral anatomy will optimize syringe therapy outcomes and lead to ideal patient satisfaction.

FURTHER READING

Ali, M. J., Ende, K., & Maas, C. S. (2007). Perioral rejuvenation and lip augmentation. *Facial Plastic Surgery Clinics of North America*, *15*(4), 491–500. https://doi.org/10.1016/j.fsc.2007.08.008. vii.

American Society of Plastic Surgeons. (2009). Women in the workforce link cosmetic surgery to success. http://www.plasticsurgery.org/Media/Press_Releases/Women_in_the_Workforce_Link_Cosmetic_Surgery_to_Success.html. Accessed June 26, 2021.

Berger, E. D. (2009). Managing age discrimination: An examination of the techniques used when seeking employment. *The Gerontologist*, *49*(3), 317–332. https://doi.org/10.1093/geront/gnp031.

Borrell, M., Leslie, D. B., & Tezel, A. (2011). Lift capabilities of hyaluronic acid fillers. *Journal of Cosmetic and Laser Therapy*, *13*(1), 21–27. https://doi.org/10.3109/14764172.2011.552609.

Braz, A., Humphrey, S., Weinkle, S., Yee, G. J., Remington, B. K., Lorenc, Z. P., et al. (2015). Lower face: Clinical anatomy and regional approaches with injectable fillers. *Plastic and Reconstructive Surgery*, *136*, 235s–257s. https://doi.org/10.1097/PRS.0000000000001836.

Carruthers, A., Carruthers, J., Hardas, B., Kaur, M., Goertelmeyer, R., Jones, D., et al. (2008). A validated grading scale for marionette lines. *Dermatologic Surgery*, *34*(suppl 2), S167–S172. https://doi.org/10.1111/j.1524-4725.2008.34366.x.

Carruthers, J., & Carruthers, A. (2003). A prospective, randomized, parallel group study analyzing the effect of BTX-A (Botox) and nonanimal sourced hyaluronic acid (NASHA, Restylane) in combination compared with NASHA (Restylane) alone in severe glabellar rhytides in adult female subjects: Treatment of severe glabellar rhytides with a hyaluronic acid derivative compared with the derivative and BTX-A. *Dermatologic Surgery*, *29*(8), 802–809. https://doi.org/10.1046/j.1524-4725.2003.29212.x.

Charles Finn, J., Cox, S. E., & Earl, M. L. (2003). Social implications of hyperfunctional facial lines. *Dermatologic Surgery*, *29*(5), 450–455. https://doi.org/10.1046/j.1524-4725.2003.29112.x.

Coleman, K. R., & Carruthers, J. (2006). Combination therapy with BOTOX and fillers: The new rejuvnation paradigm. *Dermatologic Therapy*, *19*(3), 177–188. https://doi.org/10.1111/j.1529-8019.2006.00072.x.

Cotofana, S., Fratila, A. A., Schenck, T. L., Redka-Swoboda, W., Zilinsky, I., & Pavicic, T. (2016). The anatomy of the aging face: A review. *Facial Plastic Surgery*, *32*(3), 253–260. https://doi.org/10.1055/s-0036-1582234.

Goodman, G. J., Swift, A., & Remington, B. K. (2015). Current concepts in the use of Voluma, Volift, and Volbella. *Plastic and Reconstructive Surgery*, *136*, 139s–148s. https://doi.org/10.1097/PRS.0000000000001734.

McKee, D., Remington, K., Swift, A., Lambros, V., Comstock, J., & Lalonde, D. (2019). Effective rejuvenation with hyaluronic acid fillers: Current advanced concepts. *Plastic and Reconstructive Surgery.*, *143*(6), 1277e–1289e. https://doi.org/10.1097/PRS.0000000000005607.

Muhn, C., Rosen, N., Solish, N., Bertucci, V., Lupin, M., Dansereau, A., et al. (2012). The evolving role of hyaluronic acid fillers for facial volume restoration and contouring: A Canadian overview. *Clinical, Cosmetic and Investigational Dermatology*, *5*, 147–158.

Perkins, N. W., Smith, S. P., Jr., & Williams, E. F., 3rd. (2007). Perioral rejuvenation: Complementary techniques and procedures. *Facial Plastic Surgery Clinics of North America*, *15*(4), 423–432, vi. https://doi.org/10.1016/j.fsc.2007.08.002.

Swift, A., Liew, S., Weinkle, S., Garcia, J. K., & Silberberg, M. B. (2021). The facial aging process from the "inside out". *Aesthetic Surgery Journal*, *41*(10), 1107–11190. https://doi.org/10.1093/asj/sjaa339.

Tezel, A., & Fredrickson, G. H. (2008). The science of hyaluronic acid dermal fillers. *Journal of Cosmetic and Laser Therapy*, *10*(1), 35–42. https://doi.org/10.1080/14764170701774901.

Weinkle, S. (2010). Injection techniques for revolumization of the perioral region with hyaluronic acid. *Journal of Drugs in Dermatology*, *9*(4), 367–371.

Wise, J. B., & Greco, T. (2006). Injectable treatments for the aging face. *Facial Plastic Surgery*, *22*(2), 140–146. https://doi.org/10.1055/s-2006-947720.

24

Soft Tissue Augmentation of the Chin and Jawline

Matthew Sandre and Vince Bertucci

SUMMARY AND KEY FEATURES

- The use of injectable soft tissue fillers in the chin and jawline is becoming increasingly popular.
- A deep knowledge of the underlying anatomy and anatomic changes that occur with age is essential to improve outcomes and minimize risk when treating the lower face.
- Hyaluronic acid-, calcium hydroxyapatite-, and poly-L-lactic acid-based injectables can all be considered for chin and jawline augmentation.
- Adjuvant therapy with neuromodulators, energy-based devices, and in some cases, surgical modalities, can help optimize aesthetic results.

INTRODUCTION

Lower face augmentation is increasing in popularity as evidenced by the American Society for Aesthetic Plastic Surgery data showing a 20% increase in mentoplasties between 2017 and 2018, with this procedure being most common in the 18- to 34-year-old age category. Historically, augmentation of the lower face was frequently addressed surgically, whereas a skilled injector can now achieve similar aesthetic results with soft tissue fillers. Despite the benefits of soft tissue filler injections, practitioners not uncommonly fail to address the lower face, possibly because of the advanced techniques required and challenging nature of treating this area. Assessment of the lower face is an important consideration in the facial aesthetics for both men and women as appropriate treatment of the chin and jawline can lead to significant improvement in global facial aesthetics.

AGING OF THE LOWER FACE

Facial aging occurs as a result of many factors including bone and fat remodeling and resorption, attenuation of facial septa, and loss of elastic tissue (Fig. 24.1). When combined with gravity, these changes result in soft tissue descent. A 2010 computed tomography (CT) scan study found many similarities between male and female skeletal changes over time, including decreased mandibular ramus height, body height, and body length and increased mandibular angle (Fig. 24.2). As a result, the mandible undergoes an anterior and inferior pattern of resorption. The chin also undergoes changes, becoming more anterior and shorter with age.

Fat pad resorption and weakening of facial ligaments and septa contribute to changes seen in the lower face. Some authors believe that the ligaments retain their strength yet the unsupported tissue between the ligaments shifts inferiorly due to gravity. In contrast, it is thought that a weakening of the mandibular septum causes the superior and inferior jowl fat pads to shift inferiorly, contributing to the appearance of jowls. No significant anterior fat pad shift occurs due to what is thought to be the retained strength of the mandibular ligament, which appears as a groove in the skin anterior to the jowl. The weak adherence of the platysma to the mandible posterior to this ligament has also been shown to contribute to jowl formation. Furthermore, Suwanchinda and colleagues demonstrated in cadaver dissections that the arrangement of subcutaneous fibroconnective tissue leads to the formation of the mental crease.

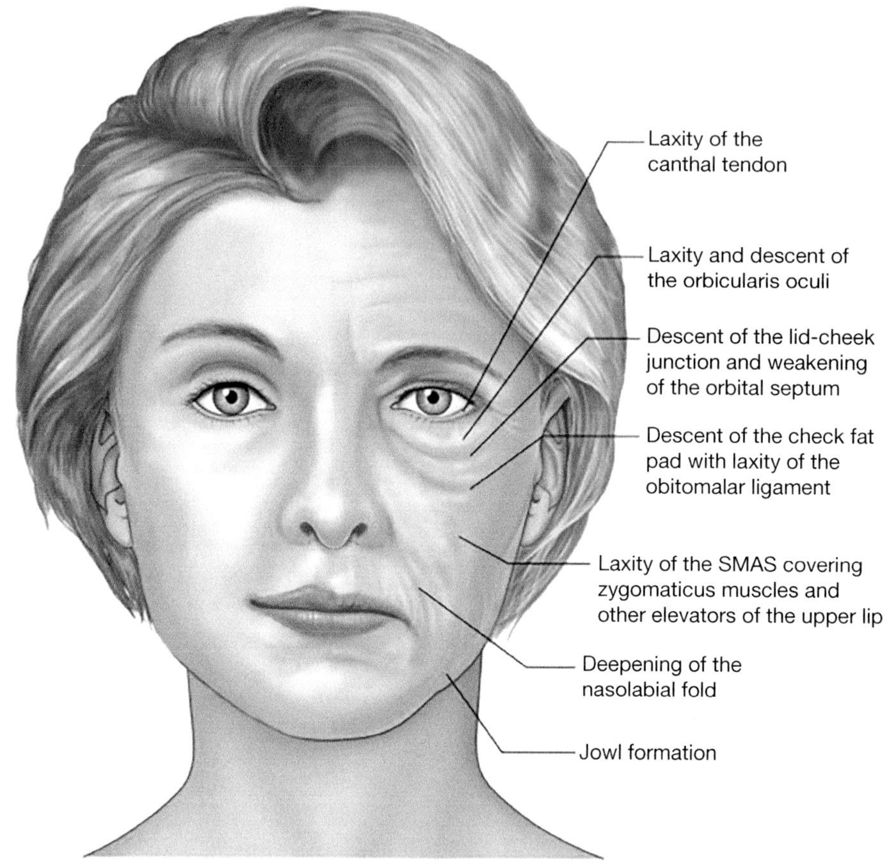

Fig. 24.1 Split-face diagram highlighting changes seen with the aging process. (From The Aging Face—ClinicalKey Fig 38.12.)

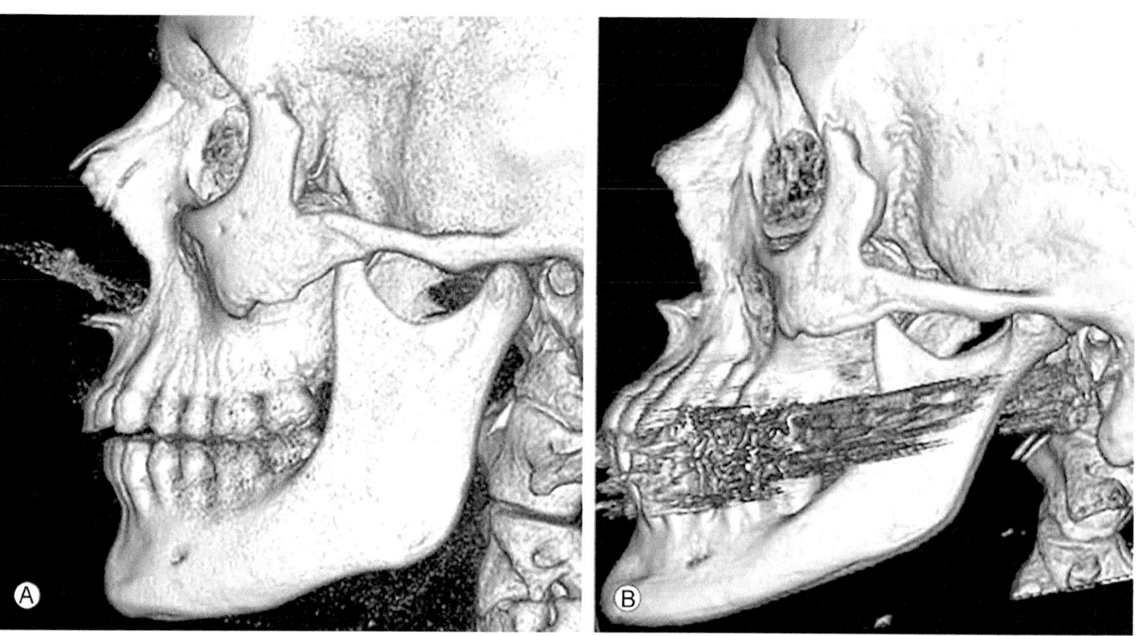

Fig. 24.2 Mandibular changes that occur with aging. (A) Young skeleton. (B) Aged skeleton. (From Rejuvenation of the aging face and skeleton with implants—ClinicalKey Fig. 13.8.)

Females tend to have more rapid soft tissue atrophy in the perimenopausal period, whereas males show a more linear decline over time. Combined with skin atrophy, these changes result in an overall loss of chin and jawline definition, leading to an aged appearance of the lower face.

IDEALS OF LOWER FACE BEAUTY

Although concepts of facial beauty and ideals have evolved somewhat over time and vary between ethnic groups, understanding global facial proportions and symmetry are still critical to achieving optimal outcomes. Furthermore, many ideals of facial beauty are shared across cultures and over time it is through an understanding of these ideals that one can understand facial beauty.

A foundational concept in achieving optimal results is that of 360 degree facial assessment. This seemingly simple concept is often overlooked by patients and injectors alike. Failure to assess the profile view carries with it the real risk of creating unnatural proportions. Similarly, it is important to assess the face both at rest and in animation.

The frontal view permits assessment of the vertical thirds and horizontal fifths of the face, which should respectively be roughly equal. Understanding these and the importance of facial proportions in general may lead the injector to plan, for example, to elongate the chin or widen the jawline to help balance facial proportions.

As seen in Fig. 24.3, a masculine facial shape is often compared to a square, where the bizygomatic to bigonial width ratio is close to 1:1. Men often have wider chins that are roughly the width of the mouth and have more well-developed lateral chin tubercles. In contrast, females often desire a more rounded and narrowed chin. The ideal overall facial shape for females can vary from patient to patient, including oval, heart, round, and angular, to name a few. It is important to note that in females, a bizygomatic-to-bigonial ratio of greater than 1:1 is desired such that the midface is wider and the lower face is narrower. However, injectors must keep in

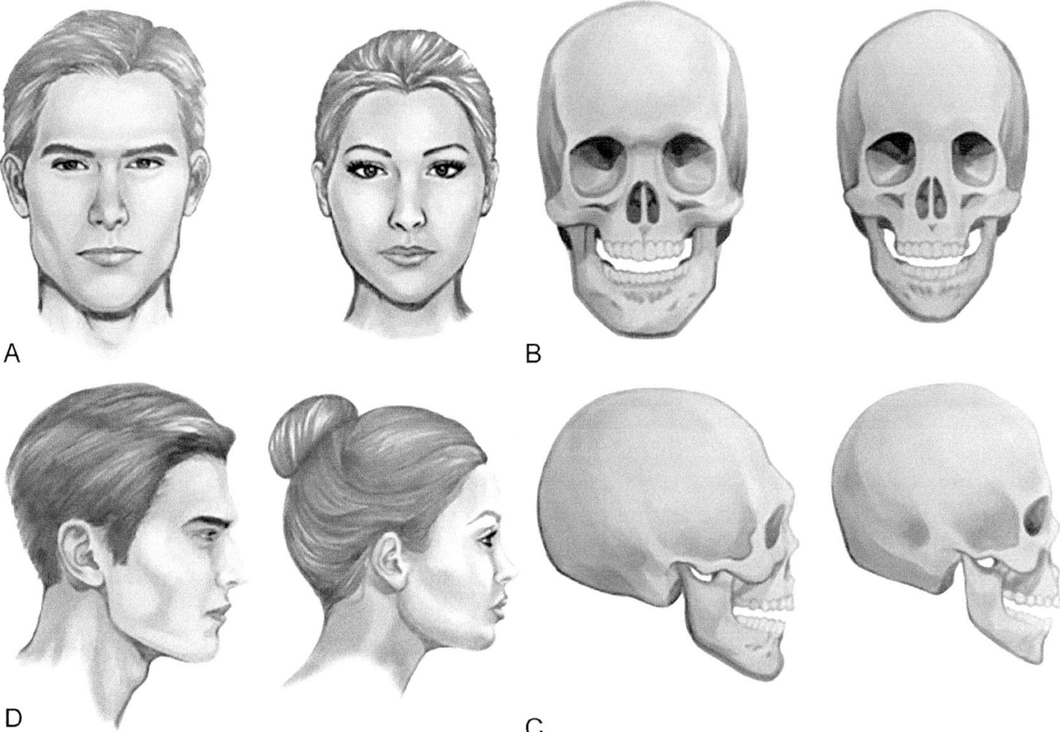

Fig. 24.3 Differences in male and female faces. (A) Frontal view. (B) Frontal skeletal view. (C) Lateral view. (D) Lateral skeletal view. (From Lower jaw recontouring in facial gender-affirming surgery—ClinicalKey.)

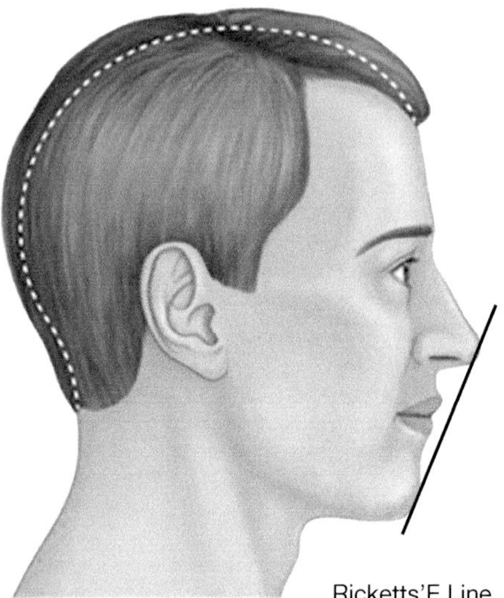

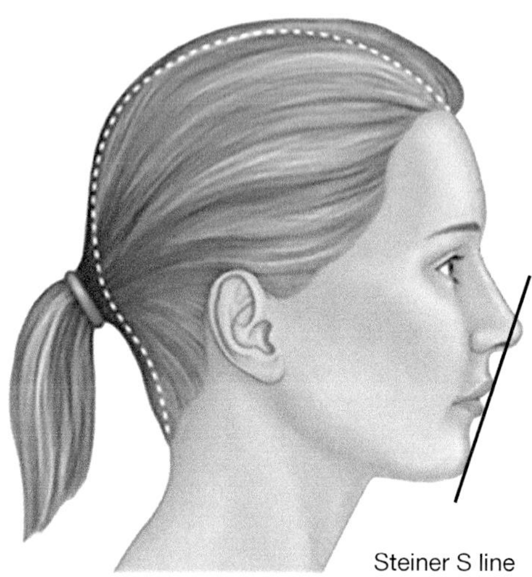

Fig. 24.4 Ricketts' E Line *(left)* and Steiner S line *(right)*. (From Aesthetic contouring of the craniofacial skeleton—ClinicalKey Figure 14.4.)

mind that the zygoma and mandible, and their ideal ratios, do not exist independently from the remainder of the midface and upper face. For example, in a patient with temporal volume loss, widening the bizygomatic width to achieve facial harmony with the bigonial width may inadvertently accentuate the skeletonized appearance of the upper face.

On the profile view, males have a more protuberant chin, whereas a feminine chin sits just posterior to the vermillion of the lower lip. Upper lip, nose, and chin projections are closely related and must be considered together in treatment planning. A number of methods for assessing soft tissue balance of the lips, nose and chin have been developed, including Ricketts E line and Steiner S line (Fig. 24.4), the latter being widely used in orthodontics. When the aforementioned structures are balanced, the lips should touch the Steiner S line, which is a line extending from the soft tissue pogonion to the middle of an S-shaped curve between the nasal tip and subnasale. Jacobson's soft tissue analysis is another useful cephalometric landmark to be aware of when assessing facial profiles (Fig. 24.5). This analysis classifies facial profiles into straight, convex, or concave categories based on the angle formed at the intersection of lines drawn from the glabella to subnasale, and subnasale to soft tissue pogonion. An angle of convexity of 8 to 16 degrees indicates a straight profile, while an increased or decreased angle represents a convex or concave profile, respectively.

Where the most inferior portion of the mandibular ramus and the most lateral portion of the mandibular body meet is termed the "mandibular angle." A 2016 internet survey on male jaw shape revealed that desirable features include a 130-degree mandibular angle and that the transition to the vertical portion of the jawline should be no lower than the lower lip and ideally in line with the oral commissure. A reduction in the mandibular angle, resulting in a smoother vertical to horizontal transition, is thought to create a more feminine jawline compared to the prominent flexure of the male jaw.

ANATOMY

Bone

The mandible is the primary bony structure of the lower face consisting of a horseshoe-like inferior body and two perpendicular mandibular rami. The mandibular bodies join at the midline mentonian symphysis. Falling near the midpupillary vertical line, the mental foramen is found between the lower and upper mandibular borders. A vertical line drawn through the second inferior premolar is another landmark used to locate the mental foramen. Both the mental nerve and artery exit from this foramen.

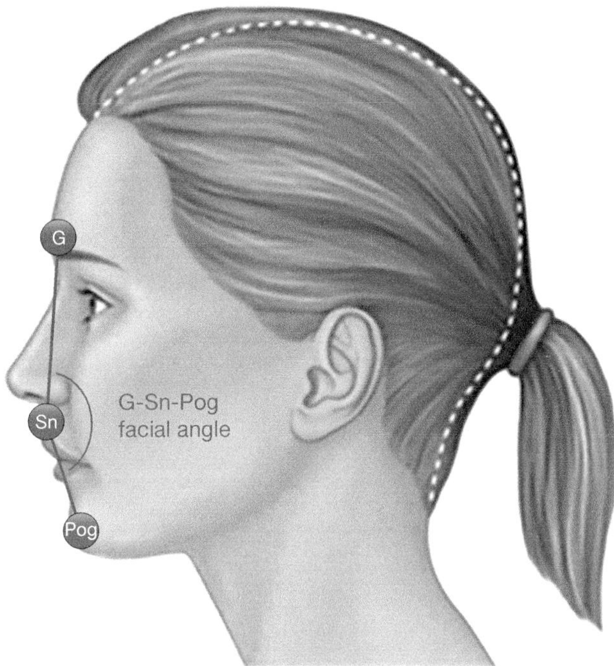

Fig. 24.5 G-Sn-Pog facial angle.

Fat Pads

As with other areas of the face, the lower face has superficial and deep fat compartments (Fig. 24.6). The mandibular region consists of four deep fat compartments: the superior and inferior mandibular fat compartments, submandibular fat compartment, and a fat compartment covering the parotid-masseteric fascia. The superficial fat pads relevant to the soft tissue augmentation of the lower fat are the lateral-temporal cheek compartment located in the preauricular area, the midcheek fat compartment, and the superior and inferior jowl fat compartments. The chin has its own superficial and deep fat pads as well that can be addressed with filler.

Ligaments and Septi

The facial septums and ligaments most relevant to soft tissue augmentation of the lower face are the mandibular septum, mandibular ligament, and masseteric cutaneous ligament (Fig. 24.7). Their possible relevance to the aging process has been discussed earlier. The mandibular septum originates approximately 1 cm superior to the mandibular border and separates the mandibular edge from the submandibular fat compartment. Some authors believe that it is an extension of the mandibular ligament. The mandibular ligament is found at the inferior border of the labiomandibular sulcus, anterior to the jowls, and traverses behind the depressor anguli oris (DAO) muscle, inserting into the dermis. The mandibular ligament reflects the most inferior portion of the facial line of ligaments. This line of ligaments is important for injectors to be aware of as placement of product lateral and medial to the line has a lifting and volumizing effect, respectively. Lastly, the masseteric cutaneous ligament is considered a vertical separation of the lateral cheek and premasseteric space. Its exact placement over the masseter appears to vary from the anterior-border to the midline of the masseter muscle itself.

Vasculature

The facial artery traverses the mandible at the antegonial notch, approximately 3 cm anterior to the mandibular angle and approximately 1 cm anterior to the anterior border of the masseter (Fig. 24.8). This vessel can often easily be palpated. Lateral and deep to the facial artery is the facial vein. Both of these vessels cross the mandible in the deep fat, deep to the platysma. The facial artery runs deep in the buccal fat, branching into the superior and inferior labial arteries near the modiolus.

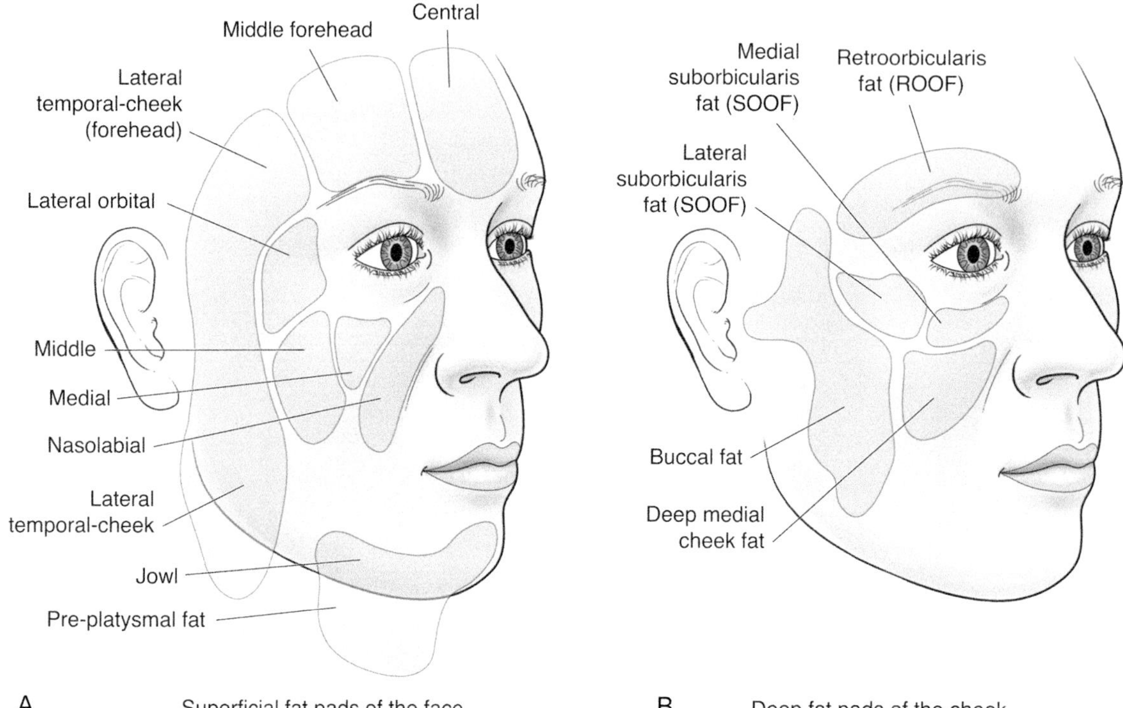

Fig. 24.6 Facial fat pads. (From Nerad, Jeffrey A., MD, FACS: Techniques in Ophthalmic Plastic Surgery. Published December 31, 2020. © 2021, Elsevier)

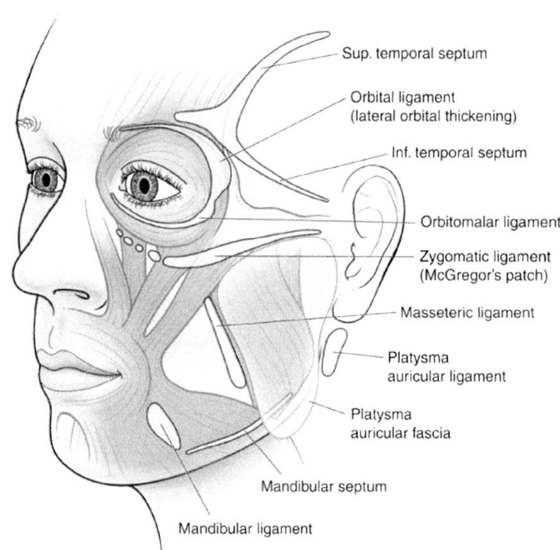

Fig. 24.7 Retaining ligaments of the face.

It is near this area that the facial artery becomes the angular artery, and changes depth to be more superficial as it moves caudally.

In the chin, the mental artery exits from the mental foramen on the lateral chin and moves medially as terminal branches. The mental nerve is a sensory nerve that also exits from the mental foramen and follows a path similar to the mental artery. The cervical branch of the facial artery branches into the submental artery. It exits under the mandible at the submandibular gland, travelling anteriorly before crossing the mandible near the mandibular symphysis.

Musculature

Expert injectors should have a deep understanding of facial muscle dynamics in areas of filler injection, as even in the absence of neurotoxins, filler may also independently alter muscle movement, a concept referred to as myomodulation.

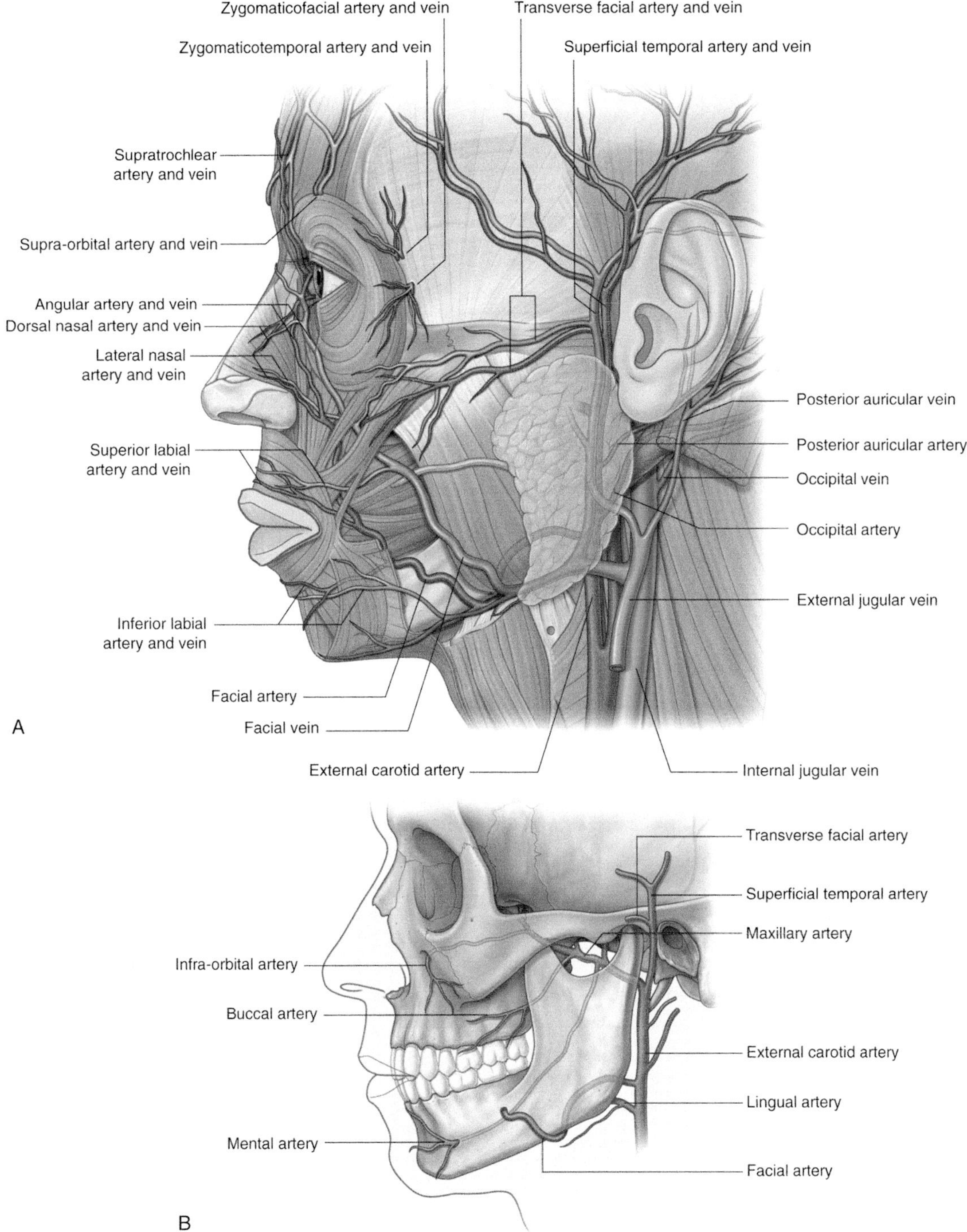

Fig. 24.8 Superficial and deep vascular anatomy of the face. (From Head and Neck—ClinicalKey Figure 8.67)

The DAO, depressor labii inferioris (DLI), mentalis, masseter, and the most superior aspects of the platysma are the five main muscles found in the lower face. Originating along the mandible and inserting at differing areas near the lower lip, the DAO, DLI, and mentalis are found in the mental area and merge inferiorly with the platysma. Fibers of the DAO, DLI, mentalis, and even the orbicularis oris are seen to intermingle at varying locations in the mental area.

The masseter is a square or rhomboid-shaped muscle that runs under the superficial fat compartments in the lateral, lower cheek, providing support to the lateral face and jawline. This muscle has both a larger superficial and a smaller deep component that originate from the zygomatic arch and insert into the mandible.

The Parotid Gland and Duct

The posterior portion of the masseter muscle is covered by the parotid gland. The parotid duct, also known as Stensen's duct, arises from the anterior portion of the gland, crosses the masseter, and penetrates into the buccinator at the anterior border of the masseter to eventually enter the oral cavity. An approximate cutaneous landmark for the path of the parotid duct is a line drawn from the earlobe to the ipsilateral oral commissure.

Tissue Layers

In the lower face, the tissue layers vary anterior and posterior to the labiomandibular sulcus. The anterior portion of the lower face moves from superficial to deep in the following order: skin, superficial fat compartments, muscle, deep labiomandibular fat/deep mental fat, periosteum. Posterior to this sulcus, the layers in order from superficial to deep are the skin, superficial fat compartments, platysma, deep fat compartments, masseteric fascia, masseter muscle, and periosteum. In this posterior area, the musculoaponeurotic layer, such as the platysma, has a weaker adhesion to its surrounding structures, making it more susceptible to the aging process.

INJECTION PLANNING AND TECHNIQUE

As with so many endeavors, careful assessment and planning are critical. Furthermore, an open discussion with the patient is essential to ensure that injector and patient goals are aligned. While seemingly simple in principle, such conversations can be challenging when there is a difference between what the patients want and what the injector believes the patient needs. The authors find that an educational approach to the consultation process is most effective in terms of arriving at a plan agreeable to both parties that gives the most aesthetically pleasing results.

Although many areas of the lower face can be safely injected with both needle and cannula techniques, the authors prefer using a cannula, especially since it was recently shown that cannula use has 77.1% lower odds of vascular occlusion than use of a needle. A 25-gauge, 2-inch cannula is typically used by the authors, providing accessibility to most areas of the lower face with minimal entry points. Products with a high G prime are often selected for use in the lower face in areas where structure, support, and definition are desirable, such as the chin and jawline. Molding the product after injection is especially important when using high-G prime products to reduce the risk of visible or palpable lumps. However, more flexible products that move with animation are preferred in areas such as the melomental region, where less definition and more flexibility are preferred. Hyaluronic acid (HA) fillers are preferred by the authors, but calcium hydroxyapatite and poly-L-lactic acid may also be effectively used in the lower face.

Chin

General Principles

Familiarizing oneself with dental occlusion patterns can help injectors convey the benefits of chin augmentation to patients (Fig. 24.9). Having an aligned bite pattern is considered a Class I occlusion pattern or orthognathia. In a Class II occlusion pattern, patients often have an overbite with resultant retrognathia and retruded chin. Lastly, an underbite, prognathia, and overprojected chin are seen in patients with a class III occlusion.

While there are many potential cannula entry points when injecting the chin, two common entry sites include the mid prejowl sulcus region just superior to the mandibular border and the area lateral to the mental crease at the height of the mental crease. Given that the chin consists of fibrous and densely compacted tissue, placing too much product in the chin during one session may lead to significant posttreatment discomfort and may adversely affect lower lip movement. The authors therefore advise against placing more than

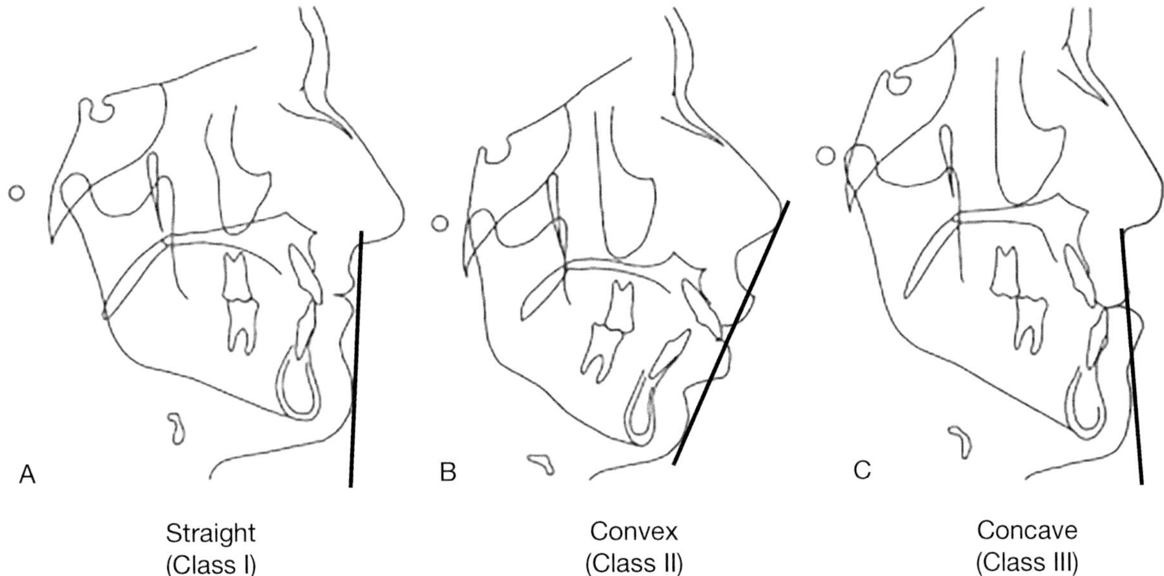

Fig. 24.9 Dental occlusion patterns.

approximately 2 mL of product into the chin during one session and instead suggest considering adding further volume at a subsequent session a few weeks later.

When treating the chin area, having patients keep their mouth slightly open during injection helps to relax the mentalis muscle, allowing easier advancement of the cannula and needle and placement of product.

Mental Crease

A deep mental crease may be addressed with a cannula or needle. One cannula entry point is sufficient to reach the entire length of the mental crease and approximately 0.5 to 1 mL of HA filler can be threaded into the subcutaneous plane. By having the patient bring their lower lip superior and posterior over the bottom teeth, the skin over the mental crease can be stretched, thus allowing one to assess for even product placement and ensure that there are no visible product accumulations. If threading product within the deeper subcutaneous plane is not sufficient to improve the mental crease, a small amount of product can be placed more superficially with a needle or cannula using a microdroplet technique. It is important to note that these more superficial injections may increase the risk of visible nodules and Tyndall effect. In addition to reducing the depth of the mental crease, a secondary benefit of filling the mental crease and decreasing the shadow in this area, is the ability to create an illusion of chin lengthening by increasing the surface area of confluent chin brightness.

Projection

Supraperiosteal boluses bilaterally at the soft tissue pogonion using a needle can address anteroposterior axis augmentation. Volumes vary widely depending on the amount of projection required. As noted previously, where large volumes are required, consideration should be given to treating over more than one session. The location of injection will vary with the contour goals. If a wider chin appearance is desired, injecting approximately 1 cm lateral to the midline is recommended. While not foolproof, the authors recommend aspiration as the mental foramen and mental arteries are often found just lateral to these injection points, with the mental arteries being in a more superficial plane. Alternatively, a single midline injection point can be used in some cases, especially if the goal is to achieve a narrow, round chin contour as is desired by some women. Approaching the chin from a lateral entry point with a cannula can also be done to inject boluses or threads of product. Pulling the chin anteriorly while advancing the cannula helps to ensure a deep injection plane. In patients that have a pronounced chin cleft and do not wish to diminish its appearance, a cotton tip applicator may be placed perpendicularly within the cleft and pressure may be applied during injection to lessen the chance of cleft effacement.

Lengthening or Rounding

In the correct patient, lengthening of the chin can significantly improve the overall facial aesthetic by improving balance and proportions. The face may appear slimmer when one increases the vertical height relative to the width. If using an entry point lateral to the mental crease, a cannula can be used to place small boluses of product at the gnathion and soft tissue menton. With an entry point just above the mandibular line, small linear threads can be placed in similar locations. Needle injections are frequently done on bone in the midline at the gnathion and in the submental/menton area but may also be placed in the subcutaneous layer. Aspiration is strongly recommended if using a needle for injection as the submental artery is located near these injection points. A volume of 0.2 to 0.3 mL of filler per side is often sufficient but each case is best assessed individually.

In males, molding the product to form a more linear inferior border helps to create the often-desired square chin shape. In contrast, a more rounded and classically feminine chin may be achieved by molding the product more centrally. Of note, botulinum toxin injections into the mentalis muscle can synergistically help lengthen the chin by relaxing the muscle and allowing the chin to unfurl.

Widening and Squaring

Chin widening is a goal often but not exclusively reserved for male patients that can be achieved by using a needle or cannula to deliver small boluses supraperiosteally on the lateral apices of the chin (Video 24.1). When planning injections in this area, it's important to recall that the ideal chin is approximately the width of the mouth in males and the width of the nose in females. Caution is advised when injecting this area as the submental artery is in the vicinity.

"Shortening"

Perception of vertical chin length is affected by the point of maximal light reflex in the area. In the authors' experience, placing the light reflex higher up on the chin can give the illusion of a shorter chin. This can be achieved by threading filler across the width of the chin at the desired vertical height, in essence creating a new, more superiorly positioned pogonion. Everything inferior to this will appear to be more shadowed, thus giving the impression of shorter chin vertical height.

Jawline

General Principles

When assessing and planning for jawline filler injections, an open discussion with patients is essential to establish their desired final appearance. For example, when asked about treatment goals, many patients pull posteriolaterally on their lower face to convey the appearance of reduced jowls and tighter skin. In these cases, setting realistic expectations is of the utmost importance as filler injection may not be able to achieve the surgical results that are desired.

Prejowl Sulcus

Treatment of the prejowl sulcus is a satisfying area as it can help attain a straighter jawline. While improvement of the prejowl sulcus can be accomplished by direct injection of the area, it is important to recognize that it can also be addressed indirectly by using lateral and forward vectors, through treatment of the lateral jawline/preauricular area, and chin, respectively. If the indirect approach is not sufficient or appropriate, then direct treatment in the prejowl area is possible. Care must be taken to assess the overall jawline and chin shape and size prior to treatment, as complete effacement of the prejowl sulci may sometimes result in squaring of the jaw or widening of the chin, leading to an undesired masculine appearance in women.

A supraperiosteal injection using a high-G prime product can be done directly into the prejowl sulcus using a needle. Alternatively, a lateral or medial entry point also allows cannula access to this area for injections in the subcutaneous plane. If jowls are present, avoiding injection of the jowl itself is important to avoid accentuating its appearance.

Jawline Contouring

Injectors often approach jawline contouring with the mindset of achieving a masculine or feminine shape. Although this division may hold true in the majority of cases, acknowledge that each individual has unique goals, and it is thus important to discuss this with the patient prior to injection to ensure alignment on aesthetic ideals and goals. Traditionally, a male jawline is considered more angular and represented by two almost perpendicular lines meeting at the angle of the mandible. In contrast, a traditional female jawline is often seen as a continuous convex downward curve extending from the antegonial notch to the inferior border of the preauricular area. Assessment of overall facial shape is also important prior to proceeding with jawline contouring as adding filler to the jawline may result in a more square and masculine appearance of the lower and midface, which may not fit with the patient's desires.

Jawline contouring can be thought of in three anatomical, although not mutually exclusive, zones: jawline proper, mandibular angle, and preauricular area. Injections in these areas are best performed using high-G prime products using either needle or cannula. The authors prefer cannulas for the jawline given that the facial artery crosses the mandible at the antegonial notch and is therefore often in the path of injection in this area. Fortunately, the facial artery can often be easily palpated and subsequently landmarked as a danger zone to avoid during injection. Furthermore, cannula use permits broad access to the region with minimal needle sticks. When using a cannula in this area, entry points differ between injectors based on factors such as injector preference, cannula length, size of the patient's face, other cosmetic areas being treated, presence or absence of jowls, and desired outcome. Quantity of filler needed for jawline contouring can vary widely between patients, and therefore realistic expectations based on budgetary restraints are important to discuss.

In patients without jowls, product can be placed along the entire length of the jawline as needed. However, if jowls are present, care must be taken to avoid injecting directly into this area so as to avoid accentuating them.

As previously noted, a traditional masculine jawline profile can be achieved by threading product in the subcutaneous plane along the length of the mandible to the mandibular angle and then changing direction to thread product along the preauricular area. A bolus at the mandibular angle can help achieve a more masculine widening of the lower face bringing the bizygomatic to bigonial ratio closer to 1:1. If using a needle to inject this bolus, the injector should palpate the mandibular angle and inject at a 90-degree angle and place the product deep on bone.

For a more traditionally feminine jawline profile, the filler can be threaded using cannula from a single-entry site posterior to the antegonial notch to the inferior border of the preauricular area in order to create a convex contour. A tip from the authors to determine if filler is needed in the preauricular area is to take note of how much of the tragus is visible when examining the patient head-on. If the entire tragus is visible, then adding filler in the preauricular region may lead to an aesthetically pleasing outcome. The authors recommend Injecting in the subcutaneous plane in the preauricular area as the parotid and parotid duct run deep and may accidentally be injured if care is not taken. Injury may result in characteristic nontender, nonecchymotic swelling in the subzygomatic region.

In some cases, lengthening of the jawline is desired. This can be achieved by adding filler posterior to the angle of the mandible with either a needle or cannula. With the latter, the ideal entry point is posterior to the angle of the mandible, where filler can be deposited on bone to extend the length of the mandible.

As previously noted, the masseter muscle provides support and structure to the lateral face and jawline. Although the focus of this chapter is injectable fillers for the lower face, injectors must also keep in mind that treatment of the masseter muscle with botulinum toxin to reduce its size can have both positive and negative effects on the overall shape of the face, especially the lower face. Botulinum toxin injections reduce masseter muscle volume, leading to a slimmer lower facial appearance, and ultimately increasing the bizygomatic to bigonial ratio. While this may be beneficial in some cases, care must be taken, especially in older patients, as reducing the size of the masseter can significantly accentuate the appearance of jowls. If the purpose of treating the masseters is to reduce jaw clenching or teeth grinding, using filler to restore lost volume along the posterior jawline caused by reduced masseter muscle bulk, is a good solution to avoid accentuation of the jowls, while still minimizing teeth clenching and teeth grinding.

CONCLUSION

With increasing awareness of the importance of the lower face in overall facial appearance, harmony, and balance, soft tissue filler use for the chin and jawline promises to play an expanding role in facial rejuvenation. It is because of this, that injectors must become knowledgeable, skilled, and confident in assessment, anatomy, treatment planning, and injection of the chin and jawline in order to create natural, aesthetically pleasing results. Furthermore, comprehensive knowledge of other treatment modalities and their role in treatment of the lower face, such as face lift surgery, energy-based devices, and neuromodulator injection, alone or in combination with dermal fillers, is essential if we are to achieve the best possible aesthetic outcomes.

FURTHER READING

Alam, M., Kakar, R., Dover, J. S., et al. (2021). Rates of vascular occlusion associated with using needle vs. cannulas for filler injection. *JAMA Dermatology*, *157*(2), 174–180. https://doi.org/10.1001/jamadermatol.2020.5102.

Alghoul, M., & Codner, M. (2013). Retaining ligaments of the face: Review of anatomy and clinical applications. *Aesthetic Surgery Journal*, *33*(6), 769–782. https://doi.org/10.1177/1090820X13495405.

Braz, A., & Aquino, B. O. (2013). Reabsorção Óssea. In M. H. L. Sandoval, & E. L. Ayres (Eds.), *Preenchedores: Guia prático de técnica e produtos* (1st ed., pp. 39–44). AC Farmacêutica.

Braz, A., & de Paula Eduardo, C. (2020). Reshaping the lower face using injectable fillers. *Indian Journal of Plastic Surgery*, *53*(2), 207–218. https://doi.org/10.1055/s-0040-1716185.

Braz, A., & de Paula Eduardo, C. (2020). The facial shapes in planning the treatment with injectable fillers. *Indian Journal of Plastic Surgery*, *54*(2), 230–243. https://doi.org/10.1055/s-0040-1715554.

Braz, A. V., & Pirmez, R. (2014). Preenchimento global ("Volumização"). In D. Steiner, & F. Addor (Eds.), *Tratado de Envelhecimento Cutâneo* (1st ed., pp. 255–260). AC Farmacêutica.

Braz, A. V., & Sakuma, T. H. (2013). Compartimentos de gordura. In M. Sandoval, & E. Ayres (Eds.), *de tecnica e produtos* (1st ed., pp. 35–38). AC Farmacêutica.

Braz, A., Humphrey, S., Weinkle, S., et al. (2015). Lower face: Clinical anatomy and regional approaches with injectable fillers. *Plastic and Reconstructive Surgery*, *136*(5 suppl), 235S–257S. https://doi.org/10.1097/PRS.0000000000001836.

Braz, A. V., Louvain, D., & Mukamal, L. V. (2013). Combined treatment with botulinum toxin and hyaluronic acid to correct unsightly lateral-chin depression. *Anais Brasileiros de Ginecologia*, *88*, 138–140. https://doi.org/10.1590/s0365-05962013000100024.

Casabona, G., Frank, K., Koban, K. C., et al. (2019). Lifting vs volumizing—The difference in facial minimally invasive procedures when respecting the line of ligaments. *Journal of Cosmetic Dermatology*, *18*, 1237–1243. https://doi.org/10.1111/jocd.13089.

Choi, Y. J., Kim, J. S., Gil, Y. C., et al. (2014). Anatomical considerations regarding the location and boundary of the depressor anguli oris muscle with reference to botulinum toxin injection. *Plastic and Reconstructive Surgery*, *134*, 917–921. https://doi.org/10.1097/PRS.0000000000000589.

Dayan, S. H., & Arkins, J. P. (2012). The subliminal difference: Treating from an evolutionary perspective. *Plastic and Reconstructive Surgery*, *129*, 189e–190e. https://doi.org/10.1097/PRS.0b013e3182365eec.

De Maio, M. (2015). Ethnic and gender considerations in the use of facial injectables: Male patients. *Plastic and Reconstructive Surgery*, *136*(5s), 40s–43s. https://doi.org/10.1097/PRS.0000000000001729.

De Maio, M. (2018). Myomodulation with injectable fillers: An innovative approach to addressing facial muscle movement. *Aesthetic Plastic Surgery*, *42*, 798–814. https://doi.org/10.1007/s00266-018-1116-z.

De Maio, M., & Rzany, B. (2009). Facial aesthetics in male patients. In *The Male Patient in Aesthetic Medicine* (pp. 1–18). Springer-Verlag.

De Maio, M., Wu, W., Goodman, G., et al. (2017). Facial assessment and injection guide for botulinum toxin and injectable hyaluronic acid fillers: Focus on the lower face. *Plastic and Reconstructive Surgery*, *140*(3), 393e–404e. https://doi.org/10.1097/PRS.0000000000003646.

Donnelly, S., Hens, S. M., Rogers, N. L., & Schneider, K. L. (1998). A blind test of mandibular ramus flexure as a morphological indicator of sexual dimorphism in the human skeleton. *American Journal of Physical Anthropology*, *107*, 363–366. https://doi.org/10.1002/(SICI)1096-8644(199811)107:3<363::AID-AJPA11>3.0.CO;2-Y.

Eslami, N., Omidkhoda, M., Shafaee, H., & Mozhdehifard, M. (2016). Comparison of esthetics perception and satisfaction of facial profile among male adolescents and adults with different profiles. *Journal of Orthodontic Science*, *5*(2), 47–51. https://doi.org/10.4103/2278-0203.179406.

Fagien, S., Bertucci, V., von Grote, E., & Mashburn, J. (2019). Rheologic and physicochemical properties used to differentiate injectable hyaluronic acid filler products. *Plastic and Reconstructive Surgery*, *143*(4), 707–720. https://doi.org/10.1097/PRS.0000000000005429.

Farhadian, J., Bloom, B., & Brauer, J. (2015). Male aesthetics: A review of facial anatomy and pertinent clinical implications. *Journal of Drugs in Dermatology*, *14*(9), 1029–1034.

Fitzgerald, R. (2018). Addressing facial shape and proportions with injectable agents in youth and age. In B. Azizzadeh, M. Murphy, C. Johnson, G. Massry, & R. Fitzgerald (Eds.), *Master Techniques in Facial Rejuvenation* (pp. 15–54). Canada: Elsevier.

Hur, M. S., Kim, H. J., Choi, B. Y., et al. (2013). Morphology of the mentalis muscle and its relationship with the orbicularis oris and incisivus labii inferioris muscles. *Journal of Craniofacial Surgery*, *24*, 602–604. https://doi.org/10.1097/SCS.0b013e318267bcc5.

Hur, M. S., Kim, H. J., & Lee, K. S. (2014). An anatomic study of the medial fibers of depressor anguli oris muscle passing deep to the depressor labii inferioris muscle. *Journal of Craniofacial Surgery*, *25*(2), 614–616. https://doi.org/10.1097/SCS.0000000000000452.

Hussain, G., Manktelow, R. T., & Tomat, L. R. (2004). Depressor labii inferioris resection: An effective treatment for marginal mandibular nerve paralysis. *British Journal of Plastic Surgery*, *57*, 502–510. https://doi.org/10.1016/j.bjps.2004.04.003.

Jacobson, A. (1995). *Radiographic cephalometry: From basics to video imaging* (1st ed.). Quintessence Publishing Co.

James, R. D. (1998). A comparative study of facial profiles in extraction and nonextraction treatment. *American Journal of Orthodontics and Dentofacial Orthopedics*, *114*, 265–276. https://doi.org/10.1016/s0889-5406(98)70208-2.

Keaney, T. (2016). Aging in the male face: Intrinsic and extrinsic factors. *Dermatologic Surgery*, *42*, 797–803. https://doi.org/10.1097/DSS.0000000000000505.

Lee, J. Y., Kim, J. N., Yoo, J. Y., et al. (2012). Topographic anatomy of the masseter muscle focusing on the tendinous digitation. *Clinical Anatomy*, *25*, 889–892. https://doi.org/10.1002/ca.22024.

Marur, T., Tuna, Y., & Demirci, S. (2014). Facial anatomy. *Clinical. Clinical Dermatology*, *32*, 14–23. https://doi.org/10.1016/j.clindermatol.2013.05.022.

Mazess, R. B., & Barden, H. S. (1990). Interrelationships among bone densitometry sites in normal young women. *Bone and Mineral*, *11*, 347–356. https://doi.org/10.1016/0169-6009(90)90030-J.

Mendelson, B. C. (1995). Extended sub-SMAS dissection and cheek elevation. *Clinics in Plastic Surgery*, *22*, 325–339. https://doi.org/10.1016/S0094-1298(20)30971-8.

Mommaerts, M. (2016). The ideal male jaw angle—An internet survey. *Journal of Cranio-Maxillo-Facial Surgery*, *44*(4), 381–391. https://doi.org/10.1016/j.jcms.2015.12.012.

Moradi, A., Shirazi, A., & David, R. (2019). Non surgical chin and jawline augmentation using calciumhydroxylapatite and hyaluronic acid fillers. *Facial Plastic Surgery*, *35*(02), 140–148. https://doi.org/10.1055/s-0039-1683854.

Morrison, S., Vyas, K., Motakef, S., et al. (2016). Facial feminization: Systemic review of the literature. *Plastic and Reconstructive Surgery*, *137*(6), 1759–1770. https://doi.org/10.1097/PRS.0000000000002171.

Naini, F., Moss, J., & Gill, D. (2006). The enigma of facial beauty: Esthetics, proportions, deformity and controversy. *American Journal of Orthodontics and Dentofacial Orthopedics*, *130*(3), 277–282. https://doi.org/10.1016/j.ajodo.2005.09.027.

Owsley, J. (1986). Superficial musculoaponeurotic system platysma face lift. In H. Dudley, D. Carter, & R. Russell (Eds.), *Operative surgery* Butterworth.

Özdemir, R., Kilinc, H., Unlu, R. E., et al. (2002). Anatomicohistologic study of the retaining ligaments of the face and use in face lift: Retaining ligament correction and SMAS plication. *Plastic and Reconstructive Surgery*, *110*, 1134–1149. https://doi.org/10.1097/01.PRS.0000021442.30272.0E.

Pessa, J. E., & Rohrich, R. J. (2012). The cheek. In J. E. Pessa, & R. J. Rohrich (Eds.), *Facial Topography, Clinical Anatomy of the Face* (pp. 47–93). Missouri: Quality Medical Publishing.

Proffit, W., Fields, H., & Sarver, D. (2007). *Contemporary Orthodontics*. Missouri: Elsevier.

Radlanski, R. J., & Wesker, K. H. (2012). The facial skeleton. In R. J. Radlanski, & K. H. Wesker (Eds.), *The face, pictorial atlas of clinical anatomy* (pp. 148–161). Quintessence Publishing.

Reece, E. M., Pessa, J. E., & Rohrich, R. J. (2008). The mandibular septum: Anatomical observations of the jowls in aging-implications for facial rejuvenation. *Plastic and Reconstructive Surgery*, *121*(4), 1414–1420. https://doi.org/10.1097/01.prs.0000302462.61624.26.

Saghiri, M., Eid, J., Tang, C. K., & Freag, P. (2021). Factors influencing different types of malocclusion and arch form—A review. *Journal of Stomatology, Oral and Maxillofacial Surgery*, *122*, 185–191. https://doi.org/10.1016/j.jormas.2020.07.002.

Schenck, T., Koban, K. C., Schlattau, A., et al. (2018). The functional anatomy of the superficial fat compartments of the face: A detailed imaging study. *Plastic and Reconstructive Surgery*, *141*(6), 1351–1359. https://doi.org/10.1097/PRS.0000000000004364.

Shaw, R., Katzel, E., Koltz, P., et al. (2010). Aging of the facial skeleton: Aesthetic implications and rejuvenation strategies. *Plastic and Reconstructive Surgery*, *127*(1), 374–383. https://doi.org/10.1097/PRS.0b013e3181f95b2d.

Steiner, C. (1953). Cephalometric for you and me. *American Journal of Orthodontics*, *39*, 729–754. https://doi.org/10.1016/0002-9416(53)90082-7.

Stuzin, J. M., Baker, T. J., & Gordon, H. L. (1992). The relationship of the superficial and deep facial fascias: Relevance to rhytidectomy and aging. *Plastic and Reconstructive Surgery*, *89*, 441–451. https://doi.org/10.1097/00006534-199203000-00007.

Stuzin, J. M., Baker, T. J., Gordon, H. L., et al. (1995). Extended SMAS dissection as an approach to midface rejuvenation. *Clinics in Plastic Surgery*, *22*, 295–311. https://doi.org/10.1016/S0094-1298(20)30969-X.

Suwanchinda, A., Rudolph, C., Hladik, C., et al. (2018). The layered anatomy of the jawline. *Journal of Cosmetic Dermatology*, *17*(04), 625–631. https://doi.org/10.1111/jocd.12728.

Swift, A., & Remington, K. (2011). BeautiPHIcation: A global approach to facial beauty. *Clinics in Plastic Surgery*, *38*, 347–377. https://doi.org/10.1016/j.cps.2011.03.012.

Thayer, Z. M., & Dobson, S. D. (2010). Sexual dimorphism in chin shape: Implications for adaptive hypotheses. *American Journal of Physical Anthropology*, *143*, 417–425. https://doi.org/10.1002/ajpa.21330.

The American Society for Aesthetic Plastic Surgery. (2018). Cosmetic (Aesthetic) Surgery National Data Bank STATISTICS [PDF file]. https://www.surgery.org/sites/default/files/ASAPS-Stats2018.pdf.

Toledo Avelar, L. E., Cardoso, M. A., Santos Bordoni, L., de Miranda Avelar, L., & de Miranda Avelar, J. V. (2017). Aging and sexual differences of the human skull. *Plastic and Reconstructive Surgery. Global Open*, *5*(4), e1297. https://doi.org/10.1097/GOX.0000000000001297.

Vanaman Wilson, M. J., Jones, I. T., Butterwick, K., & Fabi, S. G. (2018). Role of nonsurgical chin augmentation in full face rejuvenation: A review and our experience. *Dermatologic Surgery*, *44*(7), 985–993. https://doi.org/10.1097/DSS.0000000000001461.

Vazirnia, A., Braz, A., & Fabi, S. G. (2019). Nonsurgical jawline rejuvenation using injectable fillers. *Journal of Cosmetic Dermatology*, *19*(9). https://doi.org/10.1111/jocd.13277.

Wysong, A., Joseph, T., Kim, D., Tang, J. Y., et al. (2013). Quantifying soft tissue loss in facial aging: A study in women using magnetic resonance imaging. *Dermatologic Surgery*, *12*, 1895–1902. https://doi.org/10.1111/dsu.12362.

Wysong, A., Kim, D., Joseph, T., et al. (2014). Quantifying soft tissue loss in the aging male face using magnetic resonance imaging. *Dermatologic Surgery*, *40*, 786–793. https://doi.org/10.1111/dsu.0000000000000035.

Yin, L., Jiang, M., Chen, W., Smales, R. J., Wang, Q., & Tang, L. (2014). Differences in facial profile and dental esthetic perceptions between young adults and orthodontists. *American Journal of Orthodontics and Dentofacial Orthopedics*, *145*, 750–756. https://doi.org/10.1016/j.ajodo.2014.01.021.

25

Lip Augmentation

Sabrina Fabi, Jean Carruthers, Susan Weinkle, and Michelle Vy

SUMMARY AND KEY FEATURES

- The lips are a defining feature of the face; enhancement of lip volume and structure through the use of fillers is a commonly requested cosmetic procedure.
- Ethnic variations and aesthetic preferences should be considered in the evaluation and treatment planning for lip augmentation.
- Hyaluronic acids are commonly used filler products for lip rejuvenation; their safety profile, coupled with their potential reversibility using hyaluronidase, makes them a frequent choice for treatment of the lips. Semipermanent and permanent fillers, such as calcium hydroxylapatite, poly-L-lactic acid, silicone, and polymethylmethacrylate, have higher incidences of nodule and granuloma formation and should therefore be avoided in the lips.
- Injection of filler product into the rolled border of the lip will produce definition of the lip. Injection of filler product along the wet–dry junction of the lip will augment the volume of the lips.
- Bruising and swelling are common, temporary side effects of lip augmentation. Small-volume injections can minimize these effects. Touch-up treatments 1 to 2 weeks later may be necessary.
- More serious complications such as vascular compromise may be prevented with a thorough understanding of anatomy, use of expert injection technique, and potential use of a duplex ultrasound.
- Multimodality treatments including soft tissue fillers, botulinum toxins, and resurfacing techniques can be incorporated into treatment of the lips and perioral area.

INTRODUCTION

The lips are a defining feature of youth and beauty. With the increasing cultural emphasis on youth and beauty, full lips are aesthetically desired because they are considered youthful. Although they may represent a small portion of the face based on size, they can have a substantial effect on a person's overall appearance. Unfortunately, as we age, lips undergo some of the most dramatic changes of the entire face. These changes are a natural part of the aging process, but they can be softened or reversed to give a more youthful and rejuvenated appearance. Understanding the normal process of aging and the anatomy and variations in anatomy, managing patient expectations, and taking into account patient's unique facial features and their ethnic racial background will create a pleasing outcome and achieve optimal cosmetic results.

THE AGING PROCESS ON THE LIPS

Although this chapter will focus specifically on the rejuvenation of the lips, it is important to consider the lips in the larger context of the perioral region, demarcated by the nasal base, cheeks, chin, and framed by the masseter muscle. Patients may have thin lips at baseline or progressively thin as part of the well described aging process. Pouty full lips are usually synonymous with youth, while the loss of these features attribute to the overall aging appearance of the face.

There are a multitude of causes and effects of the aging process in the lower face. It is important to consider the following aging changes that contribute to lip size and position: maxillary bone resorption, increased prominence of the pyriform fossa, and mandibular bone resorption. With the former, there is an associated alveolar tooth loss and loss of the maxillary arch, causing posterior displacement of the nasal base and upper lip. Additionally, there is a loss of elevator muscles and soft tissue, resulting in redundancy, which causes increased upper lip length and loss of anterior projection of the upper lip. With mandibular bone resorption, this leads to loss of support of the lip depressors, which inevitably causes less lower lip show and decreased incisor show. In addition to intrinsic aging, ultraviolet radiation can cause photoaging of the skin, resulting in mottled dyspigmentation and irregular texture. Collagen fibers diminish, elastic tissue is degraded, and there is a loss of subcutaneous fat and bone. These changes result in an overall drooping of the perioral region, which may call attention to the lips. Therefore, to truly rejuvenate the lips, it may be necessary to address the entire perioral region, including the nasolabial folds, melomental creases, and chin. These topics are covered elsewhere in this book but should be considered in any cosmetic consultation.

> **PEARL 1** When rejuvenating the lips, it may be necessary to address other components of the perioral region. Multimodality approaches, including the use of soft tissue fillers, botulinum toxin, and resurfacing, may be necessary to achieve the best outcomes.

The lips specifically are dramatically redefined by an overall loss of lip volume and structure throughout the aging process: the upper lip becomes thin and elongated, and the lower lip becomes thin and rolls inward. There is blunting of the appearance of the pink vermilion of the lip and a sagging of the corners of the mouth, which is further accentuated by the activity of the depressor anguli oris muscle. Sagging in the perioral region causing descent of the upper mouth over the bottom lip can result in an entity named "lateral lip festoon." The overall result is a loss of show of the upper teeth, with an increase in the show of the lower teeth. The Cupid's bow—the area defined by the two high arched points of the upper lip—becomes effaced and flattened; the two philtral columns of the upper lip also loose definition. Over time, the beautiful, defined, arched structure of the upper lip is lost, and in its place a thin, poorly defined upper lip develops. In conjunction with the overall loss of lip volume, there is also the chronic effect of activity of the orbicularis oris muscle, leading to the formation of radiating deep perioral rhytides. Patients often complain that these rhytides cause "bleeding lipstick" lines and are a frequent issue of discussion in cosmetic consultations. Given that the aging process is multifactorial, the goal of lip rejuvenation includes diminishing fine lines, diminishing length of the upper lip, redefining the Cupid's bow and vermilion border, eversion of the vermilion, and improving the volume within the oral commissures that may contribute to the "lateral lip festoons."

Multiple assessment scales have been developed to quantify these changes. Validated scales include the 5-point Medicis Lip Fullness Scale (MLFS) by Carruthers et al. (Fig. 25.1), the five-point Allergan Lip Fullness Scale by Werschler et al., the Perioral Lines at Rest (POL), Perioral Lines at Maximum Contraction (POLM) and Oral Commissures Severity (OCS) scales by Cohen et al., the facial fold assessment scale by Narins et al., the Catherine-Knowles-Clarke (CKC) scale by Downie et al. (Table 25.1), and the photonumeric grading scale for assessing lip volume and thickness by Rossi et al. These scales may be of benefit in the initial assessment of patients and their clinical improvement following lip augmentation.

When done well, lip augmentation and rejuvenation can dramatically address many of these changes associated with aging lips to both replace the volume loss and redefine the lip structure. Numerous studies have shown that for a majority of patients, injection of HA fillers to the lips produces significant improvement in lip fullness and investigator- and patient-assessed global appearance (via the Global Aesthetic Improvement Scale [GAIS]).

However, in some cases, simply injecting soft tissue fillers into the lips alone may not achieve the best results. Low-dose botulinum toxins around the lips may improve perioral rhytides, whereas botulinum toxin injections into the depressor anguli oris muscles may reduce the down turning of the oral commissures and enhance the longevity of the fillers. In addition to soft tissue fillers, the "lip flip"—where botulinum toxin is

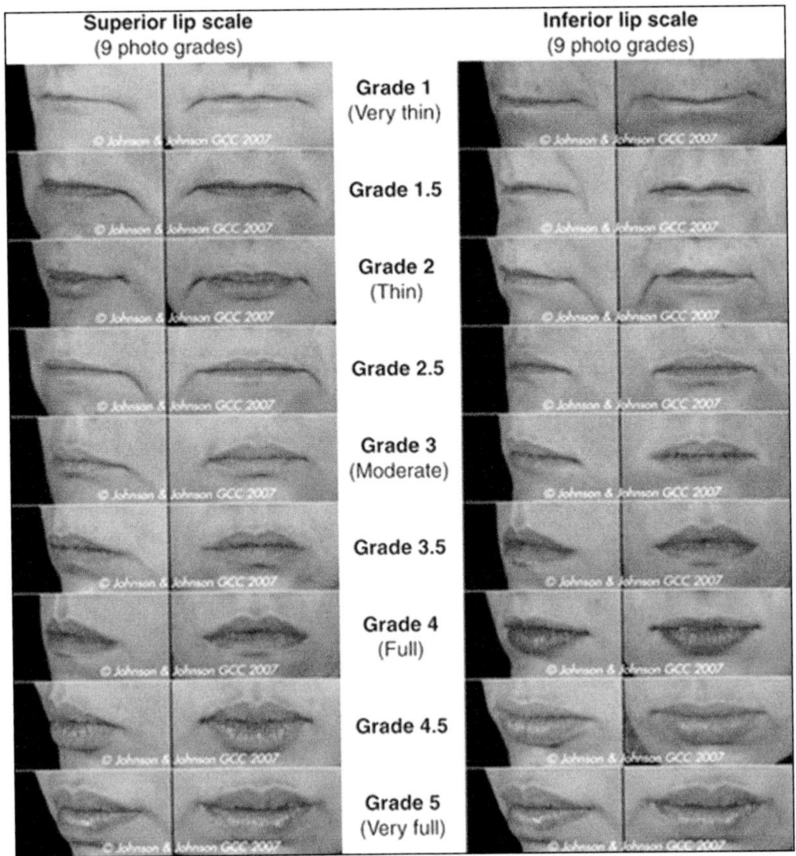

Fig. 25.1 Validated lip fullness grading scale. (Reprinted with permission from Carruthers A, Carruthers J, Hardas B, et al. A validated lip fullness grading scale. *Dermatologic Surgery.* 2008;34(suppl 2):S161–S166.)

injected at the vermilion border—has been shown to improve lip contour, eversion, and fullness. However, although reported in the literature, these are off-label uses of botulinum toxin not approved by regulatory authorities, such as the US Food and Drug Administration (FDA), Health Canada, or European regulatory authorities. In severe cases, resurfacing of the perioral skin with lasers or chemical peels may be necessary. Although this chapter will focus on the use of soft tissue fillers, in many cases, a multimodality approach may be beneficial for patients to achieve optimal rejuvenation.

AN APPROACH TO PATIENT EVALUATION

The first issue to address with lip augmentation is to determine the treatment goals of the patient. Does the patient seek enhancement or restoration of the lips? Younger patients typically seek enhancement in lip volume, and their desire may stem from what is seen in modern celebrity pop culture and social media platforms. Older patients typically seek rejuvenation to treat signs of aging by recreating youthful shape and ratio, with subtle enhancement as a platform for their lipstick, and to diminish vertical lines. With regard to women versus men, Ramaut et al. reported that women have up to a 31.79% thinner upper lip than their same-age male counterparts.

Is the patient seeking enhancement of the lips, are they satisfied with their existing lip shape but desire fuller lips, or is the patient seeking an entirely different shape of his or her lips? It is then important to perform a careful assessment of the appropriateness of that desired look in proportion to the rest of the patient's face.

TABLE 25.1 The Catherine-Knowles-Clarke Lip Evaluation Scale

SIZE			
Score	**Letter**	**Description**	
−2	V	Very thin	≤1:15
−1	T	Thin	1:15 to 1:10
0	M	Medium sized	1:10 to 1:7
1	F	Full	1:7 to 1:4
2	E	Extremely full	>1:4

VERMILION BODY	
Score	**Description**
−1	Tight almost unlined
0	Rounded with natural lines
1	Less rounded with fine lines
2	Flattening with moderate wrinkles
3	Severe wrinkles

VERMILION BORDER	
Score	**Description**
−1	Protruding and/or creating perioral shadow
0	Distinct and intact, with/without shadow from mid–lower lip
1	Distinct but broken by fine lines, with/without shadow from mid–lower lip
2	Indistinct and broken by moderate lines with/without shadow from mid–lower lip
3	Indistinct and severely lined, with/without shadow from mid–lower lip

Reprinted with permission from Downie J, Mao Z, Lo WR, et al. A double-blind, clinical evaluation of facial augmentation treatments: a comparison of PR 1, PR 2, Zyplast® and Perlane®. *J Plast Reconstr Aesthet Surg.* 2009;62:1636–1643.

Surek et al. suggest three defined areas of potential enhancement:

1. The white roll, which is the junction between cutaneous lip and dry vermilion. This is responsible for determining the lip profile.
2. The vermilion lip, which is between the white and red rolls. This determines the lip projection.
3. The red roll, which is the invagination of the orbicularis oris muscle and wet mucosa. This correlates to lip augmentation.

Lip volume enhancement not only increases the vertical height of the vermilion but also increases lip volume circumferentially, potentially resulting in the undesirable "duck lip" appearance. To prevent an unnatural look, the forward projection of the lip should barely graze a line drawn from the midcolumella to the chin (Steiner line), not projecting beyond 1 to 2 mm beyond the top of the lower lip. We advocate small-volume treatments, especially for first-time treatments, with potential touch-up procedures 1 to 2 weeks later to achieve the best outcome and limit the potential for overcorrection.

For patients seeking lip restoration, it is important to determine their specific concerns. Are the lips asymmetric at baseline? Has the patient lost the overall structure of the lips? Are they having trouble with "lipstick bleed?" A single concern may necessitate multiple treatments, while at times, one treatment may achieve various objectives. Treatments do not need to occur in a single session; indeed, it is often better to schedule multiple visits with gradual treatments in order to better assess the effects of previous sessions on the overall restoration goal.

Aside from individual preferences, morphologic differences between racial groups and ethnic variations should also be considered to optimize results and achieve patient satisfaction. Many ethnic patients seek lip augmentation based on their cultural and racial background rather than obtaining a more Westernized appearance. African Americans and Hispanics tend to have fuller lips. African Americans tend to have more maxillary and mandibular resorption, so consideration of the bony support can help provide the lip with a better framework. Individuals of African descent tend to have fuller lips and shorter philtral columns, but as they age, volume loss occurs, particularly of the upper lip. Therefore, the goal of lip augmentation would focus more on upper lip enhancement rather than on upper and lower lip restoration. Kar et al. reported that African American patients genetically do have greater upper lip volume; however, they are less prone to solar elastosis, so consequently, they rarely develop radial rhytides and have retained volume in the vermilion. Hispanic people naturally have larger lips than White people. Although there has not been much research with regard to the detailed preferred lip measurements for Hispanic people, Kollipara et al. reported that the upper and lower lips of Mexican-American peoples were 2 to 3 mm and 0.6 to 2.4 mm more protrusive, respectively, compared to those of European descent. The authors mentioned that this is likely due to teeth-related factors, but more so due to the greater soft tissue thickness found in Mexican American peoples. Heidekrueger et al. showed that compared with laypersons in all other demographic groups, those in Latin America favored the largest size lips.

Asian people tend to have fuller lips, thus necessitating a different approach to lip injection. Peng et al. discussed the differences in anatomical and aesthetics between Asian and White people and reported that Asian people tend to have a longer cutaneous upper and lower lip, fuller upper and lower vermilion lip, more upper lip volume, and more common have bimaxillary protrusion and a retruded chin. Furthermore, this study proposes four categorizations of Asian lips for injection approaches, which includes young lips with good proportionality, disproportionated lips of any age, well-proportioned lips with dryness or wrinkling, and lastly, aging lips.

Oftentimes, examination of symmetry, movement, overall shape, and volume can be done during normal conversation, and assessing this dynamic nature can be very helpful for knowing what needs to be done. An important part to the evaluation also involves assessing a patient's occlusion prior to injection. A class II or a class III malocclusion can create a challenge in providing appropriate proportions and balance on profile and can cause an upper lip pseudoaugmentation or a lower lip pseudoaugmentation, respectively. From discussion goals during the pretreatment consultation, existing asymmetries should be pointed out and frontal, oblique, and lateral photos taken before any intervention is performed. It is prudent to set expectations with what can be achieved before treatment to avoid disappointment; understand the patient's aesthetic ideals and goals. Counsel the patient on expected side effects and downtime.

FILLER PRODUCTS

When performing lip rejuvenation, temporary fillers are the treatment of choice. Historically, collagen was the gold standard product for lip augmentation. Collagen is no longer commercially available in the United States, and HA products have become the most frequently used products for lip rejuvenation. These HA fillers are cross-linked to extend their longevity to 6 to 12 months. Restylane (Galderma Laboratories, L.P. Fort Worth, TX), Restylane-L, Restylane Silk, Juvéderm Ultra XC (Allergan Inc., Irvine, CA), Juvéderm Volbella XC, and Restylane Kysse were approved by the FDA for lip enhancement in patients older than 21 years of age in 2011, 2012, 2014, 2015, 2016, and 2020, respectively. Restylane Silk, Restylane Kysse, Juvéderm Ultra XC, and Juvéderm Volbella XC, in addition to Belotero Balance (Merz North America, Greensboro, NC), are also FDA approved for perioral rhytids. Most of these products are premixed with lidocaine to reduce discomfort during injections. The future of soft tissue augmentation is exciting given there are other HA products undergoing clinical trials for FDA approval for lip augmentation.

In 2007, a multidisciplinary group of experts in aesthetic treatments (the Facial Aesthetics Consensus Group) developed recommendations for lip augmentation and rejuvenation. Of the available HA products, the faculty typically used Restylane, Juvéderm Ultra, or Juvéderm Ultra Plus for lip and perioral rejuvenation. The majority of the faculty (67%) used 1.0 mL of HA, while the remainder (33%) used 2.0 mL to reshape the vermilion border and rejuvenate the lips. In a study of Restylane, Glogau et al. showed that using more than 3 mL of filler was associated with a significant increase in moderate-to-severe adverse events.

Although a full discussion of filler properties is beyond the scope of this chapter, a few notable differences should be considered. Restylane and Restylane Silk are biphasic particulate gels that create a greater surface area for water binding, which may result in more postprocedure edema. Restylane Silk is even more hydrophilic than Restylane and Restylane-L because it has a greater number of particles, which are also smaller. Juvéderm Ultra and Juvéderm Ultra Plus are nonparticle monophasic gels that contain long-chain HA cross-linked via Hylacross technology. In contrast, Juvéderm Voluma, Volbella, and Volift are viscous nonparticle gels made using Vycross technology, which incorporate both long and short chains of HA, producing more cross-linking and longer duration in tissue. In addition, their lower HA concentration results in less water absorption.

Semipermanent fillers, such as calcium hydroxylapatite and poly-L-lactic acid, can be used to rejuvenate the perioral area, including the nasolabial folds and jowls, but have an increased risk of adverse effects and nodule formation. Permanent fillers, such as polymethylmethacrylate and liquid injectable silicone, have been used for lip rejuvenation. However, these permanent fillers have an increased risk of granulomas, foreign body reaction, extrusion, recurrent chronic inflammation, and possible permanent scarring when injected into the lips.

As a result, semipermanent and permanent fillers are not recommended for lip augmentation.

INJECTION TECHNIQUES FOR LIP REJUVENATION

To provide the best outcome and minimize complications with lip fillers, it is judicious to have detailed knowledge of facial anatomy, particularly the areas that could be associated with complications. The superior and inferior labial arteries arise from the facial artery, approximately 1.5 mm superolateral to oral commissure. Cotofana et al. noted that anatomic variations of the arteries are common and vary among three positions. The superior labial artery (SLA) is located most commonly between the orbicularis oris and oral mucosa (78.1%), intramuscularly (17.6%), and between skin and muscle (2.6%). The inferior labial artery (ILA) is located most commonly between the orbicularis oris and oral mucosa (78.1%), intramuscularly (17.3%), and between skin and muscle (1.7%). These arteries form a circular network periorally and are located posterior to the wet–dry border. Because the SLA is frequently more superficial in the midline, more caution should be given for treatment of the Cupid's bow area. In both the lower and upper lip, the median regions are noted as danger zones, while the paramedian areas are typically safer for superficial injection. Superficial injections are usually the safer choice given that SLA and ILA tend to run in deeper planes; however, it has been shown that these arteries could run through any depth given individual variations and with evidence from previous cadaver studies. In addition to individual variations, the authors have also shown variability in the depth of the labial arteries even between two different sides, within one person. Trévidic et al. showed in 20 hemifacial dissections of 10 cadavers that the safe areas for fillers free of SLA, ILA, or their branches were located 3 to 4 mm above the vermilion mucosal junction of the upper lip and 3 to 5 mm below the vermilion mucosal junction of the lower lip. Lee et al. examined the course of the SLA in 36 cadavers. They found that in most cases, the artery ran superior to the lateral vermilion border under the orbicularis oris muscle at a minimum depth of 3 mm. Prior to approaching the peak of Cupid's bow, the artery courses inferior to the vermilion border. Twenty-one percent of the superior labial arteries examined contained a nasal septal branch that ramified in the sagittal midline and coursed above the orbicularis muscle. The authors concluded that to safely treat the upper lip, injections should not be deeper than 3 mm. Because the ILA courses in the cutaneous lower lip between the orbicularis oris and the lip depressors, injections above the muscle are considered safe.

There are many different techniques for injecting soft tissue fillers, including tunneling, serial puncture, threading, cross-hatching, and fanning. In our experience, the exact location and volume of product injected are most important to the outcome (Video 25.1).

Most patients feel mild to moderate discomfort during lip injections. Although HA products premixed with lidocaine can reduce the discomfort, some patients may still prefer to have either topical anesthesia or a small nerve block. The nerve block should be placed near the infraorbital foramen (midpupillary line, lateral to nasal ala) and the mental foramen (angle of jawline, inferior to the corners of the mouth) and can be injected via an intraoral approach or through the skin. Alternatively, a small amount of lidocaine can be placed as a bleb at the junction where the gum and mucosa join. It is important to remember that if lidocaine is used, the minimal amount of lidocaine should be injected to avoid distorting the lip architecture, which would make the aesthetic correction more difficult to assess. In our experience, these blocks are often not necessary.

> **PEARL 2** In general, injections in the rolled border of the lip produce definition, whereas injections in the body will augment the volume of the lips. Pushing in an anterograde fashion or "tunneling" the filler in a single injection from lateral to medial and allowing it to "flow" into the potential space just under the dermis can result in a smooth effect and avoid lumpiness associated with serial injections.

Lip aesthetics have changed through history, and among different racial and ethnic groups. The "ideal" vertical height ratio of the upper lip to the lower lip, also known as the "golden ratio" or the "Fibonacci proportion," is 1:1.6 in whites. In Asian females, Peng et al. suggest that the ideal ratio is roughly 1:1.2 to 1:1.36. African American patients may require greater volume injections into the upper lip than in the lower lip to achieve their ideal outcome. A previous survey study by Keramidas et al. done in 2008 showed that the majority (70%) preferred a ratio of 0.85:1, while 20% chose the 1:1 ratio. Heiderueger et al. published a survey study in 2017 showing that the current contemporary trend preferred female lip ratio of 1:1 in white women. The Popenko et al. study in 2017 showed that the majority in this survey study prefers the 1:2 ratio, while interestingly the ratio of 2:1 was deemed the least attractive. Overall, many patients require slightly more volume in the lower lip than in the upper lip, but the exact volume and proportions must be individualized for each patient.

There are numerous techniques when approaching lip augmentation that can result in the enhancement of lip aesthetics. Typically, when rejuvenating the upper lip, the vermilion border is treated first to define the Cupid's bow and vermilion border prior to volumizing the body of the lip (Fig. 25.2). The needle or cannula is inserted at the lateral edge of the upper lip and tunneled lateral to medial along the vermilion border to the G-K points in the Cupid's bow. A small amount of filler is placed into the Cupid's bow to define this area. The remainder of the product is then injected in a retrograde fashion as the needle is withdrawn. Alternatively, the filler can be "pushed" anterograde along the border in the superficial to mid dermis. Applying gentle traction to the surrounding skin can make needle insertion more comfortable. Injection should be stopped before the needle exits the skin to prevent filler from being placed too superficially. Although most physicians use hypodermic needles, Fulton et al. showed that blunt-tip microcannulas can be used to inject the vermillion border of the lips. The authors in the study recommend a 38-mm, 27-gauge microcannula for this area.

If the patient's philtral columns are poorly defined, the filler can also be used to redefine these points. A highly cross-linked cohesive filler will be best for the philtral columns. The needle should be inserted at the G-K points and then advanced superiorly along the philtral column in a mid-dermal plane. Again, the product is placed with a retrograde injection technique. A small amount of filler is sufficient to redefine each column; a slightly greater amount of the filler should be placed toward the inferior aspect to maintain the natural contour and appearance of the philtral column. If the patient desires volume enhancement of the upper lip, filler can be placed along the body of the lip using a serial puncture or linear threading technique, focusing on maintaining the fullness of the tubercles by adding more product in these areas. After any injection, it is important to palpate the treated area and massage any lumps to create a smooth contour.

The lower lip is similarly treated. We recommend inserting the needle at the lateral edge of the lower lip and then either pushing the filler in an anterograde fashion in the subdermal space or tunneling the needle along the vermilion border to the midpoint of the lower lip and injecting in a linear retrograde fashion. If augmentation is also desired, product can be injected along the body of the lower lip.

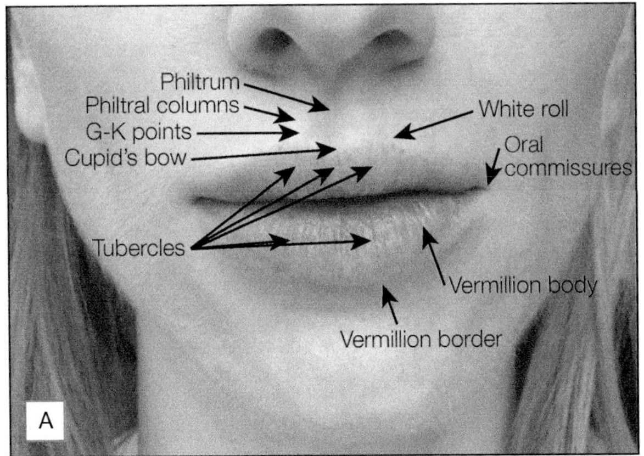

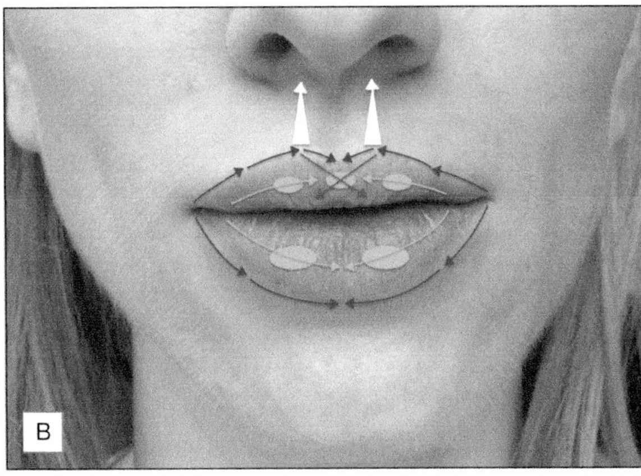

Fig. 25.2 (A) Anatomic landmarks of the lips. (B) Location of injections for the lips. *Blue lines* represent the vermillion border. *White lines* signify the philtral columns; more filler should be placed in the inferior aspect. *Pink lines* indicate injection technique for the medial upper lip. *Green lines* denote the area of injection of the body of the lips; more filler should be placed in the tubercles (*green circles*).

With regard to the oral commissures and the lateral lip festoons, injection of HA in this area could help with structural support and lift the corners of the mouth. Weinkle suggests a serial puncture technique for the deeper depressions and linear threading technique for the shallower grooves. To start, the needle should be inserted into the modiolus, at the mid-dermal plane. The patient's mouth should be slightly open, and product should be slowly injected to form a strut as the needle goes from inferior to superior. For patients with deeper depression requiring more correction, a cross-hatching or multidirectional approach is recommended and allows maximal filler coverage to the treatment area.

If the patient's lips are symmetric prior to augmentation, it is important to ensure that an equal amount of product is placed into each side of the lip to maintain this symmetry. Frequently, patients have asymmetrical lips requiring a slightly different amount to be injected to each side of the lips. It should be noted that, sometimes, a small amount of filler (0.1–0.3 mL) can make an enormous difference in the appearance of the lips.

Several studies have been published in recent years reporting various novel lip injection techniques that resulted in a safe and effective lip augmentation with improved outcomes. Sahan et al. reported a technique called the "four-point injection technique." The authors divided the lips equally into right and left side, and four entry points were made above the vermilion border for the upper lip and below the vermilion border for the lower lip. They administered the filler via a fanning technique through each entry point and found that 90% of the patients (45 out of 50) were satisfied or extremely satisfied with their lip enhancement procedures. The authors had no serious complications and report that this technique reduces the risk of complications and allows easy access to injection sites with good outcomes. Surek et al. published a "No-Touch" technique for lip enhancement. The authors performed lip analysis via anthropometric measurements and evaluation of patient smile attractiveness, teeth, gingiva, ethnic characteristics, white roll, vermilion, and wet–dry junction. This technique focuses on seeking an anatomy-based stepwise approach to determine the aesthetic needs of a patient and describes a method that does not violate the lip mucosa. The authors report that this method of tailoring lip treatment toward lip profile, projection, and/or augmentation with minimal mucosal trauma allows for a predictable and reproducible outcome for proper lip enhancement. Trévidic et al. published a technique named the "French kiss technique" (FKT). The authors proposed a novel approach to identifying locations where lip eversion using fillers would be well tolerated, with results showing that the novel FKT has produced a marked natural lip plumping effect. This method allows for lip eversion but will not treat perioral rhytides or increase overall lip volume. The technique is relevant to mainly White patients. Although most studies and authors recommend against injecting fillers deeply under the orbicularis oris, the authors injected small amounts of fillers in the submucosal plane based on their anatomical findings, to achieve lip eversion. They assessed 20 hemifaces from cadavers to reveal "safe areas" for filler injections, which was shown to be in the submucosal plane 3 to 4 mm above the vermilion–mucosa junction of the upper lip and 3 to 5 mm below the vermilion–mucosa junction of the lower lip. The authors concluded that the FKT injection technique allows for good cosmetic outcomes, lower pain intensity, and without any major reported complications. However, further evaluation of the approach is needed, and studies in a more diverse cohort with different ethnic backgrounds are recommended. Last, the most recent reported lip injection technique named the "step-by-step phi technique" was published by Keramidas et al. in 2021. This technique uses a specific caliper with the "golden ratio" guide of 1:1.618 to identify the proper points for injection, and they never inject more than 1 to 1.5 mL of HA in a single session. Using the specific caliper, they identify three to four points in each upper half of the lip. To restore volume, a 30-gauge needle is inserted at a 30-degree angle, with small boluses of 0.01 to 0.05 mL of HA injected slowly in each of the points, from the vermilion border into the vermilion, taking care not to go more than 2.5 mm deep to avoid lip vessels. The authors suggest bending the needle at 2.5 mm to ensure the depth. The same is done for the lower lip. To restore shape, the same injection points are used, but injection is performed into the vermillion border at a parallel angle (rather than 30 degrees). If necessary, patients are seen in follow-up sessions at an interval of 15 to 30 days. The authors reported that 92.4% of patients marked results as exceptional on the GAIS 5-point scale. Overall, the authors describe the "step-by-step phi technique" as a safe, easy-to-learn/perform method to providing natural and improved results in lip augmentation.

In addition to rejuvenating the lips themselves, it is often necessary to buttress the corners of the mouth to prevent or reverse downturned corners of the lips. This can be easily accomplished by injecting filler product underneath the lateral corners of the mouth, providing a scaffolding to support the remainder of the lips. This effect can be further enhanced by injecting botulinum toxin into the depressor anguli oris muscles to help turn the corners of the mouth up, thereby rejuvenating the lips and mouth.

Finally, the patient may desire treatment of perioral rhytides. These lines can be improved with soft tissue augmentation. The needle should be inserted at one end of the rhytides, and then tunneled along the depression. Very small amounts of filler are placed in a relatively superficial plane. Alternatively, microdroplets can be injected along the line using a microdroplet technique. Botulinum toxin can also be administered to relax the orbicularis oris muscle and to help prevent or reduce these rhytides. In severe cases, a chemical peel, laser resurfacing, or radiofrequency microneedling may be necessary to provide better improvement.

PEARL 3 Place filler inferior to the commissures of the mouth to provide a buttress to elevate and turn up the corners of the mouth, which relax and turn downward with age.

POTENTIAL SIDE EFFECTS

Stojanovic et al. published a systemic review on the use of HA-based fillers for the lips, and looking at patient satisfaction and safety data from 2000 to 2017, they found that majority of patients are satisfied with their lip improvement. However, a wide range of adverse events have been reported, with the most common being local injection site reactions including swelling, bruising, pain, redness, and itching. Most patients reported treatment-related adverse events as mild (71%–88%) or moderate (11%–16%) in severity and majority resolving within 2 weeks. Some studies have shown that Fitzpatrick skin type IV/V/VI tends to have a lower incidence of adverse events than those with Fitzpatrick skin

CASE STUDY 1

A patient presented for lip rejuvenation (Fig. 25.3A). On examination, the upper lip is thin and flat, with a loss of the Cupid's bow. The philtral columns are not well defined. There are multiple perioral radiating rhytides. The lower lip is also small and lacks definition.

The patient underwent lip rejuvenation with 1 mL of HA product (see Fig. 25.3B). Following the augmentation, note the reshaped and defined Cupid's bow; there is also greater definition of the inferior aspects of the philtral columns. The overall volume of the upper and lower lips is increased slightly as well. Finally, there is a reduction in the appearance of the radiating perioral rhytides.

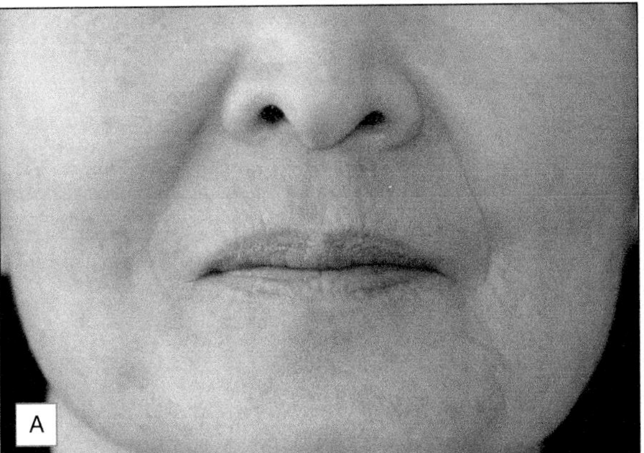

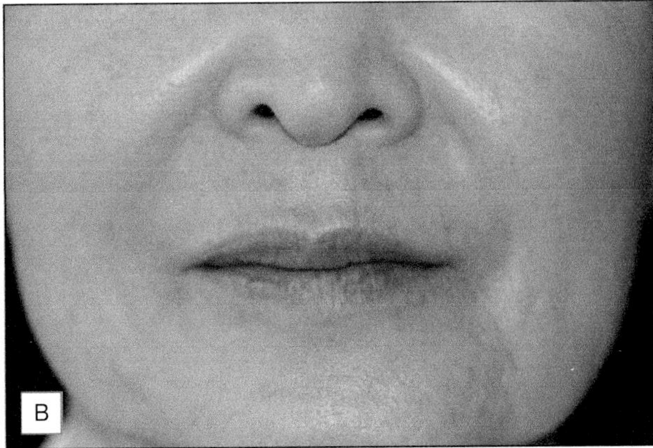

Fig. 25.3 (A) A patient presented complaining of thin lips, a loss of structure and shape on the upper lip, and radiating perioral rhytides. (B) Following lip rejuvenation with 1 mL of hyaluronic acid product, note the defined Cupid's bow and vermilion border of the lip. There is also enhanced volume and a reduction in the appearance of the radiating perioral rhytides.

type I/II/III. There is no evidence of the risk of postinflammatory pigment alterations, hypertrophic scarring, or keloid formation in ethnic patients following treatment. Although rare, there are reports of filler migration to the surrounding perioral skin, herpes simplex virus reactivation, and late-onset nodule and granuloma formation, even with HA fillers.

Serious complications of filler treatment include vascular compromise, leading to skin necrosis, or in rarer cases, blindness. Oftentimes, patients who develop vascular compromise and necrosis will have blanching of the lip and pain as the most common sign. Beleznay et al. described their clinical experiences over a 10-year period with a total of 12 cases of vascular compromise, out of a total of 14,335 filler injections in that time. Of those 12 cases, three patients had vascular complications of the lip. Numerous other studies looking at cases of blindness due to soft tissue fillers have been published by Beleznay et al., Chatrath et al., and Lazzeri et al. These studies report that the high-risk areas for blindness include the nasal region and the glabellar complex. Lazzeri et al. did a systematic review finding 32 patients that had cases in which blindness was a direct consequence of filler injections. Of the 32 cases, 3 had blindness after injections were done into the lower part of the face (they grouped this as nasolabial folds, lips, and chins) with autologous fat injections. Among these studies, there is at time of writing no reported case of blindness from lip injections with HA.

The mild complications (swelling and bruising) typically self-resolve within the first 2 weeks. Although massaging after injections can help with lumps and bumps, too much of a vigorous massage may lead to more intense swelling. Typically, short duration of icepacks immediately after treatment may help with swelling. Patients should be advised to maintain head of bed position while resting and avoid significant exercise, particularly the head-down position for 24 hours postinjection. For complications like herpes simplex virus reactivation, a short course (7–10 days) of antiviral with valacyclovir or acyclovir can be given. For vascular complications of the lip, Belaznay et al. recommend the following treatment: warm compresses; massage; nerve block if necessary (without epinephrine); hyaluronidase if HA filler was used—keeping in mind that one injection may not be sufficient and multiple hyaluronidase may be warranted for treatment; aspirin 325 mg under the tongue immediately after and 81 mg daily thereafter; oral prednisone at 20 to 40 mg daily for 3 to 5 days; and lastly hyperbaric oxygen therapy, especially with impending tissue loss. Schelke et al. proposed using ultrasound guidance to inject hyaluronidase directly into the filler deposit, which allows for more precision and improved outcomes when treating adverse events from lip filler injections.

IMPROVED SAFETY TECHNIQUES/ PREVENTION

While mild complications from lip injections are common and fortunately the more serious complications are rare, steps should be taken to maximize outcome and minimize any adverse events. As vessels are not visible clinically and given the anatomic variations among individuals, understanding the anatomy and steps toward prevention of complications is extremely important. Guidelines advise using cannulas to inject slowly small volumes to reduce these mild side effects and the likelihood of overcorrection and asymmetry; potential touch-up procedures 1 to 2 weeks after the initial treatments can be performed as needed.

Pavicic et al. showed that cannulas resulted in more precise injection of materials compared to needles. Additionally, the authors found that cannulas in all measured sizes except 27 gauge requires greater forces for intraarterial penetration compared with corresponding needle sizes, which supports the improved safety of 22- and 25-gauge cannulas. Blunt tip cannulas have been shown to minimize risk of intravascular injection, and van Loghem et al. reported that 71% of 58 expert injectors agreed that cannulae are safer than needles for injecting fillers at the periosteum. Murad et al. recently did a retrospective cohort study showing the rates of vascular occlusion using needles vs. cannulas for filler injections. The authors showed that the overall risk of intravascular occlusion events was very low with either needles or cannulas and the risk of occlusion with microcannulas was significantly less than with needles. Importantly, they showed that the majority of the vascular occlusion events were minor and resolved without scarring or other significant injury. Schelke et al. showed the use of ultrasound/ duplex can minimize risk by identifying underlying muscles, veins, and arteries. The authors are able to identify structures and filler substances base on echogenicity and showed that anatomical mapping of these clinically nonvisible vessels are possible. Therefore, they suggest the use of duplex ultrasound in clinics when using HA based fillers for improve safety and minimization of complications.

CASE STUDY 2

A 40-year-old female patient presents for lip augmentation. The upper lip is augmented with 0.3 mL of HA to define the rolled border. The lower lip is augmented with 0.5 mL of HA, with injections along the rolled border and into the wet–dry junction of the lip. At the conclusion of the procedure, the lips are slightly swollen but appear symmetric. Two days later, the patient calls the office upset that her lips are "huge and overcorrected." She requests treatment with a reversing agent to undo the augmentation. What should the treating physician do next?

The patient should be reassured and instructed to return to the office. Swelling following the augmentation is very common and may require several days to resolve. Hyaluronidase will remove the product but will not improve bruising or swelling associated with the injections themselves. Patients often benefit from massage of the area to smooth down any nodules or lumpiness. Patients should then be instructed to ice the areas and wait for any swelling associated with the procedure to resolve before judging the final result. Translucent lumps still present after swelling has subsided can represent superficial collections of filler. An 18- or 22-gauge needle can be used to pierce the center of the collection and manually express filler. The patient in this case study returned to the office, had a good response to massage, and 1 week later was thrilled with the appearance of her augmentation.

CONCLUSIONS

The lips are a dramatic and defining feature of the face. Unfortunately, the aging process denies patients of the beautiful structure and volume of the lips. Lip rejuvenation and augmentation is a safe, simple, and effective procedure to reverse these changes. HA fillers are the treatment of choice to both redefine and restore volume to the lips. In more advanced cases, a multimodality approach may be necessary to complete the rejuvenation of the perioral area.

FURTHER READING

Alam, M., Gladstone, H., Kramer, E. M., with the Guidelines Task Force., et al. (2008). ASDS guidelines of care: Injectable fillers. *Dermatologic Surgery, 34*, S115–S148. https://doi.org/10.1111/j.1524-4725.2008.34253.x.

Alam, M., Kakar, R., Dover, J. S., et al. (2021). Rates of vascular occlusion associated with using needles vs cannulas for filler injection. *JAMA Dermatology, 157*(2), 174–180. https://doi.org/10.1001/jamadermatol.2020.5102.

Beer, K., Glogau, R. G., Dover, J. S., et al. (2015). A randomized, evaluator-blinded, controlled study of effectiveness and safety of small particle hyaluronic acid plus lidocaine for lip augmentation and perioral rhytides. *Dermatologic Surgery, 41*(suppl 1), S127–S136. https://doi.org/10.1097/DSS.0000000000000199.

Beleznay, K., Humphrey, S., Carruthers, J. D., et al. (2014). Vascular compromise from soft tissue augmentation: Experience with 12 cases and recommendations for optimal outcomes. *The Journal of Clinical and Aesthetic Dermatology, 7*(9), 37–43.

Beleznay, K., Carruthers, J. D., Humphrey, S., et al. (2015). Avoiding and treating blindness from fillers: A review of the world literature. *Dermatologic Surgery, 41*(10), 1097–1117. https://doi.org/10.1097/DSS.0000000000000486.

Carruthers, J., Glogau, R., Blitzer, A., & Facial Aesthetics Consensus Group Faculty. (2008). Advances in facial rejuvenation: Botulinum toxin type A, hyaluronic acid dermal fillers, and combination therapies—Consensus recommendations. *Plastic and Reconstructive Surgery, 121*(suppl 5), S5–S30. https://doi.org/10.1097/PRS.0b013e31816de8d0.

Chatrath, V., Banerjee, P. S., Goodman, G. J., & Rahman, E. (2019). Soft-tissue filler-associated blindness: A systematic review of case reports and case series. *Plastic and Reconstructive Surgery. Global Open, 7*(4), e2173. https://doi.org/10.1097/GOX.0000000000002173.

Cohen, J. L., Thomas, J., Paradkar, D., et al. (2014). An interrater and intrarater reliability study of 3 photographic scales for the classification of perioral aesthetic features. *Dermatologic Surgery, 40*(6), 663–670. https://doi.org/10.1111/dsu.0000000000000008.

Cotofana, S., Steinke, H., Schlattau, A., et al. (2017). The anatomy of the facial vein: Implications for plastic, reconstructive, and aesthetic procedures. *Plastic and Reconstructive Surgery, 139*, 1346–1353. https://doi.org/10.1097/PRS.0000000000003382.

Custis, T., Beynet, D., Carranza, D., et al. (2010). Comparison of treatment of melomental fold rhytides with cross-linked hyaluronic acid combined with onabotulinumtoxinA and cross-linked hyaluronic acid alone. *Dermatologic Surgery, 36*(suppl 3), S1852–S1858. https://doi.org/10.1111/j.1524-4725.2010.01741.x.

Dayan, S., Bruce, S., Kilmer, S., et al. (2015). Safety and effectiveness of the hyaluronic acid filler, HYC-24L, for lip and perioral augmentation. *Dermatologic Surgery, 41*(suppl 1), S293–S301. https://doi.org/10.1097/DSS.0000000000000540.

DeJoseph, L. M., Agarwal, A., & Greco, T. M. (2018). Lip augmentation. *Facial Plastic Surgery Clinics of North America, 26*(2), 193–203. https://doi.org/10.1016/j.fsc.2017.12.005.

Eccleston, D., & Murphy, D. K. (2012). Juvéderm® VolbellaTM in the perioral area: A 12-month prospective, multicenter, open-label study. *Clinical, Cosmetic and Investigational Dermatology, 5*, 167–172. https://doi.org/10.2147/CCID.S35800.

Fulton, J., Caperton, C., Weinkle, S., et al. (2012). Filler injections with the blunt-tip microcannula. *Journal of Drugs in Dermatology, 11*(9), 1098–1103.

Glogau, R. G., Bank, D., Brandt, F., et al. (2012). A randomized, evaluator-blinded, controlled study of the effectiveness and safety of small gel particle hyaluronic acid for lip augmentation. *Dermatologic Surgery, 38*(7 pt 2), 1180–1192. https://doi.org/10.1111/j.1524-4725.2012.02473.x.

Heidekrueger, P. I., Juran, S., Szpalski, C., et al. (2017). The current preferred female lip ratio. *Journal of Cranio-Maxillo-Facial Surgery, 45*(5), 655–660. https://doi.org/10.1016/j.jcms.2017.01.038.

Ibher, N., Kloepper, J., Penna, V., Bartholomae, J. P., & Stark, G. B. (2008). Changes in the aging upper lip—A photomorphometric and MRI-based study (on a quest to find the right rejuvenation approach). *Journal of Plastic, Reconstructive & Aesthetic Surgery, 61*, 1170–1176. https://doi.org/10.1016/j.bjps.2008.06.001.

Kar, M., Muluk, N. B., Bafaqeeh, S. A., et al. (2018). Is it possible to define the ideal lips? *Acta Otorhinolaryngologica Italica, 38*(1), 67–72. https://doi.org/10.14639/0392-100X-1511.

Keramidas, E., Rodopoulou, S., & Gavala, M. I. (2021). A safe and effective lip augmentation method: The Step-by-Step Φ (Phi) Technique. *Plastic and Reconstructive Surgery. Global Open, 9*(2), e3332. https://doi.org/10.1097/GOX.0000000000003332.

Kollipara, R., Walker, B., & Sturgeon, A. (2017). Lip measurements and preferences in Asians and Hispanics: A brief review. *The Journal of Clinical and Aesthetic Dermatology, 10*(11), 19–21.

Lazzeri, D., Agostini, T., Figus, M., Nardi, M., Pantaloni, M., & Lazzeri, S. (2012). Blindness following cosmetic injections of the face. *Plastic and Reconstructive Surgery, 129*(4), 995–1012. https://doi.org/10.1097/PRS.0b013e3182442363.

Lee, S. H., Gil, Y. C., Choi, Y. J., Tansatit, T., Kim, H. J., & Hu, K. S. (2015). Topographic anatomy of the superior labial artery for dermal filler injection. *Plastic and Reconstructive Surgery, 135*(2), 445–450. https://doi.org/10.1097/PRS.0000000000000858.

Melo, A. R., Conti, A. C. C. F., Almeida-Pedrin, R. R., Didier, V., Valarelli, D. P., & Capelozza Filho, L. (2017). Evaluation of facial attractiveness in black people according to the subjective facial analysis criteria. *Dental Press Journal of Orthodontics, 22*(1), 75–81. https://doi.org/10.1590/2177-6709.22.1.075-081.oar.

Narins, R. S., Carruthers, J., Flynn, T. C., et al. (2012). Validated assessment scales for the lower face. *Dermatologic Surgery, 38*, 333–342. https://doi.org/10.1111/j.1524-4725.2011.02247.x (2 spec no).

Pavicic, T., Frank, K., Erlbacher, K., et al. (2017). Precision in dermal filling: A comparison between needle and cannula when using soft tissue fillers. *Journal of Drugs in Dermatology, 16*(9), 866–872.

Pavicic, T., Webb, K. L., Frank, K., et al. (2019). Arterial wall penetration forces in needles versus cannulas. *Plastic and Reconstructive Surgery, 143*(3), 504e–512e. https://doi.org/10.1097/PRS.0000000000005321.

Peng, J. H., & Peng, H. P. (2020). Classifications and injection strategy for lip reshaping in Asians. *Journal of Cosmetic Dermatology, 19*(10), 2519–2528. https://doi.org/10.1111/jocd.13635.

Popenko, N. A., Tripathi, P. B., Devcic, Z., et al. (2017). A quantitative approach to determining the ideal female lip aesthetic and its effect on facial attractiveness. *JAMA Facial Plastic Surgery, 19*, 261–267. https://doi.org/10.1001/jamafacial.2016.2049.

Ramaut, L., Tonnard, P., Verpaele, A., et al. (2019). Aging of the upper lip: Part I: A retrospective analysis of metric changes in soft tissue on magnetic resonance imaging. *Plastic and Reconstructive Surgery, 143*(2), 440–446. https://doi.org/10.1097/PRS.0000000000005190.

Rossi, A. B., Nkengne, A., Stamatas, G., & Bertin, C. (2011). Development and validation of a photonumeric grading scale for assessing lip volume and thickness. *Journal of the European Academy of Dermatology and Venereology, 25*(5), 523–531. https://doi.org/10.1111/j.1468-3083.2010.03816.x.

Sahan, A., & Funda, T. (2018). Four-point injection technique for lip augmentation. *Acta Dermatovenerologica Alpina, Pannonica, et Adriatica, 27*(2), 71–73.

San Miguel Moragas, J., Reddy, R. R., Hernández Alfaro, F., et al. (2015). Systematic review of "filling" procedures for lip augmentation regarding types of material, outcomes and complications. *Journal of Cranio-Maxillo-Facial Surgery, 43*(6), 883–906. https://doi.org/10.1016/j.jcms.2015.03.032.

Schelke, L. W., Decates, T. S., & Velthuis, P. J. (2018). Ultrasound to improve the safety of hyaluronic acid filler treatments. *Journal of Cosmetic Dermatology, 17*(6), 1019–1024. https://doi.org/10.1111/jocd.12726.

Shahrabi Farahani, S., Sexton, J., Stone, J. D., et al. (2012). Lip nodules caused by hyaluronic acid filler injection: Report of three cases. *Head and Neck Pathology*, *6*(1), 16–20. https://doi.org/10.1007/s12105-011-0304-9.

Stojanovič, L., & Majdič, N. (2019). Effectiveness and safety of hyaluronic acid fillers used to enhance overall lip fullness: A systematic review of clinical studies. *Journal of Cosmetic Dermatology*, *18*(2), 436–443. https://doi.org/10.1111/jocd.12861.

Surek, C. C., Guisantes, E., Schnarr, K., Jelks, G., & Beut, J. (2016). "No-Touch" technique for lip enhancement. *Plastic and Reconstructive Surgery*, *138*(4), 603e–613e. https://doi.org/10.1097/PRS.0000000000002568.

Tansatit, T., Apinuntrum, P., & Phetudom, T. (2014). A typical pattern of the labial arteries with implication for lip augmentation with injectable fillers. *Aesthetic Plastic Surgery*, *38*(6), 1083–1089. https://doi.org/10.1007/s00266-014-0401-8.

Teixeira, J. C., Ostrom, J. Y., Hohman, M. H., et al. (2021). Botulinum toxin type-A for lip augmentation: "Lip flip". *The Journal of Craniofacial Surgery*, *32*(3), e273–e275. https://doi.org/10.1097/SCS.0000000000007128.

Trévidic, P., & Criollo-Lamilla, G. (2020). French kiss technique: An anatomical study and description of a new method for safe lip eversion. *Dermatologic Surgery*, *46*(11), 1410–1417. https://doi.org/10.1097/DSS.0000000000002325.

van Loghem, J. A. J., Humzah, D., & Kerscher, M. (2017). Cannula versus sharp needle for placement of soft tissue fillers: An observational cadaver study. *Aesthetic Surgery Journal*, *38*(1), 3–88. https://doi.org/10.1093/asj/sjw220.

Votto, S. S., Read-Fuller, A., & Reddy, L. (2021). Lip augmentation. *Oral and Maxillofacial Surgery Clinics of North America*, *33*(2), 185–195. https://doi.org/10.1016/j.coms.2021.01.004.

Weinkle, S. (2010). Injection techniques for revolumization of the perioral region with hyaluronic acid. *Journal of Drugs in Dermatology*, *9*(4), 367–371.

Werschler, W. P., Fagien, S., Thomas, J., Paradkar-Mitragotri, D., Rotunda, A., & Beddingfield, F. C. (2015). Development and validation of a photographic scale for assessment of lip fullness. *Aesthetic Surgery Journal*, *35*(3), 294–307. https://doi.org/10.1093/asj/sju025.

26

Soft Tissue Augmentation of Lip Lines

Farah Moustafa, Omer Ibrahim, and Jeffrey S. Dover

SUMMARY AND KEY FEATURES

- Intrinsic and extrinsic factors contribute to the appearance of aging skin.
- Vertical lip lines or perioral rhytides contribute to the aged appearance of the perioral area and are a significant cosmetic concern for patients.
- Women exhibit perioral lines much more frequently and more severely than men.
- Lines are caused by repeated contraction of the orbicularis oris muscle, along with loss of collagen and elastin fibers over time.
- Prior to treatment, proper counseling with the patient must occur to discuss realistic treatment expectations and outcomes.
- The treatment of perioral lines is multimodal and often requires a combination of modalities to yield optimal results. These include neuromodulator, fillers, and laser resurfacing.
- Soft tissue augmentation with hyaluronic acid-based fillers provides a valuable tool in improving the appearance of lip rhytides giving an overall rejuvenated appearance to the perioral area.
- Finer, lower G-prime hyaluronic acid fillers should be used at just the minimum quantities to give the desired effects. Permanent, semipermanent, and non-hyaluronic acid fillers should be avoided.
- With treatment, patients can expect bruising and swelling, and with good technique, patients can expect modest, natural-appearing results.
- Risk of more serious complications such as vascular occlusion can be minimized with an intimate knowledge of anatomy and precise, effective technique.

BACKGROUND

Aging of the skin occurs via a multitude of offending processes that ultimately lead to cutaneous fine lines, deeper wrinkles, dyschromia, and laxity. Intrinsic factors such as inherent physiology and genetic makeup contribute only marginally to the aging process. On the other hand, extrinsic (environmental) influences including solar radiation and pollution account for the vast majority of factors that cause cutaneous aging and rhytid formation. Fine lines and wrinkles can affect almost any part of the face, and the perioral area is no exception. Lip lines can be especially bothersome and notoriously difficult to treat. In this chapter, we will discuss the anatomical basis of lip lines, proper counseling and approach to the problem, and safe and effective treatment guidelines.

PATHOGENESIS OF LIP LINES

Perioral lines arise from a combination of repeated contraction of the orbicularis oris muscle and the natural epidermal and dermal atrophy, as well as collagen and elastin loss as a result of aging. The numerous muscle fibers of the orbicularis oris muscle originate from the medial aspect of the maxilla and mandible, perioral skin, and modiolus (Fig. 26.1). The upper and lower

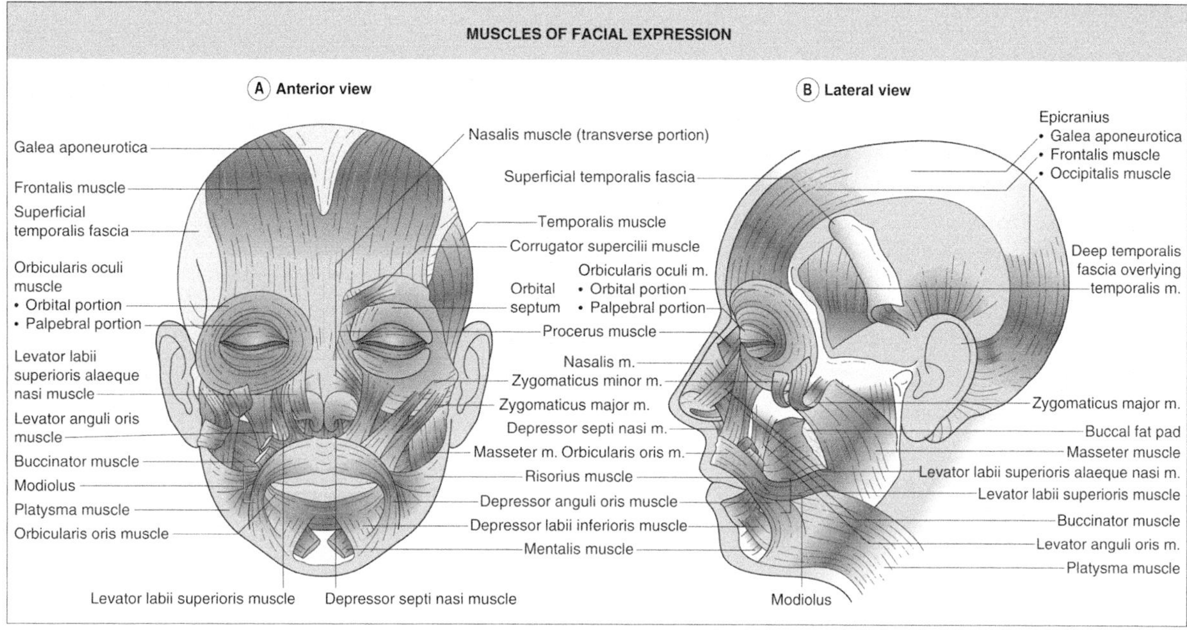

Fig. 26.1 Muscles of facial expression.

portions of the muscle insert into the deep dermis of the lip mucosa. This intricate arrangement allows for closure of the mouth and puckering or pursing of the lips. The repeated dynamic contraction of this muscle group results in radial lines projecting vertically outward from the vermillion border of the upper and lower lip (perpendicular to the direction of muscle contraction). These lines are more prominent in individuals with marked photoaging due to other intrinsic and extrinsic factors and in those who frequently pucker their lips or forcibly exhale (smokers, certain woodwind instrumentalists, etc.).

There are other global changes that transpire in the face that can exacerbate the aged appearance of the lips and perioral area. Structural loss occurs due to bony resorption and subcutaneous fat atrophy, which results in flattening of the lower face and the appearance of the jowl and accentuation of the labiomandibular fold (marionette lines). The corners of the mouth, which are upturned in youth, begin to turn downward with age, creating the appearance of a resting frown and a chronically sad facial expression. This is exacerbated by the activity of the depressor anguli oris (DAO), which further depresses the corners of the mouth. Although outside the scope of this chapter, these are important factors that are prudent to address at the time of consultation for perioral lip lines, as a holistic approach yields the most aesthetically pleasing results.

LIP LINES: DOES THE PATIENT'S SEX MATTER?

Historically, more women than men seek correction of perioral rhytids. This may be due partly to the fact that women seek cosmetic treatments more frequently than men do. However, histological studies have confirmed key anatomical differences between men and women that predispose the latter to more severe lip lines. In the perioral area, men exhibit a higher number of sebaceous glands and sweat glands, with a significantly higher sebaceous gland count per hair follicle, although the number of hair follicles do not differ. Men display more blood vessels, thicker epidermis, and more robust connective tissue in the dermis. Finally, the distance between the dermis and the orbicularis oris muscle was significantly larger in men; that is, the orbicularis oris muscle attaches closer to the dermis in women than it does in men. These anatomical differences seen on histology may explain why women express more severe perioral rhytids.

CONSULTATION

Optimal patient selection helps to ensure satisfactory outcomes. While studies suggest that a grade of "3" or "moderate" on the Lemperle or Perioral Lines at Rest scale is appropriate to treat, this determination is based on the patient's desire and the physician's ability to improve the undesired findings. Although these validated tools are helpful, a practical consideration for patient assessment is (1) whether the patient has sufficient depth to the individual rhytid at rest (perhaps 1 mm or more), (2) the number of vertical rhytides in the area (to assess amount of product or limitations of treatment), and (3) the overall perioral anatomy, with particular focus on the upper cutaneous lip. Patients who have significantly elongated upper lip or with significant maxillary prognathism should be approached cautiously, as soft tissue augmentation of vertical lip lines could result in further imbalance in the overall facial harmony by adding volume to the upper portion of the mouth. Augmentation of lower facial structures such as the chin and jawline could be helpful in these patients who still desire treatment. Prior to any cosmetic intervention, discuss the goals of treatment and manage patient expectations. Clearly communicate that the goal is a softening of the perioral lines and not complete effacement. Discussing balance between softening the lines, maintaining a natural appearance, and avoiding excess filler placement that is not aesthetically pleasing and may cause functional impairment are essential. Patients who do not have realistic expectations are not ideal candidates for treatment. During the discussion, assess the patient's availability for downtime and any contraindications that may preclude treatment. Bruising is common with filler injection in this area and should be noted. Finally, discuss cost of treatment as well as the need for maintenance treatment for optimal long-term results. The clinician and patient should work together to prioritize interventions based on budget, availability for downtime, and availability for repeat treatments if necessary.

PLANNING

Prior to any intervention, take a series of high-quality photographs with adequate lighting. We recommend capturing at least three views for clinical photographs—facing forward, as well as at a 45-degree angle on each side. Additionally, consider including dynamic photographs such as having the patient pucker and smile. Capturing animation photos not only allows for a more complete documentation of the patient's anatomy but also documents subtleties in the patient's dynamic movements in case before and after comparisons must be made later on. Obtain written informed consent and include detailed risks and benefits of the planned procedure. Finally, assess the need for preintervention topical anesthesia.

At the consultation, it is best to determine the depth, width, type, and severity of the lip lines. This helps to guide the approach to treatment. The basis to treating dynamic lip lines is regular injections of neuromodulators. Very low doses injected fairly frequently (as often as every 6 weeks) yield the best improvement. Lines at rest and loss of volume in the lip are best addressed with hyaluronic acid filler. Finally, laser resurfacing, with or without drug delivery, is best reserved for individuals with extensive photoaging and elastosis.

SOFT TISSUE AUGMENTATION OF LIP LINE INJECTION TECHNIQUE

Injections of the vertical lip lines should be superficial to correct the appearance of the line with the least amount of product and avoid a heavy and unnatural look. The ideal plane of injection is in the papillary and upper reticular dermis. The injector should still be able to see the needle through the skin. The superior and inferior labial arteries that lie in the submucosal layer are branches of the facial artery and supply the upper and lower lips. As injections are kept superficial, the risk of cannulation of these vessels is small. Enhancing lip volume is described in Chapter 25.

Patient position is up to the individual injector. Some prefer to have the patients sitting up in the exam chair, while others prefer the patient lying supine for injections. Bending the needle 15 degrees can allow for more superficial injections. Insert the needle at the superior edge of the rhytid and advance inferiorly. As you retract the needle, inject retrograde. It is helpful to have the patient pucker and relax to further elucidate the area that should be injected. Superficial injections allow for not only better effacement of the linear rhytides but also result in less use of product and a less bulky final result.

Another injection technique for upper lip lines employs the depot method, in which small aliquots of filler are deposited along the length of the line (Video 26.1).

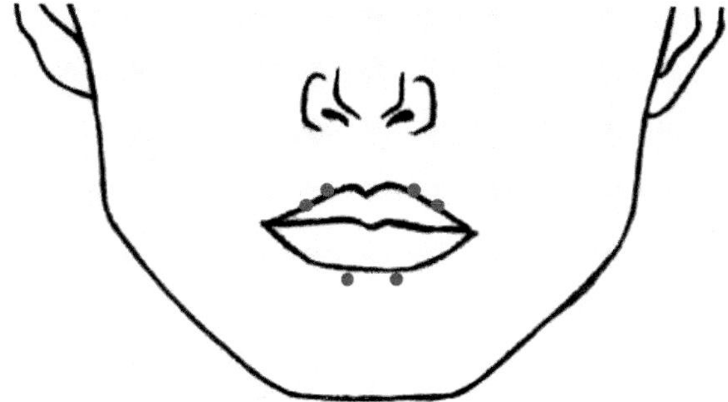

Fig. 26.2 Botulinum toxin injection points. (From Moustafa, Farah, MD; Ibrahim, Omer, MD; Dover, Jeffrey S., MD, FRCPC. Published May 31, 2020. Volume 3, Issue 1. Pages 89–98. © 2020.)

If the wrinkles are especially prominent, the entire area may need buttressing using the cross-hatching method, in which a series of threads, or multiple fans, at slightly different angles, are injected in order to deposit a very thin sheet of filler superficially (Video 26.2). Overcorrection can lead to an unnatural appearance. Regardless of the technique, following injection, it is important to press or "mold" the gel to avoid any ridging or unevenness between the injected and the noninjected area (Fig. 26.2).

FILLER SELECTION

Generally, fillers chosen for this area are thin, hyaluronic acid-based fillers, which are safe and reversible. Fillers approved for the perioral area include Juvederm Ultra, Volbella, Restylane-L, Restylane Refyne, Restylane Silk, Belotero, and RHA2. Products blended with xylocaine plain or with epinephrine, such as Juvederm Ultra, Volbella, Restylane-L, Restylane Refyne, are also frequently used for fine vertical lip like filling. In the authors' experiences, flexible, small gel particle HAs are ideal in this area. Belotero and Restylane Silk are great choices for these superficial injections. When using Restylane products, it is important to be mindful of the possibility of Tyndall due to the particulate nature of the hyaluronic acid gel. Thicker hyaluronic acid-based fillers that are not flexible (Voluma, Restylane Lyft, Restylane Defyne, and RHA4) are not suitable choices for this area. We recommend against the use of injection of permanent or non-hyaluronic acid base fillers such as calcium hydroxylapatite (Radiesse) or poly-L-lactic acid (PLLA) (Sculptra) due to the higher risk of nodule formation of these products.

PAIN MANAGEMENT/TREATMENT CONSIDERATIONS

Injections in this area are painful and some patients may request topical anesthesia. We recommend topical anesthesia in the most sensitive patients and not as a routine part of the procedure as topical anesthesia may cause some localized soft tissue swelling in the treatment area. In lieu of topical anesthesia, the application of ice immediately prior to and after injection can help mitigate discomfort.

ANTICIPATED SIDE EFFECTS

Clinicians must counsel patients on the associated immediate side effects of treatment. Bruising is fairly common, and in some patients unavoidable. Adequate application of pressure during the procedure can help reduce the extent of bruising. Vascular laser treatment immediately after treatment and up to 48 hours postprocedure may accelerate the clearance of the bruising. Postprocedural swelling can be significant as well and may last for 2 to 5 days. Ice, antihistamines, and, only if absolutely necessary, oral corticosteroids can ameliorate swelling.

COMPLICATIONS

As with any filler injections, the risk of vascular cannulation and occlusion must be acknowledged and respected. Superficial injections with small aliquots greatly decrease the risk of vascular compromise. If occlusion is suspected, the clinician must promptly initiate the "rescue protocol" discussed in the vascular compromise chapter in this text (see Chapter 36).

Delayed-onset nodules after hyaluronic acid filler occur at a reported rate of 0.02%–4.25% and largely vary based on the type of hyaluronic acid filler, cross-linking technology, and location of filler placement. Vycross cross-linking technology has been reported to result in more delayed-onset filler nodules compared to other fillers. Nodules tended to occur in the perioral area. For this reason, our authors do not select these fillers as first-line treatment for upper lip lines, especially in those patients who are immunologically sensitive or have a prior history of delayed nodule formation. Prompt recognition and appropriate treatment are required for resolution of these nodules. In the authors' practice for noninflammatory delayed-onset nodules, injection of a small amount of hyaluronidase with plain lidocaine in a

1:1 ratio along the area where nodule is palpable is recommended as an initial treatment. Reevaluate the patient in 3-to-4-week intervals to assess for improvement and possible reinjection. Addition of injectable triamcinolone at a concentration of 5 mg/mL (1:1 with hyaluronidase) can also be added at subsequent injections.

Inflammatory nodules are more complicated in nature and require empiric antibody therapy, culture, and biopsy, where applicable, and intralesional steroid injections once infectious etiologies have been eliminated.

COMPLIMENTARY TECHNIQUES FOR IMPROVEMENT OF LIP LINES

Neuromodulators

Although perioral neuromodulators will be discussed at length in a separate chapter in this series, the subject merits mention here for the sake of completion, as clinicians often combine neuromodulator and soft tissue fillers in this area to optimize results. Commercially available neurotoxins include onabotulinumtoxinA (Botox), abobotulinumtoxinA (Dysport), incabotulinumtoxinA (Xeomin), and most recently, prabotulinumtoxinA (Jeuveau). Neurotoxin injected into the orbicularis oris can decrease the appearance of perioral rhytids (Fig. 26.2).

LASER RESURFACING AND LASER-ASSISTED DRUG DELIVERY OF POLY-L-LACTIC ACID

In addition to injectables, ablative and nonablative resurfacing lasers alone can be employed to further improve the appearance of the perioral area. Laser treatment can be personally tailored to the patient depending on their desired results and availability for downtime. Most recently, combination therapy with low-density fractionated carbon dioxide (CO_2) and topical PLLA has been shown to improve the appearance of upper lip wrinkles. With the understanding that laser-assisted PLLA has been used to successfully treat atrophic scars, a recently published study demonstrated the safety and efficacy of laser-assisted PLLA delivery in the treatment of upper lip wrinkles in a cohort of 10 patients. Ibrahim et al. described one pass of the fractionated CO_2 (Fraxel Re:Pair) with a spot size of 135 mm, an energy level of 70 mJ (depth of 1579 mm), and a density of 10%, followed by topical application of PLLA onto the treatment area. The authors demonstrated an almost 50% reduction in the appearance of upper lip lines after three treatments (Fig. 26.3A and B). This approach utilizes the combined benefits of both interventions for perioral rejuvenation, while mitigating the risk of nodule formation and prolonged downtime.

- Laser-assisted drug delivery PLLA—Video 26.3.

CONCLUSIONS

Perioral rhytids are a significant concern for many patients and are notoriously difficult to treat. Given that each treatment modality may offer limited results, clinicians must often use a combination of modalities to optimize outcomes. Within the realm of soft tissue fillers, the plethora of available hyaluronic acid fillers on the market, as well as varied evidence-based techniques, have allowed clinicians to safely and effectively

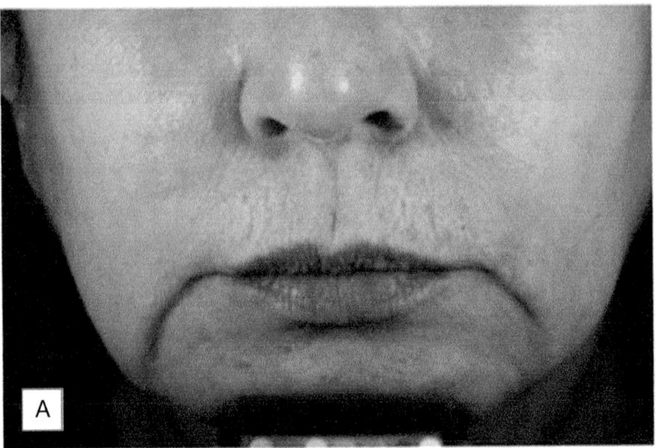

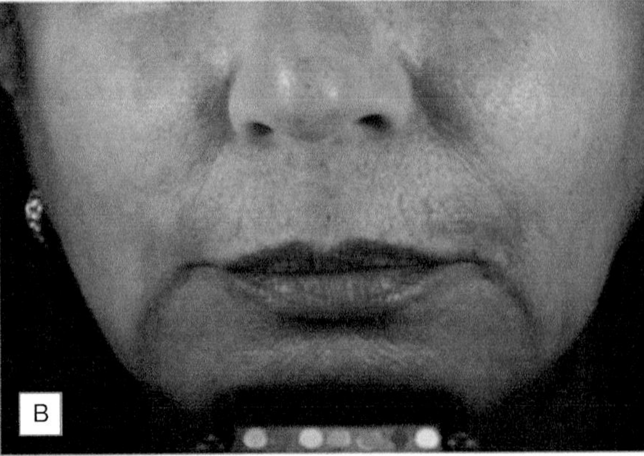

Fig. 26.3 Before (A) and after (B) three sessions of carbon dioxide laser-assisted delivery of topical poly-L-lactic acid in the treatment of upper lip wrinkles. (Copyrights reserved by Omer Ibrahim, MD.)

incorporate injectable fillers in the treatment of perioral wrinkles. With an appropriate knowledge of anatomy and precise, purposeful technique, injectors can implement these fillers safely and effectively in the patient's treatment regimen.

FURTHER READING

Barbarino, S. C., Woodward, J. A., Levine, J., & Fezza, J. (2021). Evaluating an incobotulinumtoxinA and Cohesive Polydensified Matrix((R)) hyaluronic acid filler combination to treat moderate-to-severe periorbital and perioral rhytids. *Journal of Cosmetic Dermatology, 20*(5), 1459–15466. https://doi.org/10.1111/jocd.13745.

Bertucci, V., Nikolis, A., Solish, N., Lane, V., & Hicks, J. (2021). Subject and partner satisfaction with lip and perioral enhancement using flexible hyaluronic acid fillers. *Journal of Cosmetic Dermatology, 20*(5), 1499–1504. https://doi.org/10.1111/jocd.13956.

Cohen, J. L., Thomas, J., Paradkar, D., Rotunda, A., Walker, P. S., Beddingfield, F. C., Philip, A., Davis, P. G., & Yalamanchili, R. (2014). An interrater and intrarater reliability study of 3 photographic scales for the classification of perioral aesthetic features. *Dermatologic Surgery, 40*(6), 663–670. https://doi.org/10.1111/dsu.0000000000000008.

Ibrahim, O., Ionta, S., Depina, J., Petrell, K., Arndt, K. A., & Dover, J. S. (2019). Safety of laser-assisted delivery of topical poly-L-lactic acid in the treatment of upper lip rhytides: A prospective, rater-blinded study. *Dermatologic Surgery, 45*(7), 968–974. https://doi.org/10.1097/DSS.0000000000001743.

Jansen, D. A., & Graivier, M. H. (2006). Evaluation of a calcium hydroxylapatite-based implant (Radiesse) for facial soft-tissue augmentation. *Plastic and Reconstructive Surgery, 118*(3 suppl), 22S–30S. discussion 31S–33S https://doi.org/10.1097/01.prs.0000234903.55310.6a.

Keni, S. P., & Sidle, D. M. (2007). Sculptra (injectable poly-L-lactic acid). *Facial Plastic Surgery Clinics of North America, 15*(1), 91–97. vii https://doi.org/10.1016/j.fsc.2006.10.005.

Lemperle, G., Holmes, R., Cohen, S., & Lemperle, S. (2001). A classification of facial wrinkles. *Plastic and Reconstructive Surgery, 108,* 1735–1750. discussion 1751 https://doi.org/10.1097/00006534-200111000-00048.

Lindsey, S., Rosen, A., Shagalov, D., & Weiss, E. (2019). Sex differences in perioral rhytides—does facial hair play a role? *Dermatologic Surgery, 45*(2), 320–323. https://doi.org/10.1097/DSS.0000000000001586.

Lorenc, Z. P., Greene, T., & Gottschalk, R. W. (2016). Injectable Poly-L-lactic acid: Understanding its use in the current era. *Journal of Drugs in Dermatology, 15*(6), 759–762.

Narurkar, V., Shamban, A., Sissins, P., Stonehouse, A., & Gallagher, C. (2015). Facial treatment preferences in aesthetically aware women. *Dermatologic Surgery, 41*(suppl 1), S153–S160. https://doi.org/10.1097/DSS.0000000000000293.

Ogilvie, P., Thulesen, J., Leys, C., Sykianakis, D., Chantrey, J., Safa, M., et al. (2020). Expert consensus on injection technique and area-specific recommendations for the hyaluronic acid dermal filler VYC-12L to treat fine cutaneous lines. *Clinical Cosmetic and Investigational Dermatology, 13,* 267–274. https://doi.org/10.2147/CCID.S239667.

Paes, E. C., Teepen, H. J., Koop, W. A., & Kon, M. (2009). Perioral wrinkles: Histologic differences between men and women. *Aesthetic Surgery Journal, 29*(6), 467–472. https://doi.org/10.1016/j.asj.2009.08.018.

Penna, V., Stark, G. B., Voigt, M., Mehlhorn, A., & Iblher, N. (2015). Classification of the aging lips: A foundation for an integrated approach to perioral rejuvenation. *Aesthetic Plastic Surgery, 39*(1), 1–7. https://doi.org/10.1007/s00266-014-0415-2.

Philipp-Dormston, W. G., Goodman, G. J., De Boulle, K., Swift, A., Delorenzi, C., Jones, D., Heydenrych, I., Trindade De Almeida, A., & Batniji, R. K. (2020). Global approaches to the prevention and management of delayed-onset adverse reactions with hyaluronic acid-based fillers. *Plastic and Reconstructive Surgery–Global Open, 8*(4), e2730. https://doi.org/10.1097/GOX.0000000000002730.

Sadeghpour, M., Quatrano, N. A., Bonati, L. M., Arndt, K. A., Dover, J. S., & Kaminer, M. S. (2019). Delayed-onset nodules to differentially crosslinked hyaluronic acids: Comparative incidence and risk assessment. *Dermatologic Surgery, 45*(8), 1085–1094. https://doi.org/10.1097/DSS.0000000000001814.

Taylor, S. C., Downie, J. B., Shamban, A., Few, J., Weichman, B. M., Schumacher, A., et al. (2019). Lip and perioral enhancement with hyaluronic acid dermal fillers in individuals with skin of color. *Dermatologic Surgery, 45*(7), 959–967. https://doi.org/10.1097/DSS.0000000000001842.

27

Soft Tissue Augmentation of the Hands

Nisrine Kawa, Nada Soueidan, and Heidi A. Waldorf

SUMMARY AND KEY FEATURES

- Aging of the hands is characterized by superficial changes as well as volume loss and prominence of underlying structures.
- Restoration of volume by means of autologous fat transfer or filler material has proven to be a safe and effective rejuvenation strategy.
- The most common fillers for the hands are calcium hydroxyapatite, hyaluronic acid, and autologous fat.
- Poly-L-lactic acid has fallen out of favor for hand augmentation because of the risk of visible nodules under lax skin.
- Use of disposable blunt-tipped cannulas has improved the ease and reduced the side effect profile for hand filling.
- Following the procedure, patients should be instructed to ice, elevate, and massage the hand.
- While soft tissue augmentation is a good option for hand rejuvenation, combination therapies, such as lasers, radiofrequency, microneedling, and platelet-rich plasma, may be synergistic and improve outcomes.

INTRODUCTION

Aging of the hand becomes appreciable as of the fourth decade of life. Following chronic exposure to ultraviolet radiation, pollutants, irritants, and mechanical stress, hands are subject to visible senescence. Superficial damage including discoloration, textural variation, and the development of neoplastic lesions is often seen. Aging of the hand involves changes to underlying structures as well. The process is characterized by loss of subcutaneous fat and increased visibility of bones, tendons, and veins. In certain diseased states, aberrant microcirculation may be an exacerbating factor.

Rejuvenation treatments for the hands have become increasingly popular. In one study on first impressions, evaluators rated images of hands that underwent soft tissue augmentation. Perception scores for social skills, academic performance, and various areas of success were significantly higher for images of treated hands in comparison to untreated ones. Blinded evaluations by experts and patients alike report the degree of volume loss and vessel prominence as major indicators of aged hands. While a number of topical and device-based therapies can target superficial damage, soft tissue augmentation is the treatment of choice for restoration of volume and reduction of laxity. A variety of grading scales such as the 5-point photonumeric grading scale, the Global Aesthetic Improvement Scale, and the Merz Grading Scale were developed to evaluate the degree of volume loss and improvement in hand rejuvenation following soft tissue augmentation. Interventions must account for local anatomical structures and mobility of the hand, in addition to safety, durability, and tolerability of injected products. Several materials have been used for this purpose, each demonstrating variable levels of success. This chapter will discuss the techniques and outcomes of different modalities, touching upon risks and benefits of each option.

SOFT TISSUE AUGMENTATION OF THE HANDS

Anatomical Considerations

Beneath the epidermal and dermal skin barrier, the dorsum of the hand is made up of three dorsal laminae, separated by fascial planes. The most superficial layer is devoid of structures and has variable fat content. In cadaveric models, higher fat volume in the superficial lamina was associated with higher body mass index. Several septal adhesions may be found within the superficial lamina and may contribute to the uneven or lumpy appearance of injected material. During tissue augmentation procedures, disruption of perforating arteries within these septal adhesions can result in bruising. Deep to the dorsal superficial fascia lies the intermediate lamina, where veins and sensory nerves are located. The extensor tendons of the hand are found deeper still, within the deep dorsal lamina. Thorough evaluation of the degree of volume loss, coupled with understanding of anatomical structures, allows injectors to adequately plan and perform volume augmentation procedures.

Preparation

Prior to proceeding with any intervention, the provider must assess the degree of volume loss, presence of concomitant superficial damage and discuss expected outcomes. Patients must be aware of the estimated longevity of each treatment modality and understand the potential associated adverse events, including possible downtime. Combination of treatment modalities may also be discussed for optimization of results. Additional procedures should be tailored to patient needs.

Some providers begin the treatment process with 30 to 40 minutes of topical anesthetic. Others forgo this step given the presence of anesthetic in the injectable products and because mild edema may ensue, leading to potential undertreatment. Before the procedure, thorough cleaning of the hands is necessary. Patients should start by washing their hands with soap and water. Next, the injector should clean the area up to and including the wrist with antiseptic. One author (NS) follows a two-step process, starting with betadine, then wiping with alcohol swabs. Another (HAW) prepares the skin first with alcohol and then stabilized hypochlorous acid 0.009%. Hands are placed in a neutral position, for example, on a drape-covered mayo stand or a firm pillow, and patients are asked to avoid making a fist or straining. For detailed procedure preparation and implementation, please refer to videos 27.1, 27.2 and 27.3.

Fat Grafting

Since its initial use in the 1980s, tissue augmentation of the hands through autologous fat transfer has evolved significantly. A variety of harvesting, processing, storage, and transplant recommendations exist. Irrespective of the preferred harvesting method, maintenance of sterility is imperative. While some methods encourage centrifugation to reduce chances of contamination, others note that this step results in damage to the fat cells, reducing viability.

Exposure of fat tissue to air for longer than 15 minutes resulted in cell lysis of more than 50% of collected sample. Similarly, use of high-pressure during injection resulted in lipocyte crushing. Overall, transplantation of samples with lysed fat cells led to suboptimal outcomes. Small-scale blinded evaluations also compared the results of hand augmentation using freshly harvested fat to previously frozen fat. During the 5- to 7-month follow-up period, results of hands injected with the frozen fat appeared to be equivalent or even better than their fresh fat counterparts, despite the potential for fat cell death at low temperatures. Comparative standards included aesthetic preference, prominence of veins, and depth of metacarpal space.

Early injection techniques described by Fournier relied on bulk deposition of collected fat into the dorsum of the hand. Digital manipulation followed, to spread transplanted fat evenly throughout the area. Coleman attempted to refine this method by using a 16-gauge sharp needle to inject multiple lumps to be dispersed in a similar fashion. Disappointing results led to abandonment of these methods. Instead, Coleman developed a novel "structural fat grafting" strategy that made use of a cannula inserted through 1- to 2-mm incisions. Sequential passes are used to deposit 0.02 to 0.1 mL aliquots, creating a projected plane. From a retention perspective, a study by Carpenela demonstrated that fat cylinders with diameters less than 3 mm produce optimal outcomes. This is due to tissue nutrients' ability to penetrate a mere 1.5 mm within the transplanted site.

Reported longevity of treatment is highly variable and depends on several factors including anesthesia type, donor site, and harvesting and processing techniques. While some sources claim maintenance of results beyond 1 year, others note that a third of injected volume is lost 6 months after treatment. Resorption of 30% to 70% is expected; however, smaller cylinders of deposited fat may minimize this loss. Overall, autologous fat transfer is a safe and viable option for patients seeking simultaneous fat reduction from a donor site. Nevertheless, touch-ups may be necessary to preserve aesthetic appearance in the long run.

Calcium Hydroxyapatite

Calcium hydroxyapatite (CaHA) filler (Radiesse, Merz Aesthetics) is a non-permanent injectable agent consisting of collagenesis-inducing microspheres (30%) suspended in gel (70%). This material was originally US Food and Drug Administration (FDA) approved for soft tissue augmentation of the face, first for HIV lipoatrophy and then for aesthetic use. In addition to its utility as a long-lasting biostimulatory filler, CaHA was an appealing choice for treatment of volume loss of the hands given its opacity and white color, which allows successful camouflaging of vessels and avoids the risk of the Tyndall effect present with hyaluronic acid (HA) gel fillers. The product was used off-label for this purpose, but its viscosity and propensity for causing pain led injectors to seek modification strategies such as preoperative injection of lidocaine.

In 2007, Busso and Applebaum described a novel dilution technique that improved product texture and reduced procedural pain. By homogenizing the then standard 1.3-cc syringe of Radiesse (the product now comes as a 1.5-cc syringe) with 0.5 cc of 2% lidocaine without epinephrine, the mixture became more malleable and the injection more tolerable. The mixing process was facilitated by use of Luer-Lock to Luer-Lock connectors. Since then, additional studies have been conducted to optimize dilution ratios. Marmur et al. describe a combination of 2.0 mL of 2% lidocaine without epinephrine per 1.3 mL syringe of CaHA as a successful option. Overall, the degree of dilution is up to the injector's discretion. Although dilution may reduce the potential for volumization due to gel dispersion, the reduction in pain, postinjection edema, and the potential for an uneven surface has made it standard of care. Greater than 1:1 dilutions (so-called "hyperdilute" CaHA) may be chosen when the primary goal is improvement in skin quality rather than tissue augmentation.

PEARL 1 Using 3 mL or greater Luer-Lock syringes allows for easier and more complete product homogenization by reducing high extrusion pressure and increasing the space available for CaHA and diluent to mix.

PEARL 2 Prime the Luer-Lock connector with diluent by pushing the plunger until the diluent fills the connector prior to connecting to the CaHA syringe to avoid incorporating air into the mixture.

PEARL 3 During homogenization, start by injecting the CaHA into the diluent. A total of 10 "passes" of product and diluent between syringes should suffice for adequate mixing. For greater dilutions, the original 1.5-mL CaHA syringe may be substituted for a 3-mL syringe or greater during mixing.

PEARL 4 Mix 1:1 or 1.5:1.0 dilution of CaHA with 1% or 2% lidocaine without epinephrine alone or in combination with saline. (HAW recommends 0.3 cc of 1% lidocaine without epinephrine plus 1.2 cc saline as diluent for a 1:1 dilution.) Saline alone may be used to prepare CaHA premixed with lidocaine (Radiesse (+) Merz Aesthetics.)

PEARL 5 In cases of severe volume loss, less dilution may be warranted and 2.6:1.0 dilution of CaHA with 1% or 2% lidocaine without epinephrine with or without saline can be used. (NS recommendation)

PEARL 6 Splitting the expected treatment into two sessions separated by 2 to 4 weeks, rather than injecting to optimal fullness in one, can significantly reduce posttreatment edema and discomfort. (HAW recommendation)

Different injection techniques have been described in the literature. A study by Figueredo et al. compared the outcomes of injecting 3 mL of diluted CaHA in deep fat lamina and in subdermal space. For the "tenting technique," a 27-gauge needle was used to inject eight boluses into the intermetacarpal deep fat tissue, below the veins. In contrast, a cannula was used for injection within the superficial lamina, above the veins. Evaluation was based on both subjective grading scales (Merz hand grading scale and Global Aesthetic Improvement Scale) and objective measurements (skin viscoelasticity, biopsy, and ultrasonography). All parameters showed significant improvement with both injection techniques with slightly greater satisfaction noted in the subdermal group. No difference was noted in pain or incidence of adverse events.

Following a pivotal study with 113 patients, CaHA received specific FDA approval for hand rejuvenation in 2015, making it the first filler with that indication in the United States. That on-label use describes blending the CaHA with 0.3 cc of 1% lidocaine without epinephrine injected as small boluses utilizing a 25-gauge needle. In current practice, it is more frequently prepared utilizing higher dilutions and injected through a 22- or 25-gauge, 1.5- or 2.0-inch disposable cannula. Both proximal and distal entry sites have been shown to be safe and effective with minimal if any risk of bruising.

Multinational studies have demonstrated a high degree of patient and physician satisfaction with results of CaHA for soft tissue augmentation of the hands. Despite significant improvements in tolerability associated with the dilution technique, adverse events may still occur. According to the FDA report, swelling, pain, redness, and bruising are the most common complaints, reported by over 70% of study participants. These adverse events were usually self-limited and generally lasted less than 2 weeks. Use of icepacks and massage is often recommended post treatment. In some instances, prescription of short-course oral corticosteroids may be warranted if edema persists or the patient reports difficulty performing activities. A double-blind sham-controlled split-hand trial conducted by Wu et al. tested the potential reduction of side effects with triamcinolone injection following the use of CaHA. In this study, 5 mL triamcinolone acetate was injected at multiple sites immediately after tissue augmentation with 1:1 saline diluted CaHA. Control groups received an equivalent volume of saline injection post procedure. Short term follow-up over a 2-week period demonstrated significant reduction in patient-reported swelling in the triamcinolone group. A trend toward reduction in other adverse events was also noted. In the long run, treatment efficacy was not compromised in the triamcinolone group.

Generally, injecting small boluses of 0.2 to 0.5 mL with a maximum injected volume of 3 mL per hand helps prevent incidence of significant swelling and makes the addition of triamcinolone unnecessary. Planning the procedure in stages at 2- to 4-week intervals is an option as well (ie using one 1.5-mL predilution syringe CaHA per visit split between two hands). Overcorrection is unnecessary as 1:1 implant to defect correction is recommended. Correction can be anticipated to last 9 to 12 months, with residual CaHA potentially lasting up to 72 weeks. Due to the biostimulatory effect of CaHA, longer-term benefit in skin quality may be seen.

Hyaluronic Acid

HA fillers are extremely popular in the cosmetic field. Available products display a range of concentrations, molecular weights, degrees of cross linking, and gel particle size, allowing versatility in use. High biocompatibility and the ability to rapidly dissolve the product with hyaluronidase make HA a highly useful tool for tissue augmentation. Early comparisons to human collagen fillers demonstrated the superiority of HA for soft tissue augmentation of the hands. Nevertheless, it was less utilized in hand rejuvenation due to the need for follow-up treatment and potential for clear gels to produce a Tyndall effect (blue hue to the skin due to the optics of a subcutaneous clear gel). In a study comparing the outcomes of HA to those of CaHA hand rejuvenation treatments, the former was found to cause less adverse events while the latter required less follow-up treatment.

In a multicenter split-hand study, large-gel particle HA with lidocaine was used for improvement in the Merz Hand Grading Scale. Total injection volumes varied from 1 to 5 mL depending on the degree of volume loss in the treated areas. Of the 89 participants enrolled, 74 required touch-up treatments at 4 weeks. At 12 weeks, participant satisfaction questionnaires indicated that 84.5% of participants would recommend treatment to a friend, and 77.4% would undergo repeat treatment in the future. Both patients and investigators demonstrated a high degree of satisfaction, with 92.8% reporting an improvement on the Global Aesthetic Improvement Scale. Based on this study, the first HA filler achieved FDA approval for hand indication in 2018 (Restylane Lyft, Galderma). Smaller studies evaluating small-gel particle HA use also demonstrated successful outcomes, with only mild adverse events (itching, swelling) and no incidence of severe event. In practice, one author (NS) notes that outcomes are equivalent irrespective of particle size.

The injection technique for HA filler volumization of hands is similar to that used for CaHA. The product may be used as is or, off-label, diluted with lidocaine and/or saline for improved moldability. Either a disposable blunt-tipped cannula (same gauge and length as for CaHA) or needle may be used. Needle techniques include multiple microinjections, fewer small bolus injections, a single large central bolus, or linear threading. Superficial microdroplet technique utilizing skin boosting HA fillers is available outside the United States where none have yet been FDA approved. Injection method and depth differ significantly, and the outcome of interest favors hydration over volume restoration. The versatility of HA fillers makes them a useful and safe tool for hand rejuvenation. Nevertheless, injectors should be mindful of the theoretical risk of Tyndall effect given the gel's clear color. Some regularly mix HA with smaller quantities of CaHA to theoretically provide increased hydration with opacity.

Poly-L-Lactic Acid

Poly-L-lactic acid (PLLA) has been used in the medical field for a variety of applications ranging from orthopedics (pins and screws) to dermatology (treatment of lipoatrophy in HIV patients). In the cosmetic realm, PLLA is used as an FDA-approved filler for facial rejuvenation. It is thought that this biodegradable polymer induces a foreign-body reaction, leading to neocollagenesis and volumization over time. PLLA has been used off-label for soft tissue augmentation of the hands, demonstrating substantial longevity of up to 2 years. Nevertheless, suboptimal results have led injectors to favor alternative products.

In two European studies, PLLA diluted with anesthetic was used for soft tissue augmentation of the hands and treatment sessions spanned over several sessions. Posttreatment massage was completed for adequate distribution of product. At follow-up evaluations, nodule formation was noted, even 1 year post intervention. Higher dilutions of water and lidocaine have also been attempted. While this modification resulted in reduced nodule formation, "unevenness" was still reported. Given the anatomic considerations of the hand, opting for greater injection depth may not be feasible.

> **PEARL 7** Combine multiple modalities, such as lasers, peels, and fillers, to get improved and sustained results in the aging hand.

COMBINATION THERAPIES

As with any cosmetic treatment, a holistic approach is highly recommended. While volume restoration through soft tissue augmentation provides substantial improvement in appearance, combination treatments can provide even greater outcomes and prolonged effects.

As chronically exposed parts of the body, the hands are subject to photoaging, and complementary treatments should address dyschromia, lentigines, and textural changes.

First and foremost, diligent sun protection must be incorporated into any treatment plan, especially for patients who perform regular outdoor activities. Mild pigmentary alterations may be addressed with light chemical peels while lentigines will benefit from laser ablation. Both nonablative and fractional modalities are effective for hand rejuvenation, with the latter providing additional textural improvement. For laxity reduction, radiofrequency devices such as Thermage can be used. It is also noted that treatments aimed at vein reduction become unnecessary when tissue augmentation is performed.

Several literature reviews and reports of personal experiences demonstrate successful treatments for hand rejuvenation. One study reported successful outcomes with combined soft tissue augmentation (CaHA), fractional resurfacing, and radiofrequency treatments, demonstrating no loss in efficacy of volumization. Providers clearly have a large armamentarium of options; however, there are insufficient studies assessing the sequence or strategic combination for optimal results.

FURTHER READING

Aboudib, J. H., de Castro, C. C., & Gradel, J. (1992). Hand rejuvenescence by fat filling. *Annals of Plastic Surgery*, *28*(6), 559–564. https://doi.org/10.1055/s-0039-1700960.

Abrams, H. L., & Lauber, J. S. (1990). Hand rejuvenation: The state of the art. *Dermatologic Clinics*, *8*(3), 553–561. https://doi.org/10.1016/S0733-8635(18)30486-8.

Bains, R. D., Thorpe, H., & Southern, S. (2006). Hand aging: Patients opinions. *Plastic and Reconstructive Surgery*, *117*(7), 2212–2218. https://doi.org/10.1097/01.prs.0000218712.66333.97.

Bank, D. E. (2009). A novel approach to treatment of the aging hand with Radiesse. *Journal of Drugs in Dermatology*, *8*(12), 1122–1126.

Bertucci, V., Solish, N., Wong, M., & Howell, M. (2015). Evaluation of the Merz Hand Grading Scale after calcium hydroxylapatite hand treatment. *Dermatologic Surgery*, *41*(suppl 1), S389–S396. https://doi.org/10.1097/DSS.0000000000000546.

Busso, M., & Applebaum, D. (2007). Hand augmentation with Radiesse (calcium hydroxylapatite). *Dermatologic Therapy*, *20*(6), 385–387. https://doi.org/10.1111/j.1529-8019.2007.00153.x.

Busso, M., Moers-Carpi, M., Storck, R., Ogilvie, P., & Ogilvie, A. (2010). Multicenter, randomized trial assessing the effectiveness and safety of calcium hydroxylapatite for hand rejuvenation. *Dermatologic Surgery*, *36*(s1), 790–797. https://doi.org/10.1111/j.1524-4725.2010.01568.x.

Bidic, S. M., Hatef, D. A., & Rohrich, R. J. (2010). Dorsal hand anatomy relevant to volumetric rejuvenation. *Plastic and Reconstructive Surgery*, *126*(1), 163–168. https://doi.org/10.1097/PRS.0b013e3181da86ee.

Butterwick, K. J. (2002). Lipoaugmentation for aging hands: A comparison of the longevity and aesthetic results of centrifuged versus noncentrifuged fat. *Dermatologic Surgery*, *28*(11), 987–991.

Butterwick, K. J. (2005). Rejuvenation of the aging hand. *Dermatologic Clinics*, *23*, 515–527. https://doi.org/10.1016/j.det.2005.04.007.

Butterwick, K. J., Bevin, A. A., & Iyer, S. (2006). Fat transplantation using fresh versus frozen fat: A side-by-side two-hand comparison pilot study. *Dermatologic Surgery*, *32*(5), 640–644. https://doi.org/10.1111/j.1524-4725.2006.32135.x.

Carruthers, A., Carruthers, J., Hardas, B., et al. (2008). A validated hand grading scale. *Dermatologic Surgery*, *34*, S179–S183. https://doi.org/10.1111/j.1524-4725.2008.34368.x.

Cohen, J. L., Dayan, S. H., Brandt, F. S., et al. (2013). Systematic review of clinical trials of small- and large-gel-particle hyaluronic acid injectable fillers for aesthetic soft tissue augmentation. *Dermatologic Surgery*, *39*(2), 205–231. https://doi.org/10.1111/dsu.12036.

Coleman, S. R. (2002). Hand rejuvenation with structural fat grafting. *Plastic and Reconstructive Surgery*, *110*(7), 1731–1744. https://doi.org/10.1097/01.PRS.0000033936.43357.08. discussion 1745–1747.

Dayan, S. H., Arkins, J. P., & Gal, T. J. (2010). Blinded evaluation of the effects of hyaluronic acid filler injections on first impressions. *Dermatologic Surgery*, *36*(3), 1866–1873. https://doi.org/10.1111/j.1524-4725.2010.01737.x.

Edelson, K. L. (2009). Hand recontouring with calcium hydroxylapatite (Radiesse). *Journal of Cosmetic Dermatology*, *8*(1), 44–51. https://doi.org/10.1111/j.1473-2165.2009.00423.x.

Fabi, S. G., & Goldman, M. P. (2012). Hand rejuvenation: A review and our experience. *Dermatologic Surgery*, *38*(7), 1112–1127. https://doi.org/10.1111/j.1524-4725.2011.02291.x.

Figueredo, V. O., Miot, H. A., Dias, J. S., Nunes, G. J., de Souza, M. B., & Bagatin, E. (2020). Efficacy and safety of 2 injection techniques for hand biostimulatory treatment with diluted calcium hydroxylapatite. *Dermatologic Surgery*, *46*(suppl 1), S54–S61. https://doi.org/10.1097/DSS.0000000000002334.

Fournier, P. F. (2009). Fat transfer to the hand for rejuvenation. *Autologous Fat Transfer*, *26*, 273–280. https://doi.org/10.1007/978-3-642-00473-5_35.

Giunta, R. E., Eder, M., Machens, H. G., Muller, D. F., & Kovacs, L. (2010). Structural fat grafting for rejuvenation of the dorsum of the hand. *Handchirurgie, Mikrochirurgie, Plastische Chirurgie*, *42*(2), 143–147. https://doi.org/10.1055/s-0030-1249039.

Goldman, M. P., Moradi, A., Gold, M. H., et al. (2018). Calcium hydroxylapatite dermal filler for treatment of dorsal hand volume loss: Results from a 12-month, multicenter, randomized, blinded trial. *Dermatologic Surgery*, *44*(1), 75–83. https://doi.org/10.1097/DSS.0000000000001203.

Graivier, M. H., Lorenc, Z. P., Bass, L. M., Fitzgerald, R., & Goldberg, D. J. (2018). Calcium hydroxyapatite (CaHA) indication for hand rejuvenation. *Aesthetic Surgery Journal*, *38*(suppl 1), S24–S28. https://doi.org/10.1093/asj/sjy013.

Gubanova, E. I., & Starovatova, P. A. (2015). A prospective, comparative, evaluator-blind clinical study investigating efficacy and safety of two injection techniques with Radiesse® for the correction of skin changes in aging hands. *Journal of Cutaneous and Aesthetic Surgery*, *8*(3), 147–152. https://doi.org/10.4103/0974-2077.167271.

Gutowski, K. A. (2009). Current applications and safety of autologous fat grafts: A report of the ASPS fat graft task force. *Plastic and Reconstructive Surgery*, *124*(1), 272–280. https://doi.org/10.1097/PRS.0b013e3181a09506.

Haq, S., Storck, R., Martine, B., et al. (2010). Multinational, multipatient study of calcium hydroxylapatite for treatment of the aging hand: European Cosmetic Physician Group on Hand Augmentation. *Dermatologic Surgery*, *36*(s1), 782–789. https://doi.org/10.1111/j.1524-4725.2010.01548.x.

Hartmann, V., Bachmann, F., Plaschke, M., Gottermeier, T., Nast, A., & Berthold, R. (2010). Hand augmentation with stabilized hyaluronic acid (Macrolane VRF20 and Restylane Vital, Restylane Vital Light). *Journal der Deutschen Dermatologischen Gesellschaft*, *8*(1), 41–44. https://doi.org/10.1111/j.1610-0387.2009.07271.x.

Jakubietz, R. G., Kloss, D. F., Gruenert, J. G., & Jakubietz, M. G. (2008). The ageing hand. A study to evaluate the chronological ageing process of the hand. *Journal of Plastic, Reconstructive & Aesthetic Surgery*, *61*(6), 681–686. https://doi.org/10.1016/j.bjps.2007.12.028.

Kühne, U., & Matthias, I. (2012). Treatment of the ageing hand with dermal fillers. *Journal of Cutaneous and Aesthetic Surgery*, *5*(3), 163. https://doi.org/10.4103/0974-2077.101369.

Lefebvre-Vilardebo, M., Trevidic, P., Moradi, A., Busso, M., Sutton, A. B., & Bucay, V. W. (2015). Hand: Clinical anatomy and regional approaches with injectable fillers. *Plastic and Reconstructive Surgery*, *136*(5 suppl). https://doi.org/10.1097/PRS.0000000000001828.

Man, J., Rao, J., & Goldman, M. (2008). A double-blind, comparative study of nonanimal-stabilized hyaluronic acid versus human collagen for tissue augmentation of the dorsal hands. *Dermatologic Surgery*, *34*(8), 1026–1031. https://doi.org/10.1111/j.1524-4725.2008.34201.x.

Marmur, E. S., Al Quran, H., De Sa Earp, A. P., & Yoo, J. P. (2009). A five-patient satisfaction pilot study of calcium hydroxylapatite injection for treatment of aging hands. *Dermatologic Surgery*, *35*(12), 1978–1984.

Moradi, A., Allen, S., Bank, D., et al. (2019). A prospective, multicenter, randomized, evaluator-blinded, split-hand study to evaluate the effectiveness and safety of large-gel particle hyaluronic acid with lidocaine for the correction of volume deficits in the dorsal hand. *Journal of the American Academy of Dermatology*, *81*(4), 586–596. https://doi.org/10.1097/PRS.0000000000006070.

Narurkar, V. (2014). Combination therapy of the aging hand using non-ablative fractional resurfacing radiofrequency and calcium hydroxylapatite in clinical practice. *Journal of Drugs in Dermatology*, *9*(4), s20–s22. https://doi.org/10.1111/iwj.13213.

Nikolis, A., & Enright, K. M. (2011). Evaluating the role of small particle hyaluronic acid fillers using micro-droplet technique in the face, neck and hands: A retrospective chart review. *Clinical, Cosmetic and Investigational Dermatology*, *11*, 467–475. https://doi.org/10.2147/CCID.S175408.

Pu, L. L., Coleman, S. R., Cui, X., Ferguson Jr, R. E., & Vasconez, H. C. (2008). Autologous fat grafts harvested and refined by the Coleman technique: A comparative study. *Plastic and Reconstructive Surgery*, *122*(3), 932–937. https://doi.org/10.1097/PRS.0b013e3181811ff0.

Redaelli, A. (2006). Cosmetic use of polylactic acid for hand rejuvenation: Report on 27 patients. *Journal of Cosmetic Dermatology*, *5*(3), 233–238. https://doi.org/10.1111/j.1473-2165.2006.00259.x.

Rendon, M. I., Cardona, L. M., & Pinzon-Plazas, M. (2010). Treatment of the aged hand with injectable poly-L-lactic acid. *Journal of Cosmetic and Laser Therapy*, *12*(6), 284–287. https://doi.org/10.3109/14764172.2010.538410.

Rivkin, A. (2016). Volume correction in the aging hand: Role of dermal fillers. *Clinical, Cosmetic and Investigational Dermatology*, *9*, 225–232. https://doi.org/10.2147/ccid.s92853.

Sadick, N. S. (2011). A 52-week study of safety and efficacy of calcium hydroxylapatite for rejuvenation of the aging hand. *Journal of Drugs in Dermatology*, *10*(1), 47–51.

Sadick, N. S., Anderson, D., & Werschler, W. P. (2008). Addressing volume loss in hand rejuvenation: A report of clinical experience. *Journal of Cosmetic and Laser Therapy*, *10*(4), 237–241. https://doi.org/10.1080/14764170802524429.

Sattler, G., Walker, T., Buxmeyer, B., & Blwer, B. (2014). Efficacy of calcium hydroxylapatite filler versus hyaluronic acid filler in hand augmentation. *Aktuelle Dermatologie*, *40*, 445–451. https://doi.org/10.1055/s-0034-1378110.

Shamban, T. (2009). Combination hand rejuvenation procedures. *Aesthetic Surgery Journal*, *29*(5), 409–413. https://doi.org/10.1016/j.asj.2009.08.003.

Villanueva, N. L., Hill, S. M., Small, K. H., & Rohrich, R. J. (2015). Technical refinements in autologous hand rejuvenation. *Plastic and Reconstructive Surgery*, *136*(6), 1175–1179. https://doi.org/10.1097/PRS.0000000000001762.

Vleggaar, D. (2006). Soft-tissue augmentation and the role of poly-L-lactic acid. *Plastic and Reconstructive Surgery*, *118*(3 suppl), 46S–54S. https://doi.org/10.1097/01.prs.0000234846.00139.74.

Werschler, P. B. M., & Busso, M. (2010). Prepackaged injectable soft-tissue rejuvenation of the hand and other nonfacial area. *Body Rejuvenation*, *7*, 221–225.

Wu, D. C., & Goldman, M. O. (2018). Randomized, double-blinded, sham-controlled, split-hand trial evaluating the safety and efficacy of triamcinolone acetate injection after calcium hydroxylapatite volume restoration of the dorsal hand. *Dermatologic Surgery*, *44*(4), 534–541. https://doi.org/10.1097/DSS.0000000000001325.

28

Soft Tissue Augmentation of the Neck and Chest

Kerry Heitmiller, Nazanin Saedi, and Nicole Y. Lee

SUMMARY AND KEY FEATURES

- Soft tissue fillers are increasingly being utilized for rejuvenation of the neck and décolletage to create a seamless transition from the rejuvenated face.
- Hyaluronic acid fillers are best used for improving the appearance of necklace lines on the neck.
- Biostimulatory fillers, such as hyperdilute CaHA and PLLA, improve fine lines and skin laxity of the neck and chest with minimal to no downtime.
- Optimal results are often observed when these soft tissue fillers are combined with other cosmetic treatments, including neuromodulators and laser, light, or energy-based devices.
- Hyaluronic acid fillers for improving the appearance of necklace lines.
- Biostimulatory fillers, such as hyperdilute CaHA and PLLA, for improving lines and skin laxity of the neck and chest with minimal to no downtime.

INTRODUCTION

The rising popularity of aesthetic procedures on the face has created an increase in demand for cosmetic treatments of nonfacial areas. The face, neck, and chest (décolletage) undergo similar patterns of aging with loss of collagen, an increase in skin laxity, and dyschromia that is either caused or accelerated by chronic ultraviolet (UV) exposure. As more time and money are spent on facial aesthetics, the signs of aging of the untreated adjacent skin of the neck and chest become more visually pronounced. As a result, it is equally important to address these areas to provide a seamless and uniform appearance.

Laser-based energy devices such as fractioned ablative or nonablative lasers and intense pulsed light lasers address the pigmentary changes as well as the texture. Fractional radiofrequency devices improve the quality and surface of the skin, while microfocused ultrasound devices target overall skin laxity. Neuromodulators can also be used to reduce the appearance of the platysma bands of the neck to provide a nonsurgical "liquid necklift." Fillers can be used to address individual rhytides as well as promote neocollagenesis to improve the overall texture and laxity of the skin. While there are multiple modalities for treatment, this chapter will focus on the use of soft tissue fillers in the rejuvenation of the neck and décolletage.

THE NECK

Aging of the neck manifests as cutaneous dyschromia, skin laxity, rhytides, loss of the mandibular contour, widening of the cervicomental angle, accumulation of submental fat, and volume loss. Additionally, rotational movement along with the upward contractions of the platysmal muscle results in prominent bands, horizontal rhytides, and sagging of the skin. Traditionally, transverse neck creases were associated with aging. However, there has been an increase in the number of younger patients presenting with horizontal necklines or "tech neck," thought to be related to the hours spent on the computer and phone. This has especially become more relevant with the recent COVID-19 pandemic and the increasing use of "Zoom" meetings and video conferencing. Given the multifactorial etiology of the aging neck, rejuvenation often requires the incorporation of a myriad of treatments for optimal results. However, as monotherapy, soft tissue fillers can be used successfully to address neck laxity and rhytides.

Horizontal Necklines

When evaluating a patient for treatment of horizontal necklines, it is important to determine the degree and severity as this will guide treatment. A validated scale has recently been created to assess transverse necklines with a standardized grading system and can be used during the patient evaluation. The current available treatment options include neuromodulators, soft tissue fillers, rhytidectomy, fractional laser therapy, fractional radiofrequency, and microfocused ultrasound. Soft tissue fillers can be used successfully to improve horizontal necklines, especially those that are mild to moderate in severity. The benefits of injectable fillers include immediate correction, favorable tolerability, minimal to no downtime, and low risk of adverse effects. However, moderate to severe horizontal necklines would benefit most when combining other therapeutic modalities with filler, and patients should be counseled accordingly prior to any procedure.

While studies are limited, hyaluronic acid (HA) fillers, calcium hydroxylapatite (CaHA), and poly-L-lactic acid (PLLA) have been shown to provide favorable outcomes in the treatment of horizontal necklines. Typically, fillers with a lower viscosity and greater cohesivity are utilized for this purpose due to the thinner quality of the skin on the neck. These products demonstrate a more seamless integration into the skin and can be placed superficially with less risk for nodule formation. However, nodules can still occur. As a result, it is important to inject filler as small aliquots and evenly into the subdermal plane in order to prevent a nodular appearance to the corrected necklines.

Most of the current studies have demonstrated the efficacy of cohesive polydensified matrix HA filler (Belotero Balance) and small particle HA filler (Restylane Vital or Restylane Silk) for the treatment of transverse necklines, with significant improvement noted at follow-up compared to baseline. Recently, Minokadeh and colleagues reported the successful use of a Vycross technology HA filler, Juvederm Volbella, in the treatment of horizontal necklines and showed similar results when compared to Belotero Balance. Mild lumpiness was observed after injection of Juvederm Volbella, which resolved spontaneously at the 12-week follow-up. Unlike many of the prior reports, these authors utilized a cannula for injection as opposed to a needle, which they argued ensured proper placement within the subdermal space, limited the number of injections required, and decreased the risk of postinjection bruising. However, others have advocated against the use of blunt-tipped cannulas, arguing that placement within the horizontal necklines requires a high degree of precision obtained only with the use of a needle (i.e., 31-gauge, 0.3-cc syringe). Alternatively, a micropuncture or serial puncture technique with small aliquots along the length of the neckline with a 27- to 30-gauge needle can be used. Lee and Kim treated 14 patients with transverse necklines with HA fillers using either a linear threading technique or a vertical (micropuncture) technique. They observed a statistically significant greater improvement as well as patient satisfaction with the vertical technique at the 2-month follow-up. They also found that the linear threading technique was more often associated with complications (i.e., moderate skin irregularity, accentuation of neck lines) than the vertical technique. The authors argued that the micropuncture technique places the filler material in vertical columns which directly oppose the vertical depressions of the horizontal necklines, resulting in better structural support to the skin. However, given the limited sample size and variability in injector technique, further studies are needed to determine whether micropuncture is truly superior to threading. The authors of this chapter have seen clinical improvement in transverse necklines when using a cohesive polydensified matrix HA filler (Belotero Balance), diluted with 0.5 mL of 2% lidocaine without epinephrine and injected with a 25- to 27-gauge cannula using a linear threading technique.

Recently, the RHA collection of HA dermal fillers made in Switzerland by Teoxane and sold in the United States by Revance (Newark, CA) and in the rest of the world by TEOXANE SA (Geneve, Switzerland) were introduced onto the market. They are the first and only HA fillers approved by the US Food and Drug Administration (FDA) for dynamic wrinkles and folds. These include RHA-2, RHA-3, and RHA-4. This unique line of HA fillers is made of products with longer HA chains, a lower degree of chemical modifications, more preserved covalent bonds, and less 1,4-butanediol diglycidyl ether (BDDE) bonds required for stabilization. Therefore, these products are more flexible, less rigid, and more closely resemble naturally occurring HA in the skin. The products contain the same concentration of HA (23 mg/mL) but each product differs in the degree of cross-linking, with RHA-2 having the lowest degree of cross-linking (3.1%) and RHA-4 having the highest (4.0%). The degree of cross-linking correlates with the strength and lift capacity of the filler. RHA-2 and RHA-3 are indicated for injection into the mid to deep dermis for correction of moderate to severe dynamic facial wrinkles and folds, and RHA-4 is indicated for injection into the deep dermis to superficial subcutaneous tissue for the correction of significant dynamic facial wrinkles and folds such as the nasolabial folds. While there are currently no formal studies on the use of RHA-2 or RHA-3 for horizontal necklines, anecdotal reports of this off-label use have described successful outcomes. However, formal studies are needed to better characterize the safety and efficacy of RHA filler products for the treatment of horizontal necklines.

CaHA (Radiesse, Merz aesthetics, Frankfurt, Germany) is a long-lasting, biodegradable filler composed of 30% CaHA microspheres suspended in a sodium carboxymethylcellulose gel carrier and will be discussed in further detail in the next section. There has only been one report describing the use of CaHA for horizontal necklines. Chao and colleagues treated a patient with CaHA in a 1:1 dilution using a 27-gauge needle, placing the product at the dermal-subdermal junction with serial puncture in a linear threading pattern around the neck. Improvement of the necklines was appreciated within 7 days and was sustained at the 16-week follow-up. The procedure was well tolerated with prominent swelling and bruising immediately after injection that resolved within 7 days of treatment. The authors argued that this product is optimal for patients without excessive drooping of neck fat or platysmal banding. This product may also have the added benefit of promoting neocollagenesis in addition to the direct fill, which may lead to continued improvement over time. Although CaHA has greater viscoelastic properties, proper dilution and injection technique with placement of the product into the subdermal space is paramount to prevent complications such as nodule formation.

Neck Laxity and Tightening

In addition to discrete horizontal rhytides in the neck, neck skin laxity can also be successfully treated with soft tissue fillers that possess biostimulatory capabilities such as CaHA and PLLA. CaHA is currently FDA approved for moderate to severe facial wrinkles, HIV-associated facial lipoatrophy, and dorsal hand augmentation. However, recently, dilute (1:1) and hyperdilute (> 1:2) formulations of CaHA have been used off-label for skin tightening and rejuvenation of nonfacial sites, including the neck, chest, arms, abdomen, thighs, and buttocks. After injection into the skin, immediate fill and lift are seen at the time of injection from the gel carrier, which then decreases over several weeks, leaving the CaHA microspheres at the site of injection. The CaHA microspheres subsequently stimulate a subclinical, inflammatory, host response acting as a scaffold for fibroplasia and new collagen and elastin formation, translating into sustained aesthetic improvements. Given its highly viscoelastic properties, CaHA is well suited for supraperiosteal, subdermal, and deep-dermal placement, especially when used for volume augmentation. CaHA, however, can be injected more superficially for dermal rejuvenation when diluted, as would be necessary in the neck. Lower dilution ratios provide both volume and dermal remodeling, whereas dilutions of greater than 1:1 may be better at providing biostimulation. Global consensus guidelines on the use of hyperdilute and dilute CaHA for skin tightening have recently been published. In the neck, hyperdilute and dilute CaHA have been shown to effectively improve skin laxity and increase dermal thickness alone and when used in combination with energy-based devices. Per the current guidelines, dilution ratios of 1:2 to 1:4 are recommended for use in the neck. However, in general, dilutions should be titrated based on skin thickness and degree of skin laxity. For dilution, bacteriostatic saline or 1% to 2% lidocaine with or without epinephrine can be used. Neuromodulators can also be added to the diluent for the added benefit of relaxing the platysmal muscle and decreasing the prominence of platysmal bands, or the neuromodulators can be injected separately. The product should be injected in the subdermal plane in a retrograde linear threading technique with a 22- to 25-gauge cannula at three to five injection points, as illustrated in Video 28.1. The short linear threading technique with a needle is an alternative option. Typically, one to two syringes per session are indicated. It is important to gently massage the treated area after injection to ensure even distribution and to prevent nodule formation. While follow-up intervals between 3 and 9 months after the initial treatment are recommended to evaluate response, more frequent follow-up at 2 to 3 months is more commonly performed. Results may be visible after one treatment, but more often, two to four treatment sessions, spaced 6 to 8 weeks apart, are required to achieve appreciable results, followed by maintenance treatments every 12 to 18 months. Patients with mild to moderate laxity and textural changes from photodamage may benefit from this treatment. Excess skin will not necessarily disappear after treatment but will become smoother in appearance as the skin tightens from neocollagenesis, as can be seen in Fig. 28.1. If needed, HA fillers can also be used in combination to soften any residual lines for optimal results.

Treatment with CaHA is typically well tolerated. Adverse effects most commonly associated with treatment are related to the injection itself, including bruising, swelling, mild pain, and induration. Edema typically resolves within 48 to 72 hours, although patients may experience delayed edema 1 week after injection that spontaneously resolves. Uncommon complications are hypersensitivity reactions, inflammatory or noninflammatory nodules, and granuloma formation. A rare xanthelasma-like reaction has also been reported following injection with CaHA, thought to be secondary to superficial placement of the product. The risk for nodule formation is associated with patient skin type and quality, injection technique, and degree of dilution. Patients with thinner and darker skin tend to be at greater risk for a lumpier appearance to the skin after treatment, as the product may be more visible after injection. Additionally, injections that are placed too

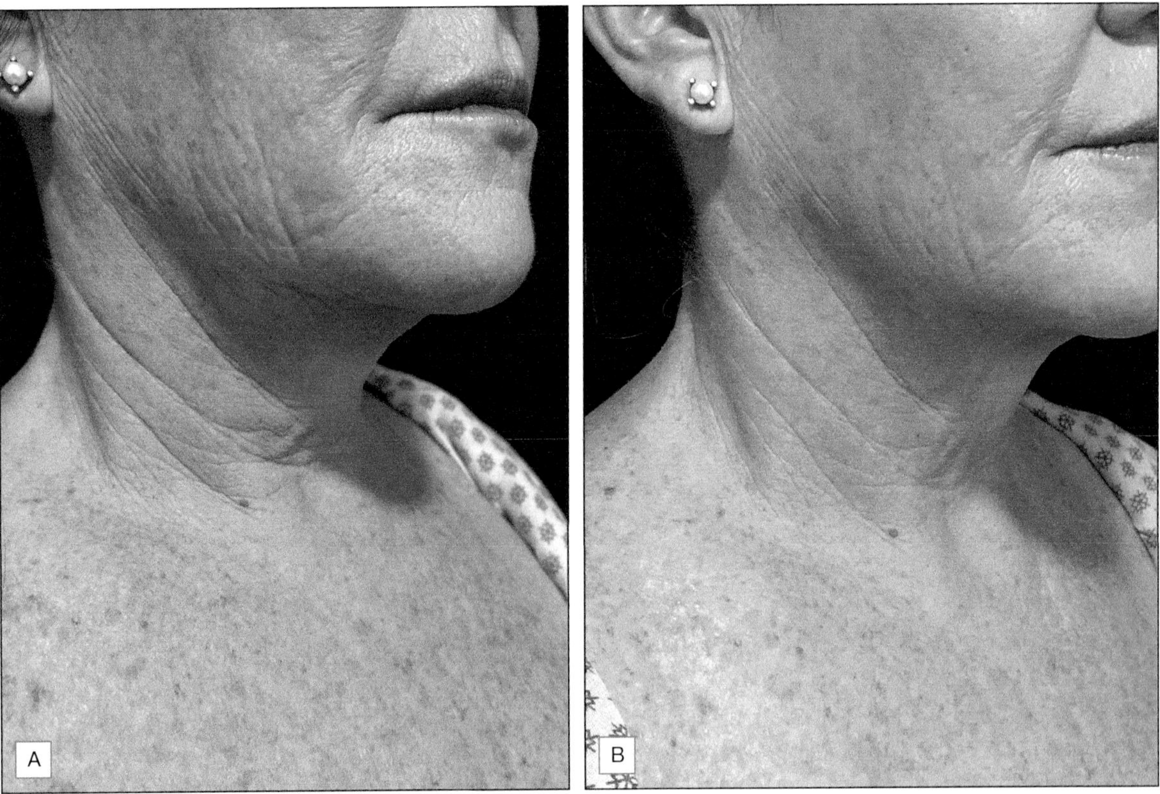

Fig. 28.1 A 62-year-old female (A) before and (B) 8 weeks after undergoing injection to the neck with two syringes of calcium hydroxylapatite with lidocaine (Radiesse) at a 1:1 dilution with 1 cc of 1% lidocaine without epinephrine and 0.5 cc of normal saline, using a 2-inch, 22-gauge cannula. (Copyrights reserved by Nicole Y Lee, MD, MPH.)

superficially and the use of less dilute CaHA increase the risk of nodule formation or a "beaded" appearance following injection. Use of a cannula may help to better ensure subdermal placement of the product. Greater dilutions help to create a less viscoelastic product that will allow for smooth and uniform placement within the thin skin of the neck. Postinjection massage can also ensure even distribution of the product. Patients can be instructed to massage the treated area twice daily for 3 to 7 days following the procedure. If nodules do develop, they can be treated with intralesional lidocaine and saline followed by vigorous massage or intralesional 5-fluorouracil, triamcinolone, or sodium thiosulfate for more recalcitrant nodules. Excision may be required for persistent nodules.

PLLA is another filler agent that has been used to successfully tighten and improve the appearance of the neck. PLLA (Sculptra, Sinclair Pharmaceuticals, Galderma Laboratories, Fort Worth, TX) is a synthetic, biodegradable polymer composed of microparticles of PLLA in a sodium carboxymethylcellulose gel. It is FDA approved for the treatment of HIV-associated facial lipoatrophy and severe wrinkles in immunocompetent individuals. However, it is being increasingly utilized off-label at higher dilutions for skin rejuvenation, volume loss, and skin tightening of the neck, chest, and other areas of the face and body. Similarly to CaHA, PLLA stimulates a host-dependent immunologic response that results in increased fibroblast activity and new collagen formation after placement into the dermal-subcutaneous junction or upper hypodermis, resulting in long-lasting cosmetic results. A limited number of studies have demonstrated the efficacy of PLLA for neck rejuvenation, and PLLA continues to be used successfully in clinical practice for this indication. However, given the paucity of data, current and standardized recommendations of PLLA for neck rejuvenation are lacking.

Based on recent consensus guidelines for neck rejuvenation, soft tissue fillers (i.e., low-viscosity HA fillers and dilute CaHA) are considered third-line agents following neuromodulators and energy-based skin tightening devices in the correction of residual, deeper neck lines, or skin laxity. However, soft tissue fillers can arguably be used as monotherapy for reducing fine wrinkling and improving skin texture of the neck with excellent cosmetic outcomes, especially in those with mild to moderate photodamage (i.e., skin atrophy, rhytides, textural changes), with a favorable risk profile.

THE CHEST (DÉCOLLETAGE)

Similar to the face and neck, the chest is susceptible to cumulative UV exposure and photodamage. Skin laxity and rhytides progressively develop on the chest from volume loss and decreased collagen due to these extrinsic factors as well intrinsic factors (i.e., aging, breast size, sleeping positions, etc.). Additionally, movement of the breasts in women often contributes to the deep, vertical cleavage lines. Contemporary women's clothing exposes the décolletage, prompting an increasing number of women to seek treatment of this area. The skin of the décolletage has a thinner epidermis and dermis compared to the face with a paucity of pilosebaceous units. Therefore, deep or ablative resurfacing treatments are associated with more adverse events as the chest heals slowly and scars easily in comparison to the face. Injectable fillers, on the other hand, offer a favorable treatment alternative as they can be used successfully for rejuvenation of the décolletage with minimal side effects and limited to no downtime.

SKIN LAXITY AND LIGHTENING

Patient evaluation and thorough counseling are paramount prior to any cosmetic treatment. Assessment of the degree of photodamage, volume loss, laxity, and wrinkles is important as this dictates the most appropriate management. Younger individuals or those with only minimal age-related changes to the décolletage may benefit simply from daily application of a broad-spectrum sunscreen and topical formulations (i.e., topical retinoids and peptides) that stimulate the production of new collagen to prevent wrinkles and improve skin tone and texture. Injectable soft tissue fillers can augment this skin care regimen for additional improvements. However, patients who present with significant photodamage, moderate to severe rhytides, and pronounced volume loss will benefit most from a multimodal approach with energy-based devices in addition to injectable fillers. It is important to discuss appropriate expectations of treatment to optimize patient satisfaction.

Injectable soft tissue fillers can be effectively used for rejuvenation of the décolletage to improve overall skin laxity and texture. Most of the current literature describes the use of biostimulatory agents such as CaHA and PLLA as being highly effective in this regard. Although HA-based filler is not typically considered first-line treatment for the chest, there are few reports demonstrating improvement of chest wrinkles and lines with HA filler. Low-viscosity HA products provide immediate correction, stimulate mild neocollagenesis, and improve cutaneous hydration, skin roughness, and elasticity. Cohen described the use of 2 to 3 mL of a nonanimal stabilized HA (NASHA) product (Restylane Vital) at a 1:4 dilution for improving chest lines. The product was injected directly with a needle using a threading technique, a mesotherapy-like approach, or a combination of the two. The procedure was well tolerated without the report of significant adverse effects. However, the clinical improvement lasted only 6 to 8 months and the authors recommended combining treatment with a laser or light-based device to optimize results. Other physicians have described the use of a monophasic polydensified HA product (Belotero Balance), or a biphasic, small particle sized HA product (Restylane Silk) diluted with 0.2 to 0.5 mL of 1% lidocaine without epinephrine with similar short-lived results. While HA fillers may provide immediate correction with a low risk profile of complications, the cosmetic benefits are not long-lasting and would require multiple treatments to maintain, which could become costly to the patient. Current consensus guidelines recommend the use of low-viscosity HA fillers via micropuncture placement of small aliquots of product throughout the treatment area for décolletage rejuvenation. It is considered a part of first-line treatment for early intervention when only mild changes, such as fine lines, wrinkles, photodamage, are present.

Injectable fillers with biostimulatory properties, such as CaHA and PLLA, are most commonly used and have consistently demonstrated improvement in the rejuvenation of the décolletage (Fig. 28.2). Similar to the neck, hyperdilute CaHA has been used off-label for the décolletage, with recommended dilutions ranging from 1:2 to 1:4. Dilutions up to 1:6 have demonstrated biostimulatory properties with an increase in collagen and elastin, although there are insufficient data to determine whether one dilution is superior to another regarding the degree of neocollagenesis. The preferred CaHA dilution for the promotion of

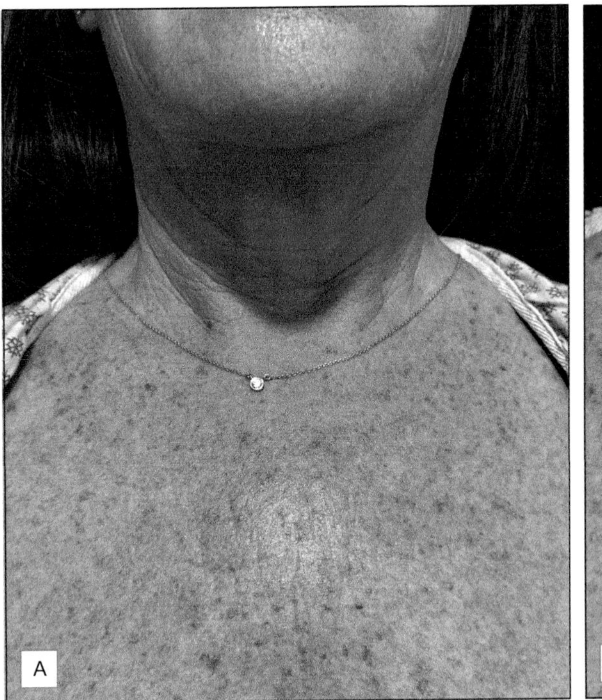

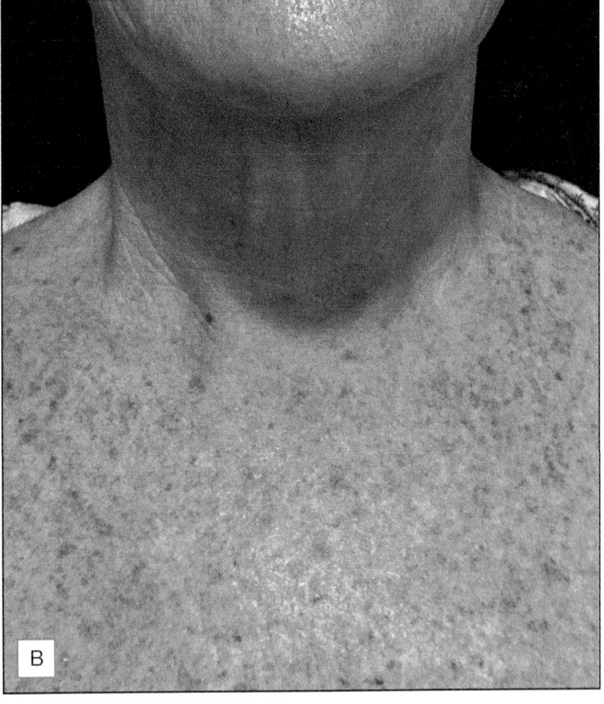

Fig. 28.2 A 62-year-old female (A) before and (B) 8 weeks after a single treatment to the chest with 3 syringes of calcium hydroxylapatite with lidocaine (Radiesse) at a 1:1 dilution with 1 cc of 1% lidocaine without epinephrine and 0.5 cc of normal saline, using a 2-inch, 22-gauge cannula. (Copyrights reserved by Nicole Y Lee, MD, MPH.)

biostimulation and skin tightening of the chest depends on the extent of skin laxity and atrophy present. Lower dilutions can be safely used in patients with thicker skin, while higher dilutions of 1:4 or more are appropriate in individuals with more extensive atrophy and laxity. It can be performed by a short linear threading technique with a needle or via a retrograde threading or fanning technique with a cannula, as is demonstrated in Video 28.2. Typically, 0.5 to 1 syringe per session is recommended, although the authors of this chapter typically use two to three syringes when treating the chest. The treatment areas should be massaged following injection to ensure even distribution of the product. Follow-up 2 to 3 months after the initial treatment to evaluate response is recommended to determine if additional treatment is needed. The authors of this chapter typically plan for one to three treatment sessions that are spaced 8 weeks apart for optimal results, followed by maintenance treatments every 12 to 18 months thereafter.

As when treating the neck, treatment with hyperdilute CaHA in the décolletage is well tolerated with a low risk of adverse effects, which include bruising, swelling, mild pain, induration, and nodule formation. However, proper injection technique, avoiding superficial injection of the product, use of appropriate dilution based on the skin thickness and degree of atrophy, and postinjection massage can help to reduce the risk of adverse events.

PLLA has consistently demonstrated improvements in the décolletage, and the current literature, while limited, supports its use. In 2009, Mazzuco and Hexel reported the first case series of the successful use of PLLA for rejuvenation of the aging neck and chest, with improvement in 81% to 100% of 21 subjects and a 92% patient satisfaction rate. Patients with mild photoaging received an average of one treatment and subjects with moderate to severe photoaging received an average of 2.38 treatments. Improvements were maintained at 18-month follow-up, with only 1 of 36 patients developing an early-onset subcutaneous nodule. Subsequent studies have demonstrated similar efficacy and safety of PLLA when injected into the décolletage for decreasing fine lines, wrinkles, and volume loss, with correction lasting up to 2 years and longer (Fig. 28.3).

Prior to use, PLLA requires reconstitution in sterile water, which is often combined with lidocaine with or without epinephrine. The manufacturer recommends use of at least 5 mL of sterile water for reconstitution 24 to 72 hours before injection. Current recommendations in the published literature describe reconstitution volumes of 5 to 10 mL. However, when treating the décolletage, larger volumes of 10 to 18 mL are recommended. Recent reviews of treatment of the aging chest describe the use of 16- to 18-mL

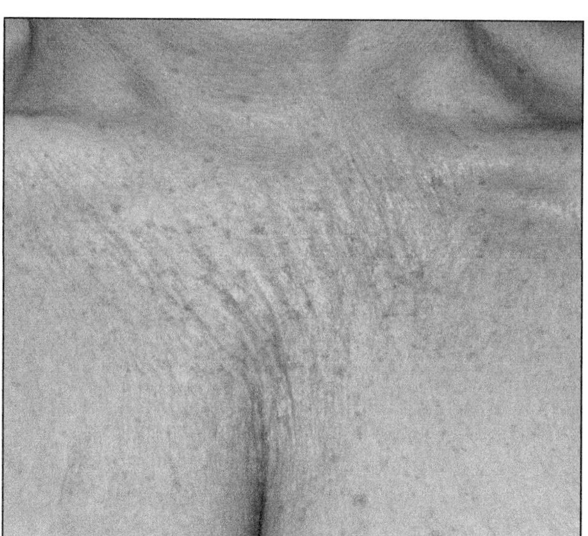

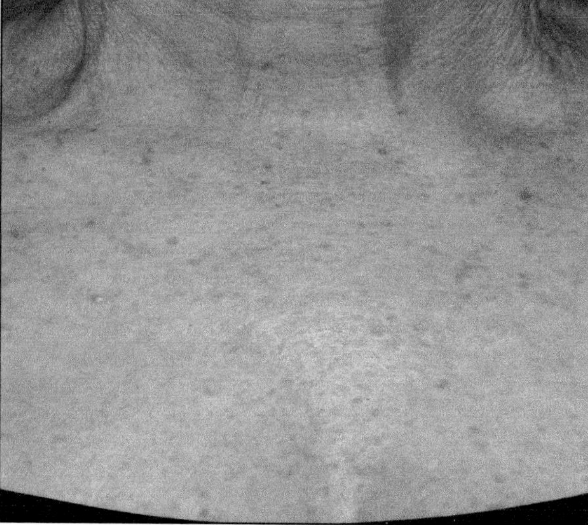

Fig. 28.3 A 49-year-old female *(left)* before and *(right)* 3 years after undergoing treatment with three vials of poly-L-lactic acid for rhytides and two intense pulsed light sessions for dyschromia.

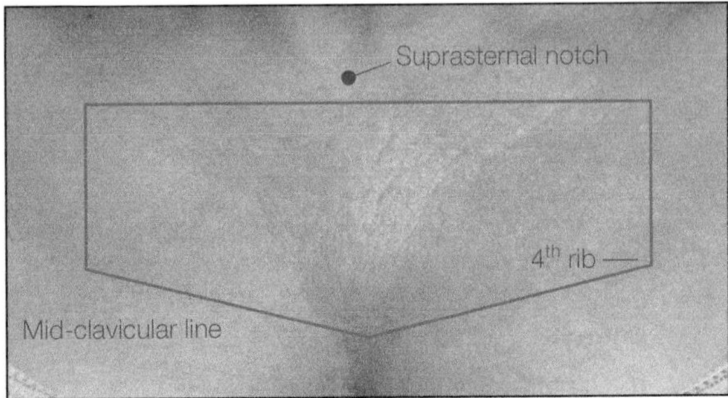

Fig. 28.4 The boundaries of the treatment area when using calcium hydroxylapatite and poly-L-lactic acid in the chest are the suprasternal notch superiorly, the midclavicular lines laterally, and the fourth rib inferiolateraly.

dilutions of PLLA. The product is evenly injected in a retrograde fanning technique into the subdermal space using a 27-gauge needle within the boundaries of the suprasternal notch superiorly, midclavicular lines laterally, and inferior sternum or 4th ribs inferiorly (Fig. 28.4). The treated area is then vigorously massaged post injection. Patients should then be instructed to massage the treated area for 5 minutes, five times a day, for 5 days after injection. Three to four treatment sessions spaced 1 month apart are recommended for optimal results.

While injection of PLLA is often well tolerated, potential adverse effects include ecchymoses, edema, pain, pruritus, hematomas, and palpable nonvisible and visible subcutaneous nodules. In particular, PLLA is known to have a relatively high incidence of subcutaneous nodule formation. In a retrospective, single-center review by Palm and colleagues, an 8.5% incidence rate of nodule formation in 130 patients treated with PLLA in facial and nonfacial sites was observed; however, no nodules developed in patients treated on the chest. Subcutaneous nodules can develop for a number of reasons, including insufficient reconstitution time of the filler material, variations in dilution and injection technique, concentration of PLLA from muscle movement, or allergic or inflammatory host responses. Patients with thinner skin may also be at greater risk of nodule formation and the use of PLLA should be avoided in these patients. Recommended techniques to decrease the risk of nodule formation with PLLA are avoidance of intradermal injection or overcorrection, use of dilutions greater than 5 mL, lengthening the time of reconstitution, separating treatment sessions at least 4 weeks apart, and postinjection massage. It is also important to instruct patients to continue massaging the treated area(s) for 5 minutes, five times a day, for 5 days after treatment (rule of "5's") to mitigate potential risk of nodule formation. Nodules that do develop often resolve spontaneously. Those that persist can be treated with intralesional 5-fluorouracil or triamcinolone. Given these potential adverse effects, it is paramount to counsel patients appropriately prior to treatment with PLLA.

Soft tissue fillers, particularly those with biostimulatory properties, successfully rejuvenate the décolletage by improving the appearance of chest lines, wrinkles, and volume loss when used as monotherapy. These biostimulatory fillers provide long-lasting effects, which make them a more favorable option than HA fillers. However, combination therapy often produces the most optimal outcomes, especially in those with more moderate to severe photodamage. Use of laser, light, or energy-based devices (i.e., nonablative modalities, radiofrequency microneedling) in combination with soft tissue fillers can lead to greater improvements in skin laxity, in addition to addressing other aspects of photoaging including dyspigmentation and telangiectasias. Therefore, it is important to discuss that, while soft tissue fillers can lead to noticeable improvement as monotherapy, the benefit may still be limited without the use of other modalities.

CONCLUSIONS

Soft tissue fillers are increasingly being utilized for rejuvenation of the neck and décolletage to create a seamless transition from the rejuvenated face. A variety of soft tissue fillers, especially those with biostimulatory capabilities, have been shown to successfully improve fine lines and wrinkles and skin laxity of the neck and chest with minimal to no downtime. While these agents have demonstrated significant success when used alone, optimal results are often observed when these soft tissue fillers are combined with other cosmetic treatments, including neuromodulators and laser, light, or energy-based devices.

FURTHER READING

Abraham, M. T., & Ross, E. V. (2005). Current concepts in nonablative radiofrequency rejuvenation of the lower face and neck. *Facial Plastic Surgery*, *21*, 65–73. https://doi.org/10.1055/s-2005-871765.

Agarwal, A., Dejoseph, L., & Silver, W. (2005). Anatomy of the jawline, neck, and perioral area with clinical correlations. *Facial Plastic Surgery*, *21*, 3–10. https://doi.org/10.1055/s-2005-871757.

Alessio, R., Rzany, B., Eve, L., Grangier, Y., et al. (2014). European expert recommendations on the use of injectable poly-L-lactic acid for facial rejuvenation. *Journal of Drugs in Dermatology*, *13*, 1057–1066.

Alexiades, M., & Berube, D. (2015). Randomized, blinded, 3-arm clinical trial assessing optimal temperature and duration for treatment with minimally invasive fractional radiofrequency. *Dermatologic Surgery*, *41*, 623–632. https://doi.org/10.1097/DSS.0000000000000347.

Apikian, M., Roberts, S., & Goodman, G. J. (2007). Adverse reactions to poly-L-lactic acid injection in the peri-orbital area. *Journal of Cosmetic Dermatology*, *6*, 95–101. https://doi.org/10.1111/j.1473-2165.2007.00303.x.

Bencini, P. L., Tourlaki, A., Galimberti, M., & Pellacani, G. (2015). Non-ablative fractionated laser skin resurfacing for the treatment of aged neck skin. *The Journal of Dermatological Treatment*, *26*, 252–256. https://doi.org/10.3109/09546634.2014.933765.

Berlin, A., Cohen, J. L., & Goldberg, D. J. (2006). Calcium hydroxylapatite for facial rejuvenation. *Seminars in Cutaneous Medicine and Surgery*, *25*, 132–137. https://doi.org/10.1016/j.sder.2006.06.005.

Berlin, A. L., Hussain, M., & Goldberg, D. J. (2008). Calcium hydroxylapatite filler for facial rejuvenation: a histologic and immunohistochemical analysis. *Dermatologic Surgery*, *34*(suppl 1), S64–S67. https://doi.org/10.1111/j.1524-4725.2008.34245.x.

Busso, M., & Voigts, R. (2008). An investigation of changes in physical properties of injectable calcium hydroxylapatite in a Carrier gel when mixed with lidocaine and with lidocaine/epinephrine. *Dermatologic Surgery*, *34*(suppl 1), S16–S23. https://doi.org/10.1111/j.1524-4725.2008.34238.x.

Casabona, G., & Teixeira, D. N. (2018). Microfocused ultrasound in combination with diluted calcium hydroxylapatite for improving skin laxity and the appearance of lines in the neck and decolletage. *Journal of Cosmetic Dermatology*, *17*, 66–72. https://doi.org/10.1111/jocd.12475.

Chao, Y. Y., Chiu, H. H., & Howell, D. J. (2011). A novel injection technique for horizontal neck lines correction using calcium hydroxylapatite. *Dermatologic Surgery*, *37*, 1542–1545. https://doi.org/10.1111/j.1524-4725.2011.02086.x.

Courderot-Masuyer, C., Robin, S., Tauzin, H., & Humbert, P. (2016). Evaluation of lifting and antiwrinkle effects of calcium hydroxylapatite filler. In vitro quantification of contractile forces of human wrinkle and normal aged fibroblasts treated with calcium hydroxylapatite. *Journal of Cosmetic Dermatology*, *15*, 260–268. https://doi.org/10.1111/jocd.12215.

Engelhard, P., Humble, G., & Mest, D. (2005). Safety of Sculptra: A review of clinical trial data. *Journal of Cosmetic and Laser Therapy*, *7*, 201–205. https://doi.org/10.1080/14764170500451404.

Fabi, S. G., Burgess, C., Carruthers, A., Day, D., Goldie, K., et al. (2016). Consensus recommendations for combined aesthetic interventions using botulinum toxin, fillers, and microfocused ultrasound in the neck, decolletage, hands and other areas of the body. *Dermatologic Surgery*, *42*, 1199–1208. https://doi.org/10.1097/DSS.0000000000000869.

Fabi, S. G., & Goldman, M. P. (2014). Retrospective evaluation of micro-focused ultrasound for lifting and tightening the face and neck. *Dermatologic Surgery*, *40*, 569–575. https://doi.org/10.1111/dsu.12471.

Fabi, S. G., Goldman, M. P., Mills, D. C., et al. (2016). Combining microfocused ultrasound with botulinum toxin and temporary and semi-permanent dermal fillers: Safety and current use. *Dermatologic Surgery*, *42*, S168–S176. https://doi.org/10.1097/DSS.0000000000000751.

Goldie, K., Peeters, W., Alghoul, M., et al. (2018). Global consensus guidelines for the injection of diluted and hyperdiluted calcium hydroxylapatite for skin tightening. *Dermatologic Surgery*, *44*, S32–S41. https://doi.org/10.1097/DSS.0000000000001685.

Goldman, M. P. (2011). Cosmetic use of poly-L-lactic acid: My technique for success and minimizing complications. *Dermatologic Surgery*, *37*, 688–693. https://doi.org/10.1111/j.1524-4725.2011.01975.x.

Gonzalez, N., & Goldberg, D. J. (2019). Evaluating the effects of injected calcium hydroxylapatite on changes in human skin elastin and proteoglycan formation. *Dermatologic Surgery*, *45*, 547–551. https://doi.org/10.1097/DSS.0000000000001809.

Hamilton, D. G., Gauthier, N., & Robertson, B. F. (2008). Late-onset, recurrent facial nodules associated with injection of poly-L-lactic acid. *Dermatologic Surgery*, *34*, 123–126. https://doi.org/10.1111/j.1524-4725.2007.34027.x.

Han, T. Y., Lee, J. W., Lee, J. H., et al. (2011). Subdermal minimal surgery with hyaluronic acid as an effective treatment for neck wrinkles. *Dermatologic Surgery*, *37*, 1291–1296. https://doi.org/10.1111/j.1524-4725.2011.02057.x.

Hart, D. R., Fabi, S. G., White, W. M., et al. (2015). Current concepts in the use of PLLA: Clinical synergy noted with combined use of microfocused ultrasound and poly-L-lactic acid on the face, neck, and décolletage. *Plastic and Reconstructive Surgery*, *136*, 180S–187S. https://doi.org/10.1097/PRS.0000000000001833.

Jeon, H., Kim, T., Kim, H., et al. (2018). Multimodal approach for treating horizontal neck wrinkles using intensity focused ultrasound, cohesive polydensified matrix hyaluronic acid, and incobotulinumtoxinA. *Dermatologic Surgery*, *44*, 421–431. https://doi.org/10.1097/DSS.0000000000001312.

Jiang, B., Ramirez, M., Ranjit-Reeves, R., et al. (2019). Noncollagen dermal fillers: A summary of the clinical trials used for their FDA approval. *Dermatologic Surgery*, *45*, 1585–1596. https://doi.org/10.1097/DSS.0000000000002141.

Jones, D., Carruthers, A., Hardas, B., et al. (2016). Development and validation of a photonumeric scale for evaluation of transverse neck lines. *Dermatologic Surgery, 42,* S235–S242. https://doi.org/10.1097/DSS.0000000000000851.

Lee, S.-K., & Kim, H. S. (2018). Correction of horizontal neck lines: Our preliminary experience with hyaluronic acid fillers. *Journal of Cosmetic Dermatology, 17,* 590–595. https://doi.org/10.1111/jocd.12382.

Loghem, J. V., Yutskovskaya, Y. A., & Werschler, W. (2015). Calcium hydroxylapatite over a decade of experience. *The Journal of Clinical and Aesthetic Dermatology, 8,* 38–49.

Lorenc, Z. P., Fitzgerald, R., Vleggaar, D., et al. (2014). Consensus recommendations on the use of injectable poly-L-lactic acid for facial and nonfacial volumization. *Journal of Drugs in Dermatology, 13*(4 suppl), s44–s51.

Marmur, E. S., Phelps, R., & Goldberg, D. J. (2004). Clinical, histologic and electron microscopic findings after injection of a calcium hydroxylapatite filler. *Journal of Cosmetic and Laser Therapy, 6,* 223–226. https://doi.org/10.1080/14764170410003048.

Mazzuco, R., & Hexsel, D. (2009). Poly-L-lactic acid for neck and chest rejuvenation. *Dermatologic Surgery, 35,* 1228–1237. https://doi.org/10.1111/j.1524-4725.2009.01217.x.

Meland, M., Groppi, C., & Lorenc, Z. P. (2016). Rheological properties of calcium hydroxylapatite with integral lidocaine. *Journal of Drugs in Dermatology, 15,* 1107–1110.

Minokadeh, A., Black, J. M., & Jones, D. H. (2018). Effacement of transverse neck lines with Vyc-15L and cohesive polydensified matrix hyaluronic acid. *Dermatologic Surgery, 44,* S53–S55. https://doi.org/10.1097/DSS.0000000000001634.

Or, L., Eviator, J. A., Massry, G. G., et al. (2017). Xanthelasma-like reaction to filler injection. *Ophthal Plast Reconstr Surg, 33*(4), 244–247. https://doi.org/10.1097/IOP.0000000000000722.

Oram, Y., & Akkaya, A. D. (2014). Neck rejuvenation with fractional CO_2 laser: Long-term results. *The Journal of Clinical and Aesthetic Dermatology, 7,* 23–29.

Palm, M. D., Woodhall, K. E., Butterwick, K. J., & Goldman, M. P. (2010). Cosmetic use of poly-L-lactic acid: a retrospective study of 130 patients. *Dermatologic Surgery, 36,* 161–170. https://doi.org/10.1111/j.1524-4725.2009.01419.x.

Peterson, J. D., & Goldman, M. P. (2011). Rejuvenation of the aging chest: A review and our experience. *Dermatologic Surgery, 37,* 555–571. https://doi.org/10.1111/j.1524-4725.2011.01972.x.

Peterson, J. D., & Kilmer, S. L. (2016). Three-dimensional rejuvenation of the decolletage. *Dermatologic Surgery, 42,* S101–S107. https://doi.org/10.1097/DSS.0000000000000758.

Robinson, D. M. (2018). In vitro analysis of the degradation of calcium hydroxylapatite dermal filler: A proof-of-concept study. *Dermatologic Surgery, 44,* S5–S9. https://doi.org/10.1097/DSS.0000000000001683.

Robinson, D. M. (2020). Commentary on the use of intralesional sodium thiosulfate to dissolve facial nodules from calcium hydroxylapatite. *Dermatologic Surgery, 46*(10), 1368–1370. https://doi.org/10.1097/DSS.0000000000002360.

Rullan, P. P., Olson, R., & Lee, K. C. (2020). The use of intralesional sodium thiosulfate to dissolve facial nodules from calcium hydroxylapatite. *Dermatologic Surgery, 46*(10), 1366–1368. https://doi.org/10.1097/DSS.0000000000002238.

Schulman, M. R., Lipper, J., & Skolnik, R. A. (2008). Correction of chest wall deformity after implant-based breast reconstruction using poly-L-lactic acid (Sculptra). *The Breast Journal, 14,* 92–96. https://doi.org/10.1111/j.1524-4741.2007.00529.x.

Streker, M., Reuther, T., Krueger, N., & Kerscher, M. (2013). Stabilized hyaluronic acid-based gel of non-animal origin for skin rejuvenation: face, hand, and décolletage. *Journal of Drugs in Dermatology, 12,* 990–994.

Succi, I. B., da Silva, R. T., & Orofino-Costa, R. (2012). Rejuvenation of periorbital area: Treatment with an injectable nonanimal non-crosslinked glycerol added hyaluronic acid preparation. *Dermatologic Surgery, 38,* 192–198. https://doi.org/10.1111/j.1524-4725.2011.02182.x.

Trindade de Almeida, A., Gonzaga da Cunha, A. L., Casabona, G., et al. (2019). Consensus recommendations for the use of hyperdiluted calcium hydroxyapatite (Radiesse) as a face and body biostimulatory agent. *Plastic and Reconstructive Surgery. Global Open, 7,* e2160. https://doi.org/10.1097/GOX.0000000000002160.

Vanaman, M., & Fabi, S. G. (2015). Decolletage: Regional approaches with injectable fillers. *Plastic and Reconstructive Surgery, 136,* 276S–281S. https://doi.org/10.1097/PRS.0000000000001832.

Vanaman, M., Fabi, S. G., & Cox, S. E. (2016). Neck rejuvenation using a combination approach: Our experience and a review of the literature. *Dermatologic Surgery, 42,* S94–S100. https://doi.org/10.1097/DSS.0000000000000699.

Vleggaar, D. (2006). Soft-tissue augmentation and the role of poly-L-lactic acid. *Plastic and Reconstructive Surgery, 118,* S46–S54. https://doi.org/10.1097/01.prs.0000234846.00139.74.

Wilkerson, E. C., & Goldberg, D. J. (2018). Poly-L-lactic acid for the improvement of photodamage and rhytids of the decolletage. *Journal of Cosmetic Dermatology, 17,* 606–610. https://doi.org/10.1111/jocd.12447.

Woodward, J. A., Fabi, S. G., Alster, T., & Colon-Acevedo, B. (2014). Safety and efficacy of combining microfocused ultrasound with fractional CO2 laser resurfacing for lifting and tightening the face and neck. *Dermatologic Surgery, 40*(suppl 12), S190–S193. https://doi.org/10.1097/DSS.0000000000000228.

Yutskovskaya, Y. A., & Kogan, E. A. (2017). Improved neocollagenesis and skin mechanical properties after injection of diluted calcium hydroxylapatite in the neck and décolletage: A pilot study. *Journal of Drugs in Dermatology*, *16*, 68–74.

Yutskovskaya, Y., Kogan, E., & Leshunov, E. (2014). A randomized, split-face, histomorphologic study comparing a volumetric calcium hydroxylapatite and a hyaluronic acid-based dermal filler. *Journal of Drugs in Dermatology*, *13*, 1047–1052.

29

Soft Tissue Augmentation and Buttocks Contouring

Inayaguassu Moura de Lavôr, Ada Regina Trindade de Almeida, and Raúl Alberto Banegas

SUMMARY AND KEY FEATURES

- A female body shape with a small waist and round buttocks is considered as the most attractive.
- Autologous fat grafting is the gold standard for volumizing the gluteal area.
- Collagen biostimulator injection into the gluteal area is indicated to correct postoperative irregularities, contour, cellulite, stretch marks, and sagging skin.

GLUTEAL AESTHETICS

The buttocks are important in sexual attraction and in the concept of body beauty for most cultures and ethnic groups. A female body shape with small waist and round buttocks is considered as the most attractive. The "universally beautiful" gluteal contour is symmetrical, rounded, with greater volume and projection between its middle and upper thirds, the latter being considered the main attribute for the buttocks' attractiveness. The transition between the lumbosacral area and the waist must be smooth. The infragluteal fold must be minimal and should not laterally surpass the posterior midline of the thighs. In the lateral view, the gluteal contour is like a smooth "C," with no depressions. The skin should have homogeneous color and be smooth, without surface irregularities, like cellulite, striae, scars, or wrinkling/sagging. Box 29.1 describes the main gluteal beauty-related aesthetic references (Fig. 29.1).

AGING

The aging and menopause processes progress with changes of the subcutaneous fat distribution—accumulation in the waist and reduction in the trochanteric area, sagging skin, muscular fascia relaxation, and sarcopenia, resulting in intergluteal fold elongation, infragluteal fold drop and elongation, flattening of the areas on the ischial tuberosities, and greater projection of the lower third, giving an old, ptotic appearance to buttocks.

The demand for procedures in the gluteal area is growing. The main motivations are volume augmentation and projection, correction of asymmetries, stretch marks, cellulite, and sagging skin.

GLUTEAL VOLUMIZATION USING AUTOLOGOUS FAT

Autologous fat grafting is considered the gold standard for volumizing the gluteal area. The advantages of autologous fat are relative abundance, low immunogenicity, natural appearance, ease of symmetry, and absence of the complications related to silicone implants.

For patient selection, the following should be considered: presence of fat (20%–30% of fat or body mass index [BMI] between 20 and 30 kg/m^2), excessive skin (absent or a low degree of ptosis), and body shape (the squared or "V" shapes anticipate lower results than those for patients with "A" or rounded shapes).

Fat Removal and Processing

There is no standard process accepted as the best to fat collection and processing. The donor areas are usually

BOX 29.1 Gluteal Aesthetic Landmarks

Lateral depressions: cavities formed in the region lateral.
Infragluteal fold: the groove under the ischial tuberosity.
Supragluteal fossettes: two cavities located on each side of the medial sacral crest.
Waist–hip ratio: ideally between 0.6 and 0.7.
Triangle or V-shaped fold: the sulcus formed by two lines originating in the gluteal crease and directed to the supragluteal fossettes.

From Che DH, Xiao ZB. Gluteal augmentation with fat grafting: literature review. *Aesthetic Plast Surg*. Nov. 20, 2020; and Roberts TL 3rd, Weinfeld AB, Bruner TW, Nguyen K. "Universal" and ethnic ideals of beautiful buttocks are best obtained by autologous micro fat grafting and liposuction. *Clin Plast Surg*. 2006;33(3):371–394.

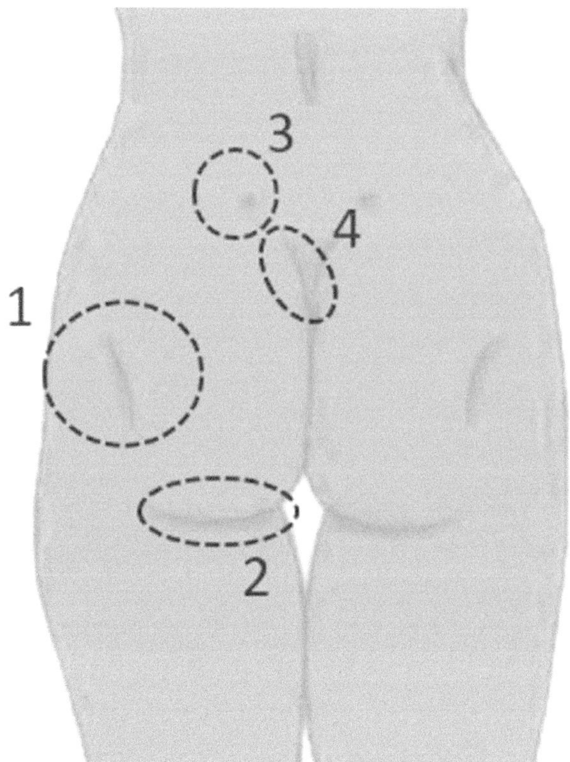

Fig. 29.1 Gluteal aesthetic references: *1*, Lateral depressions; *2*, infragluteal fold; *3, supragluteal fossettes*; *4*, V-shaped fold.

those close to the gluteal area. A systematic review showed the following: liposuction alone with a vacuum machine (40%), associated with a syringe (26.7%), syringe alone (20%), and liposuction with ultrasound (6.7%). The most used fat processing techniques were decantation (58%), high- or low-speed centrifugation (21%), and washing (16%).

Injection Technique

Incisions in the infragluteal area should be avoided. Typically, fat should be injected into the superficial planes in the upper mid and lateral buttock regions to promote elevation and contribute to the hourglass figure. The danger area should be avoided: it contains the main neurovascular structures (Fig. 29.2).

There is no consensus on the safe amount of fat to be injected, although studies suggest 400 to 550 mL per gluteus per session. The procedure must be stopped before whitening skin or fat leakage through the incision are observed. Safety recommendations suggested are subcutaneous fat grafting only, avoiding muscular injections; the use

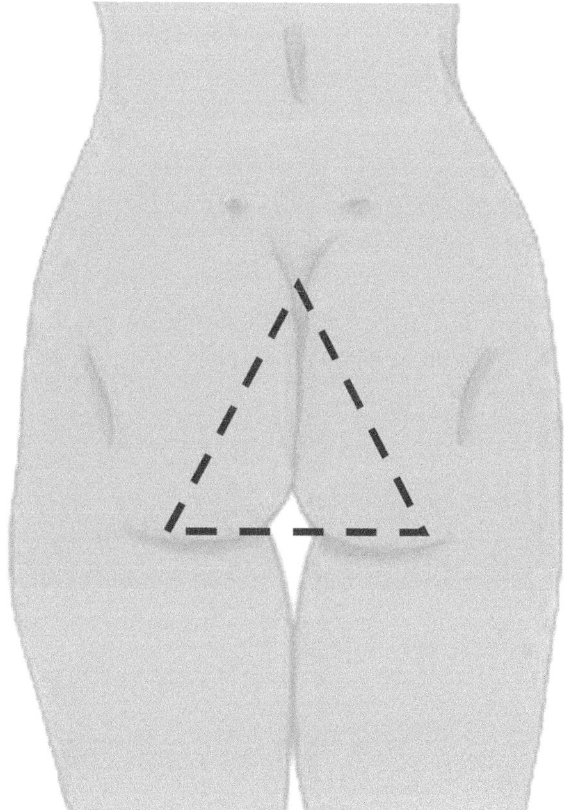

Fig. 29.2 "Danger area": triangle with apex in the intergluteal cleft and base in the medial and lower one third of the buttocks. (From O'Neill RC, Abu-Ghname A, Davis MJ, Chamata E, Rammos CK, Winocour SJ. The role of fat grafting in buttock augmentation. *Semin Plast Surg*. 2020;34(1):38–46.)

of thicker cannulas 4 mm or larger, avoid the use of lidocaine in the locally infiltrated solution when under general or locoregional anesthesia (risk of systemic toxicity).

PEARL 1 The main safety recommendation is to inject fat in the subcutaneous plane ONLY.

PEARL 2 Stop fat injection:
- Skin whitening
- Fat leakage through the incision

Postoperative Care and Complications

The use of compression garments for 4 to 8 weeks is recommended in most studies. The complication rate associated is estimated at 7% to 10%, with serious events representing less than 1% of total cases. The most feared one, fat embolism, may occur through two mechanisms: adipocyte emboli in the pulmonary vessels (pulmonary fat embolism) and fat embolism syndrome (pulmonary inflammatory and systemic reaction caused by fatty acid micro emboli) (Fig. 29.3).

GLUTEAL REJUVENATION WITH BIOSTIMULATORS

Poly-L-Lactic Acid

Poly-L-lactic acid (PLLA) is a biocompatible and biodegradable synthetic polymer from the family of alpha-hydroxy-acids. The injectable form, marketed as

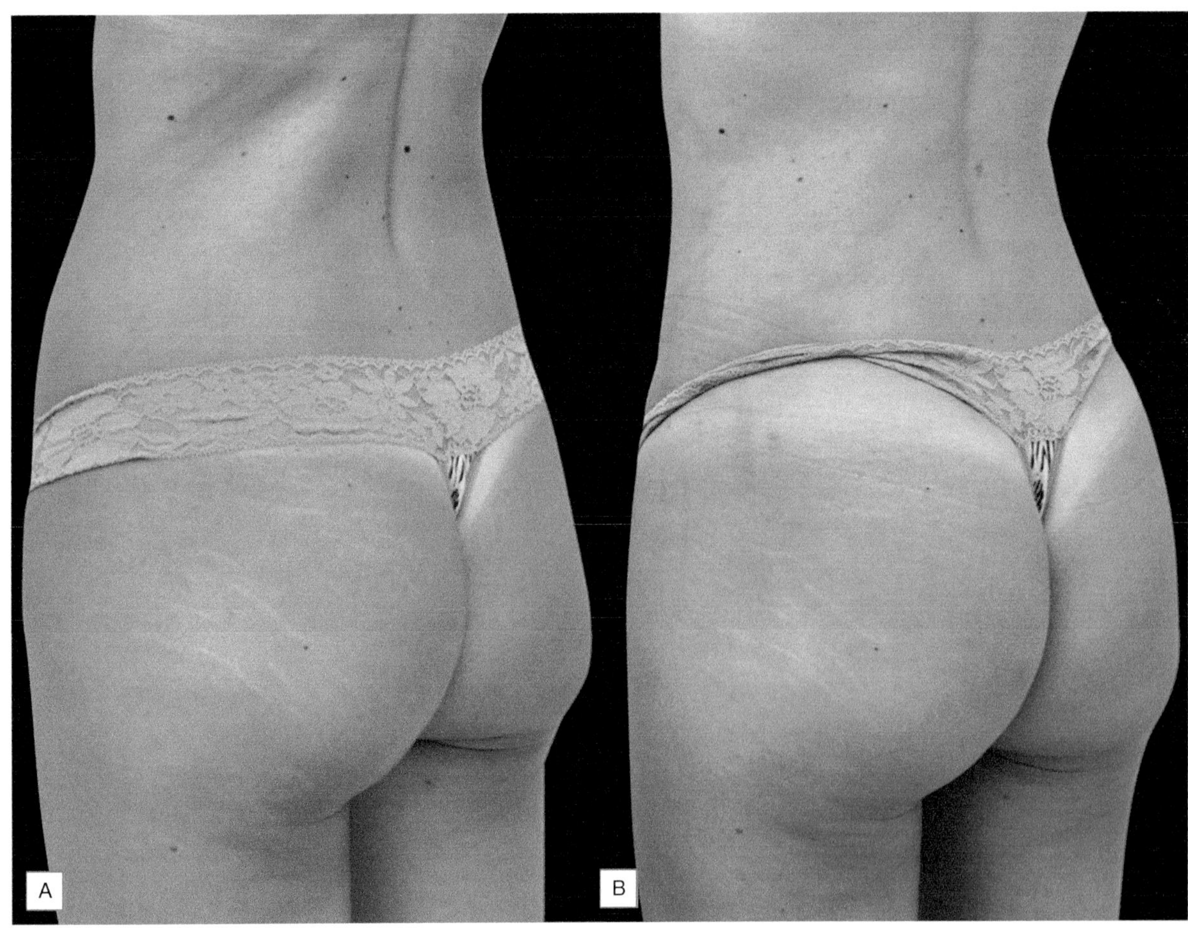

Fig. 29.3 Before (A) and 90 days after (B) lipofilling with 420 cc of fat grafting per side. (Courtesy of Dr. Raul Banegas, MD, Argentina.)

Sculptra Aesthetic (Galderma Pharma AS/Galderma SA, Lausanne, Switzerland), is a lyophilized powder composed of PLLA microparticles, sodium carboxymethylcellulose, and mannitol.

After injection, a mechanical tissue expansion occurs, which disappears at the end of the first week following reabsorption of the carrier solution. PLLA's mechanism of action begins as a subclinical inflammatory response, followed by particle encapsulation and subsequent fibroplasia. It is a foreign body reaction with increased fibroblastic activity and neocollagenesis with collagen type I and III deposition.

The final result begins 3 to 4 weeks later and becomes clear 3 months after. At 6 months, the implant degraded by 58% to 82% and the capsule is almost totally filled with collagen. The result lasts 18 to 24 months, with reports of persistence for up to 3 years.

The literature describes PLLA injection for buttock volumization, correction of postoperative irregularities, contouring, cellulite, stretch marks, and sagging skin. The best results are expected in under 60-year-old physically active individuals with a BMI of 20 kg/m^2 (or under) and minimal excessive fat (a relative contraindication for autologous lipografting), seeking mild to moderate gluteal augmentation, and not willing to undergo surgical procedures.

PLLA may be an alternative treatment for cellulite on the buttocks. Mazzuco R described good results and good cost-effectiveness with the combination of Subcsion with PLLA for patients with moderate to severe cellulite associated with sagging skin on the gluteal area.

Preparation and Dilution

Sterile water for injection is the most commonly used diluent, with hydration time between 24 and 72 hours and a minimum time of 2 hours.

PLLA must be shaken before use to produce an even and translucent solution. This may be done manually, with a vortex or a back-and-forth (connector between two syringes) movement method. The latter resulted in homogeneous suspension without precipitation even after 30 minutes of rest. The final solution is transferred to smaller syringes (1 or 3 mL) before injection.

Different dilutions have been described in the literature for injection into buttocks, ranging from 12 mL to 16 mL to 30 mL of the final solution. Immediately before injection, 2% lidocaine (with or without epinephrine) is often added to the suspension.

Injection and Number of Sessions

The volume injected is defined by the size of the area to be treated. For body regions, some authors recommend the use of one vial per session per area equivalent to a sheet of A4 paper, while others reported using between 40 and 240 mL per side per session, three sessions, 6 weeks apart, totaling up to 48 vials.

The injection may be performed with a needle (26–27 G) in a short linear or fanning technique or with a cannula (22–23 G, 50 mm) in a fanning manner, into the subcutaneous plane, depositing aliquots of 0.05 to 0.1 mL/cm^2. Aspiration before injection is recommended to avoid intravascular placement of the product.

> **PEARL 3** The objective of the poly-L-lactic acid injection is to evenly distribute the product with the formation of a subcutaneous sheet in the treated area.

> **PEARL 4** One Sculptra vial is recommended for an area equivalent to a sheet of A4 paper, per session.

Posttreatment Care

Massage after PLLA injection is essential for optimizing results and preventing nodules.

Immediately after, it helps homogeneous distribution of the product. At home, patients are advised to follow the 5–5–5 rule: vigorous massage for 5 minutes, five times a day, for 5 days (Fig. 29.4).

> **PEARL 5** After Sculptra injection, massage is essential for optimizing results and preventing nodules.

Complications and Management

Complications due to technical failure, nodules and papules due to product accumulation, disappear over time. Real complications are vascular (occlusion and ischemia) and inflammatory (clinical granulomas due to the host's exacerbated response). They appear in several treated areas and respond well to intralesional or systemic steroids, whether associated or not with intralesional 5-fluorouracil.

Calcium Hydroxyapatite

Calcium hydroxyapatite (CaHA; Radiesse, Merz Pharmaceuticals GmbH, Frankfurt, Germany) consists of 30% microspheres of synthetic CaHA in an aqueous gel of water, glycerin, and carboxymethylcellulose.

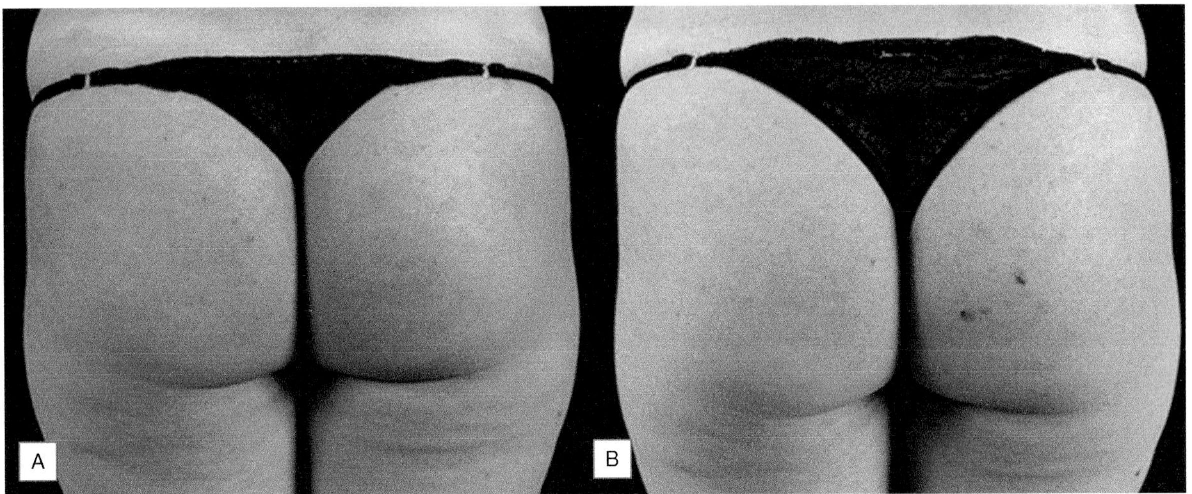

Fig. 29.4 Poly-L-lactic acid (16 mL dilution), before (A) and after (B) 3 months of four vials injected in one session. (Courtesy of Dr. Maria Paula Del Nero, MD, São Paulo, Brazil.)

The microspheres are identical in composition to the mineral component of bones and teeth.

CaHA stimulates dermal remodeling with formation of elastin and physiological neocollagenesis where collagen type I gradually replaces collagen type III. The peak deposition of collagen and elastin occurs at four and stabilizes after 9 months. While microspheres are absorbed within one year, neocollagenesis effect induces clinical response duration of 12 to 18 months.

The main indications for CaHA into buttocks are sagging skin and contour irregularities (cellulite and stretch marks). When treating cellulite, the result is enhanced by the association with the use of microfocused ultrasound with visualization (MFU-V). For stretch marks, CaHA injection increases the quantity and quality of collagen and elastic fibers.

Preparation and Dilution

CaHA is available as a viscoelastic material with a milky appearance in 1.5-mL syringes. Diluted CaHA is defined as the original formulation reconstituted with 2% lidocaine (with or without epinephrine) or saline at a 1:1 ratio (see Video 29.1). It is considered hyperdiluted with reconstitutions of 1:2 or more.

A minimum of 20 passes between two syringes is recommended for solution homogeneity. It must be used immediately after reconstitution. For treatment of skin laxity and surface irregularities of the buttocks, CaHA can be used in dilutions ranging from 1:2 to 1:6, according to the thickness of the dermis. Usually, one syringe (1.5 mL) is used to treat a 100- to 300-cm^2 area.

PEARL 6 The skin thickness is the main criterion when choosing the dilution of CaHA (Radiesse).

PEARL 7 >
One CaHA syringe (1.5 mL) is used to treat a 100- to 300-cm^2 area.

Injection and Number of Sessions

The injection may be performed using needles (27–30 gauge) or cannulas (22–25 gauge). Injection with cannulas resulted in greater accuracy when compared to needles.

When injecting with a cannula, the amount injected is 0.1 to 0.2 mL, and with a needle, it is 0.1 mL per pass, 2 cm apart between linear injections. For sagging buttocks, the fanning technique with a cannula or asterisk-like injection is suggested, with 1:1 to 1:4 dilutions (1.5–6 mL of diluent), mainly injecting the superior and lateral portions (see Video 29.2).

In cellulite depressions, smaller dilutions (1:1 or 1:2) may be used with a short linear technique using a needle (Fig. 29.5) (see Video 29.3 and Video 29.4).

The treatment of stretch marks may be performed using the intradermal or subdermal microbolus technique

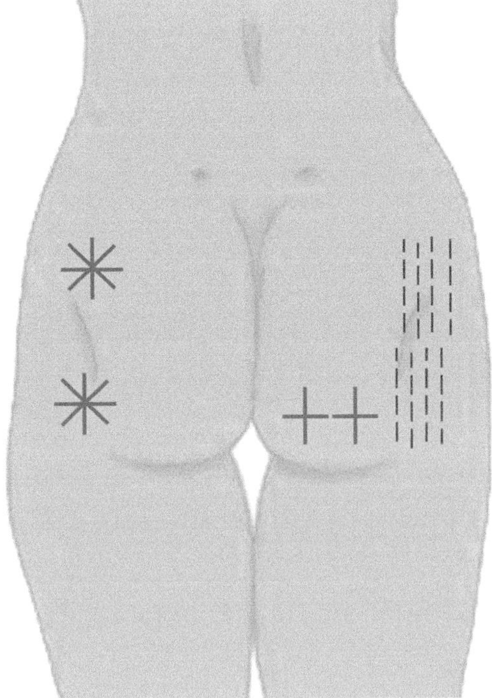

Fig. 29.5 All bioestimulators (poly-L-lactic acid, calcium hydroxyapatite, or polycaprolactone) are suggested to be injected in superficial fanning, linear (*red dashed lines*), asterisk like (*blue star*) or cross-hatching (*blue crosses*) techniques using needles or cannulas.

("pearl necklace"), depositing 0.05 mL per site at the center of the lesion or with the retrograde linear technique (0.5 mL per lesion).

One to three sessions in the first year are recommended, at 3- to 4-month intervals. Maintenance injections are to be given every 12 to 18 months (Fig. 29.6).

Posttreatment Care

Perform an initial massage after the procedure for a homogeneous distribution of the product. Patients are advised to massage the sites twice a day during the first week.

Complications

In long-term studies of CaHA, the adverse events were mild and mostly related to the injection (erythema, ecchymosis, edema, and inflammation). Pain and pruritus were also reported.

The formation of noninflammatory nodules is associated with injection into areas with great muscle movement (lips) or the superficial injection of the product. In most cases, the nodules were not visible and resolved spontaneously. It may be treated with lidocaine or saline infiltration followed by vigorous massage.

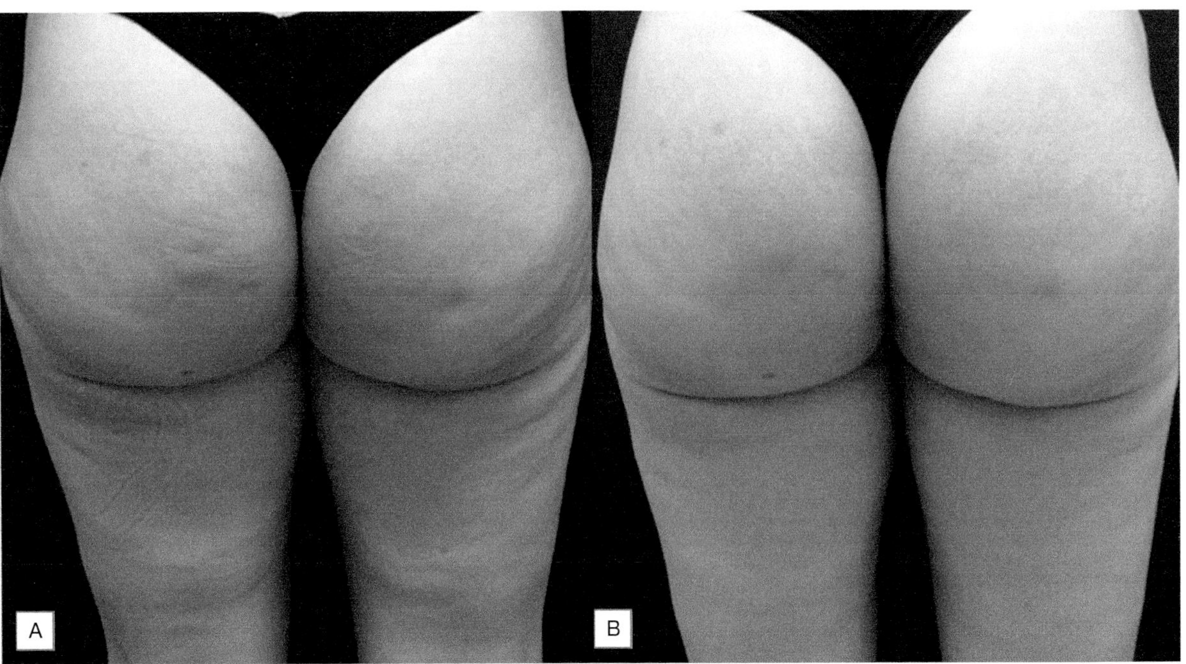

Fig. 29.6 Before (A) and 3 months after (B) the third session with hyperdiluted (1:2) Radiesse (one syringe per gluteal side per session). (Courtesy of Dr. Ada Trindade de Almeida, MD, São Paulo, Brazil.)

Late events, such as granulomas and infections, were not reported.

Polycaprolactone

Marketed since 2009 in Europe, Ellansé (Sinclair Pharma, London, UK) is a collagen biostimulator composed of polycaprolactone (PCL) microspheres. It is a biocompatible, biodegradable, and bioabsorbable polyester, used as a component of suture threads (Monocryl Ethicon, Inc., New Jersey) and encapsulated drug delivery systems such as contraceptives and oncology drugs.

The neocollagenesis mechanism of PCL biostimulator is similar to that of CaHA. In both products, the particles (30%) are suspended in carboxymethylcellulose (70%). The differences are observed in the tissue reaction intensity and longevity of the particles. Histological evaluation shows that the dermal longevity of this filler is superior to 4 years.

The product is available in 1-mL syringes with preparations that differ in terms of duration of action: Ellansé-S, 18 months; Ellansé-M, 24 months; Ellansé-L, 3 years; and Ellansé-E, 4 years.

The product is indicated for facial and hand rejuvenation. Despite the off-label use for body treatments, medical publications for this indication are scarce. Into the buttocks, it is suggested to inject the product pure or adding 0.1 mL lidocaine for each milliliter, in subdermal injections using the retrograde linear technique with a 27 G needle or 25 G cannula, in a fanning manner.

Further research studies on the use of PCL for body injection are needed.

CONCLUSIONS

The buttocks are important for body beauty and sexual attraction in different cultures and ethnicities, with a growing demand for aesthetic procedures. Options for aesthetic improvement include lipografting for volume augmentation and projection and the use of collagen biostimulators to improve contour and correct irregularities such as cellulite, stretch marks, and sagging skin.

FURTHER READING

Amselem, M. (2015). Radiesse: A novel rejuvenation treatment for the upper arms. *Clinical, Cosmetic and Investigational Dermatology*, *9*, 9–14. https://doi.org/10.2147/CCID.S93137.

Baspeyras, M., Dallara, J. M., Cartier, H., Charavel, M. H., & Dumas, L. (2017). Restoring jawline contour with calcium hydroxylapatite: A prospective, observational study. *Journal of Cosmetic Dermatology*, *16*(3), 342–347. https://doi.org/10.1111/jocd.12335.

Breithaupt, A., & Fitzgerald, R. (2015). Collagen stimulators: Poly-L-lactic acid and calcium hydroxyl apatite. *Facial Plastic Surgery Clinics of North America*, *23*(4), 459–469. https://doi.org/10.1016/j.fsc.2015.07.007.

Cansancao, A. L., Condé-Green, A., Gouvea Rosique, R., Junqueira Rosique, M., & Cervantes, A. (2019). "Brazilian butt lift" performed by board-certified Brazilian plastic surgeons: Reports of an expert opinion survey. *Plastic and Reconstructive Surgery*, *144*(3), 601–609. https://doi.org/10.1097/PRS.0000000000006020.

Cárdenas-Camarena, L., Silva-Gavarrete, J. F., & Arenas-Quintana, R. (2011). Gluteal contour improvement: Different surgical alternatives. *Aesthetic Plastic Surgery*, *35*(6), 1117–1125. https://doi.org/10.1007/s00266-011-9747-3.

Centeno, R. F., Sood, A., & Young, V. L. (2018). Clinical anatomy in aesthetic gluteal contouring. *Clinics in Plastic Surgery*, *45*(2), 145–157. https://doi.org/10.1016/j.cps.2017.12.010.

Che, D. H., & Xiao, Z. B. (2021). Gluteal augmentation with fat grafting: Literature review. *Aesthetic Plastic Surgery*, *45*(4), 1633–1641. https://doi.org/10.1007/s00266-020-02038-w.

Chen, S. Y., Chen, S. T., Lin, J. Y., & Lin, C. Y. (2020). Reconstitution of injectable poly-L-lactic acid: Efficacy of different diluents and a new accelerating method. *Plastic and Reconstructive Surgery. Global Open*, *8*(5), 28–29. https://doi.org/10.1097/GOX.0000000000002829.

Christen, M. O., & Vercesi, F. (2020). Polycaprolactone: How a well-known and futuristic polymer has become an innovative collagen-stimulator in esthetics. *Clinical, Cosmetic and Investigational Dermatology*, *13*, 31–48. https://doi.org/10.2147/CCID.S229054.

Condé-Green, A., Kotamarti, V., Nini, K. T., et al. (2016). Fat grafting for gluteal augmentation: A systematic review of the literature and meta-analysis. *Plastic and Reconstructive Surgery*, *138*(3), 437–446. https://doi.org/10.1097/PRS.0000000000002435.

Cuenca-Guerra, R., & Quezada, J. (2004). What makes buttocks beautiful? A review and classification of the determinants of gluteal beauty and the surgical techniques to achieve them. *Aesthetic Plastic Surgery*, *28*(5), 340–347. https://doi.org/10.1007/s00266-004-3114-6.

de Almeida, A. T., Figueredo, V., da Cunha, A. L. G., et al. (2019). Consensus recommendations for the use of hyperdiluted calcium hydroxyapatite (Radiesse) as a face and body biostimulatory agent. *Plastic and Reconstructive Surgery*, *7*(3), e2160. https://doi.org/10.1097/GOX.0000000000002160.

Fitzgerald, R., Bass, L. M., Goldberg, D. J., Graivier, M. H., & Lorenc, Z. P. (2018). Physiochemical Ccharacteristics of Ppoly-L-Llactic Acid (PLLA). *Aesthetic Surgery Journal, 38*, S13–S17. https://doi.org/10.1093/asj/sjy012.

Goldie, K., Peeters, W., Alghoul, M., et al. (2018). Global consensus guidelines for the injection of diluted and hyperdiluted calcium hydroxylapatite for skin tightening. *Dermatologic Surgery, 44*, S32–S41. https://doi.org/10.1097/DSS.0000000000001685.

Gonzalez, R. (2006). Etiology, definition, and classification of gluteal ptosis. *Aesthetic Plastic Surgery, 30*(3), 320–326. https://doi.org/10.1007/s00266-005-0051-y.

Haddad, A., Menezes, A., Guarnieri, C., et al. (2019). Recommendations on the use of injectable poly-L-lactic acid for skin laxity in off-face areas. *Journal of Drugs in Dermatology, 18*(9), 929–935.

Kadouch, J. A. (2017). Calcium hydroxylapatite: A review on safety and complications. *Journal of Cosmetic Dermatology, 16*(2), 52–161. https://doi.org/10.1111/jocd.12326.

Keni, S. P., & Sidle, D. M. (2007). Sculptra (injectable poly-L-lactic acid). *Facial Plastic Surgery Clinics of North America, 15*(1), 91–97. https://doi.org/10.1016/j.fsc.2006.10.005.

Kim, J. S. (2019). Changes in dermal thickness in biopsy study of histologic findings after a single injection of polycaprolactone-based filler into the dermis. *Aesthetic Surgery Journal, 39*(12), 484–494. https://doi.org/10.1093/asj/sjz050.

Kim, J. A., & Van Abel, D. (2015). Neocollagenesis in human tissue injected with a polycaprolactone-based dermal filler. *Journal of Cosmetic and Laser Therapy, 17*(2), 99–101. https://doi.org/10.3109/14764172.2014.968586.

Lacombe, V. (2009). Sculptra: A stimulatory filler. *Facial Plastic Surgery, 25*(2), 95–99. https://doi.org/10.1055/s-0029-1220648.

Lam, S. M., Azizzadeh, B., & Graivier, M. (2006). Injectable poly-L-lactic acid (Sculptra): Technical considerations in soft-tissue contouring. *Plastic and Reconstructive Surgery, 118*(3), 55–63. https://doi.org/10.1097/01.prs.0000234612.20611.5a.

Lee, E. I., Roberts, T. L., & Bruner, T. W. (2009). Ethnic considerations in buttock aesthetics. *Seminars in Plastic Surgery, 23*(3), 232–243. https://doi.org/10.1055/s-0029-1224803.

Lin, M. J., Dubin, D. P., Goldberg, D. J., & Khorasani, H. (2019). Practices in the usage and reconstitution of poly-L-lactic acid. *Journal of Drugs in Dermatology, 18*(9), 880–886.

Mazzuco, R. (2020). Subcision plus poly-lL-lactic acid for the treatment of cellulite associated to flaccidity in the buttocks and thighs. *Journal of Cosmetic Dermatology, 19*(5), 1165–1171. https://doi.org/10.1111/jocd.13364.

Mazzuco, R., Dal'Forno, T., & Hexsel, D. (2020). Poly-L-lactic acid for nonfacial skin laxity. *Dermatologic Surgery, 46*, S86–S88. https://doi.org/10.1097/DSS.0000000000002390.

Mazzuco, R., & Sadick, N. S. (2016). The use of poly-L-lactic acid in the gluteal area. *Dermatologic Surgery, 42*(3), 441–443. https://doi.org/10.1097/DSS.0000000000000632.

O'Neill, R. C., Abu-Ghname, A., Davis, M. J., Chamata, E., Rammos, C. K., & Winocour, S. J. (2020). The role of fat grafting in buttock augmentation. *Seminars in Plastic Surgery, 34*(1), 38–46. https://doi.org/10.1055/s-0039-3401038.

Rios, L., & Gupta, V. (2020). Improvement in Brazilian butt lift (BBL) safety with the current recommendations from ASERF, ASAPS, and ISAPS. *Aesthetic Surgery Journal, 40*(8), 864–870. https://doi.org/10.1093/asj/sjaa098.

Roberts, T. L., 3rd, Weinfeld, A. B., Bruner, T. W., & Nguyen, K. (2006). "Universal" and ethnic ideals of beautiful buttocks are best obtained by autologous micro fat grafting and liposuction. *Clinics in Plastic Surgery, 33*(3), 371–394. https://doi.org/10.1016/j.cps.2006.05.001.

Vleggaar, D., Fitzgerald, R., & Lorenc, Z. P. (2014). Understanding, avoiding, and treating potential adverse events following the use of injectable poly-L-lactic acid for facial and nonfacial volumization. *Journal of Drugs in Dermatology, 13*, s35–s39.

Wong, W. W., Motakef, S., Lin, Y., & Gupta, S. C. (2016). Redefining the ideal buttocks: A population analysis. *Plastic and Reconstructive Surgery, 137*(6), 1739–1747. https://doi.org/10.1097/PRS.0000000000002192.

30

Earlobe Rejuvenation

Courtney Gwinn, Murad Alam, and Jeffrey S. Dover

SUMMARY AND KEY FEATURES

- The earlobe is a site of adornment and a reflection of beauty across world cultures.
- With increasing interest in facial and neck rejuvenation, the earlobes have emerged as a site of cosmetic concern.
- Like other sun-exposed areas of skin, the earlobes may exhibit signs of age, including pigmentary and vascular changes, increased laxity, loss of volume, and elongation (ptosis).
- Volume loss of the earlobes can be corrected safely and effectively using injectable fillers.
- The quality of the earlobe skin can be improved with laser and other light-based devices.

INTRODUCTION

With a growing interest in minimally invasive cosmetic procedures, a new anatomic site is gaining increasing attention: the earlobes. Like sun-exposed areas of the face, chest, neck, and hands, the ears can show significant signs of aging. These may include wrinkling, dyspigmentation, and elongation (ptosis) due to chronic exposure to ultraviolet light, loss of elastic fibers and collagen, and natural aging. Such changes can be exacerbated by the use of heavy earrings. Earlobe restoration is indicated in patients with ptosis or other signs of lobule aging; those who have undergone cosmetic procedures on the face and neck and desire similarly youthful earlobes; and those with piercing holes that have stretched or were initially suboptimally placed such that the lobule cannot adequately support earrings. Soft tissue augmentation using injectable fillers can safely restore volume and minimize sagging and wrinkling. Lasers and other energy-based treatments can improve skin dyspigmentation and the overall quality of the earlobe skin.

PEARL 1 Earlobes can exhibit signs of aging and can become elongated as a result of gravity, photoaging, and the pull of heavy earrings.

PEARL 2 With volume loss, the earlobes become thin and wrinkled and can lose the ability to adequately support earrings.

ANATOMY AND CLASSIFICATION OF EARLOBES

The earlobe is composed of tough areolar and adipose tissue and can have a natural shape that is round, flat, or triangular. Lobules are generally smooth but occasionally exhibit creases. Creased or crumpled earlobes can suggest an underlying genetic disorder, such as Beckwith-Wiedemann syndrome or congenital contractural arachnodactyly, respectively. Diagonal earlobe creases, also known as Frank's sign, extending from the lateral cheek toward the inferior helix have been reported as a risk factor for myocardial infarction, ischemic heart disease, and cerebrovascular disease. However, earlobes lack the firmness and elasticity of the rest of the pinna and can become creased and elongated with age even in the absence of heart disease.

Elongated earlobes increase a person's perceived age and negatively impact perceived attractiveness, according to a study by Forte et al. Pendulous earlobes, which do not adhere to the lateral cheek, are most likely to elongate and become asymmetric with time (Fig. 30.1). These are inherited in autosomal dominant fashion. Nonpendulous earlobes, attached to the lateral cheek, are less likely to elongate with age and are inherited in a recessive pattern (see Fig. 30.1).

The earlobe is commonly measured from the intertragal notch to the subaurale (Fig. 30.2). Ptosis has been defined as an elongated free caudal segment (otobasion inferius to the subaurale), whereas pseudoptosis refers to elongation of the attached cephalic segment (intertragal notch to otobasion inferius) (see Fig. 30.2). In 1972, Loeb observed the natural range of the cephalic segment to be 1 to 2.5 cm and advocated for surgical correction when this segment (pseudoptosis) exceeds 2.0 cm. A more recent study describes pseudoptosis as cephalic segment length exceeding 1.5 cm. Mowlavi (2003) reported increased incidence of earlobe ptosis and pseudoptosis following facelift surgery, highlighting the need to address signs of earlobe aging at the time of facial rejuvenation.

Using another means of evaluating the ear, in a randomized, prospective study of 547 men and women aged 20 to 80 years, Azaria et al. measured earlobe length using a line of balance through the long axis of the ear (intertragic notch to caudal tip) (Fig. 30.3). The authors demonstrated that the left earlobe is shorter than the right, on average (1.97 cm vs. 2.01 cm; mean difference 0.4 mm). Earlobe size and symmetry varied by race (individuals of African descent had the shortest earlobes, and Ashkenazi and Sephardic Jews had relatively long left earlobes), and earlobe length increased slightly with heavier body weight among women. Earlobe length increased by 30% to 35% between the youngest and oldest age groups, but no significant change was noted in women aged 40 years and older. Prior to treatment, it is beneficial to discuss ear size and any natural asymmetry with the patient and offer anticipatory guidance about earlobe changes based on age and body habitus.

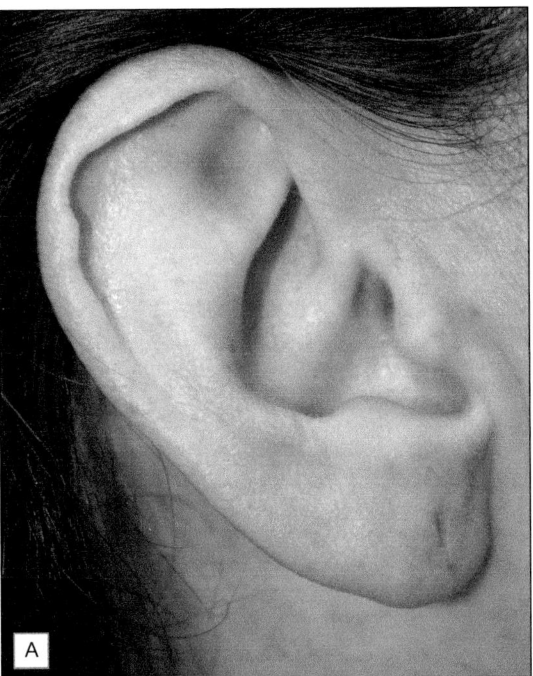

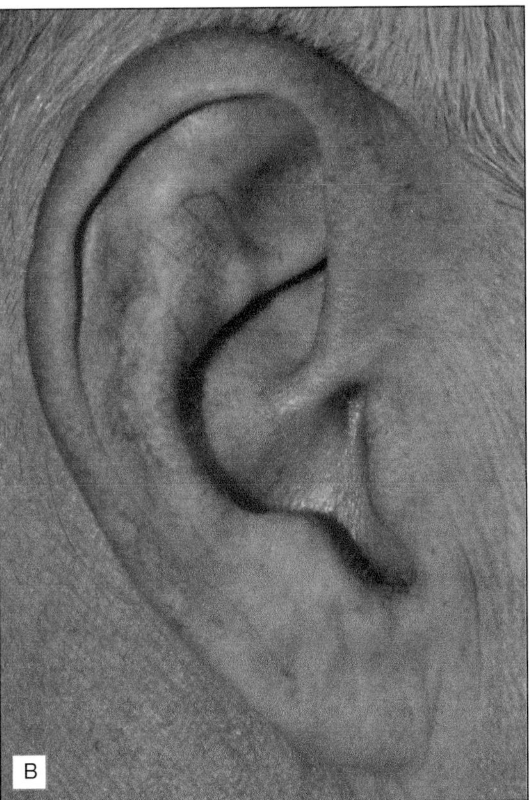

Fig. 30.1 Anatomic shape of earlobes: (A) unattached and (B) attached.

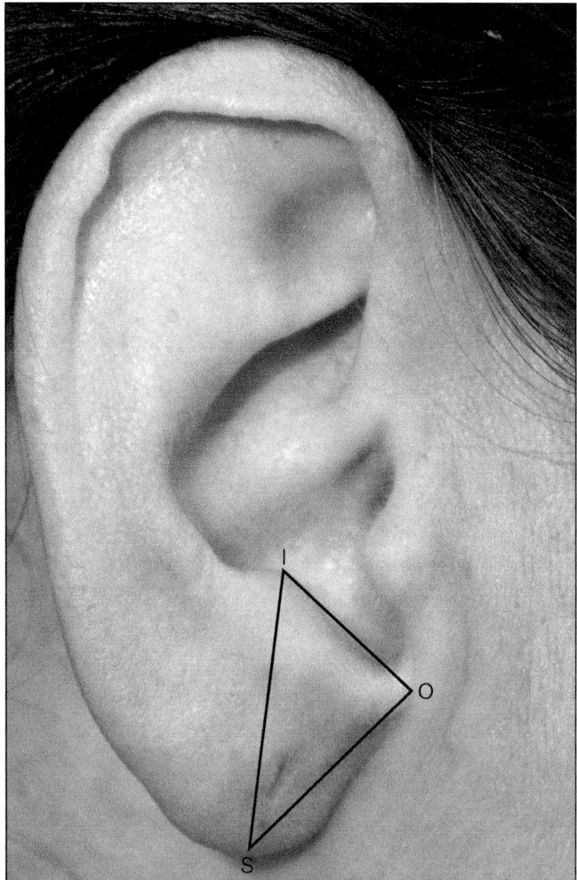

Fig. 30.2 The anatomic landmarks of the *I*, *O*, and *S* are labeled. Earlobe height parameters are defined with respect to the attached cephalic segment (*I to O segment*) and the free caudal segment to *S* segment). *I*, Intertragal notch; *O*, otobasion inferius; *S*, subaurale.

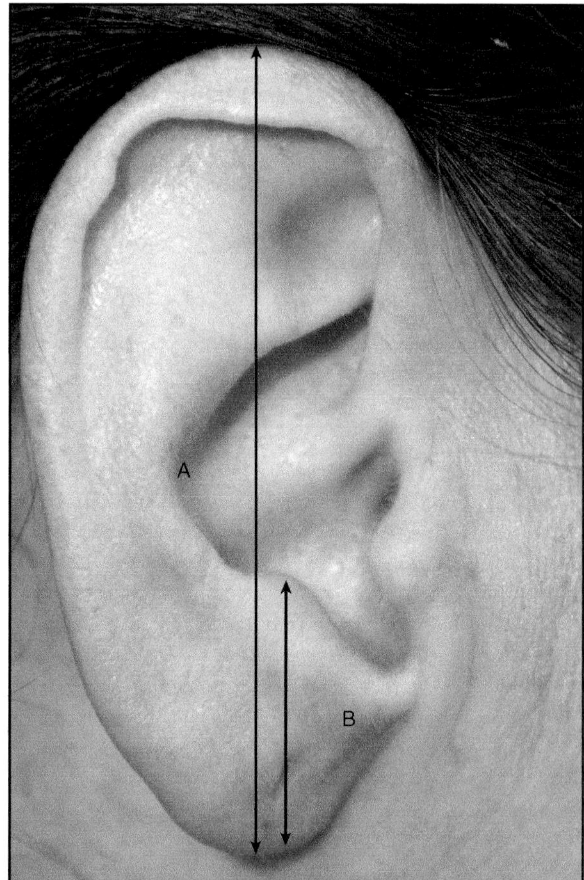

Fig. 30.3 Measurement technique of earlobes: line of balance (*line A*) and earlobe length (*line B*).

Before considering modification of the earlobe, it is important to understand general aesthetic optimal ratios and lengths. In general, the length of the lobe should be between 25% and 30% of the total length of the ear. The ideal length of the free or caudal segment of the lobe (anterior earlobe crease to subauricular point) ranges from 1 to 5 mm.

FILLERS FOR EARLOBE REJUVENATION

Soft tissue augmentation using fillers is a safe, effective, and increasingly popular means of restoring volume to the earlobes. A variety of different filler classes and types have been used to effectively fill thinned earlobes. These include hyaluronic acid (HA) fillers such as Restylane, Restylane Lyft, Restylane Silk, Restylane Refyne, Restylane Defyne, and Restylane Kysse (Galderma, Fort Worth, TX); Hylacross technology fillers Juvéderm Ultra, Juvéderm UltraPlus, and Vycross technology fillers, including Volbella, Vollure, and Voluma (Allergan Inc., Irvine, CA) and RHA 2, RHA 3, and RHA 4 (Revance, Nashville, TN). Longer-lasting fillers, such as calcium hydroxyapatite (Radiesse, Merz Aesthetics, San Mateo, CA) and poly-L-lactic acid (Sculptra, Galderma, Fort Worth, TX) have been used, although their use for earlobe rejuvenation has not been reported in the literature.

The earlobe is a small anatomic site but can require 0.3 to 1.0 mL or more to correct volume loss. Depending on the filler, 25-, 27-, and 30-gauge needles are used. Topical anesthesia or ice can be applied prior

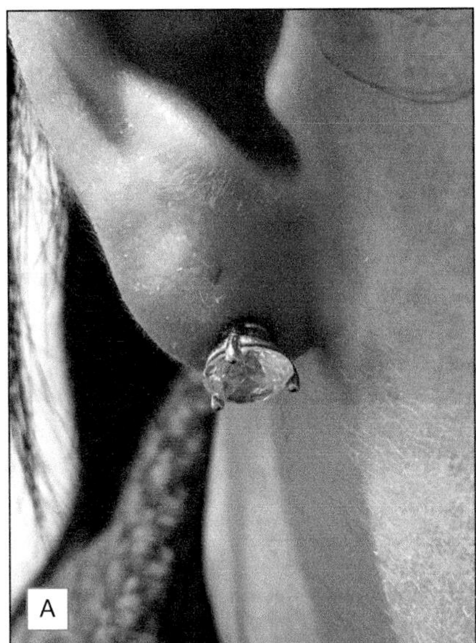

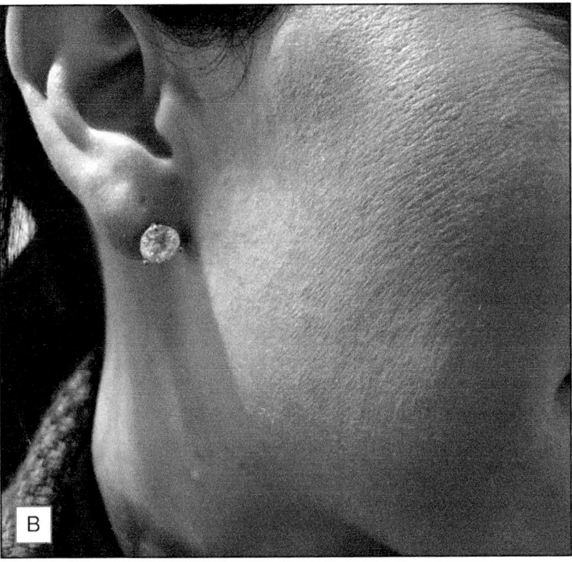

Fig. 30.4 The earlobe of a young woman before (A) and after (B) injections using Juvéderm Voluma (Allergan Inc., Irvine, CA). Note how the earring is better supported by the lobule and oriented anteriorly (rather than downward) in the after photo.

to injections, but this is often unnecessary, particularly with HA formulations containing lidocaine for anesthesia. After cleansing the area with an antiseptic of choice, the clinician may grasp the earlobe firmly between the thumb and index finger and direct the needle into the mid-dermis at a 0- to 45-degree angle. Serial injections can be used to deliver small aliquots of filler; some authors have proposed making injections in a circular pattern around the hole of a pierced ear (Video 30.1). This method helps to tighten the diameter of the piercing while allowing filler to be massaged outward to fill the entire lobule, ultimately providing better support for earrings (Fig. 30.4). With a threading or tunneling technique, the needle may be inserted into the inferior pole of the lobule, and a depot of filler is injected as the needle is withdrawn (Fig. 30.5). Firm pressure can be applied for 1 minute afterward to help to reduce the risk of bruising and edema, and the lobule may be gently massaged to distribute the product.

PEARL 3 Fillers can be delivered by making serial injections of small aliquots into the earlobe or by placing a depot of filler through the inferior pole of the lobule. Either method can restore volume and allow the lobule to better support earrings.

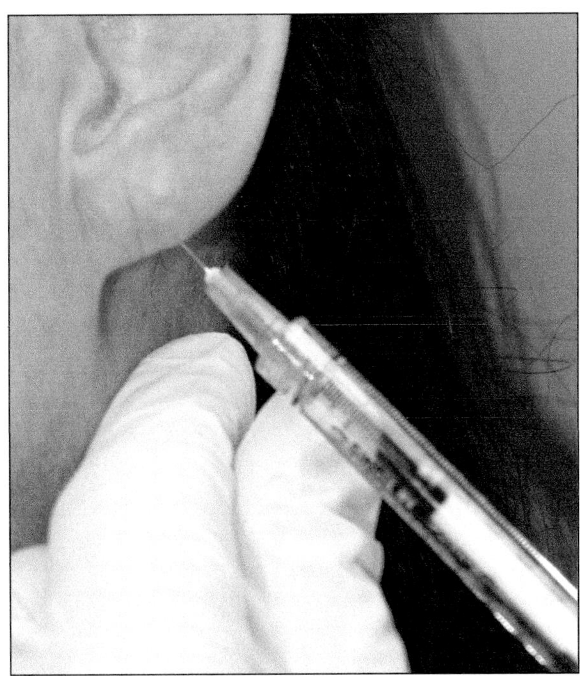

Fig. 30.5 Injection technique using Restylane (Galderma, Fort Worth, TX) to restore volume from the inferior aspect of the earlobe in a patient who has previously had earlobe repair surgery.

As with soft tissue augmentation of other sites, there is a risk of bruising, swelling, and erythema following injections. Because of the earlobe's rich vascularity, the lobule can appear red and edematous for a prolonged period. Patients can resume wearing earrings immediately after the procedure, and the earlobe can be reassessed after 2 weeks to consider the need for more product. HA filler has been noted to last longer in the earlobes relative to the face, but repeat injections are needed to maintain results. Per study by Di Gregorio et al., filler typically lasts 14 months on average in the earlobe.

In the author's experience, overfilling pendulous earlobes can lead to a "paddle-like" appearance of the ear lobe. Caution to avoid overfilling should be taken.

PEARL 4 As with any injection of filler, there is a risk of bruising, edema, and erythema that may be more pronounced on the earlobe due to its rich vascularity. Repeat injections are needed to maintain results but the benefit is often long lasting.

Little has been written on treatments for earlobe photoaging, but wrinkling and discoloration are common in this site among patients who are middle aged and older. The skin of the earlobes responds well to laser and light devices used for retexturing and for treating dyschromia. Q-switched lasers, 1927-nm thulium nonablative laser, and intense pulsed light (IPL) treatments are among the therapies that can be effective for sun-induced earlobe dyspigmentation, whereas 1550-nm erbium glass nonablative and ablative fractional lasers can help to improve earlobe texture. If treating the face, one must not forget the earlobe.

PEARL 5 The use of HA fillers for earlobe rejuvenation is safe, effective, and well tolerated.

CONCLUSIONS

As more patients elect to undergo cosmetic treatments for the face and neck, earlobe restoration is garnering increasing attention. Research on soft tissue rejuvenation of this anatomic site remains in its nascent stages. However, empiric use of injectable fillers can safely and effectively improve the appearance of elongated or wrinkled ears, can help to support earrings in lobules with excess laxity or poorly placed piercing holes, and can prevent a discordant appearance between the ears and a rejuvenated face and neck. Laser and other energy-based treatments can further improve the quality of the earlobe skin.

FURTHER READING

Azaria, R., Adler, N., Silfen, R., Regev, D., & Hauben, D. J. (2003). Morphometry of the adult human earlobe: A study of 547 subjects and clinical application. *Plastic and Reconstructive Surgery*, *111*(7), 2398–2402. https://doi.org/10.1097/01.PRS.0000060995.99380.DE.

Christoffersen, M., Frikke-Schmidt, R., Schnohr, P., Jensen, G. B., Nordestgaard, B. G., & Tybjærg-Hansen, A. (2014). Visible age-related signs and risk of ischemic heart disease in the general population. *Circulation*, *129*, 990–998. https://doi.org/10.1161/CIRCULATIONAHA.113.001696.

De Oliveria Monteiro, E. (2006). Hyaluronic acid for restoring earlobe volume. *Skin Medicine*, *5*(6), 293–294. PMID: 17085997.

Di Gregorio, C., & D'Arpa, S. (2019). Nonsurgical treatment of earlobe aging in Mowlavi stages I and II earlobe ptosis with Hyaluronic acid fillers. *Journal of Cosmetic Dermatology*, *18*(2), 508–510. https://doi.org/10.1111/jocd.12688.

Farkas, L. G. (1990). Anthropometry of the normal and defective ear. *Clinics in Plastic Surgery*, *17*, 213. https://doi.org/10.1016/S0094-1298(20)31238-4.

Friedlander, A. H., López-López, J., & Velasco-Oretga, E. (2012). Diagonal ear lobe crease and atherosclerosis: A review of the medical literature and dental implications. *Medicina Oral, Patologia Oral y Cirugia Bucal*, *17*(1), e153–e159. https://doi.org/10.4317/medoral.17390.

Forte, A. J., Andrew, T. W., Colasante, C., & Persing, J. A. (2015). Perception of age, attractiveness, and tiredness after isolated and combined facial subunit aging. *Aesthetic Plastic Surgery*, *39*, 856–869. https://doi.org/10.1007/s00266-015-0553-1.

Hotta, T. (2011). Earlobe rejuvenation. *Plastic Surgical Nursing*, *31*(1), 39–40. https://doi.org/10.1097/PSN.0b013e31820f53fc.

Jemec, B. I. (1986). Earlobe augmentation. *Aesthetic Plastic Surgery*, *10*, 35–36. https://doi.org/10.1007/BF01575265.

Loeb, R. (1972). Earlobe tailoring during facial rhytidoplasties. *Plastic and Reconstructive Surgery*, *49*, 485–488. https://doi.org/10.1097/00006534-197205000-00001.

Mowlavi, A., Meldrum, G., Kalkanis, J., Wilhelmi, B. J., Russell, R. C., & Zook, E. G. (2005). Surgical design and algorithm for correction of earlobe ptosis and pseudoptosis deformity. *Plastic and Reconstructive Surgery*, *115*(1), 290–295. https://doi.org/10.1097/01.PRS.0000146705.10277.EE.

Mowlavi, A., Meldrum, D. G., Wilhelmi, B. J., & Zook, E. G. (2004). Effect of face lift on earlobe ptosis and pseudoptosis. *Plastic and Reconstructive Surgery, 114*(4), 988–991. https://doi.org/10.1097/01.prs.0000133172.28160.6f.

Mowlavi, A., Meldrum, D., Wilhelmi, B., & Zook, E. G. (2004). Incidence of earlobe ptosis and pseudoptosis in patients seeking facial rejuvenation surgery and effects of aging. *Plastic and Reconstructive Surgery, 113*(2), 712–717. https://doi.org/10.1097/01.PRS.0000101505.66716.DF.

Murray, C. A., Zloty, D., & Warshawski, L. (2005). The evolution of soft tissue fillers in clinical practice. *Dermatologic Clinics, 23*, 343–363. https://doi.org/10.1016/j.det.2004.09.009.

Saedi, N., Kaminer, M. S., & Dover, J. S. (2012). Earlobe rejuvenation. In J. Carruthers, & A. Carruthers (Eds.), *Soft tissue augmentation: procedures in cosmetic dermatology* (3rd ed., pp. 166–169). London, England: Elsevier.

31

Hyaluronic Acid Microdroplet Injection for Skin Quality Enhancement

Daniel Yanes and Shannon D. Humphrey

SUMMARY AND KEY FEATURES

- Skin quality encompasses visual, tactile, and mechanical attributes including hydration, smoothness, elasticity, and radiance of the skin. Healthy skin is an essential component of perceived beauty.
- Treatment of skin quality is an important yet often-overlooked aesthetic treatment.
- Hyaluronic acid microdroplet injection for skin quality is an effective, well-tolerated procedure with high patient satisfaction.
- Proper technique allows for predictable results without socially relevant downtime.
- Patients perceive improvement within days, with duration of results depending on the product.

INTRODUCTION

Traditionally, dermal filler has been used for volumetric augmentation of soft tissue, providing a means to counteract the bony resorption and atrophy of fat associated with aging. However, volumetric augmentation alone is insufficient to account for changes in complexion associated with the aging face. Hyaluronic acid (HA) microdroplet injection (micro) for skin quality enhancement is a procedure that is rapidly gaining popularity globally for treatment of the face, neck, and décolleté. Although these products are composed of HA, they are not used for volumetric augmentation but rather aim to improve nonvolumetric skin quality measures associated with aging, such as skin texture, elasticity, hydration, and radiance.

SKIN QUALITY

Skin quality is a poorly studied yet incredibly important component of attractiveness. Flawless skin is difficult to define yet almost universally desired and intuitively understood. Improvement of skin quality is gaining traction as a motivation for patients seeking aesthetic treatments, regardless of age.

Skin quality is inherently linked to perception of beauty and, as such, inherently has a psychosocial impact on individuals and how they interact with the world around them.

Effectively, "skin quality" is a term that captures the subjective smoothness, hydration, elasticity, and radiance of the skin. High-quality skin is smooth, radiant, pliable, and well hydrated. In contrast, roughness, dullness, prominent pores, crepiness, dryness, and laxity are features associated with poor skin quality. It is well described that some measures of skin quality, such as elasticity and smoothness, decline with age, yet poor skin quality is not necessarily synonymous with age-related change. Although much of aesthetic literature focuses on counteracting age-related change, it is essential to consider global skin quality and appearance of the skin in the approach to the aesthetic patient to ensure optimal outcomes.

PATIENT SELECTION, EXPECTATIONS, AND SATISFACTION

HA micro for skin quality enhancement provides predictable, natural results as a field treatment and is suitable across all patient skin types (Fig. 31.1). Physician

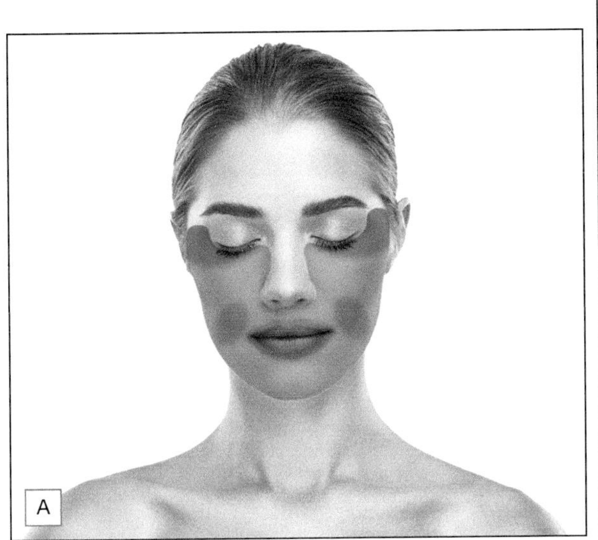

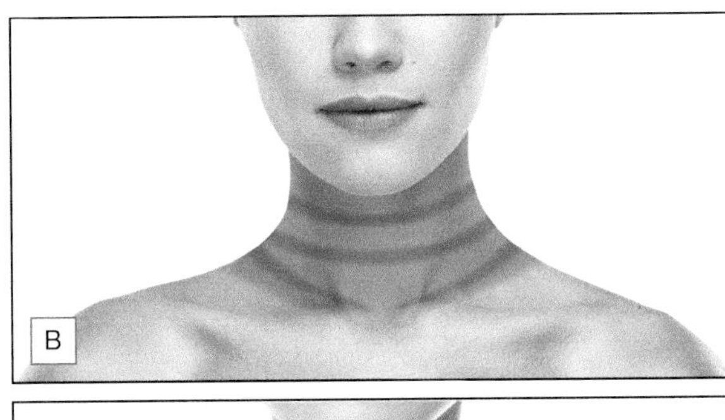

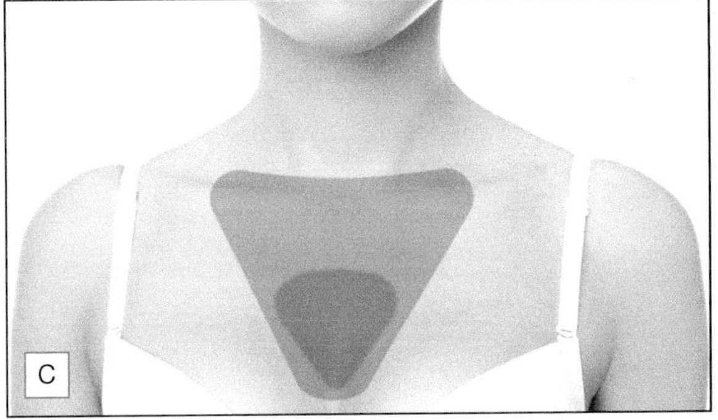

Fig. 31.1 Common sites for hyaluronic acid microdroplet injection. Light gray represents the entire treatment zone, whereas dark gray represents the treatment zone with increased density of injections for greater improvement. (A) Face. (B) Neck. (C) Chest.

and patient expectations must align. This is an injectable treatment to improve skin quality parameters, not for use in volumetric augmentation as a low G' filler. The treatment is additive and complementary to other cosmetic procedures designed to prevent or reduce signs of aging and is not meant to replace other procedures in the overall armamentarium. Patient satisfaction with these procedures is excellent, provided that expectations of treatment align with realistic outcomes. HA micro works well as a combination therapy with other procedures as part of a comprehensive aesthetic dermatology treatment plan (Fig. 31.2). Optimal combination strategies and safety have not been well studied.

The ideal patient for HA micro is one seeking youthful and healthier-appearing skin. The goal of the procedure is to improve skin luminosity, hydration, firmness, smoothness, and elasticity. As these are desirable skin quality goals for virtually every patient seeking cosmetic treatment, all patients are candidates for this procedure. The authors have identified specific patient archetypes that are well suited to HA micro. These include younger patients seeking "prejuvenation," preventing or impeding the changes associated with aging skin (i.e., as well as older patients hoping for gracefully aging skin). Notably, the treatment is well received by patients who are averse to dermal fillers. These patients should be counseled that although HA micro is composed of HA, these products function differently from filler for volumetric enhancement and are not used as such, except in specific circumstances when a low-viscosity HA with minimal lift is necessary. Lastly, HA micro is an appealing treatment for cosmetically motivated patients desiring an additional treatment while still avoiding unnatural appearing outcomes.

Injectable skin quality enhancement is well received as an initial treatment for those with skin quality concerns, as well as an additive procedure as part of a comprehensive treatment plan. These products have also been shown to be of value in treating small, distensible acne scars, with or without botulinum toxin, subscision, and adjunctive energy-based treatments. Patients with dry or rough skin respond well to the treatment. Patients with advanced photoaging, thicker skin, or darker skin and males may require an increased volume or number of treatment sessions. The volume of product needed depends on the skin quality of the patient, as those with more visible photodamage may require more volume.

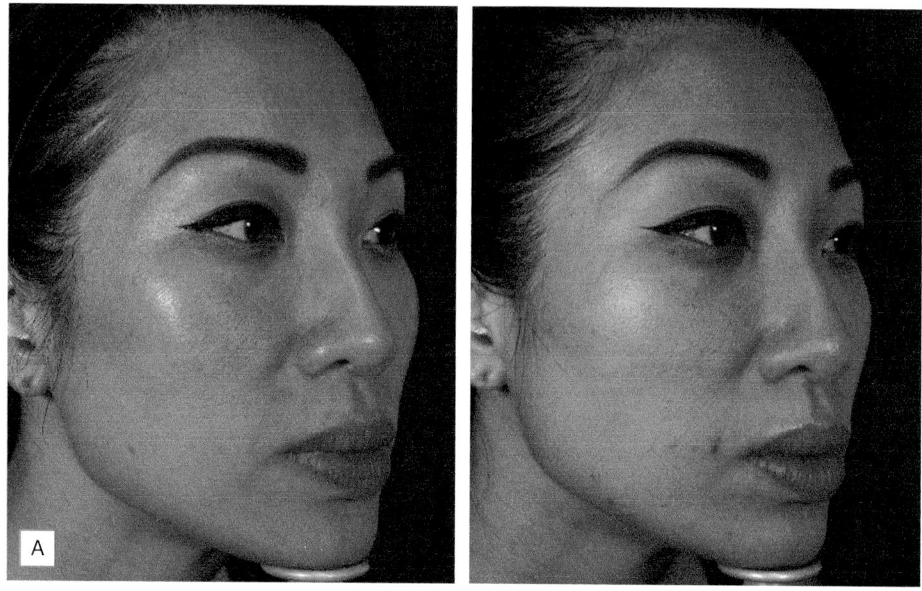

Dr. Shannon Humphrey
Cosmetic Dermatology

Before **After**

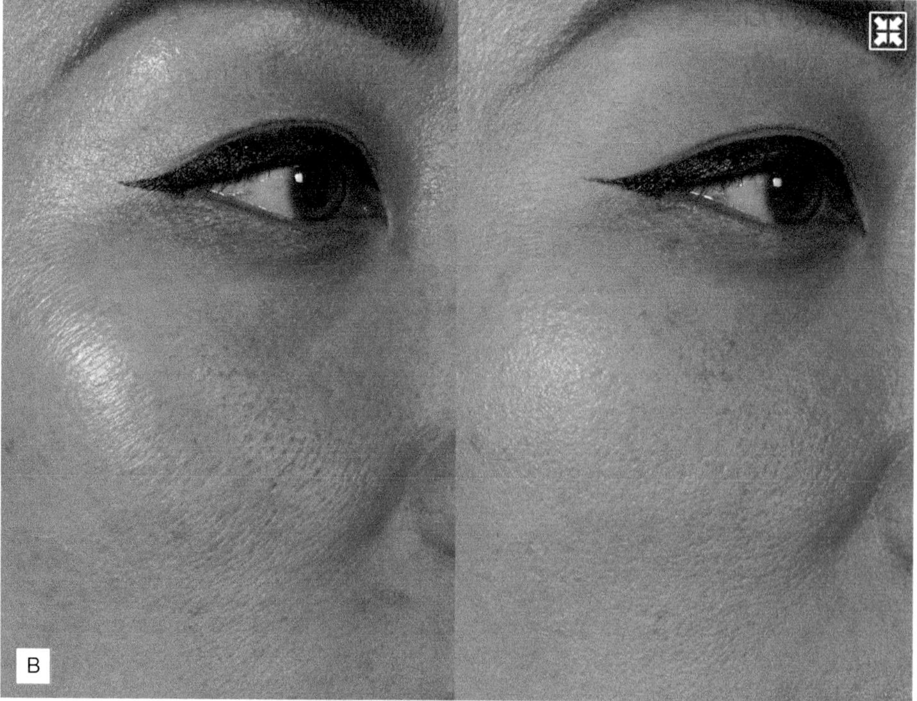

Dr. Shannon Humphrey
Cosmetic Dermatology

Before **After**

Fig. 31.2 Before and 7 weeks after treatment with 1 mL of Juvederm Volite to the (A) zygomatic and (B) malar cheek. (Please note 2–3 mL is recommended for best results.)

PRODUCT AND MECHANISM OF ACTION

HA micro is performed using low-G' HA gel and has been shown to be effective in skin quality enhancement of the face, neck, and décolleté. There are several available products available on the market, each with a unique formulation (Table 31.1). Note that the quality and study design of HA micro formulations vary greatly, including sample size, number of treatments, and duration of response. Studies of Juvéderm Volite have demonstrated effective, durable results after a single treatment session. Of note, these products are widely used globally but have not yet been granted regulatory approval in the United States at the time of this publication.

There are numerous proposed mechanisms of action of HA micro in improving skin quality and complexion, as summarized in Box 31.1. HA is known to be a hydrophilic molecule and subsequently is capable of improving hydration and skin turgor by nature of this property. Yet there are numerous other ways in which the product acts, which are somewhat less straightforward. HA micro is capable of stimulating neocollagenesis and also promotes synthesis of the extracellular matrix. These properties help to counteract the loss of skin elasticity, smoothness, and radiance associated with aging. Direct intradermal filling provides benefit to superficial cutaneous defects. In addition, the procedure itself involves numerous injections in a grid-like pattern that further serves to stimulate neocollagenesis.

TABLE 31.1 Products Available for Injectable Skin Quality Enhancement

Product	Company	Hyaluronic Acid Formulation
Juvéderm Volite	Allergan (Dublin, Ireland)	12 mg/mL Vycross HA
Restylane Skinboosters Vital	Galderma (Lausanne, Switzerland)	20 mg/mL nonanimal stabilized HA
Restylane Skinboosters Vital Light	Galderma (Lausanne, Switzerland)	12 mg/mL nonanimal stabilized HA
Belotero Revive	Merz (Frankfurt, Germany)	20 mg/mL Cohesive Polydensified Matrix HA 17.5 mg/mL glycerol
Teosyal Puresense Redensity 1	Teoxane (Geneva, Switzerland)	15 mg/mL RHA resilient HA

HA, Hyaluronic acid.

BOX 31.1 Proposed Mechanisms of Action of Hyaluronic Acid Microdroplet Injection

- Hydrophilic molecular structure
- Stimulation of neocollagenesis
- Cutaneous microfilling
- Microneedling effect

TECHNICAL CONSIDERATIONS

Preparation: The product is dispensed in 1-mL syringes. Treatment of the face typically requires 2 mL or more, depending on skin quality at baseline (Fig. 31.3). Off-face treatment requires higher volumes and/or treatment sessions. Prior to injection, ice or topical anesthesia can be applied to the treatment area. The treatment area should be cleansed thoroughly with a topical antiseptic solution such as 70% isopropyl alcohol or 4% chlorhexidine. The authors prefer on-label injection with several 32 G, ½-inch needles to allow for more accurate and precise delivery of product, customized to the patient's unique treatment plan, goals, and cutaneous anatomy. A 32 G needle is ideal for injection because they allow for excellent comfort and minimal bruising; however, it should be noted that they will dull quickly and require frequent changing throughout the procedure.

Injection technique differs greatly from traditional HA filler. The treatment itself is straightforward; however, correct placement of the product is essential to ensure optimal outcomes and avoid complications (Box 31.2). The product should be injected intradermally into the deep dermis or the immediate subdermis. To ensure appropriate placement, the skin should be stretched taut, and the needle should penetrate at a 0- to 45-degree angle to the skin to visualize the needle depth during injection (Video 31.1). Superficial placement should be avoided, as it will lead to bleb formation, which may not resolve on its own. Injection should be

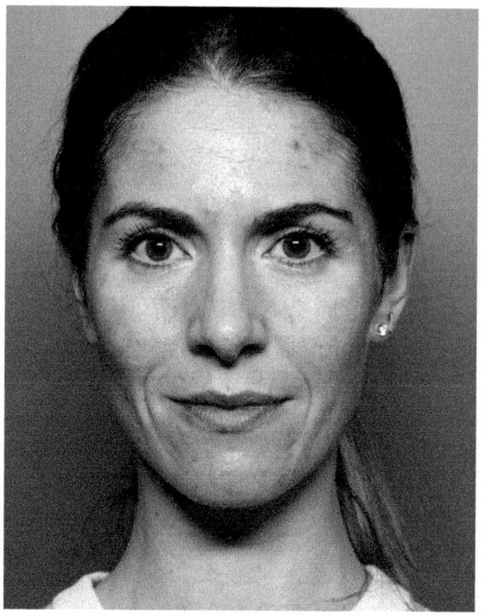

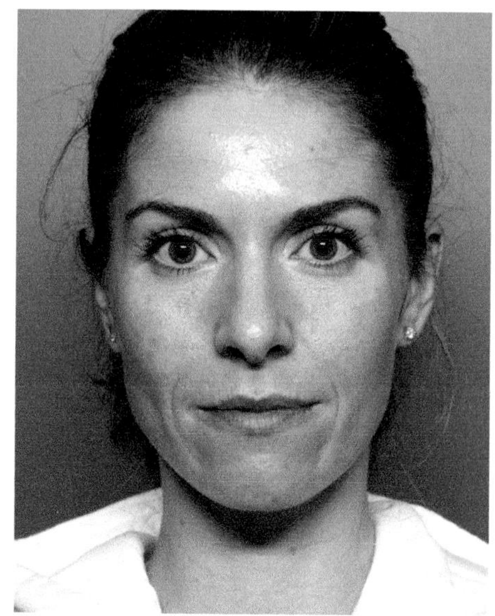

H Dr. Shannon Humphrey Cosmetic Dermatology

Fig. 31.3 Before and 4 weeks after combination treatment with 2 mL Juvederm Volite to the Cheeks, 30u Onabotulinumtoxin A to the upper face, and a low powered fractional 1927-nm diode laser treatment using the "high" setting (Clear + Brilliant Permea, Solta Medical, Hayward, CA).

BOX 31.2 Summary of the Hyaluronic Acid Microdroplet Injection Technique

- 32 G ½" needle penetrating at a 0- to 45-degree angle
- 0.01–0.05 mL per injection in deep dermis or immediate subdermis
- 2–3 mL for the entire face
- Increased density of droplets in areas requiring greater degree of improvement (i.e. perioral lines, lateral canthal lines, large pores, etc.)
- Consider starting injections on lateral face to allow for calibration of extrusion force

ceased prior to withdrawing the needle to avoid superficial placement. If a bleb is visualized, immediate massage should be performed.

Using a 32 G, ½-inch needle, microdepot injections of 0.01 to 0.05 mL are performed in a grid-like fashion every 0.5 to 1 cm evenly across the targeted area. The authors prefer performing the initial injection into the lateral malar cheek to allow for calibration of technique and extrusion force in a less painful and less visible region of the face. Following this, more targeted injections can be performed if there are notable areas with textural anomalies. Frequent needle changes should be performed throughout the procedure as described earlier. More damaged skin may require more closely spaced injections or more volume. Injection techniques utilizing cannulae or stamping devices/injection guns have been described but are less well studied. Stamping devices and injection guns do, however, present a potentially appealing way to reliably deliver equidistant microdroplets at the appropriate depth. With experience and a clinical assistant available to aid with sharp needle exchange, the procedure takes 5 to 10 minutes on average.

COMPLICATIONS AND MANAGEMENT

With frequent needle changes and measures to ensure patient comfort, the procedure is very well tolerated. There is typically minimal bruising and swelling, and there is no significant downtime associated with the procedure. Postprocedural counseling is similar to that of HA dermal filler. Patients should be counseled that the effect of the product is not immediate and is expected to appear gradually over 5 to 10 days. Although further study is required to characterize, studies suggest that peak improvement is achieved weeks to months after the initial injection, which is corroborated by the authors' experience. Effect duration is dependent on the formulation of HA micro. Patients may continue treatments at regular intervals for maintenance. It is important to recognize that given the nature of the procedure in improving overall skin quality rather than augmenting volume or facial features, the results of the treatment require consistent high-quality clinical photography. In our experience, patients readily appreciate tactile improvements in hydration and smoothness.

Bruising, swelling, and mild discomfort are the most common adverse events. Late-onset papules are rare but can occur. As with any injectable HA gel, intravascular injection can lead to cutaneous vascular compromise. Proper placement of the product intradermally will reduce the risk of nodules and vascular compromise. As aforementioned, blebbing of the skin should be avoided as they do not always spontaneously self-resolve. Blebs should be massaged immediately at the time of treatment should they form.

CONCLUSIONS

In the comprehensive approach to managing aging skin of the neck, face, and décolleté, it is important to consider hydration, luminosity, texture, and elasticity of the skin in addition to volume. HA micro for skin quality enhancement is a growing procedure worldwide that addresses these often-neglected factors.

FURTHER READING

Cavallini, M., Papagni, M., Ryder, T. J., & Patalano, M. (2019). Skin quality improvement with VYC-12, a new injectable hyaluronic acid: Objective results using digital analysis. *Dermatologic Surgery*, *45*(12), 1598–1604. https://doi.org/10.1097/DSS.0000000000001932.

Hertz-Kleptow, D., Hanschmann, A., Hofmann, M., Reuther, T., & Kerscher, M. (2019). Facial skin revitalization with CPM®-HA20G: An effective and safe early intervention treatment. *Clinical, Cosmetic and Investigational Dermatology*, *12*, 563–572. https://doi.org/10.2147/CCID.S209256.

Humphrey, S., Manson Brown, S., Cross, S., & Mehta, R. (2014). Defining skin quality: Clinical relevance, terminology, and assessment. *Dermatologic Surgery*, *47*(7), 974–981. https://doi.org/10.1097/DSS.0000000000003079.

Kerscher, M., Bayrhammer, J., & Reuther, T. (2008). Rejuvenating influence of a stabilized hyaluronic acid-based gel of nonanimal origin on facial skin aging. *Dermatologic Surgery*, *34*(5), 720–726. https://doi.org/10.1111/j.1524-4725.2008.34176.x.

Lee, B. M., Han, D. G., & Choi, W. S. (2015). Rejuvenating effects of facial hydrofilling using Restylane Vital. *Archives of Plastic Surgery*, *42*(3), 282–287. https://doi.org/10.5999/aps.2015.42.3.282.

Lim, H. K., Suh, D. H., Lee, S. J., & Shin, M. K. (2014). Rejuvenation effects of hyaluronic acid injection on nasojugal groove: Prospective randomized split face clinical controlled study. *Journal of Cosmetic and Laser Therapy*, *16*(1), 32–36. https://doi.org/10.3109/14764172.2013.854620.

Niforos, F., Ogilvie, P., Cavallini, M., et al. (2019). VYC-12 injectable gel is safe and effective for improvement of facial skin topography: A prospective study. *Clinical, Cosmetic and Investigational Dermatology*, *12*, 791–798. https://doi.org/10.2147/CCID.S216222.

Ogilvie, P., Safa, M., Chantrey, J., et al. (2020). Improvements in satisfaction with skin after treatment of facial fine lines with VYC-12 injectable gel: Patient-reported outcomes from a prospective study. *Journal of Cosmetic Dermatology*, *19*(5), 1065–1070. https://doi.org/10.1111/jocd.13129.

Proietti, I., Skroza, N., & Potenza, C. (2021). Improving skin quality in patients with dermatologic conditions using the hyaluronic acid filler VYC-12. *Italian Journal of Dermatology and Venereology*, *156*(6), 720–721. https://doi.org/10.23736/S2784-8671.19.06453-8.

Wang, F., Garza, L. A., Kang, S., et al. (2007). In vivo stimulation of de novo collagen production caused by cross-linked hyaluronic acid dermal filler injections in photodamaged human skin. *Archives of Dermatology*, *143*(2), 155–163. https://doi.org/10.1001/archderm.143.2.155.

32

Filler Injection Techniques

Omer Ibrahim, Elizabeth Kream, and Jeffrey S. Dover

SUMMARY AND KEY FEATURES

- The most common techniques for filler injection include linear threading, bolus, serial puncture, fanning, and cross-hatching.
- A combination of techniques, as well as layering of various techniques and fillers, is often employed to address both volume defects and superficial wrinkles.
- The proper technique reduces side effects such as pain, swelling, and bruising and yields better results and happier patients.
- While injections with needles and cannulas are both relatively safe, cannula-delivered injections are associated with a lower risk of vascular compromise and thus should be considered in high-risk areas.
- When cannulas are smaller than 25 gauge, they behave more like needles, and thus the protective benefit of cannulas is not afforded.

INTRODUCTION

The placement of soft tissue fillers can be likened to four-dimensional sculpture, with the fourth dimension representing dynamic movement. With this analogy in mind, rather than a hammer and chisel, an injector's toolbox includes needles and cannulas. Both art forms involve a few basic techniques that can be combined to lead to a tailored result; instead of casting and modeling, filler injection hinges on techniques like threading and fanning. The artist injector must have a detailed knowledge of anatomical structures, as the appropriate "canvas" or injection plane, changes depending on the anatomic site, injectable material, injection instrument, and desired result. In this chapter, we discuss the instruments used for injection and the fundamental techniques commonly employed to deliver soft tissue filler.

GENERAL INJECTION PRINCIPLES

Despite a myriad of stylistic approaches, safe and efficacious filler injection rests on a bedrock of good practice principles. Patient selection should ensure that the injection site is free from infection or recent procedures. Even a distant history of surgery, which can lead to vascular aberrancies, should indicate a pause in the procedure, especially in risk-prone sites like the nose. While patients may be fixated on a single fold or wrinkle, the clinician must determine if the requested injection will indeed add harmony to the patient's appearance. The patient's desired endpoint may require injection of a different anatomic site or be better achieved using a laser or energy-based modality. Once the patient is deemed an appropriate candidate and a mutual goal is shared by the patient and injector, enthusiastic written and verbal consent should be obtained. In addition to consent, pretreatment photographs not only are informative for the follow-up appointment but also serve as a safeguard in the case of medico-legal issues. The patient should be free of makeup and the skin cleansed with an appropriate antiseptic such as chlorhexidine, isopropyl alcohol, povidone-iodine, or hypochlorous acid solution. The patient should be positioned in a comfortable upright position, with lighting placed in a fashion that properly showcases the defect.

The syringe is often held near the barrel flange between the second and third fingers of the dominant hand, with the first digit in contact with the plunger thumb rest. Adducting the arms toward the trunk and resting the injecting hand on the nondominant hand minimize additional pivot points, so that movement is limited to the dexterous joints of the injecting hand (Video 32.1). Sometimes, the skin surrounding the injecting site may need to be stretched or pressure must be applied to surrounding vascular structures, and in these situations, the extra hands of a trained assistant are invaluable.

Prior to filler injection, aspiration is a maneuver that involves retracting the plunger to around 0.2–0.3 mL, holding this position for a minimum of 5 to 8 seconds, and assessing for a flash of blood entering the syringe. The presence of this flash indicates that the needle has mistakenly been placed within a vessel, and the injector must withdraw and establish a different injection point. While specific, this safety checkpoint is not sensitive; the absence of a flash does not guarantee that the injection will be extravascular. Examples where a flash may not be observed include the use of highly viscous fillers and small needles, unintentionally pinning a vessel down to the supraperiosteal plane, or cases where the needle has inadvertently changed position. Due to the likelihood of false-negatives, the practice of aspiration is highly debated. Still, aspiration is advised in high-risk areas.

A recent study proposed a revised method for aspiration, where the needle is loaded with saline before being attached to the filler syringe. The authors hypothesized that aspirating with a saline-loaded needle would "open" a path of less resistance for blood to travel into the syringe. In vitro head-to-head testing of the traditional and saline-loaded aspiration techniques using 27- and 29-gauge needles with six different hyaluronic acid fillers found that traditional aspiration was positive only in a few trials with the 27-gauge needle and false in all 29-gauge needles. In contrast, aspiration with a saline-loaded needle resulted in positive aspiration with all needle sizes and fillers, along with exhibiting a significantly shorter time to flash. In addition to aspiration, some injectors may elect to use Doppler ultrasound or other imaging devices to help avoid intravascular injection. Still, no safeguard is totally reliable, nor do they replace an intimate knowledge of anatomy and injection technique.

Depending on filler viscosity, a degree of extrusion force must be applied to the plunger for the filler to plastically deform and begin to flow as a fluid. When injecting, it is important to use minimal force. Devastating vascular complications may involve retrograde flow of product through the arterial system, which requires a forceful injection that overcomes systolic blood pressure. It has been observed that typical injection pressures are fortunately lower than that required to cause propagation of filler intravascularly; however, the required force for intravascular propagation is only 50% to 75% the reserve strength of the fingertip and 5% to 10% that of the thenar eminence. Because the strength of the fingers could theoretically propagate a column of filler through an artery, injectors should never overcome met resistance by increasing injection force; rather, the injector should withdraw and reposition the instrument so that injection with minimal force can occur. Certain practices can help reduce extrusion forces. Analogous to the difference in fuel required to drive a car on an open road versus stop-and-go traffic, less force is required for continuous injection compared to injecting after every stop. Mixing fillers with lidocaine/epinephrine or normal saline reduces viscosity and thus lowers the required extrusion force. The addition of lidocaine/epinephrine can also obviate the need for additional anesthesia, and epinephrine may reduce the risk of bruising and vascular compromise.

The quantity of filler injected and rate of injection are additional variables related to successful injection. Even if a vessel is perforated, a slow injection will deliver a forward force less than the back pressure in the lacerated vessel, thus preventing introduction of filler into the lumen. Moreover, a slow injection rate allows tissue to equilibrate, which results in less pain. Limiting both the number of syringes per treatment and the amount of filler delivered per needlestick decreases the risk of intravascular and extravascular occlusion, along with the risk of biofilm formation. Generally, no more than 0.2 mL should be injected per individual thread or bolus. For example, if a 0.5 mL bolus of filler is desired to augment the lateral cheek, the injection should be divided into two smaller bolus injections. Too much filler, especially in areas like the tear trough, can lead to poor aesthetic outcomes such as the Tyndall effect and malar edema. It is better to undercorrect and follow up with a touch-up treatment several weeks after edema has resolved.

Because static rhytids form over underlying vasculature, such as the nasolabial crease over the angular artery and glabella lines over the supratrochlear and dorsal nasal artery anastomoses, rhytids can serve as a compass for needle placement. Needle placement parallel to rhytides increases the chance of residing within the arterial system compared to a perpendicular alignment. In contrast, parallel insertion with a blunt cannula is safer. A study examining different insertion angles of a 25-gauge cannula in relation to the superficial temporal artery found that perforation is most common when the cannula is aligned with a trajectory perpendicular to the neighboring artery. When injecting in high-risk areas such as the glabella or nasolabial folds, it is especially important to keep the injection instrument in constant movement. If blanching is observed or the patient reports pain, the injection must be immediately stopped and a prompt transition must be made to prevent or mitigate vascular compromise. Avoiding and managing vascular compromise are detailed in other chapters.

Cannulas and Needles

Although many soft tissue fillers come prepackaged with two suggested needles, many practitioners opt for different injection instruments depending on the anatomic site to be treated, type of filler, goal of treatment, injector's training, and patient factors (e.g., age, history of procedures in the area, current medications/supplements, etc.). Needles are stainless-steel cylinders that come to a sharp angular point, often coated in silicone, to allow a smooth penetration into the skin. A needle's sharpness varies, based on the length and angle of the bevel. The central lumen allows for the aspiration and delivery of fluids, and the lumen's size is known as the gauge. Needles are available in different lengths and gauges, the latter of which is easily denoted by the color of the needle hub (Fig. 32.1). Commonly used needles for soft tissue filler range from 25 to 32 gauge and from ½ to 1¼ inches in length.

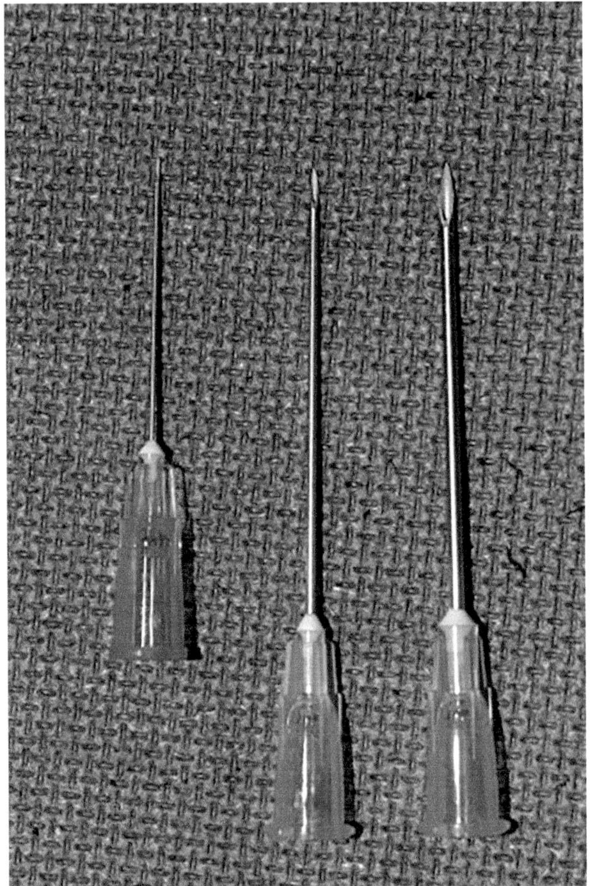

Fig. 32.1 Hypodermic needles of varying gauge sizes. (Courtesy of Nextra Health. https://www.nextrahealth.com/store/syringes-and-needle-supplies/BD305195.html?gclid=Cj0KCQjw9YWDBhDyARIsADt6sGYbdIrowrxEtwlgHfuq-M3jBhJjpkQGrxNApc5x5bK1T9HjxE8h3y8aArYeEALw_wcB.)

Since the 1950s, cannulas have been employed for the safe delivery of intravenous fluids; however, in the early 2000s, their use extended to cosmetic procedures, specifically to deliver fat for autologous fat transfer. Over the last decade, cannulas have been increasingly used to deliver soft tissue filler. Cannulas are bendable blunt-tipped metal tubes, with a delivery port approximately 1 to 2 mm proximal to the blunt tip (Fig. 32.2). For soft tissue filler delivery, cannulas are usually longer than needles, with common lengths ranging from 1½ to 2 inches and gauge ranging from 22 to 27. Because of the

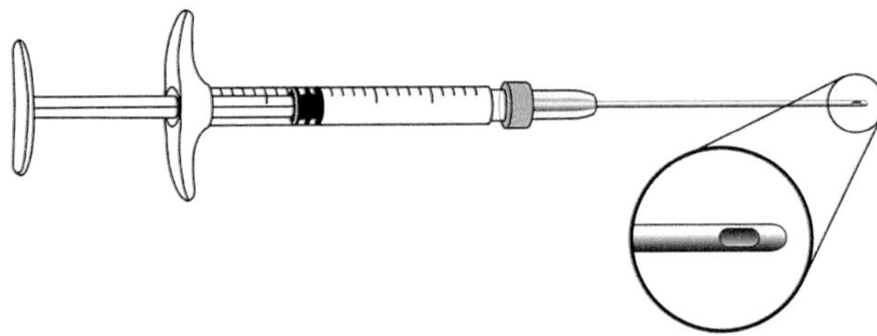

Fig. 32.2 Blunt-tipped cannula with side injection port. (Modified from Alam M, Tung R. Injection technique in neurotoxins and fillers: indications, products, and outcomes. *J Am Acad Dermatol*. 2018;79:423–435.)

blunt tip, cannulas require an entry point to be created by a needle that is 1 to 2 gauges larger than the cannula (e.g., a 23-gauge needle is often used to create an entry point for a 25-gauge cannula). The cannula is then obliquely tunneled through the entry point and glided through a horizontal injection plane.

The shift to using cannulas for soft tissue filler was galvanized by the concept that rather than piercing through neurovascular structures, cannulas would instead slide around the respective structures. Less tissue trauma translates to a decrease in both common adverse events like bruising and rare adverse events like vascular compromise. Although the protective benefit of cannulas has been acknowledged by many clinicians, Alam et al. recently quantified the degree of risk reduction when using cannulas over needles. They performed a large retrospective cohort study of 370 board-certified dermatologists, with a total of 7000 person-years of experience and 1.7 million syringes of filler injected. Participants entered deidentified data of volume statistics pertaining to patients undergoing filler procedures for the preceding 10 years. The study concluded that the risk of vascular occlusion per syringe of filler is very low with either cannulas or needles (fewer than 1 per 5000 syringes) and fortunately most occlusions remit without even a scar. However, occlusion risk was less with cannulas (1 per 40,882 1-mL syringe for cannulas and 1 per 6410 for needles), with a 77.1% lower odds ratio of occlusion. The authors concluded that cannulas are associated with a lower occlusion risk, and their use should be considered for high-risk areas such as the nasolabial folds, glabella, and nose, when practical. In accordance with this study, a 2019 literature review of filler-associated blindness identified 60 unique cases, and of 20 cases that reported injection techniques, 70% (14/20) employed needles. Of course, these safety data were gleaned from skilled physicians who perform a high volume of injections, and thus, data cannot be applied to settings where untrained physicians or nonphysicians perform injections.

An argument against using cannulas is that they provide less precision. However, if precision is defined as filler remaining in the plane of intended implantation, recent cadaveric studies demonstrate that cannulas are more precise. Both studies involved injection with needles and cannulas intended for the supraperiosteal plane of various facial sites. In one study, fluoroscopy analyses revealed that needle injection resulted in a 33.3% displacement of filler to more superficial layers. While cannulas still have backflow, the backflow generally remains within the horizontal plane, due to the cannula's traditionally oblique insertion. If needles are inserted at an angle, rather than perpendicular, their precision could approach that of cannulas; however, this would require a longer needle trajectory and thus increase tissue trauma.

In practice, maneuvering cannulas on a supraperiosteal plane can be technically difficult and uncomfortable for patients. Another cadaveric study comparing precision of filler placement of the vermilion lip using 27-gauge cannulas and 30-gauge needles found no statistical difference in precision and found that while cannulas showed a uniform injection, material was deposited in an unintended deeper intramuscular plane, rather than the intended submucosal plane. This study implies that when the intended plane is superficial, needles may be more accurate.

Although cannulas have a blunt tip and side injection port, they should not be viewed as completely atraumatic. Pavicic et al. demonstrated in a cadaveric study involving penetration procedures of the facial and superficial temporal arteries using needles and cannulas of varying sizes that as cannulas decrease in size to 27 gauge, they behave similar to needles of the corresponding size, in terms of force required to penetrate an artery. Another cadaveric study involving force testing of cannulas ranging in size from 18 to 27 gauge revealed that a low amount of force is required to penetrate the facial artery when cannulas smaller than 22 gauge are used. A significant direct correlation between decreasing gauge size and required force for arterial penetration was also observed. Compared to needles, decreased tactile sensation with cannulas makes it difficult to discriminate between the resistance of a fibrous septum and that of an artery. Thus, when resistance is encountered, reinsertion is preferred over forcing the cannula through. Needles may be indicated for injection sites with increased fibrous septae, such as the lower face of a patient with acne scarring or a history of rhytidectomy.

Neither needles nor cannulas ensure absolute safety or efficacy, and providers must be aware of other variables that can modulate a treatment's outcome. The importance of recognizing other risk factors is illuminated by a recently reported tragic case of hyaluronic acid filler-associated cerebral infarction and death. Despite a cannula being used to inject the nose, a high-risk area, an excessive amount of filler (2 mL) was injected, and the patient was still healing from another procedure performed in the same area. This devastating case underscores that even when using cannulas, safety is not guaranteed, and it is paramount to be vigilant of all variables.

INJECTION TECHNIQUES

A variety of techniques exist for placing soft tissue fillers. The most common techniques are discussed here. Site-specific applications of these techniques are also discussed in other chapters. In practice, multiple techniques are often combined. Stacking or layering involves injecting thinner fillers superficially and more viscous fillers at deeper layers to concurrently address superficial lines and deeper volume loss.

Linear Threading

In retrograde threading, the needle or cannula is inserted at an oblique (< 90 degrees) angle and is advanced, and filler is deposited in a retrograde fashion as the cannula or needle is retracted (Fig. 32.3) (Video 32.2).

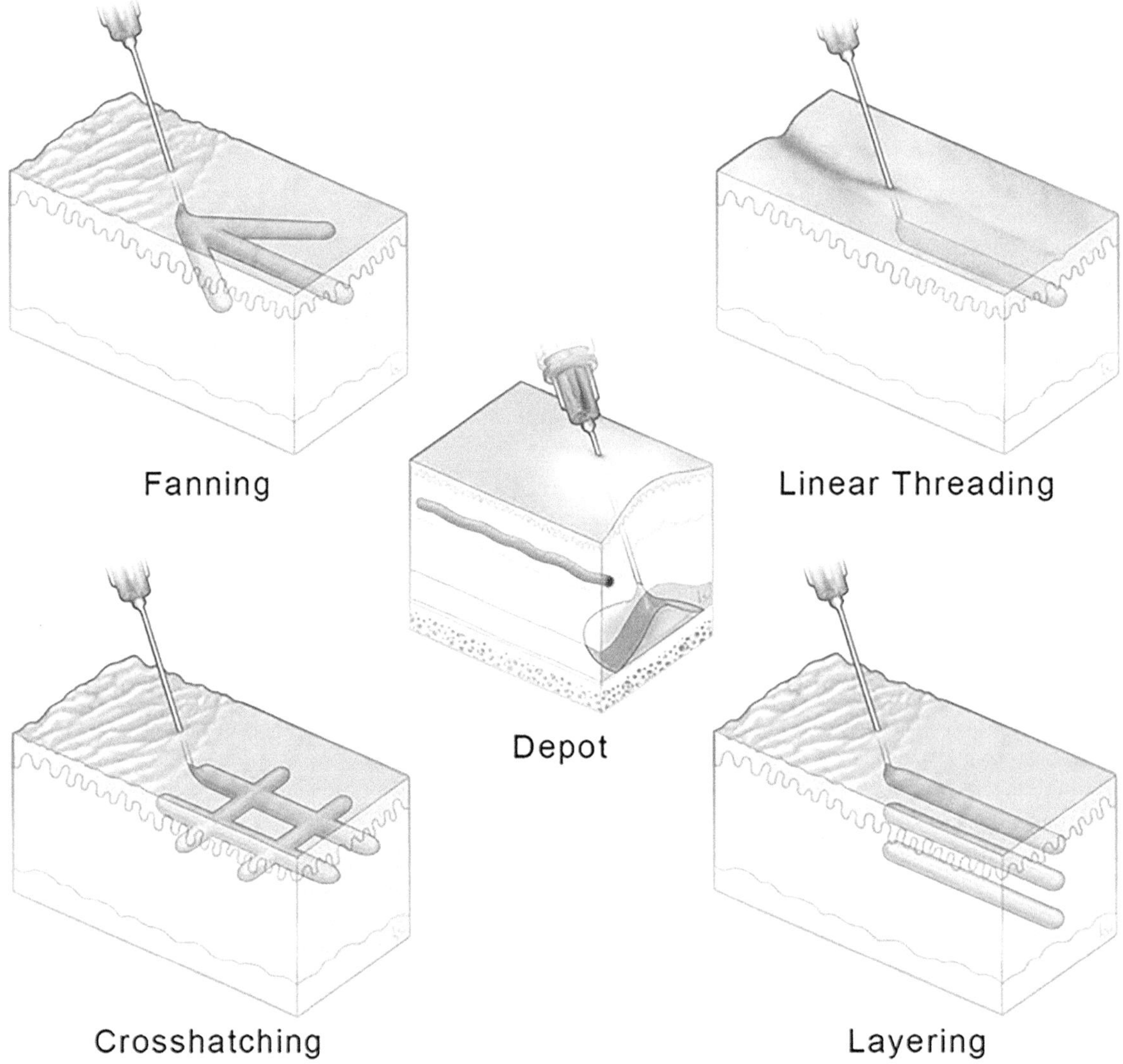

Fig. 32.3 Various injection techniques employed for soft-tissue filler delivery. (Modified from Akinbiyi T, Othman S, Familusi O, Calvert C, Card EB, Percec I. Better results in facial rejuvenation with fillers. *Plast Reconstr Surg Glob Open*. 2020;8:e2763.)

With constant pressure, this movement ultimately creates a linear "thread" of filler. Anterograde threading also results in a "thread" of filler; however, injection commences upon instrument insertion, so that filler is deposited ahead of the advancing needle or cannula. Rather than the instrument creating a tunnel for injection, anterograde threading allows hydrodissection of tissue due to the cleaving pressure of the deposited filler. Therefore, tissue trauma may be reduced with anterograde threading. Still, many prefer retrograde filler because the artificial tunnel created by the injecting instrument allows for less injection pressure and more reliability of filler placement. In sensitive sites like the vermillion lip, anterograde threading may be more comfortable for the patient.

The threading technique is frequently employed to define the philtral columns and vermillion border and to fill in superficial rhytides such as the "barcode lines" on the upper cutaneous lip. The tear troughs are sometimes filled using a threading technique with cannula. Retrograde linear threading with diluted calcium hydroxylapatite or low-viscosity hyaluronic acid along skin tension lines is a modality to treat the crepiness of nonfacial sites such as the neck, décolleté, and abdomen.

Bolus

When targeting deeper volume deficits, a bolus technique is often employed. The cannula or needle if often inserted at a 60- to 90-degree angle to deliver a depot of filler to the supraperiosteal plane or deep fat pads (Fig. 32.3) (Video 32.3). The deep filler implantation acts as a structural pillar. During injection, some recommend using the noninjecting hand to lift or gently pinch the skin, thereby increasing resistance to discourage superficial backflow. The amount of filler deposited ranges from a microaliquot (0.01–0.05 mL) to a small bolus (0.3 mL). Following injection, the area is massaged to spread the product uniformly. Because only a few injections are required, the bolus technique may be associated with less pain and bruising. Even with hyaluronic acid fillers, which are traditionally thought to create an effect for 12 to 18 months, bolus injection at the periosteal level may have an enduring volumization effect, due to neocollagenesis mediated by fibroblast stretching and possible ossification induction.

When a needle is used, the injector must ensure that the bolus is being deposited in a known avascular area (e.g., bone). While it is good practice to change needles and cannula frequently, it is especially important when bone is touched. The temporal hollows are commonly treated with one or two boluses injected at a point 1 cm superior to the brow along the lateral fusion line and one centimeter posterior to this, followed by massage with a cotton-tip applicator. The lateral cheek can be volumized with a few boluses placed deep under the malar fat pad or at the supraperiosteal plane. Other facial sites treated with the bolus technique include the mandibular angle, mental protuberance, and alar bases. Hand rejuvenation can be approached by injecting a bolus of diluted calcium hydroxylapatite or low-viscosity hyaluronic acid in three sites on the dorsal hand and massaging until fully blended and smooth.

Serial Puncture

In the serial puncture technique, multiple small injections of filler are deposited in close proximity so that the material coalesces into a smooth implantation (Fig. 32.4) (Video 32.4). This technique is used in very specific circumstances such as a "touch up" after an adjunct technique or to deliver discrete amounts of filler to define small areas such as the Cupid's bow. Some may employ the serial puncture technique to efface static rhytids, by injecting microdroplets into the superficial subcutis along the track of the rhytid. The serial puncture technique may be considered for the glabella area. Serial

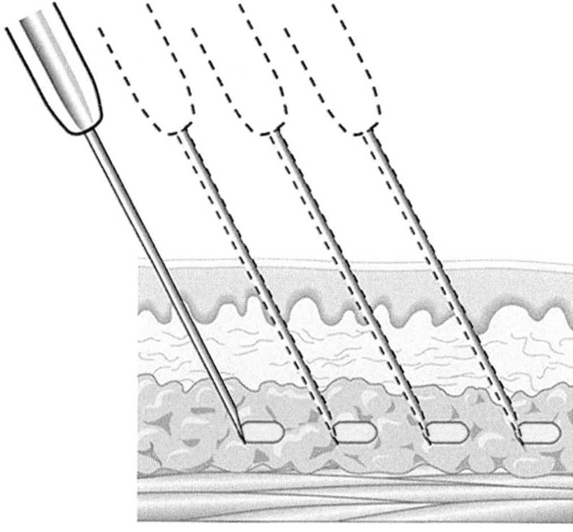

Fig. 32.4 The serial puncture technique. (Modified from Alam M, Tung R. Injection technique in neurotoxins and fillers: planning and basic technique. *J Am Acad Dermatol.* 2018;79:407–419.)

puncture using microdroplets (0.02–0.04 mL) of diluted calcium hydroxylapatite or low-viscosity hyaluronic acid may be considered to address nonfacial fine wrinkling, such as on the neck. Unlike threading, the instrument is oriented at a more vertical (approaching 90 degrees) angle and there is little lateral movement; thus, there may be less trauma. A downside to this technique is that it requires multiple needlesticks, and there is a risk of filler being placed too superficially, in the intradermal layer, leading to unnatural results.

Fanning

In the fanning technique, the cannula or needle is inserted through a single entry point, a thread is injected, and then the instrument is retracted and redirected at a slightly different angle to inject additional threads (Fig. 32.3) (Video 32.5). This process results in a radial or arc-like deposition of filler. The advent of cannulas resulted in increased use of the fanning technique. The cheeks are commonly volumized using the fanning technique with the cannula inserted in the superficial subdermal plane. A recently published algorithm for injecting the infraorbital hollows involves a combination of supraperiosteal bolus injections and fanning at the level of the suborbicularis oculi fat pad with a cannula. Mandibular augmentation can be achieved with fanning using a cannula inserted at the dorsum of the mandibular angle. Other common areas include the nasolabial folds, temporal fossa, and the triangular depressions lateral to the labiomental groove. A benefit of fanning is that a large area can be treated with less entry points. While all techniques can result in bruising, the fanning technique may be associated with more bruising.

Cross-hatching

The cross-hatching technique builds on the threading or fanning techniques discussed earlier. A series of threads, or multiple fans, at slightly different angles, are injected (Fig. 32.3). Cross-hatching results in a grid pattern of filler that provides structural support. This technique is an excellent method to treat skin redundancy such as an overhanging inferomedial cheek at the nasolabial fold or to buttress the oral commissures (Fig. 32.5). The technique can also be used to augment the angle of the mandible. When the "bar code" lines of the cutaneous lip are exceptionally prominent, the addition of cross-hatching can help to soften the area.

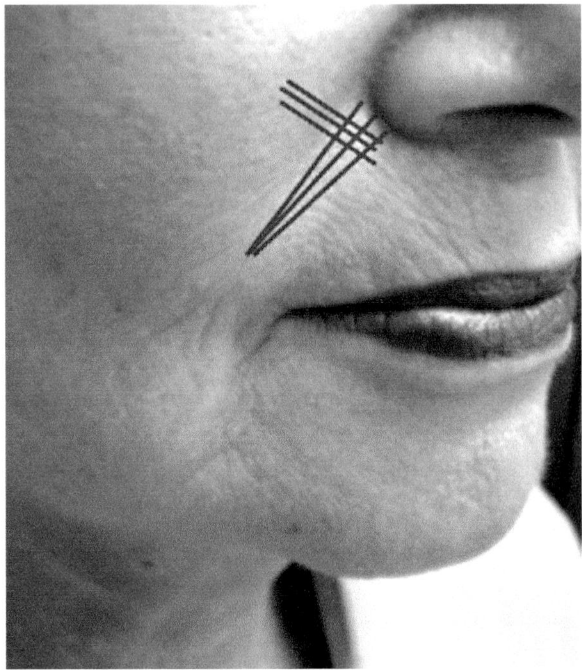

Fig. 32.5 Fanning and cross-hatching techniques are often used to correct the nasolabial fold. (Modified from Bass LS. Injectable filler techniques for facial rejuvenation, volumization, and augmentation. *Facial Plast Surg Clin North Am*. 2015;23:479–488.)

CONCLUSIONS

The abundance of "How We Do It" publications underscores that soft tissue filler techniques can be employed and combined in many effective ways. Regardless of injection instrument or technique, the literature shows that experience and frequency of performing soft tissue filler injections contribute to safe outcomes. Like any art, the importance of practice cannot be emphasized enough. Injectors must recognize their strengths and weaknesses and not let the patient or popular trends sway them to perform an injection they are uncomfortable with. Equipped with a thorough knowledge of the basic principles and techniques discussed, clinicians can adopt a meticulous and systematic way of evaluating and treating their patients, so that both safety and efficacy are optimized.

FURTHER READING

Alam, M., & Tung, R. (2018). Injection technique in neurotoxins and fillers: Indications, products, and outcomes. *Journal of the American Academy of Dermatology*, *79*, 423–435.

Alam, M., & Tung, R. (2018). Injection technique in neurotoxins and fillers: Planning and basic technique. *Journal of the American Academy of Dermatology*, *79*, 407–419.

Alam, M., Kakar, R., Dover, J. S., et al. (2021). Rates of vascular occlusion associated with using needles vs cannulas for filler injection. *JAMA Dermatology.*, *157*(2), 174–180.

Bass, L. S. (2015). Injectable filler techniques for facial rejuvenation, volumization, and augmentation. *Facial Plastic Surgery Clinics of North America*, *23*, 479–488.

Beer, K. R. (2014). Safety and effectiveness of injection of calcium hydroxylapatite via blunt cannula compared to injection by needle for correction of nasolabial folds. *Journal of Cosmetic Dermatology*, *13*, 288–296.

Bhatia, A., Arndt, K. A., Dover, J. S., Kaminer, M., & Rohrer, T. E. (2005). Bacterial sterility of stored non-animal stabilized hyaluronic acid based cutaneous filler. *Archives of Dermatology*, *141*, 1317.

Blandford, A. D., Hwang, C. J., Young, J., Barnes, A. C., Plesec, T. P., & Perry, J. D. (2018). Microanatomical location of hyaluronic acid gel following injection of the upper lip vermillion border: Comparison of needle and microcannula injection technique. *Ophthalmic Plastic and Reconstructive Surgery*, *34*, 296–299.

Braz, A., Humphrey, S., Weinkle, S., Yee, G. J., Remington, B. K., Lorenc, Z. P., et al. (2015). Lower face: Clinical anatomy and regional approaches with injectable fillers. *Plastic and Reconstructive Surgery*, *136*, 235S–257S.

Breithaupt, A. D., Jones, D. H., Braz, A., Narins, R., & Weinkle, S. (2015). Anatomical basis for safe and effective volumization of the temple. *Dermatologic Surgery*, *41*(suppl 1), S278–S283.

Casabona, G., Bernardini, F. P., Skippen, B., Rosamilia, G., Hamade, H., Frank, K., et al. (2020). How to best utilize the line of ligaments and the surface volume coefficient in facial soft tissue filler injections. *Journal of Cosmetic Dermatology*, *19*, 303–311.

De Boulle, K. (2004). Management of complications after implantation of fillers. *Journal of Cosmetic Dermatology*, *3*, 2–15.

de Maio, M., DeBoulle, K., Braz, A., & Rohrich, R. J. (2017). Alliance for the future of aesthetics consensus committee. Facial assessment and injection guide for botulinum toxin and injectable hyaluronic acid fillers: Focus on the midface. *Plastic and Reconstructive Surgery*, *140*, 540e–550e.

Donofrio, L. M. (2005). Panfacial volume restoration with fat. *Dermatologic Surgery*, *31*, 1496–1505.

Fabi, S. G., Burgess, C., Carruthers, A., Carruthers, J., Day, D., Goldie, K., et al. (2016). Consensus recommendations for combined aesthetic interventions using botulinum toxin, fillers, and microfocused ultrasound in the neck, décolletage, hands, and other areas of the body. *Dermatologic Surgery*, *42*, 1199–1208.

Galadari, H., Mariwalla, K., Delobel, P., & Mengual, E. S.-V. (2020). Pain and bruising levels after lip augmentation: A comparison of anterograde and retrograde techniques using an automated motorized injection device. A blinded, prospective, randomized, parallel within-subject trial. *Dermatologic Surgery*, *46*, 395–401.

Gladstone, H. B., & Cohen, J. L. (2007). Adverse effects when injecting facial fillers. *Seminars in Cutaneous Medicine and Surgery*, *26*, 34–39.

Kogan, I., Korolik, P., Cartier, H., Adhoute, H., & Liberzon, A. (2020). In vitro evaluation of aspiration of hyaluronic acid filler with a new saline flashing method. *Journal of Cosmetic Dermatology*, *19*, 2513–2518.

Kontis, T. C., Bunin, L., & Fitzgerald, R. (2018). Injectable fillers: Panel discussion, controversies, and techniques. *Facial Plastic Surgery Clinics of North America*, *26*, 225–236.

Mashiko, T., Mori, H., Kato, H., Doi K, Kuno S, Kinoshita K, et al. (2013). Semipermanent volumization by an absorbable filler: Onlay injection technique to the bone. *Plastic and Reconstructive Surgery. Global Open*, *1*(1), e4–e14. https://doi.org/10.1097/GOX.0b013e31828c66b0.

Mckee, D., Remington, K., Swift, A., Lambros, V., Comstock, J., & Lalonde, D. (2019). Effective rejuvenation with hyaluronic acid fillers: Current advanced concepts. *Plastic and Reconstructive Surgery*, *143*, 1277e–1289e.

Murthy, R., Eccleston, D., Mckeown, D., Parikh, A., & Shotter, S. (2021). Improving aseptic injection standards in aesthetic clinical practice. *Dermatologic Therapy*, *34*, e14416.

Pavicic, T. (2015). Complete biodegradable nature of calcium hydroxylapatite after injection for malar enhancement: An MRI study. *Clinical, Cosmetic and Investigational Dermatology*, *8*, 19–25.

Pavicic, T., Frank, K., Erlbacher, K., Neuner, R., Targosinski, S., Schenck, T., et al. (2017). Precision in dermal filling: A comparison between needle and cannula when using soft tissue fillers. *Journal of Drugs in Dermatology*, *16*, 866–872.

Pavicic, T., Webb, K. L., Frank, K., Gotkin, R. H., Tamura, B., & Cotofana, S. (2019). Arterial wall penetration forces in needles versus cannulas. *Plastic and Reconstructive Surgery*, *143*, 504e–512e.

Peng, J.-H., & Peng, P. H.-L. (2020). HA filler injection and skin quality-literature minireview and injection techniques. *Indian Journal of Plastic Surgery*, *53*, 198–206.

Quan, T., Wang, F., Shao, Y., Rittié, L., Xia, W., Orringer, J. S., et al. (2013). Enhancing structural support of the dermal microenvironment activates fibroblasts, endothelial cells, and keratinocytes in aged human skin in vivo. *The Journal of Investigative Dermatology*, *133*, 658–667.

Ramesh, S., Le, A., Katsev, B., & Ugradar, S. (2020). The force required to inject a column of filler through facial arteries. *Dermatologic Surgery*, *46*, e32–e37.

Signorini, M., Liew, S., Sundaram, H., De Boulle, K. L., Goodman, G. J., Monheit, G., et al. (2016). Global aesthetics consensus: Avoidance and management of complications from hyaluronic acid fillers-evidence- and opinion-based review and consensus recommendations. *Plastic and Reconstructive Surgery*, *1379*, 61e–971e.

Smith, S. R., Lin, X., & Shamban, A. (2013). Small gel particle hyaluronic acid injection technique for lip augmentation. *Journal of Drugs in Dermatology*, *12*, 764–769.

Sorensen, E. P., & Council, M. L. (2020). Update in soft-tissue filler-associated blindness. *Dermatologic Surgery*, *46*, 671–677.

Sundaram, H. (2009). Perfect timing: Short-notice strategies for combining hyaluronic acid and collagen fillers. *Practical Dermatology*, *2*, 60–63.

Tansatit, T., Apinuntrum, P., & Phetudom, T. (2017). A dark side of the cannula injections: How arterial wall perforations and emboli occur. *Aesthetic Plastic Surgery*, *41*, 221–227.

Tezel, A., & Fredrickson, G. H. (2008). The science of hyaluronic acid dermal fillers. *Journal of Cosmetic and Laser Therapy*, *10*, 35–42.

Ugradar, S., & Hoenig, J. (2019). Measurement of the force required by blunt-tipped microcannulas to perforate the facial artery. *Ophthalmic Plastic and Reconstructive Surgery*, *35*, 444–446.

van Loghem, J. A. J., Humzah, D., & Kerscher, M. (2017). Cannula versus sharp needle for placement of soft tissue fillers: An observational cadaver study. *Aesthetic Surgery Journal*, *38*, 73–88.

Vedamurthy, M., & Vedamurthy, A. (2008). Dermal fillers: Tips to achieve successful outcomes. *Journal of Cutaneous and Aesthetic Surgery*, *1*, 64–67.

Yang, Q., Lu, B., Guo, N., Li, L., Wang, Y., Ma, X., et al. (2020). Fatal cerebral infarction and ophthalmic artery occlusion after nasal augmentation with hyaluronic acid-a case report and review of literature. *Aesthetic Plastic Surgery*, *44*, 543–548.

Yutskovskaya, Y. A., Sergeeva, A. D., & Kogan, E. A. (2020). Combination of calcium hydroxylapatite diluted with normal saline and microfocused ultrasound with visualization for skin tightening. *Journal of Drugs in Dermatology*, *19*, 405–411.

Zeichner, J. A., & Cohen, J. L. (2012). Use of blunt tipped cannulas for soft tissue fillers. *Journal of Drugs in Dermatology*, *11*, 70–72.

33

Soft Tissue Filler for the Transgender Patient

David Kim, Omer Ibrahim, and Lauren Meshkov Bonati

INTRODUCTION

There are approximately 1.4 million self-identifying transgender individuals in the United States as of the year 2016. Many of these individuals suffer from gender dysphoria, a condition of psychological distress described by the *Diagnostic and Statistical Manual of Mental Disorders, Fifth Edition* (*DSM-V*) as an incongruence between gender identity and sex assigned at birth. Transgender individuals may choose to pursue social, legal, medical, or surgical affirmations of their gender through an extensive process called "transition."

Difficulty accessing healthcare providers who are knowledgeable and culturally sensitive to transgender concerns may hinder the transition process. This has led to reports of transgender youth and adults seeking "back-alley" procedures from unlicensed providers who administer unspecified or unapproved materials such as silicone, paraffin, and oils. Such substances are injected into various parts of the face and body for the purpose of enhancing masculine or feminine features. This may lead to disfigurement or life-threatening complications.

Compounded with poor access to health care, the transgender population is at higher risk for substance abuse, suicide, and other health comorbidities. However, dermatologists are uniquely positioned to provide safe, ethical, and aesthetically appropriate care for the transgender population. Culturally competent, transition-related care has been shown to vastly improve quality of life and may include the use of soft tissue fillers for enhancing gendered features. In this chapter, we will review gender differences in facial anatomy and offer recommendations for transgender-specific treatment strategy with soft tissue fillers.

ANATOMY

There are distinctly masculine or feminine features of the upper, mid, and lower face. Each anatomic location will be reviewed, but overall, the male face is more angular with stronger muscle mass, a thicker dermis, and higher density of hair follicles and sebaceous glands. The female face is more tapered and contains less muscle mass, fewer hair follicles and sebaceous glands, but more subcutaneous fat.

Upper Part of the Face

In males, the forehead is larger and flatter when compared to female anatomy. The eyebrow is also flat and directly superimposed on a prominent supraorbital ridge. The female eyebrow is more arched, especially in the lateral third of the eyebrow, and sits on a less prominent supraorbital ridge. The female forehead is rounder, with a mild anterior projection, whereas the procerus and corrugator muscles are wider and more prominent in males. Lastly, the male orbit is larger and rounder in shape compared to the ovoid shape seen in females.

Midface

The midface differs significantly between males and females. Across many cultures, the male nose is broad compared to the female nose, which is narrow and straight. The female nasal tip is more elevated with a nasolabial angle of 95 to 100 degrees compared to 90 to 95 degrees in men. On the cheek, males have a more prominent and broader zygomatic arch with a flatter medial cheek when compared to females. The ratio between medial to lateral cheeks in men is 1.1:1, compared to 1.5:1 in women. Women have fuller, rounder cheeks with more anterior projection, which is one of the defining features of a feminine face.

The aging pattern of soft tissue loss differs between males and females as well. In females, the thickness of soft tissue in the temporal, medial cheek, lateral cheek, and infraorbital areas declines precipitously from the fourth to sixth decade of life and does not change drastically thereafter. On the other hand, men have a much more gradual decline in soft tissue thickness throughout the third to ninth decades in all facial locations without any precipitous decline.

Lower Face

The lower face is defined by the lips, mandible, and chin. In males, the jawline is much more pronounced and angular with a prominent flexure of the mandibular ramus. Men also have significantly larger masseter muscles resulting in a wider, square face. The male chin is also larger and wider, with greater anterior projection. The female mandible and chin are less prominent and less angulated, resulting in a softer configuration that resembles an inverted triangle. Lastly, in males, the lower lip is larger than the upper lip, whereas in females, the difference is more subtle.

PATIENT SELECTION AND INJECTION STRATEGY

With a solid understanding of characteristically male versus female facial features, the experienced injector can strategically influence gender perception.. Such filler-induced changes in transgender patients have been shown to reduce self-consciousness, improve relationships, and instill ease in pursuing social, leisure, and work activities, and overall improve quality of life.

While not a replacement for gender affirmation surgery, the small changes achieved with filler may serve as an adjunct or stepping stone for those not ready, able, or currently interested in undergoing more invasive, permanent procedures. Like all cosmetic procedures, patients should be counseled to align their expectations with realistic outcomes. Modest reshaping and facial contouring is possible, but dramatic changes in skeletal structure will require surgery.

It should also be discussed that transgender patients typically require a combination of treatment modalities to maximize outcomes. Fillers are best used in conjunction with neuromodulators, laser hair removal, and other medical and cosmetic treatments that are beyond the scope of this chapter.

The following recommendations for facial gender enhancement with fillers are based on general anatomical differences. Exact technique and strategy may differ based on variability in facial characteristics amongst individuals and ethnicities. Furthermore, many of the filler uses discussed later are considered off-label. Explicit understanding of relevant anatomy and slow injections of small volumes will help avoid unintentional vascular compromise, decrease risk of infection, and reduce risk of bruising. While area-specific best practices are discussed in further detail in other chapters in this series, we will discuss general principles that can be employed in order to achieve optimal results in the transgender patient.

Upper Face

Filler may be cautiously placed in the upper face to achieve modest changes in the forehead, including reflation and curvature that creates a soft, more feminine look in male-to-female (MTF) patients. Use of a thin, more delicate filler is recommended to not cause excess bulkiness. While this approach may be useful, facial feminization surgery may ultimately be required for overall skeletal changes.

Age-related volume loss in the periorbital and temporal regions may be remedied with filler placed in the temporal fossa. Restoring lateral volume will better frame the eyes and help older MTF patients achieve a more heart-shaped face rather than the more masculine square or trapezoid shape. The use of neuromodulator to create a more laterally arched brow is an excellent adjunct.

Conversely, female-to-male (FTM) patients may benefit from filler augmentation of the supraorbital ridge, which creates a more prominent and masculine brow. Strategically and lightly dosed neuromodulator will help flatten the characteristically female arch of the brow and further masculinize its appearance.

Of note, there are currently 158 cases worldwide of filler-related blindness, most stemming from injections in the upper face. Anatomical knowledge and extreme caution must be exercised when attempting to fill these regions.

Midface

Midface filler injections are a highly effective way to feminize facial contour. Overall, larger filler volumes are used in MTF patients in order to lift and increase the angle of vectors along the cheek bones. Filler placement on the lateral portion of the zygomatic arch, inferolateral to the lateral canthus, will approximate the female apex and provide a contoured, volumized cheek (Fig. 33.1).

In FTM patients who already have a high and lateral zygomatic prominence, filler may be placed uniformly along the inferior zygomatic arch. In particular, filler placed directly inferior to the malar prominence will widen the malar base and minimize anterior projection of the higher female apex.

Any filler product may be used in this region, but those with rheologically higher G-primes may be more effective at lifting in MTF patients. The use of poly-L-lactic acid, hyaluronic acid, or calcium hydroxyapatite is appropriate, although poly-L-lactic acid may stimulate more collagen growth over time.

Small amounts of delicately placed filler along the nasal dorsum may be used in FTM patients seeking a strong, broad, and more angular nose. Again, the risk of vascular occlusion and subsequent blindness in this area is well established and extreme caution should be used when treating the area. In MTF patients, filler may be used to create an illusion of a slender dorsum and upturned nasal tip, and surgical intervention is typically required to permanently reduce nasal volume and create a slender, more upturned feminine nose.

Lower Face

There is ample opportunity in the lower face to enhance or minimize gendered features. The lips may be filled according to gender, with augmentation of the lower lip

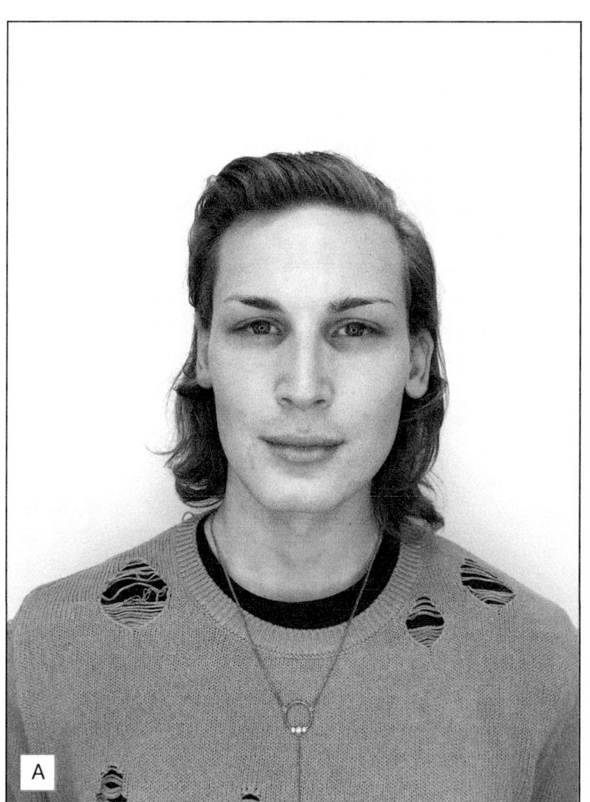

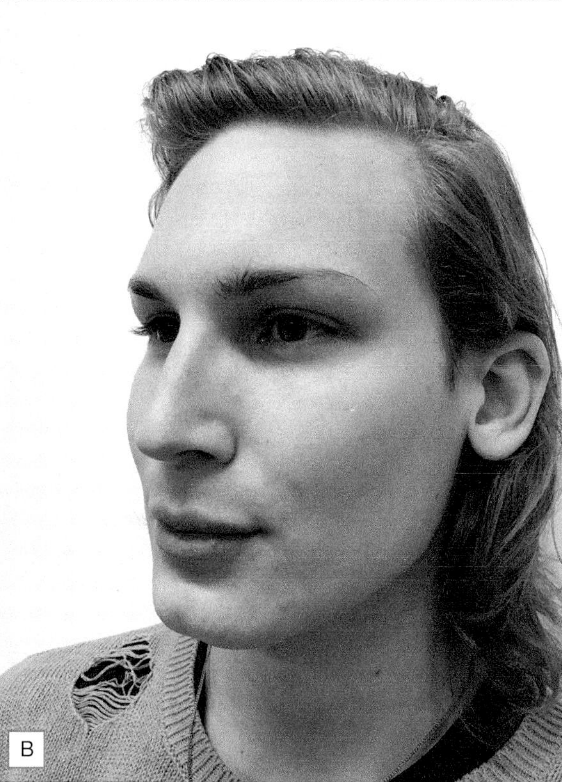

Fig. 33.1 Before and after a combination of hyaluronic acid fillers and neuromodulators in the treatment of a trans-woman. (A) Baseline masculine features before treatment include flat eyebrows and a strong jawline, large masseter muscles, and almost 90-degree angles squaring off the chin. (B) Lateral view of baseline male features.

Continued

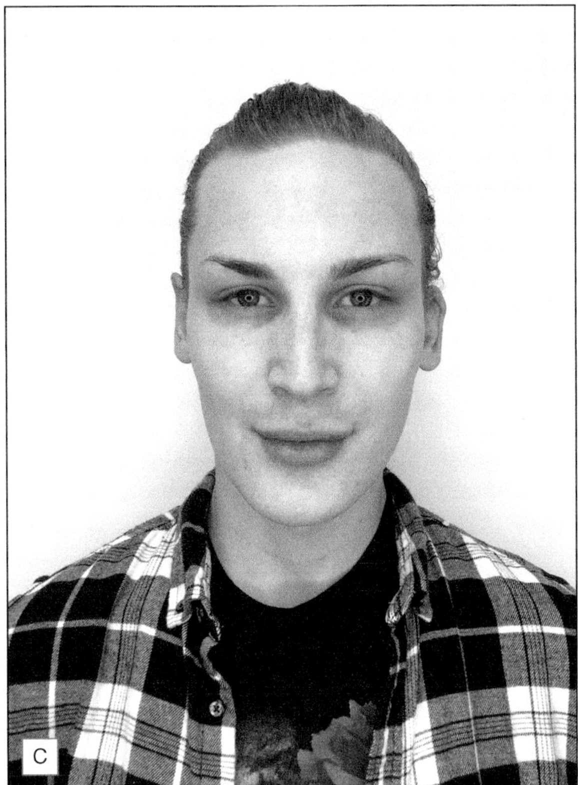

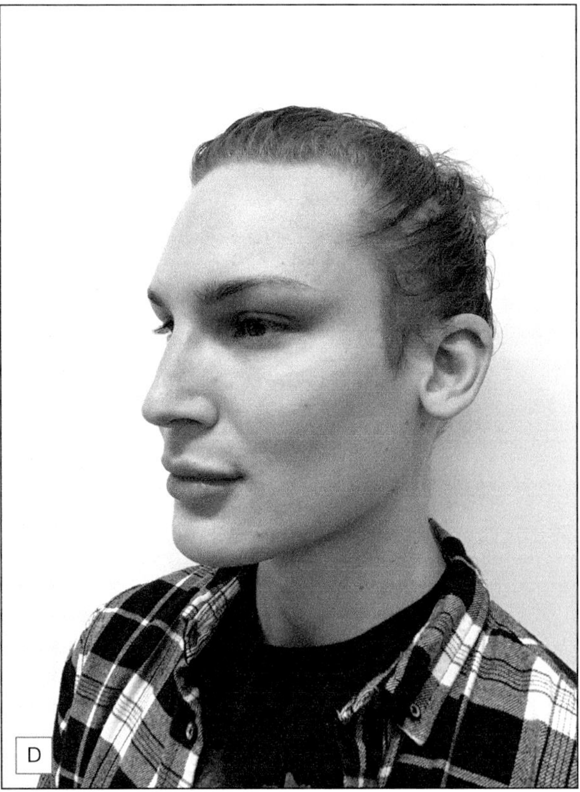

Fig. 33.1,cont'd (C) Feminization of features after treatment. Treatment included filler injection to straighten the nasal bridge, plump the lips, lift the eyebrows, and define, while tapering, the chin. Neuromodulator was used to atrophy the masseters and further slim the jawline. (D) Lateral view of feminization of features after treatment. (Copyright Omer Ibrahim, MD.)

in FTM patients and augmentation of both lower and upper lip in MTF patients. However, lip filler should only be placed in accordance with the overall facial structure of each individual, regardless of gender identity, in order to avoid distortion or disfigurement. A more gendered lip should never be done at the expense of over-filling.

To soften the jawline in MTF patients, neuromodulator may be used over a series of treatments to atrophy the masseter muscle. In FTM patients, filler augmentation of the chin, jawline, mandibular angle, and preauricular area will accentuate a more prominent and angular lower part of the face (Videos 33.1 and 33.2). Further chin and jawline definition may be achieved with deoxycholic acid injections, cryolipolysis, or liposuction of the submental region.

CONCLUSIONS

Experienced injectors may have significant impact on the well-being of transgender individuals seeking physical affirmations of their gender identity. Anatomic gender differences should guide filler treatment strategy with the knowledge that more invasive measures may be required in the future.

SUMMARY AND KEY FEATURES

Soft tissue filler is useful for enhancing certain facial features that are associated with gender. As such, transgender patients may benefit from these noninvasive and reversible procedures when performed with expert technique and special attention is given to specific patient goals.

FURTHER READING

Beer, K., & Avelar, R. (2014). Relationship between delayed reactions to dermal fillers and biofilms: Facts and considerations. *Dermatologic Surgery*, *40*(11), 1175–1179.

Beleznay, K., Carruthers, J., Humphrey, S., et al. (2015). Avoiding and treating blindness from fillers: A review of the world literature. *Dermatologic Surgery*, *41*(10), 1097–1117.

Bonati, L. M., Petrell, K., MacGregor, J., et al. (2021). Neurotoxin and soft tissue filler for influencing gender perception in transgender individuals: A pilot prospective survey-based study. *Journal of the American Academy of Dermatology*, *86*(6).

Brown, E., & Perrett, D. I. (1993). What gives a face its gender? *Perception*, *22*(7), 829–840.

Buckingham, E. D., Glasgold, R., Kontis, T., et al. (2015). Volume rejuvenation of the lower third, perioral, and jawline. *Facial Plastic and Surgery*, *31*(1), 70–79.

Carruthers, J., & Carruthers, A. (2015). Three-dimensional forehead reflation. *Dermatologic Surgery*, *41*(suppl 1), S321–S324.

Dallara, J. M., Baspeyras, M., Bui, P., Cartier, H., Charavel, M. H., & Dumas, L. (2014). Calcium hydroxylapatite for jawline rejuvenation: Consensus recommendations. *Journal of Cosmetic Dermatology*, *13*(1), 3–14.

Dempf, R., & Eckert, A. W. (2020). Contouring the forehead and rhinoplasty in the feminization of the face in male-to-female transsexuals. *Journal of Cranio-Maxillo-Facial Surgery*, *38*(6), 416–422.

Dhingra, N., Bonati, L., Wang, E., Chou, M., & Jagdeo, J. (2019). Medical and aesthetic procedural dermatology recommendations for transgender patients undergoing transition. *JAAD*, *80*(6), 1712–1721.

Farhadian, J., Blood, B., & Brauer, J. (2015). Male aesthetics: A review of facial anatomy and pertinent clinical implications. *Journal of Drugs in Dermatology*, *14*(9), 1029–1034.

Flores, A. R., Herman, J. L., Gates, G. J., & Brown, T. N. T. (2016). *How many adults identify as transgender in the United States?*. Los Angeles, CA: The Williams Institute.

Gart, M. S., & Gutowski, K. A. (2016). Overview of botulinum toxins for aesthetic uses. *Clinics in Plastic Surgery*, *43*(3), 459–471.

Gorin-Lazard, A., Baumstarck, K., Boyer, L., Maquigneau, A., Gebleux, S., Penochet, J. C., Pringuey, D., Albarel, F., Morange, I., Loundou, A., Berbis, J., Auquier, P., Lançon, C., & Bonierbale, M. (2012). Is hormonal therapy associated with better quality of life in transsexuals? A cross-sectional study. *Journal of Sexual Medicine*, *9*(2), 531–541.

Green, J., & Keaney, T. (2017). Aesthetic treatment with botulinum toxin: Approaches specific to men. *Dermatologic Surgery*, *43*, S153–S156.

Hage, J. J., Kanhai, R. C., Oen, A. L., van Diest, P. J., & Karim, R. B. (2001). The devastating outcome of massive subcutaneous injection of highly viscous fluids in male-to-female transsexuals. *Plastic and Reconstructive Surgery*, *107*, 734–741.

Jones, D. H., Carruthers, J., Joseph, J. H., et al. (2016). REFINE-1, a multicenter, randomized, double-blind, placebo-controlled, phase 3 trial with ATX-101, an injectable drug for submental fat reduction. *Dermatologic Surgery*, *42*(1), 38–49.

Keaney, T. (2015). Male aesthetics. *Skin Therapy Letter*, *20*(2), 5–7.

Kobrak, P., & White, B. (2010). *Transgender women and HIV prevention in New York City; A needs assessment*. New York, NY: NYC Health.

Lee, D. H., Jin, S. P., Cho, S., et al. (2013). RimabotulinumtoxinB versus onabotulinumtoxinA in the treatment of masseter hypertrophy: A 24-week double-blind randomized split-face study. *Dermatology*, *226*(3), 227–232.

Murariu, D., Holland, M. C., Gampper, T. J., & Campbell, C. A. (2015). Illegal silicone injections create unique reconstructive challenges in transgender patients. *Plastic and Reconstructive Surgery*, *135*(5), 932e–933e.

Rohrich, R. J., Janis, J. E., & Kenkel, J. M. (2003). Male rhinoplasty. *Plastic and Reconstructive Surgery*, *112*(4), 1071–1085. quiz 1086.

Rossi, A., Fitzgerald, R., & Humphrey, S. (2017). Facial soft tissue augmentation in males: An anatomical and practical approach. *Dermatologic Surgery*, *43*, S131–S139.

Sorensen, E. P., & Council, M. L. (2020). Update in soft tissue filler associated blindness. *Dermatologic Surgery*, *46*(5), 671–677.

Thayer, Z. M., & Dobson, S. D. (2010). Sexual dimorphism in chin shape: Implications for adaptive hypotheses. *American Journal of Physical Anthropology*, *143*(3), 417–425.

Whitaker, L. A., Morales, L., Jr., & Farkas, L. G. (1986). Aesthetic surgery of the supraorbital ridge and forehead structures. *Plastic and Reconstructive Surgery*, *78*(1), 23–32.

Wierckx, K., Van Caenegem, E., Elaut, E., et al. (2011). Quality of life and sexual health after sex reassignment surgery in transsexual men. *Journal of Sexual Medicine*, *8*(12), 3379–3388.

Wierckx, K., Van de Peer, F., Verhaeghe, E., et al. (2014). Short- and long-term clinical skin effects of testosterone treatment in trans men. *Journal of Sexual Medicine*, *11*(1), 222–229.

Wysong, A., Joseph, T., Kim, D., Tang, J., & Gladstone, H. (2013). Quantifying soft tissue loss in facial aging: A study in women using magnetic resonance imaging. *Dermatologic Surgery*, *39*(12), 1895–1902.

Wysong, A., Kim, D., Tim, J., MacFarlane, D., Tang, J., & Gladstone, H. (2014). Quantifying soft tissue loss in the aging male face using magnetic resonance imaging. *Dermatologic Surgery*, *40*(7), 786–793.

34

Combinations

Omer Ibrahim and Jeffrey S. Dover

SUMMARY AND KEY FEATURES

- There are a multitude of factors that contribute to skin aging, including volume loss, dyspigmentation, fine wrinkles, and changes in skin texture.
- A multifaceted approach targeting the various aspects of aging is often required to effectively rejuvenate the skin and ensure patient satisfaction.
- A combination of treatments with fillers, neurotoxins, and light- and energy-based devices is both safe and provides synergistic beneficial effects for the treatment of aging skin.
- Further investigation into the efficacy, mechanisms of action, and optimal techniques is essential to advancing the treatment of photoaged skin.

INTRODUCTION

Soft tissue fillers are but a single tool in the physician's arsenal in the treatment of aging skin. To effectively treat the patient and yield desirable results, the physician, as an artist, must globally visualize the entire subject and face as a whole. The physician must not only examine the types of lines and wrinkles, the fine or deep, static or dynamic, but also they must look past the mere lines and wrinkles to assess volume deficits created with the passage of time. The clinician must also study skin texture changes, telangiectasias, pigmentation, and skin laxity in the assessment of the patient. In this chapter, we discuss the efficacy and safety of combining fillers with different treatment modalities in the management of this multifaceted process of skin aging.

COMBINING SOFT TISSUE FILLERS WITH NEUROTOXINS

The use of injectable medications has revolutionized the treatment of facial rhytides and age-associated volume loss. Neurotoxins such as onabotulinumtoxinA (onaBot), abobotulinumtoxinA (aboBot), incobotulinumtoxinA (incoBot), and prabotulinumtoxinA (praboBot) have become mainstays in the treatment of dynamic wrinkles, not only of the upper face but also in the perioral skin and the neck and jaw line. To many patients, neuromodulators are the starter or "gateway" treatments on their road to facial rejuvenation. Starting with neuromodulators alone is a good starting point, but knowledge of the efficacy and safety of combining neurotoxins with soft tissue fillers is essential to more advanced techniques and better results. As early as 2003, Carruthers and Carruthers demonstrated the superiority of combining hyaluronic acid (HA) filler and botulinum toxin in the treatment of severe glabellar rhytides. Thirty-eight female subjects were randomized to either treatment with HA alone or with HA and onaBot. The combination group showed a better response both at rest and maximum frown, and this response was maintained for an average of 14 weeks longer than the HA group. No differences in adverse effects were noted. In a randomized split-face study by Dubina et al., patients' glabellar/forehead wrinkles were treated with aboBot alone on one side and aboBot and HA filler on the other side. Blinded ratings demonstrated longer-lasting effects and greater static and dynamic wrinkle reduction in the combination group without differences in side effects. Subjects also favored combination treatments over toxin alone. These studies suggest that HA fillers and neurotoxins act synergistically in alleviating skin wrinkles. The effect of the toxin results in muscle relaxation and, therefore, slower breakdown of the HA. The effect of the HA filler results in a softer, more natural return to baseline once the toxin wears off.

Since this seminal work was done, many have taken advantage of the synergistic effects of botulinum toxins and filler for glabellar creases. Often performed at the same visit for time efficiency and optimization of results, both the neuromodulator and especially the filler seem to last longer than when done alone. Often, complete correction can be achieved in deep glabellar creases with results that last for months to several years.

The combination of HA fillers and neurotoxins have been applied to other areas of the face (Video 34.1). In one study by Beer et al., aboBot was placed into the glabella and crow's feet and HA filler into the temples and glabella. Investigators noted significant improvements in glabellar rhytids, periorbital areas, crow's feet, and temporal hollowing. Furthermore, 64% of patients who received toxin alone in the past preferred combination treatments. Carruthers et al. assessed the combination of HA and toxin in the lower face and perioral region. Ninety female subjects were randomized to receive either HA filler alone, onaBot alone, or HA and onaBot in combination. Subjects in all three groups demonstrated statistically significant investigator-rated improvements in lower face appearance. The combination group had greater improvement from baseline than either modality alone. Adverse events were mild, transient, and typical of the procedures performed. Unique untoward side effects from combining treatments were not noted. Similar studies have shown comparable high rates of patient satisfaction and efficacy when fillers were combined with neurotoxins in up to 13 facial zones. In addition to treating aging skin, some investigators have used HA and neurotoxin to reshape aspects of the face in lieu of more traditional invasive cosmetic surgery. One such example is the combination of HA and toxin to redefine the contour of the nose.

The combination of filler and neurotoxin appears to be safe and effective and may lead to enhanced patient retention. However, the physician must be aware that the majority of reports and studies on this subject have used HA fillers, and reports on other types of fillers are scarce. A firm grasp of facial anatomy including the vasculature is imperative in order to achieve desirable results and minimize adverse effects.

COMBINING SOFT TISSUE FILLERS WITH LIGHT- AND ENERGY-BASED DEVICES

Lasers and light-based treatments have gained popularity as noninvasive techniques to improve the appearance of aging skin, including color and texture. The high degree of improvement, low rates of adverse events, and minimal downtime associated with laser/light-based therapies have made them favorable options. Because these technologies target different aspects of the aging process than soft tissue fillers, investigators have studied whether concomitant use of these therapies with soft tissue augmentation can be performed safely and effectively to treat the various facets of photoaging. Many studies have suggested that combining fillers with devices such as ablative and nonablative lasers, intense pulsed light (IPL), radiofrequency (RF), and ultrasound is safe and efficacious in treating photoaged skin (Fig. 34.1).

RF devices are used to tighten and contour skin; however, their ability to restore volume loss is limited. Several studies have examined the utility of combining RF therapy with fillers. England et al. demonstrated that RF treatment 2 weeks after injections with fillers does not influence the rate of side effects or adversely affect filler duration. A follow-up study concluded that RF treatment over fillers increased the inflammatory, foreign body, and fibrotic responses seen on histology. However, these findings contrast with subsequent histologic reports by Alam et al. No histopathologic changes were appreciated in patients treated with either HA filler or calcium hydroxyapatite followed by treatment with a monopolar RF device. Studies have not only demonstrated that combining RF devices with fillers appears to be safe, but more recent work has suggested that combining RF therapy with HA fillers, on the same day, may work synergistically and provide long-lasting effects for the improvement of age-related volume loss.

IPL is a nonablative device that targets melanin and hemoglobin, treating vascular and pigmented lesions

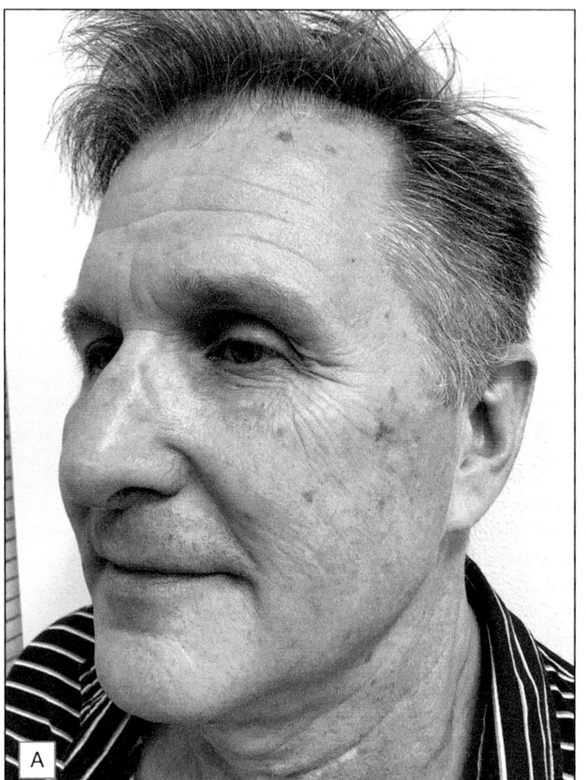

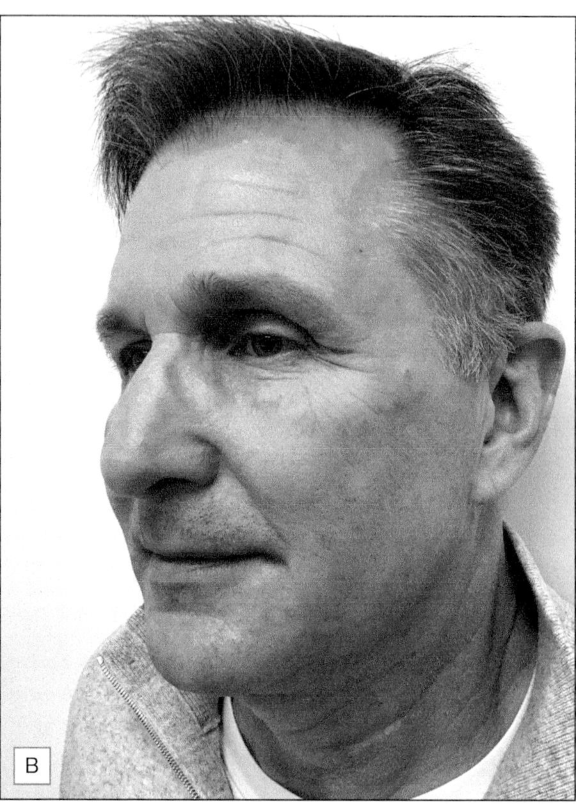

Fig. 34.1 Before (A) and after (B) a series of 1927 nm thulium laser treatments in combination with one session calcium hydroxylapaptite filler to the jawline, to safely achieve a lifted profile and smoother, clearer texture. (Copyright Omer Ibrahim, MD.)

seen in sun-damaged skin. Fabi et al. examined 90 patients treated with the IPL immediately before or as early as 6 days after poly-L-lactic acid (PLLA) injection. Some 86.7% of subjects reported at least mild photorejuvenating effects from the combination of treatments. There were no significant complications including nodule formation after IPL treatment. They concluded that a combination of PLLA injection and IPL for facial photorejuvenation is effective and does not result in increased adverse events than with each treatment modality alone.

In addition to RF devices and IPL, focused ultrasound is employed to improve skin laxity. Friedmann and colleagues reviewed their experience with combination therapy with IPL, PLLA, and microfocused ultrasound (MFUS). They reported that all three photorejuvenation modalities can be safely performed in a single treatment session. They recommend that PLLA injections be performed last to avoid blood contamination of the MFUS or IPL equipment. Similar improvements in skin laxity have been reported with the concomitant use of hyperdilute calcium hydroxylapatite and MFUS. Combining hyperdilute calcium hydroxylapatite and MFUS can also improve the appearance of atrophic acne scars.

Lasers, such as the 1,320-nm neodymium-doped yttrium aluminum garnet (Nd:YAG) laser and the 1450-nm diode laser, are thought to stimulate new collagen formation in the dermis. Goldman et al. performed a randomized trial to evaluate the effect of therapy with monopolar RF, IPL, 1320-nm Nd:YAG laser (14 to 16 J/cm^2, cooling 15 ms before, 10 ms during, 15 ms after; or 16 to 17 J/cm^2, 10 ms before, 5 ms during, and 10 ms after), or 1450-nm diode laser (6-mm spot, 12 to 14 J/cm^2 energy density) on HA injection. They concluded that HA filler can be combined with either modality without altering efficacy or safety. Ribé et al. examined whether injections with HA followed immediately by fractional 1440-nm Nd:YAG laser for neck skin rejuvenation would have clinical and histological effects. They reported improvement in skin tightness, texture, and fine lines after combination therapy. Based on biopsy specimens, they concluded that the fractional nonablative laser produced favorable epidermal and superficial changes, whereas the HA led to favorable changes deeper in the dermis.

Farkas et al. examined the histological specimens from porcine models that were treated with HA fillers followed by different lasers 2 weeks later. Based on histologic examination, the fillers were not affected by IPL, nonablative lasers, or very superficial ablative treatments. However, the deep ablative therapies (such as deep carbon dioxide or erbium:YAG lasers) demonstrated interactions with the HA filler, such as migration of fillers into the ablated microchannels. These authors suggest that if deep resurfacing is planned, laser treatments should be performed before filler injections or on different days in order to optimize outcomes and limit side effects. In fact, combining ablative laser therapy with HA filler treatments may synergistically lead to enhanced effects of the HA filler as measured by epidermal thickening.

COMBINING SOFT TISSUE FILLERS

The realm of soft tissue fillers is ever growing and evolving. More and more products with varying constituents, concentrations of HA, degrees of cross-linking, flow characteristics, and tissue lifting abilities surface on the market every year, expanding the physician's repertoire of injectables. With the advent of a more global or comprehensive approach to facial aging, the use of combinations of different types of fillers to address different aspects of aging has become commonplace (Figs. 34.2 and 34.3).

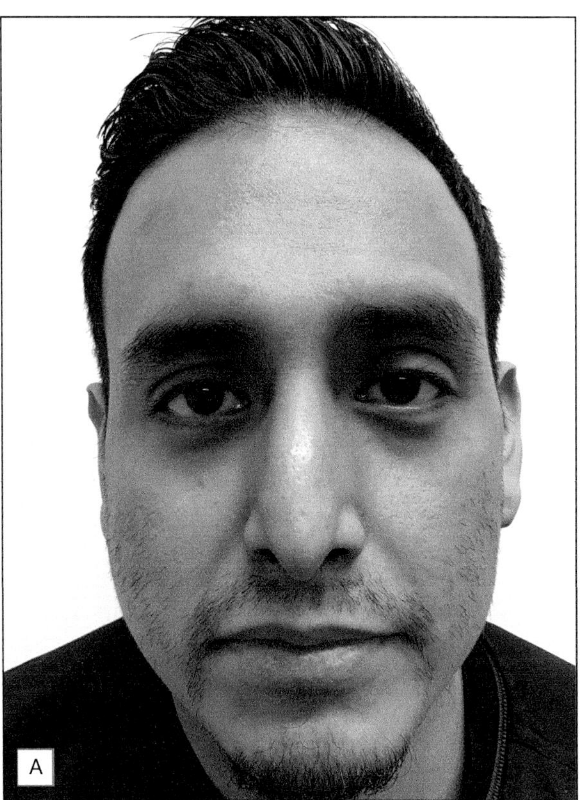

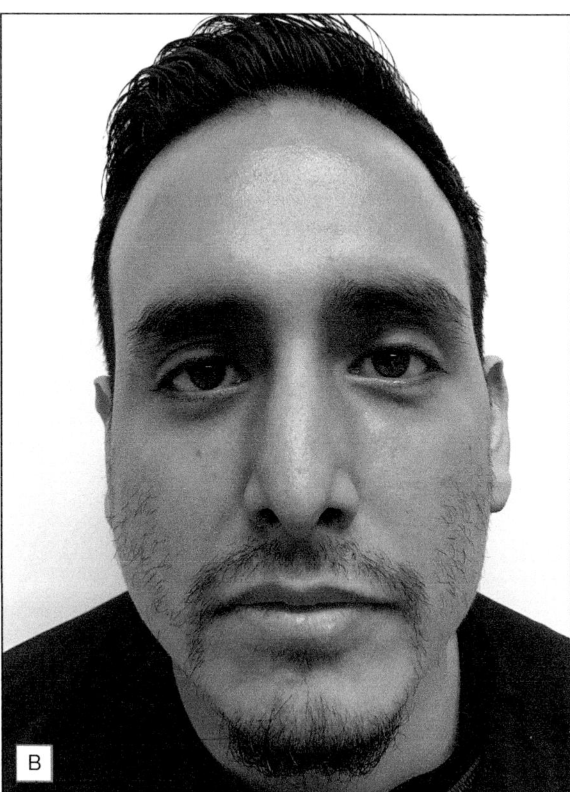

Fig. 34.2 Deep placement of higher G-prime hyaluronic acid (HA) filler in the malar cheeks combined with more superficial placement of softer, lower G-prime HA filler in the tear troughs to yield comprehensive midface rejuvenation. (A) Patient's baseline. (B) Two weeks after deep placement of higher G-prime hyaluronic acid (HA) filler in the malar cheeks combined with more superficial placement of softer, lower G-prime HA filler in the tear troughs. (Copyright Omer Ibrahim, MD.)

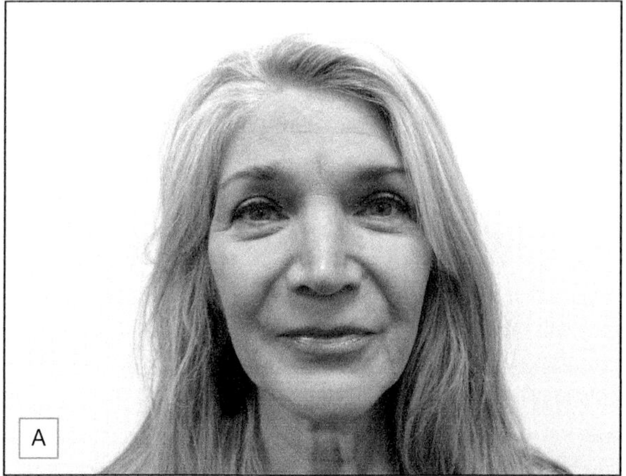

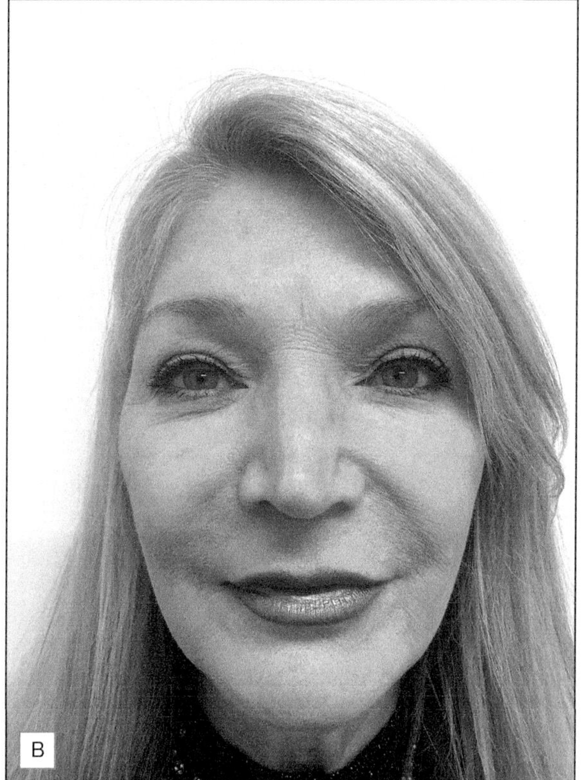

Fig. 34.3 Combination of higher G-prime hyaluronic acid (HA) fillers along the malar cheeks and lateral jawline with lower G-prime HA fillers in the nasolabial folds and marionettes to achieve a global aesthetic improvement. (A) Patient's baseline. (B) Two weeks after combination of higher G-prime hyaluronic acid (HA) fillers along the malar cheeks and lateral jawline with lower G-prime HA fillers in the nasolabial folds and marionettes. (Copyright Omer Ibrahim, MD.)

Fillers can be roughly divided into those that add volume, those that fill lines, those that provide lift, and those that are able to buttress. These different fillers can be combined in the same location, on top of the other, or in different locations to achieve desirable effects. Of note, there is broad overlap of these products, and in some cases, a single versatile filler can be used for different indications, with or without dilution or blending with xylocaine. Blending filler with lidocaine or xylocaine, with or without epinephrine, decreases the viscosity and extrusion force of the filler and increases patient comfort but may compromise the filler's integrity and homogeneity. Therefore, thicker fillers more suited for deeper placement within tissue can be softened with blending to allow for easier flow and filling of fine lines such as in the medial cheek or feathering along the edge of a filled area, increasing the filler's versatility and applicability to different areas of the face.

Among the many changes that develop over time, the disappearance of the malar fat pad with resultant drooping of the midface is one of the more prominent. Thicker HA products with a higher degree of cross-linking or calcium hydroxyapatite injected deep into the malar area can help lift the skin back closer to its original youthful state. However, not addressing the perioral lines with softer products retains an aged look. Therefore, softer, lighter, less or differently cross-linked HA products can be injected into perioral lines, marionette lines, and superficial lip lines to concurrently rejuvenate the perioral area. Thicker, more durable products or injectables that induce collagen formation can also be used to fill voids in the temples, cheeks, and jawline. Once the cheeks, malar areas, and perioral area are rejuvenated, the glabella, tear troughs, and lips can be restored with even lighter HA fillers, especially in people with thinner skin.

In addition to combining fillers geographically on the face, they can be combined temporally. Products with shorter lifespans can be placed at the patient's first visit, to test the patient's response and satisfaction with the filler. Once a patient is content, longer-lasting fillers can be injected at subsequent visits to achieve the same effects for longer duration.

CONCLUSIONS

Injectable soft tissue fillers have revolutionized the management of aging skin. While they can tackle some aspects of volume deficit, skin laxity, and static wrinkles, they fall short of addressing the multitude of factors that contribute to the aged face, especially changes in color and texture. This has necessitated the coupling of soft tissue fillers with a multitude of modalities to radically rejuvenate the skin. Through literature ranging from randomized controlled trials to expert opinion, it has become apparent that combining fillers with one another as well as with neurotoxins and light- and energy-based devices is effective and safe in treating the aging patient and yielding superior results.

FURTHER READING

Alam, M., & Tung, R. (2018). Injection technique in neurotoxins and fillers: Indications, products, and outcomes. *Journal of the American Academy of Dermatology, 79*(3), 423–435.

Alam, M., Levy, R., Pajvani, U., Ramierez, J. A., Guitart, J., Veen, H., et al. (2006). Safety of radiofrequency treatment over human skin previously injected with medium-term injectable soft-tissue augmentation materials: A controlled pilot trial. *Lasers in Surgery and Medicine, 38*(3), 205–210.

Alexiades, M. (2020). Microneedle radiofrequency. *Facial Plastic Surgery Clinics of North America, 28*(1), 9–15.

Beer, K. (2009). Dermal fillers and combinations of fillers for facial rejuvenation. *Dermatologic Clinics, 27(4), 427–432,* v.

Beer, K. R., Julius, H., Dunn, M., & Wilson, F. (2014). Remodeling of periorbital, temporal, glabellar, and crow's feet areas with hyaluronic acid and botulinum toxin. *Journal of Cosmetic Dermatology, 13*(2), 143–150.

Carruthers, J., & Carruthers, A. (2003). A prospective, randomized, parallel group study analyzing the effect of BTX-A (Botox) and non-animal sourced hyaluronic acid (NASHA, Restylane) in combination compared with NASHA (Restylane) alone in severe glabellar rhytides in adult female subjects: Treatment of severe glabellar rhytides with a hyaluronic acid derivative compared with the derivative and BTX-A. *Dermatologic Surgery, 29*(8), 802–809.

Carruthers, J., Carruthers, A., Monheit, G. D., & Davis, P. G. (2010). Multicenter, randomized, parallel-group study of onabotulinumtoxinA and hyaluronic acid dermal fillers (24-mg/ml smooth, cohesive gel) alone and in combination for lower facial rejuvenation: Satisfaction and patient-reported outcomes. *Dermatologic Surgery, 36*(suppl 4), 2135–2145.

Carruthers, A., Carruthers, J., Monheit, G. D., Davis, P. G., & Tardie, G. (2010). Multicenter, randomized, parallel-group study of the safety and effectiveness of onabotulinumtoxinA and hyaluronic acid dermal fillers (24-mg/mL smooth, cohesive gel) alone and in combination for lower facial rejuvenation. *Dermatologic Surgery, 36*(suppl 4), 2121–2134.

Cartier, H., Heden, P., Delmar, H., Bergentz, P., Skoglund, C., Edwartz, C., et al. (2020). Repeated full-face aesthetic combination treatment with abobotulinumtoxinA, hyaluronic acid filler, and skin-boosting hyaluronic acid after monotherapy with abobotulinumtoxinA or hyaluronic acid filler. *Dermatologic Surgery, 46*(4), 475–482.

Casabona, G. (2018). Combined use of microfocused ultrasound and a calcium hydroxylapatite dermal filler for treating atrophic acne scars: A pilot study. *Journal of Cosmetic and Laser Therapy, 20*(5), 301–306.

Cuerda-Galindo, E., Palomar-Gallego, M. A., & Linares-Garciavaldecasas, R. (2015). Are combined same-day treatments the future for photorejuvenation? Review of the literature on combined treatments with lasers, intense pulsed light, radiofrequency, botulinum toxin, and fillers for rejuvenation. *Journal of Cosmetic and Laser Therapy, 17*(1), 49–54.

Dayan, S. H., Ho, T. T., Bacos, J. T., Gandhi, N. D., Kalbag, A., & Gutierrez-Borst, S. (2018). A randomized study to assess the efficacy of skin rejuvenation therapy in combination with neurotoxin and full facial filler treatments. *Journal of Drugs in Dermatology, 17*(1), 48–54.

Dubina, M., Tung, R., Bolotin, D., Mahoney, A. M., Tayebi, B., Sato, M., et al. (2013). Treatment of forehead/glabellar rhytide complex with combination botulinum toxin A and hyaluronic acid versus botulinum toxin A injection alone: A split-face, rater-blinded, randomized control trial. *Journal of Cosmetic Dermatology, 12*(4), 261–266.

England, L. J., Tan, M. H., Shumaker, P. R., Egbert, B. M., Pittelko, K., Orentreich, D., et al. (2005). Effects of monopolar radiofrequency treatment over soft-tissue fillers in an animal model. *Lasers in Surgery Medicine, 37*(5), 356–365.

Fabi, S. G., & Goldman, M. P. (2012). The safety and efficacy of combining poly-L-lactic acid with intense pulsed light in facial rejuvenation: A retrospective study of 90 patients. *Dermatologic Surgery, 38*(7 pt 2), 1208–1216.

Fagien, S. (2010). Variable reconstitution of injectable hyaluronic acid with local anesthetic for expanded applications in facial aesthetic enhancement. *Dermatologic Surgery, 36*, 815–821.

Fagien, S., & Cassuto, D. (2012). Reconstituted injectable hyaluronic acid: Expanded applications in facial aesthetics and additional thoughts on the mechanism of action in cosmetic medicine. *Plastic and Reconstructive Surgery, 130*(1), 208–217.

Farkas, J. P., Richardson, J. A., Brown, S., Hoopman, J. E., & Kenkel, J. M. (2008). Effects of common laser treatments on hyaluronic acid fillers in a porcine model. *Aesthetic Surgery Journal*, *28*(5), 503–511.

Friedmann, D. P., Fabi, S. G., & Goldman, M. P. (2014). Combination of intense pulsed light, Sculptra, and Ultherapy for treatment of the aging face. *Journal of Cosmetic Dermatology*, *13*(2), 109–118.

Goldman, M. P., Alster, T. S., & Weiss, R. (2007). A randomized trial to determine the influence of laser therapy, monopolar radiofrequency treatment, and intense pulsed light therapy administered immediately after hyaluronic acid gel implantation. *Dermatologic Surgery*, *33*(5), 535–542.

Goldman, M. P., Few, J., Binauld, S., Nunez, I., Hee, C. K., & Bernardin, A. (2020). Evaluation of physicochemical properties following syringe-to-syringe mixing of hyaluronic acid dermal fillers. *Dermatologic Surgery*, *46*(12), 1606–1612.

Humphrey, S., de Almeida, A. T., Safa, M., Heydenrych, I., Roberts, S., Chantrey, J., et al. (2021). Enhanced patient retention after combination vs single modality treatment using hyaluronic acid filler and neuromodulator: A multicenter, retrospective review by The Flame Group. *Journal of Cosmetic Dermatology*, *20*(5), 1495–1498.

Huth, L., Marquardt, Y., Heise, R., Fietkau, K., Baron, J. M., & Huth, S. (2020). Biological effects of hyaluronic acid-based dermal fillers and laser therapy on human skin models. *Journal of Drugs in Dermatology*, *19*(9), 897–899.

Ko, E. J., Kim, H., Park, W. S., & Kim, B. J. (2015). Correction of midface volume deficiency using hyaluronic acid filler and intradermal radiofrequency. *Journal of Cosmetic and Laser Therapy*, *17*(1), 46–48.

Molina, B., David, M., Jain, R., Amselem, M., Ruiz-Rodriguez, R., Ma, M. Y., et al. (2015). Patient satisfaction and efficacy of full-facial rejuvenation using a combination of botulinum toxin type A and hyaluronic acid filler. *Dermatologic Surgery*, *41*(suppl 1), S325–S332.

Redaelli, A. (2008). Medical rhinoplasty with hyaluronic acid and botulinum toxin A: A very simple and quite effective technique. *Journal of Cosmetic Dermatology*, *7*(3), 210–220.

Ribe, A., & Ribe, N. (2011). Neck skin rejuvenation: Histological and clinical changes after combined therapy with a fractional non-ablative laser and stabilized hyaluronic acid-based gel of non-animal origin. *Journal of Cosmetic and Laser Therapy*, *13*(4), 154–161.

Rohrich, R. J., & Pessa, J. E. (2007). The fat compartments of the face: Anatomy and clinical implications for cosmetic surgery. *Plastic and Reconstructive Surgery*, *119*(7), 2219–2227. discussion 2228–2231.

Sadick, N. S., Manhas-Bhutani, S., & Krueger, N. (2013). A novel approach to structural facial volume replacement. *Aesthetic Plastic Surgery*, *37*(2), 266–276.

Shaw, R. B., Jr., & Kahn, D. M. (2007). Aging of the midface bony elements: A three-dimensional computed tomographic study. *Plastic and Reconstructive Surgery*, *119*(2), 675–681. discussion 682–683.

Shumaker, P. R., England, L. J., Dover, J. S., Ross, E. V., Harford, R., Derienzo, D., et al. (2006). Effect of monopolar radiofrequency treatment over soft-tissue fillers in an animal model: Part 2. *Lasers in Surgery Medicine*, *38*(3), 211–217.

Urdiales-Galvez, F., Martin-Sanchez, S., Maiz-Jimenez, M., Castellano-Miralla, A., & Lionetti-Leone, L. (2019). Concomitant use of hyaluronic acid and laser in facial rejuvenation. *Aesthetic Plastic Surgery*, *43*(4), 1061–1067.

Vanaman, M., Fabi, S. G., & Cox, S. E. (2016). Neck rejuvenation using a combination approach: Our experience and a review of the literature. *Dermatologic Surgery*, *42*(suppl 2), S94–S100.

Yutskovskaya, Y. A., Sergeeva, A. D., & Kogan, E. A. (2020). Combination of calcium hydroxylapatite diluted with normal saline and microfocused ultrasound with visualization for skin tightening. *Journal of Drugs in Dermatology*, *19*(4), 405–411.

35

Complications of Temporary Fillers

Shraddha Desai, Katherine Given, Ming Lee, Mona Sadeghpour, and Murad Alam

SUMMARY AND KEY FEATURES

- Soft tissue augmentation with temporary fillers continues to be among the most commonly performed cosmetic procedures.
- A large variety of temporary dermal fillers are in production, with an ever-increasing number coming to market.
- It is imperative that the aesthetic physician injecting dermal fillers has proper training in filler selection and use and understands the differences among products.
- Although generally safe, complications can occur with injection of temporary fillers; physicians need to recognize and manage these complications.
- Always acquire an appropriately thorough patient history, including history of bleeding diathesis, immunocompromised state, autoimmune or granulomatous disease, herpes simplex infections, infectious complications with prior injections, or history of keloids or hypertrophic scarring.
- Periprocedural adverse events including bruising, swelling, and pain are common and usually resolve in less than 7 days.
- Proper injection technique is crucial to minimize visible and/or symptomatic papules and nodules.
- Injectors should consider preinjection skin preparation with chlorhexidine and/or 70% isopropyl alcohol, to minimize the risk of infection and biofilm formation.
- Granuloma formation after filler injection is likely multifactorial. Possible etiologies include a true foreign body reaction to particulate or gelatinous filler, or the emergence of a biofilm.
- Early initiation, and often a prolonged course of antibiotics, is important when a patient presents with inflammatory papules and nodules.
- Prompt identification of impending necrosis after injection is critical, and subsequent management with hyaluronidase, topical nitroglycerin, and/or massage may be required.
- Understanding of normal facial anatomy and physiologic changes related to aging allow for judicious and strategic use of injectables.
- Virtually every facial injection site poses a risk for blindness as the vascular supply of the face is comprised of a rich anastomotic network with connecting branches of both the external and internal carotid arteries and access to the retinal circulation, but anatomic regions such as the glabella and nose may be higher risk than others.
- Due to an increasing number of nonaesthetic physicians and midlevel, nonphysician providers injecting fillers, one may expect to see more potential complications.

INTRODUCTION

In recent years, soft tissue fillers have become a mainstay in aesthetic medicine, continuing to grow in popularity, with increased access and a variety of applications. Fillers can be used for facial rejuvenation (e.g., filling wrinkles and prominent folds), restoration of age-related volume loss, sculpting of facial structure, and correcting defects such as scars and disease- or medication-induced lipoatrophy or asymmetries. The demand for these interventions increases as patients prioritize less invasive approaches to facial rejuvenation, with immediate results, limited to no recovery time, and minimal morbidity. In 2014, approximately 5.5 million injections of temporary filler agents were performed worldwide, a significant increase from previous years. A survey from the American Society for Dermatologic Surgery (ASDS) revealed that dermatologist members alone performed at least 1.6 million soft tissue filler procedures in 2017, which was a 21% increase from comparable procedures in the year prior. Despite their impressive safety record, as the number of patients seeking treatment with fillers increases, so do the reports of complications and adverse events. In particular, as the number of untrained or insufficiently trained physician and nonphysician injectors has risen, board-certified and trained physicians are seeing more complications and sequelae in our offices, even if we were not performing the original injection procedures.

In 2013, there were over 160 filler products available, by over 50 different manufacturers.[2] Materials approved for soft tissue augmentation are divided into biodegradable, semibiodegradable, and nonbiodegradable products. These classifications correlate with duration of effect, specifically temporary (~6–12 months), semipermanent (duration ≥18 months), or permanent fillers, respectively (Box 35.1). As more fillers come to market, it is imperative to understand the differences among products, possible complications of each, and how to best identify and treat complications when they arise.

PEARL 1 Physicians must be familiar with the potential complications that may occur from use of currently available fillers, and how to manage and treat these issues. As filler procedures increase worldwide and new products are approved, we expect to see an increased incidence of complications.

Experts stress the importance of understanding the types and frequency of adverse events related to filler injections as this may help physicians guide patient counseling, better target patient histories, and increase awareness about the procedure and associated risks. Complication risk depends on many factors, including injector skill, location of filler placement, site of injection, and type of filler used. Regardless, understanding that complications associated with temporary soft tissue fillers can be categorized by the time of onset (Box 35.2), specifically acute or delayed reactions, can aid in rapid diagnosis and implementation of appropriate intervention, as indicated. Acute, or early, reactions are most often related to procedural errors, injection technique, or reaction to the product itself. These adverse events are usually transient and frequently manifested by erythema, edema, ecchymosis, pruritus, or pain occurring in the first week after injection. Although blindness and hearing impairment are catastrophic potential acute complications, these risks are exceedingly low. Delayed reactions are most often due to the host's response to the injected material, or a reaction to the product itself. These adverse events frequently present with persistent erythema, swelling, nodule formation, and/or indurations developing months to years after

BOX 35.1 Historical and Currently Available Dermal Fillers

- Temporary
  - Bovine collagen (Zyderm, Zyplast)—no longer available.
  - Porcine collagen (Fibrel, Evolence)—no longer available.
  - Human-derived collagen (CosmoDerm, CosmoPlast)—no longer available.
  - Hyaluronic acid (Restylane, Restylane Lyft, Restylane Silk, Restylane Refyne, Restylane Defyne, Restylane Kysse, Juvéderm Ultra, Juvéderm Ultra Plus, Voluma, Volbella, Vollure, Volift, Volite, Belotero Hydro, Belotero Soft, Belotero Intense, Belotero Volume, Belotero Balance, Emervel Touch, Emervel Classic, Emervel Lips, Emervel Deep, Emervel Volume, Elevess/Hydrelle, Captique, Hylaform, Prevelle Silk, RHA 1–4).
  - Calcium hydroxylapatite (Radiesse).
  - Autologous fat.
- Semipermanent
  - Poly-l-lactic acid (Sculptra).
  - Autologous fibroblasts (Fibrocell).
- Permanent
  - Collagen + polymethylmethacrylate (Artecoll/Artefill/Bellafill).
  - Silicone (Adato SIL-OL 5000, NY; Silikon 1000).
  - Hydroxyethylmethacrylate/ethylmethacrylate fragments and hyaluronic acid (Dermalive).
  - Polyacrylamide hydrogel (Aquamid).

BOX 35.2 Onset of Adverse Events

Acute (occurring up to 1 week after treatment)
- Injection site reactions.
- Nodules.
- Infection.
- Hypersensitivity.
- Tissue necrosis.
- Blindness.

Delayed (occurring from weeks to years after treatment)
- Infection.
- Biofilm formation.
- Granuloma formation.

product placement. The nature of these reactions and their treatments will be summarized in this chapter.

IMMEDIATE AND EARLY-ONSET DERMAL FILLER COMPLICATIONS

Injection Site Reactions

According to the US Federal Drug Administration (FDA), some of the most common adverse events associated with fillers are local injection site reactions. These reactions are manifested by tenderness, erythema, and edema and are typically mild, localized, and transient, resolving within 4 to 7 days. Many injectors consider these reactions adverse sequelae rather than true complications. Irrespective of the type of filler used, injection of the product alone will cause a local tissue injury response due to the stretch, vasodilation, and increased permeability of the blood vessels in the treated area, leading to redness, swelling, and bruising. Despite this, there are actions that can be taken to minimize these effects, including excellent injection technique and post-procedure icing.

PEARL 2 Most patients develop a local injection site reaction after filler placement, such as erythema, edema, or ecchymosis. These reactions are usually transient and resolve within 1 day to 1 week. Nonetheless, patients should be made aware of these risks beforehand. The use of gentle pressure and cold compresses can help minimize development and hasten resolution of these sequelae.

Pain

Pain during injection is a commonly reported adverse event associated with filler agents. Pain is often attributable to hydrostatic dissection of tissue during injection, as well as the discomfort of numerous needle punctures during the implantation of the product. Certain anatomic sites, including the lips and perioral region, are more sensitive as these sites harbor increased sensory innervation. Regardless of the treatment area, a number of techniques may be used to minimize the pain associated with injections. These include the use of topical anesthetics, local anesthetics ("numbing dots"), application of ice before and after injection, and vibratory distraction. The latter can be achieved with an assistant tapping the patient's skin or with the use of handheld massagers. When treating the perioral region, some clinicians use infraorbital and mental nerve blocks or place small aliquots of lidocaine in a few points along the gingival sulcus to minimize pain associated with lip injections. However, local anesthesia is also uncomfortable. Most products are now packaged with the filler syringe premixed with lidocaine to alleviate pain as the treatment progresses. Pain can also be reduced with excellent injection technique. In a blinded, prospective, randomized study by Galadari et al., subjects were found to have less pain with anterograde injections compared to retrograde injections when using an automated motorized injection device for lip augmentation. These participants also had less bruising and fewer injection site reactions when the anterograde technique was employed. Other strategies to reduce pain include use of a smaller gauge needle or prioritization of fewer insertion points through use of a blunt-tipped cannula. In a prospective, case control, single-center study by de Felipe et al., 72% of subjects reported less pain when treated with a cannula in comparison to needles. Similar results were noted in a comparative study whereby subjects graded pain as a 3 (mild) for cannula injections and 6 (moderate) for needle injections, using the visual analog scale (VAS) for pain assessment.

PEARL 3 Topical application of a mixture of lidocaine alone or benzocaine, lidocaine, and tetracaine (BLT) 30 minutes prior to treatment and/or ice just before treatment minimizes pain associated with injections.

Edema and Ecchymosis

Bruising and swelling occur due to local trauma from the injection and are common postprocedural events (Fig. 35.1). Bruising can be severe, particularly in patients taking anticoagulation or antiplatelet agents, such as irreversible cyclooxygenase inhibitors like aspirin or adenosine diphosphate (ADP) receptor inhibitors like clopidogrel (Fig. 35.1). With regard to hyaluronic acid (HA), a phenomenon of delayed bruising can occur in some patients. HA is a member of the glycosaminoglycan (GAG) polysaccharide family, which includes heparin. Structural similarity of the HA molecule to heparin is important as it has been shown to weakly interact with the coagulation cascade and possibly lead to the phenomenon of delayed bruising in some patients. Reviewing all medications and supplements that a patient is taking and stopping any unnecessary agents prior to their procedure can minimize the degree and duration of edema and ecchymosis. Most supplements should be held at least 5 to 7 days before treatment, including garlic and *ginkgo biloba*, which have an inhibitory effect on platelets, as well as vitamin E, niacin (vitamin B_3), omega-3 fish oils, glucosamine, ginger, ginseng, green tea, chamomile, St. John's wort, and celery root, all of which can inhibit coagulation pathways. While avoidance of agents that interfere with coagulation is recommended, patients should continue any medically necessary medications, as risk of holding these (e.g., stroke, blood clot) outweighs any procedure-related bleeding risks. Finally, recent alcohol consumption should be reviewed prior to injection, as alcohol-induced vasodilation can, theoretically, exacerbate bruising.

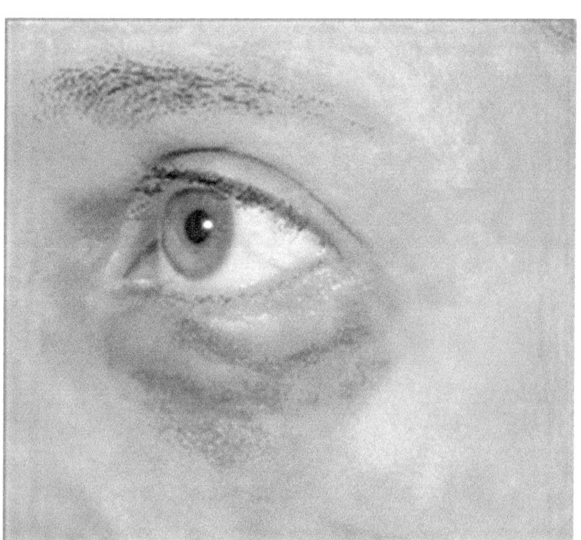

Fig. 35.1 Severe periocular ecchymosis 7 days following injection of hyaluronic acid deep into the supraperiosteal fat pads.

PEARL 4 Avoiding anticoagulants that are not medically necessary and a thorough pretreatment review of all supplements will minimize posttreatment ecchymosis and edema. Prescribed therapeutic aspirin or other anticoagulants, such as warfarin, clopidogrel, apixaban, or dabigatran, should not be discontinued prior to filler injection.

Similar to pain-reduction strategies, bruising can be minimized by reducing the number of injection points, using a smaller-gauge needle when possible, and adjusting the direction and speed of the injection. Some injectors incorporate blunt-tipped cannulas in certain treatment areas, which may reduce the risk of traumatizing blood vessels and negate the need for multiple injection points. In de Felipe's study, the incidence of bruising was lower in the cannula group (7% cannula vs. 17.4% needle), and this finding was reproduced in Fulton's study.

It has also been suggested that the direction of needle insertion into the skin is key. Perpendicular insertion reduces the length of the dermal track and the duration of time the needle is in the dermis, thereby minimizing the likelihood of vessel transection. Similarly, slow infiltration of product decreases tissue distortion and trauma. Conversely, fanning, a technique commonly used to provide structural support to overlying skin, causes increased dissection of the subepidermal plane and may increase risk of ecchymosis.

Filler type may also impact the development of ecchymoses. Although collagen-based fillers were less likely to cause bruising secondary to their inherent platelet-aggregating properties, they are no longer commercially available for a variety of reasons including their associated relatively high risk of allergic reaction.

When postinjection bruising does occur, there are several options to minimize its degree and duration, including supplements and laser and light treatment. Supplements such as bromelain, homeopathic arnica, or topical vitamin K may help reduce the incidence and length of posttreatment ecchymosis. In animal models, bromelain has been shown to decrease vascular permeability by lowering the levels of bradykinin, which may result in less edema, pain, and inflammation. Helenalin, an extract of arnica, has anti-inflammatory effects and inhibits platelet function in vitro. However, clinical studies of these compounds have demonstrated conflicting results, with some reporting a decrease in posttreatment bruising while others showed no statistically different effect. A comprehensive review by Ho et al. concluded that there are insufficient data to routinely support use of arnica and bromelain to prevent and/or treat postprocedure ecchymosis and edema. Their review included published clinical trials using oral and topical arnica and oral bromelain. The beneficial effects of these agents, if observed, were best demonstrated when administered preoperatively and continued 1 to 4 days postoperatively. Further investigations are recommended to substantiate their efficacy and the safety of these supplements.

Finally, vascular lasers and light sources at subpurpuric treatment settings hasten resolution of posttreatment bruising. It is important that the patient understands that laser/light treatment will accelerate bruise resolution but will not make it disappear immediately. Settings vary for each device, but in general, subpurpuric settings are achieved with lower fluences, and pulse durations between 3 and 10 ms. Although variations exist, useful settings for the 585/595 nm pulsed dye laser (PDL) (Vbeam Perfecta, Syneron Candela) include a 10 mm spot size, 6.0 to 7.5 J/cm^2 fluence, and 6 ms to 10 pulse duration with dynamic cooling (40/30 or 30/20) for one to two passes. When a bruise is dark purple, stacking pulses is not recommended due to concern for bulk heating and subsequent damage to surrounding tissues. With milder bruising, pulses may be stacked with a 2- to 3-second delay in between. PDL can be used immediately after onset of ecchymosis, including on the same day as filler treatment, but studies demonstrate that results are best when performed 1 day after onset of bruising. Laser treatments are effective within the first few days after bruising onset, as long as the bruise is still purple in color, indicating the presence of deoxyhemoglobin, a target chromophore of the laser. As the ecchymosis fades to green (biliverdin) and then orange-yellow (bilirubin), the target chromophore is lost, and PDL is no longer effective. Other modalities for postinjection bruising include 532 nm potassium titanium phosphate (KTP) and lithium triborate (LBO) lasers and intense pulsed light (IPL). In our practice, we use KTP (Excel V, Cutera) with similar settings to PDL: 10 mm spot, 7.0 to 8.4 J/cm^2 fluence, and 6 to 7 ms pulse duration with contact cooling for one to two passes. IPL with the Max G handpiece (Icon Pulsed Light System, Cynosure Inc., Westford, MA) was found to be effective in 15 patients with bruising within 24 to 48 hours after filler injection (28 J/cm^2 fluence, 30 ms pulse duration). The mean reduction in bruising was 85% within 72 hours of treatment. Caution should be taken with use of IPL devices, which have varying absorption filters, particularly in darker skin types. PDL and KTP are considered safe in most skin types, although longer pulse durations and lower fluences are generally recommended for Fitzpatrick skin types IV to VI. The long-pulsed neodymium-doped yttrium aluminum garnet (Nd:YAG) laser is an excellent alternative in darker Fitzpatrick skin types, as this wavelength still treats ecchymoses but has less absorption by epidermal melanin, reducing the risk of laser-associated pigmentary changes.

Incorrect Filler Placement

Inappropriate placement of fillers may result in the development of subcutaneous nodules and papules. The majority of these are manifested as palpable and/or visible bumps under the skin. Injecting too superficially can lead to lumps of visible product or bluish bumps under the skin explained by the Tyndall effect with HA fillers (Fig. 35.2). Such reactions can for the most part be prevented by use of correct technique. Treatment of visible

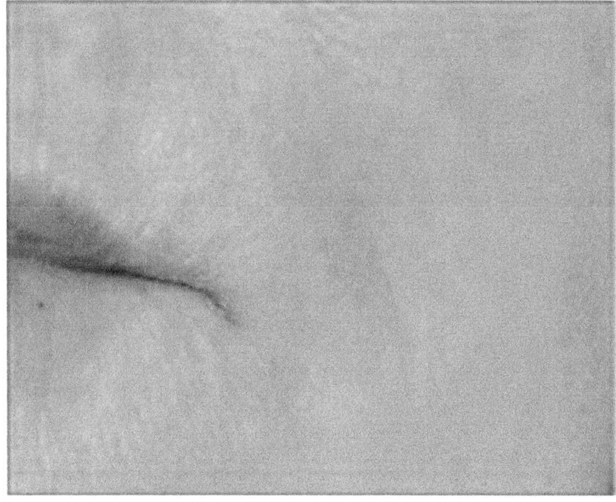

Fig. 35.2 The Tyndall effect is shown following injection of the hyaluronic acid Restylane intradermally in the superior modiolus.

papules can often be accomplished by firm digital pressure, by aspiration, or by incision and drainage. When persistent papules and nodules are due to the use of a HA filler, the enzyme hyaluronidase can be used to treat them. Small amounts of hyaluronidase (10–12 units for each 0.1 mL of biphasic or monophasic HA product, respectively) can be injected locally to dissolve the HA.

PEARL 5 When using hyaluronidase derived from an ovine or bovine source for nonemergent complications, such as overcorrection, superficial implantation, or inflammatory reactions, skin testing is recommended because there have been reports of sensitivity to the animal-derived enzyme. For emergent complications, such as vascular occlusion, hyaluronidase manufactured from a human recombinant source (Hylenex, Halozyme Therapeutics, Inc.) is the safest product to use because immediate, larger volumes are typically required, and a pretest is not an issue.

Infection

Infections after injection of temporary soft tissue fillers can occur due to the required breach in the structural integrity of the skin to place the product. While the vast majority of infections in this setting are bacterial, other reported etiologies include fungal, viral, or polymicrobial sources. In one study that looked at 3782 reported adverse events secondary to temporary filler placement, infection was the second most commonly reported complication (488 reports, or 12.9% of adverse events).

Infectious complications can be stratified into early (< 14 days) or late events. Early, or acute, bacterial reactions are hypothesized to be due to direct, traumatic inoculation of skin surface microbes during injection and may result in localized skin infections, cellulitis, or abscess. The most commonly implicated organisms are *Staphylococcus* and *Streptococcus*, which are also the most common skin commensals. Late or delayed bacterial complications arise, in part, because filler acts as indwelling foreign material and may serve as a nidus for chronic infection. Infection in this manner can occur due to hematogenous spread of a systemic infection with seeding of the filler material or from a more indolent infection or colonization (perhaps again through traumatic inoculation during initial injection) with or without subsequent biofilm or foreign body granuloma formation, both of which will be discussed in greater detail in following sections.Notably, delayed infectious complications are more likely to involve atypical organisms, such as *Mycobacteria* or *Escherichia coli.* There have been reports of an *Mycobacterium chelonae* outbreak after soft tissue augmentation with an HA-based filler. It is not clear whether the injected material was contaminated with the *Mycobacteria* during the manufacturing process or whether the patient was inoculated during the injection procedure. Contamination of filler agents is an emerging concern as non–US Food and Drug Administration (FDA)–approved or counterfeit products have been illegally imported outside of approved US distributors at increasing rates.

Prevention of infection is preferable, and many recommend a more formal sterile surgical preparation of the skin using 70% isopropyl alcohol or chlorhexidine to minimize the risk of infection. Other strategies include delayed application of makeup (up to 4 hours after injection), use of smaller-gauge needles to reduce trauma, and use of cannulas to decrease the number of skin punctures, although there is an absence of randomized trials evaluating the efficacy of these suggestions. High-risk patients, including patients with diabetes or those with compromised immune systems, require special attention. Additionally, patients with chronic sinusitis or chronic dental issues may have a greater tendency to develop infections after a filler injection in the periorbital area or central face. In these cases, it is often recommended to avoid filler implantation until 2 weeks after any dental work has been performed or wait 4 weeks after filler placement to perform any dental work.

If an infection is suspected, management and treatment should be driven by the patient's clinical presentation. In the acute setting, patients often present with a single or multiple tender erythematous and/or fluctuant nodules, with or without accompanying systemic symptoms, such as fever and fatigue. In the setting of a possible abscess, the lesion should be drained and cultured and the patient should be started on empiric, broad-spectrum antibiotic therapy. Cultures should assess for aerobic and anaerobic microorganisms, with an extended culture incubation period (3–4 weeks) to evaluate for atypical organisms. Initial antibiotic therapy recommendations in the literature vary; however, multidrug therapy with macrolides and quinolones is often recommended while awaiting culture sensitivities. In delayed cases, patients may present with noninflammatory nodules, which have a broader differential diagnosis, thereby increasing the difficulty of accurate diagnosis and management. Tissue sampling may be helpful in such cases, as more sensitive technologies including polymerase chain reaction (PCR) and fluorescence in situ hybridization (FISH) are better at identifying more elusive organisms. Tissue can also be cultured for bacteria, fungi, and acid-fast bacilli. Common pitfalls in management include administration of steroids (systemic or intralesional) for presumed hypersensitivity reaction or the use of hyaluronidase in the setting of nodule formation prior to an appropriate antibiotic course, both of which may worsen the underlying infection or allow bacterial spread into neighboring tissues.

While bacterial infections are the most common infectious complications of dermal filler injections, there have been numerous reports of herpes virus reactivation within the first 24 to 48 hours after filler injection. Triggers include local trauma, inflammatory reaction after filler placement, or systemic stress or immunosuppression. Herpes outbreaks usually arise where the filler was directly injected, often in the perioral region or nasolabial folds. Therefore, in patients with a history of herpes outbreaks (>3 outbreaks per year), prophylactic antiviral treatment is recommended, especially if the site of augmentation is high risk (e.g., perioral, vermilion lip). Notably, a standard prophylactic antiviral regimen does not exist, although many authors recommend 400 mg acyclovir three times daily for 5 to 7 days or 1 g valacyclovir daily for 1 day prior and 3 days following the procedure. Additionally, injections should be delayed if the patient is undergoing an active flare.

DELAYED AND LATE-ONSET DERMAL FILLER COMPLICATIONS

Delayed Inflammatory Reactions

The rise in popularity and use of soft tissue fillers has resulted in increased incidence of adverse inflammatory reactions associated with these procedures. Different terminology has been used in the literature to refer to these inflammatory reactions. For the purpose of the discussion in this chapter, the term "delayed inflammatory reactions" (DIRs) will be used, consistent with the most recent 2020 Artzi et al. expert panel recommendation. DIRs can manifest as discoloration (including erythema), pain, nodule formation, induration, tissue hardening, and solid edema. Both HA and non-HA fillers are subject to potential development of DIRs.

Hyaluronic Acid–Based Filler Reactions

Unlike collagen, HA is generally considered a nonimmunogenic molecule given its lack of protein epitopes. However, this notion juxtaposes the clinical finding of inflammatory-mediated delayed-onset nodules, which can form months to years after injection of HA fillers. In fact, the advent of newer crosslinking technology of HA fillers, which has increased the longevity of these products, has also led to a rise in DIRs. There has been increasing clinical and scientific evidence to support the proinflammatory role of HA which may predispose susceptible individuals to immune-mediated reactions following injection. Increased incidence of these DIRs has recently been reported with the use of the class of HA filler products that utilize a novel and proprietary Vycross crosslinking technology. In studies by Sadeghpour et al. and Artzi et al., within the Vycross family of fillers, HA-Volbella is associated with the highest risk of delayed-onset nodule formation, with the incidence varying between 1.4% and 4.2% per patient. The largest retrospective study for Vycross-related reactions was performed by Humphrey et al., where the incidence of delayed-onset nodules in 4500 patients who had received 9324 syringes of HA-Voluma over the course of 9 years was estimated to be 0.98% per patient. Similar to the findings of Sadeghpour et al., median time to onset of symptoms from the most recent injection was 4 months. Authors have found these reactions to either be self-limited, resolving on their own, or more persistent requiring treatment. The most successful treatment regimens for the management of DIR associated with the Vycross family of fillers involve a limited oral corticosteroid course (prednisone 30 mg × 5–7 days), followed by intralesional injection of combined hyaluronidase and triamcinolone injections (which may need to be performed over repeated sessions for full resolution). Although oral antibiotics have not been found to be as helpful clinically in management of delayed nodules associated with Vycross family fillers, it is important to rule out infection as an underlying cause and institute appropriate antimicrobial therapy as needed when initially evaluating and treating these reactions. Fig. 35.3 summarizes an international expert panel's latest proposed algorithm for treating DIRs secondary to HA filler injections.

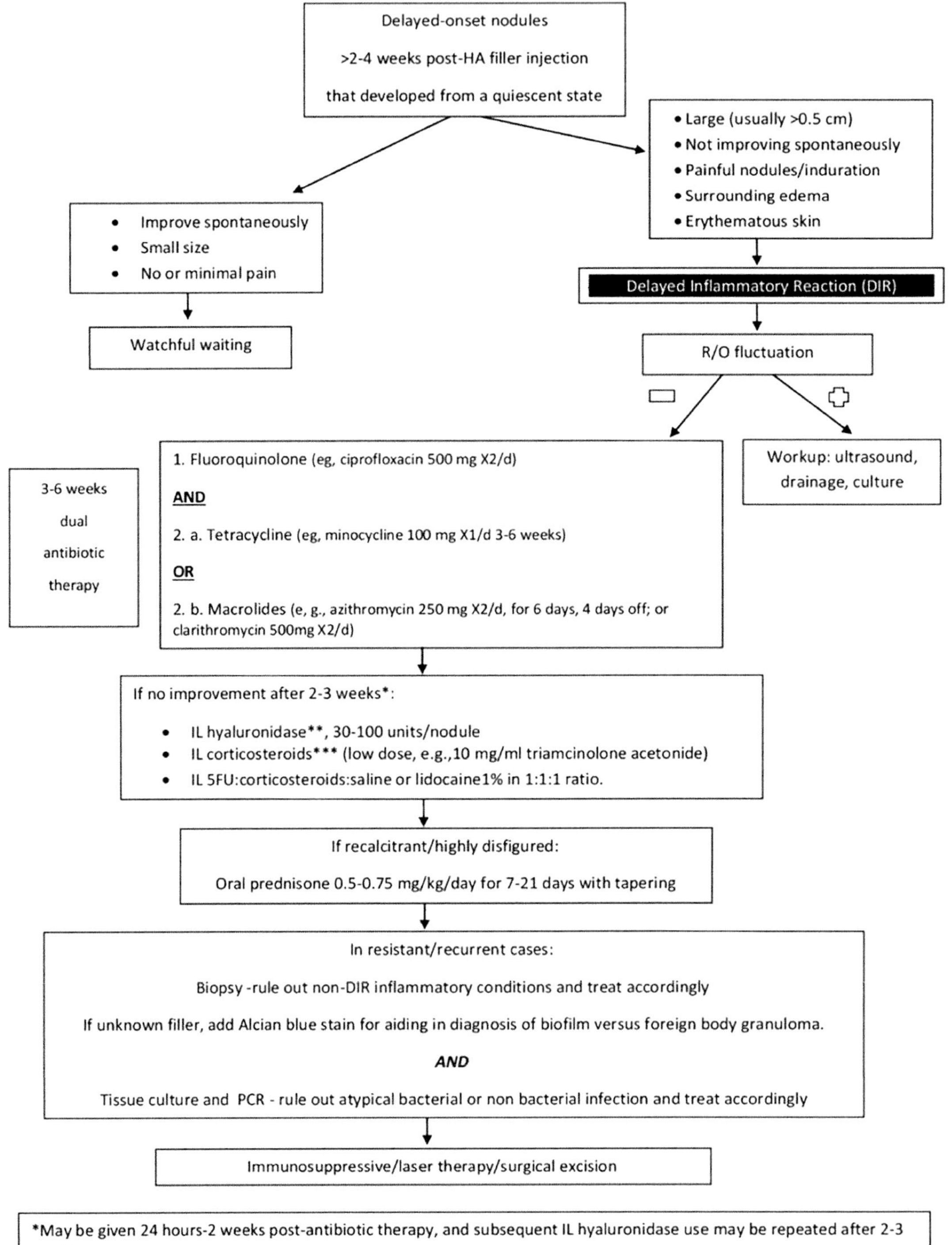

Fig. 35.3 Algorithm for treating delayed inflammatory reactions secondary to hyaluronic acid filler injections. (Clinical, Cosmetic and Investigational Dermatology 2020 13: 371-378. Originally published by and used with permission from Dove Medical Press Ltd.)

Although an investigation is currently underway, it is thought that these reactions, including swelling and nodules formation, may be the aftermath of the newer crosslinking processes that incorporate both high-molecular-weight HA (HMW-HA) and low-molecular-weight HA (LMW-HA) compared to prior crosslinking processes that used only HMW-HA. Studies suggest that different molecular weight HAs may exert variable effects on the immune system.[22–24] Whereas HMW-HA exerts a primarily anti-inflammatory effect, LMW-HA is proinflammatory and can serve as an endogenous danger signal activating the innate immune system. HA fragments of low-to-intermediate size have been shown to activate macrophages and dendritic cells and deliver costimulatory signals to T cells via their primary cell surface receptor, CD44, or TLR4. Theoretically, the presence of these proinflammatory HA fragments and LMW-HA can then prime the immune system to develop inflammation and hypersensitivity at the site of injected fillers in setting of an immunologic triggering event. Immunogenic stimuli that can trigger these delayed reactions include viral or bacterial infections, vaccinations (such as the flu or COVID-19 vaccination), facial injury or trauma, or dental work. Fortunately, the incidence of such reactions with HA remains to be low, especially when compared to other types of fillers.

Incidence of Delayed Inflammatory Reactions During the COVID-19 Pandemic

During the COVID-19 pandemic, rare cases of DIRs with HA fillers were reported in patients in setting of community-acquired COVID-19 infection, as well as COVID-19 vaccinations including both the mRNA-1273 vaccination (Moderna, Cambridge, MA) and following BNT162b2 vaccine (Pfizer, New York, NY). The reaction presents as swelling, erythema, pain, and induration at the site of previously injected soft tissue fillers occurring days to weeks following the COVID-19 infection or vaccination. The reaction is thought to be triggered by exposure to the COVID-19 spike protein. According to the FDA data from the mRNA-1273 vaccination trial (Moderna), 3 patients out of 15,184 participants developed facial or lip swelling related to dermal filler placement. However, these reactions were initially reported to be associated with the Moderna vaccine; in more recent reports by Munavalli et al., three patients developed the reaction following the Pfizer vaccine. Most interestingly, it was also demonstrated that low-dose angiotensin-converting enzyme (ACE) inhibitor therapy was successful in the management of DIR developed in patients following either the Moderna or Pfizer COVID-19 vaccination (Fig. 35.4). They found lisinopril 5 mg daily to be a good starting point for DIR therapy in these patients, titrating up to 10 mg daily if minimal improvement is observed after the initial dose. Authors found that all patients responded to therapy duration of 3 to 5 days, or 1 to 2 days after reduction of visible swelling. Thankfully, these reactions have thus far been relatively rare. Other proposed effective treatments have included oral corticosteroids or intralesional hyaluronidase.

Non-Hyaluronic Acid Filler Nodule Reactions

Collagen

Prior to the FDA approval of HAs in 2003, the most common agent for soft tissue augmentation was bovine collagen in the form of Zyderm 1, Zyderm 2, and Zyplast. Given its animal source, these products had immunogenic potential resulting in allergic reactions. Two separate skin tests were recommended to test for sensitivity. To avoid the risk of inflammatory reactions to bovine collagen, human-based collagen was then generated for injection. Obtained from human donor tissues, CosmoDerm and CosmoPlast were the most frequently used agents within this class, which were associated with fewer cases of inflammatory reactions. Given that these collagen products are no longer used in today's market, they will not be discussed further in this chapter.

Poly-l-Lactic Acid

Historically, the incidence of injection site nodules from non-HA based fillers appears to be higher in patients receiving poly-l-lactic acid (PLLA; Sculptra), particularly in the human immunodeficiency virus (HIV)–infected population. In early clinical studies conducted in Europe, nodules at the site of injection that were asymptomatic and palpable but generally not visible were described in approximately 30% to 50% of patients, and without treatment, they tended to persist for months to years. Subsequent studies in the United States reported a lower incidence of PLLA papules and nodules, occurring in approximately 6% to 13% of patients. In a later study comparing PLLA with collagen for the correction of nasolabial fold rhytides in non-HIV-infected patients, papules less than 5 mm in diameter occurred in 8.6% of patients receiving PLLA and 3.4% of those receiving

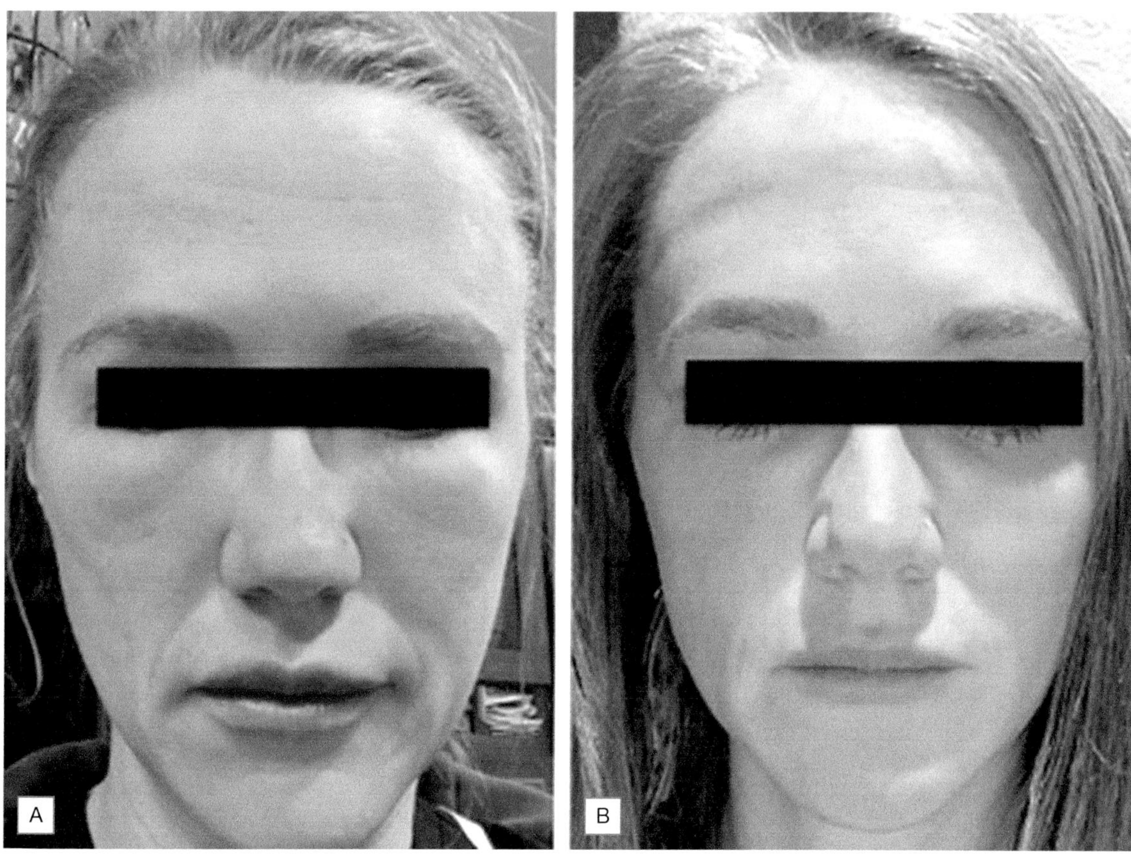

Fig. 35.4 Delayed inflammatory reaction after COVID-19 vaccination. Micrograph A, 48 hours post first Moderna vaccine injection. Micrograph B, 24 hours post 5 mg of oral lisinopril.

collagen. Nodules greater than 5 mm diameter occurred in 6.9% of subjects receiving PLLA and 6.0% of subjects receiving collagen. The literature now reveals that most of the early problems encountered with PLLA resulted from suboptimal methodology, in part from inadequate on-label reconstitution with 5 mL sterile water for injection (SWFI), short powder hydration times, and subsequent injection of highly concentrated product.

Narins and others have recommended changes in the protocol for product reconstitution, hydration, and administration that have helped mitigate this potential complication. Current consensus recommendations state that PLLA should be reconstituted 24 hours or more prior to injection with approximately 7 to 8 mL of SWFI or bacteriostatic water, with 1 to 2 mL of lidocaine added at the time of injection. Dilution in this volume range leads to even PLLA distribution, easier injection, reduced risk of needle blockage, and decreased incidence of papules and nodules. Product placement in the appropriate deep injection planes will also help minimize nodules. Fig. 35.5 shows a visible periocular papule following too-superficial placement of PLLA using an older dilution technique. For injection of the cheek, preauricular area, nasolabial folds, and lower face, injection should be into the deeper subcutaneous plane. For treatment of the temples, PLLA should be injected beneath the temporalis fascia, and for injection of the zygoma, maxilla, and mandibular regions, depot injection in the subperiosteal plane is desired. Care should be taken not to inject the precipitate at the end of the syringe. Following implantation, vigorous massage of the treatment area with instructions for the patient to massage at home is recommended. The posttreatment "rule of 5s" is easy for the patients to remember: massage 5 times daily for 5 minutes for a duration of 5 days. However, data supporting posttreatment massage are

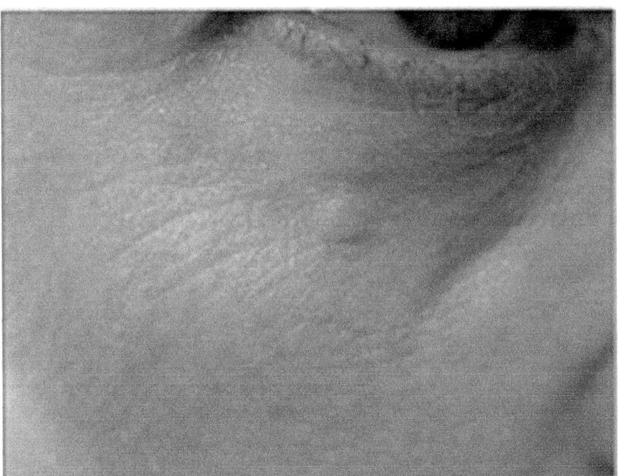

Fig. 35.5 An obvious small noninflamed papule in the periocular region following injection of poly-l-lactic acid (PLLA). An older, more concentrated dilution technique was used and the product placed too superficially. This nodule was subsequently excised and showed particles of PLLA and no inflammation.

limited and may be of less concern with the updated consensus recommendations for reconstitution and administration.

Even with recent alterations in protocol to minimize this complication, papules and nodules may still occur, as illustrated by a case report of a woman who developed numerous nodules 3 years after PLLA injections. This reaction may have been more likely due to a delayed foreign body reaction or a reaction to a latent infectious process rather than to product placement. It is important to note that the incidence of nodules is greater in areas where PLLA is able to aggregate in the muscle, which include highly mobile or dynamic areas, such as the perioral and periocular regions, as well as the hands and neck because of the proximity between the platysma and the skin; therefore, differences in regional thickness of skin should be considered when injecting PLLA. Diligence is needed when injecting these sites, and treatment should not be performed by novice injectors.

Calcium Hydroxylapatite

Similar to other soft tissue fillers, calcium hydroxylapatite (CaHA) can be associated with a risk of nodule formation. CaHA (Radiesse) injected too superficially can result in visible white nodules. These can usually be treated by puncturing the nodules with a no. 11 blade or needle and then expressing the contents. As a result of the thin skin in the tear trough, a higher incidence of nodule formation may occur when treating the nasojugal sulcus. Furthermore, there is increasing evidence to support the use of intralesional sodium thiosulfate (STS) as a dissolving agent for CaHA nodules. STS has been shown to decrease the formation of kidney stones and to decrease deep cutaneous lesions in uremic calcifying arteriopathy (calciphylaxis). Recently, in a prospective, single-center, proof-of-concept study of 12 cadaveric porcine skin samples Robinson demonstrated successful use of intralesional STS injection alone or in conjunction with topical sodium metabisulfite in completely dissolved CaHA in the skin samples. The exact mechanism of action for STS is not yet confirmed but is likely to be multifactorial. One proposed mechanism includes STS's chelation of calcium into a calcium thiosulfate salt whose solubility is 250- to 100,000-fold higher than CaHA.

Hypersensitivity Reactions

HA is one of the components of the extracellular matrix of the dermis and has no organ or species specificity. When introduced to the market, nonanimal stabilized HA (NASHA) compounds were thought to be nonimmunogenic. Indeed, in spite of its frequent use for cosmetic reasons, there are very few descriptions of hypersensitivity reactions secondary to injections of HA. A case of circulating antibodies against HA in patients after several injections was reported; however, these findings could not be confirmed by other investigators. In a randomized clinical trial using Restylane and Perlane (now known as Lyft), researchers failed to detect clinical or laboratory evidence for elicitation of humoral (type I hypersensitivity) or cell-mediated (delayed type IV hypersensitivity) immunity to NASHA in the majority of patients treated. At most, it is estimated by some experts that 1 in every 10,000 individuals undergoing augmentation with these materials reports a clinical hypersensitivity reaction. Many now feel, based on their clinical course and response to treatment, that a number of these reported hypersensitivity reactions are likely due to an infectious process.

Severe systemic hypersensitivity reactions secondary to injections of HA fillers are even more rare than local side effects. In 2009, a case was reported of a patient who developed acute facial angioedema accompanied by generalized urticarial lesions, pruritus, and fever 3 weeks after implantation of 1 mL of NASHA (Restylane) in her nasolabial folds. The patient subsequently developed palpable purpura on the trunk and extremities and had a biopsy that was consistent with leukocytoclastic vasculitis. Whether this was a true immunologic reaction in this specific case is questionable. However, it is important to be cognizant that there may be coincidental or idiosyncratic reactions with the use of dermal fillers.

In cases where there have been reports of clinical hypersensitivity reactions, it is postulated that the reactions were caused by residual proteins or impurities resulting from the manufacturing process rather than by the HA itself. There were two sources for industrial production of the HA used as agents for soft tissue augmentation: an animal HA produced from rooster combs (Hylaform) and a NASHA produced by bacterial fermentation from specific strains of streptococci (Restylane family, Juvéderm family, and Belotero). Some studies have shown that LMW fragments obtained from different preparations of HA stimulated the synthesis of interleukin-12 and tumor necrosis factor alpha in monocytes and that these findings might explain the rare reports of delayed hypersensitivity reactions in patients treated with HA injections. Others have postulated that when the cross-linked HA is broken down, the components used to stabilize the HA molecules might lead to inflammation or precipitate an immunologic response. In early European use of NASHA, delayed hypersensitivity reactions were reported at relatively low incidences, 0.15% to 0.42%. Since then, manufacturing processes have become even more stringent, subsequently reducing the protein load by sixfold and virtually eliminating the incidence of implant-site hypersensitivity reactions.

> **PEARL 6** The documented incidence of allergic reactions to NASHA gel remains extremely low. However, with the surge in popularity of these fillers, this risk may increase. It is incumbent upon physicians to discuss with patients not only the benefits but also the risks of a potential for an allergic response.

Although the incidence is low, there have been case reports of localized and generalized hypersensitivity reactions, immune-mediated granuloma formation, and sarcoidosis-like disease following injection with temporary soft tissue fillers. A rare but dramatic type of reaction that was reported in 2005 was an angioedema-type hypersensitivity to 1 mL of Restylane following injection into the upper lip. One hour after injection, the patient developed an angioedema-type swelling of the upper lip without systemic complaints. The patient was treated with intramuscular corticosteroids, with stabilization of swelling occurring 2 hours later, and was subsequently treated with an oral steroid taper with complete resolution of edema within 5 days.

Biofilms

Biofilms can contribute to delayed nodule formation or late infectious complications related to dermal filler injection. Biofilms arise when microorganisms form heterogeneous, largely immobile, densely packed, and quiescent colonies that adhere to inert surfaces and encapsulate themselves in a protective, self-developed polymeric extracellular matrix. Organisms can be introduced directly during injection, or through seeding of foreign material via hematologic or contiguous spread. Biofilms employ a number of virulence mechanisms that make them extremely difficult to eradicate, once established. Their complex scaffolding allows for evasion of immune system interference by physically limiting mobility of immune cells into the biofilm and subsequent phagocytosis of microbes. Additionally, studies have shown that altered gene expression in biofilms allows for active development of anti-infective resistance mechanisms. As an example, bacteria in biofilms have been shown to exhibit enhanced penicillin resistance through impaired penetration of the antibiotic through its matrix itself and rapid efflux of the antibiotic through pumps in the bacteria cell walls. Biofilm communities may require up to 1000-fold higher concentrations of antibiotic therapy for efficacy compared to their free-floating counterparts.

Biofilm formation therefore appears to be a critical step in pathogenesis for many subacute and chronic bacterial infections. Commonly commensal species, including *Staphylococcus aureus*, *Staphylococcus epidermidis*, *Pseudomonas aeruginosa*, and *Enterococcus* species, are often implicated in biofilm formation and are responsible for approximately two thirds of infections reported in the setting of indwelling foreign material. Less commonly, biofilms may also be composed of other microorganisms, such as *Candida* species. Biofilm-related infections are a well-known problem in medicine and have been reported with implantation of orthopedic devices, heart valves, indwelling catheters, and stents and have more recently been described in the setting of filler use for soft tissue augmentation.

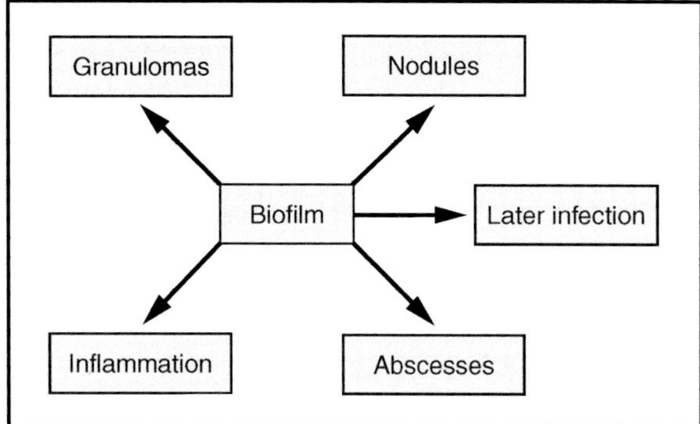

Fig. 35.6 Potential complications from biofilms.

Biofilm formation has been reported with most filler types; however, reports suggest that this occurrence is most prominent when permanent nondegradable gels such as silicone or polyacrylamide gel are used. Clinical presentation of biofilms can be acute or late (up to years after injection), usually with onset of erythematous papules and nodules (Fig. 35.6). However, biofilm-induced nodules can also present as inert granulomas, increasing diagnostic ambiguity. While biofilms may remain indolent for long periods of time, they can become activated in the setting of trauma or repeat injection at sites of previous filler placement, even years after they are established, resulting in active local infections, sepsis, or chronic inflammation with granulomatous responses. A classic presentation that should increase suspicion of biofilm formation is recurring, often pyogenic infections after "successful" past treatment as the biofilms can continue to seed local tissue.

PEARL 7 Biofilms may account for a number of today's delayed-onset complications, including granulomas, nodules, inflammation, and abscesses. Prolonged antibiotic use may be necessary even when cultures do not reveal a definitive organism.

Work-up and management are similar to that discussed in the prior section; however, when biofilms are suspected, more sensitive diagnostic technologies such as PCR and FISH should be prioritized as biofilm colonies are frequently culture negative. Macrolides are particularly useful in the treatment of biofilms because they are lipophilic and accumulate in the fat (often where the filler resides), and they can inhibit quorum sensing, which biofilm organisms use to communicate with each other and regulate their environment. Many authors recommend clarithromycin or minocycline for a 2- to 6-week course. If a patient's nodules are noninflammatory and do not respond to an appropriate course of antibiotics, trials of oral or intralesional steroids as well as intralesional 5-fluorouracil have been carried out, with some success. If these strategies do not clear the nodule(s), especially in the setting of long-lasting particulate fillers, excision should be considered as a last resort (Box 35.3).

BOX 35.3 Key Prevention and Management Strategies to Avoid Blindness

- Prevention
  - Know the location and depth of facial vessels.
  - Inject slowly and with minimal pressure.
  - Inject in small increments (0.1 mL aliquots).
  - Move the needle tip while injecting to prevent large deposit in one location.
  - Aspirate prior to injection (efficacy controversial but recommended, especially with poly-l-lactic acid [PLLA]).
  - Use a small-diameter needle (necessitates slower injection).
  - Smaller syringes are preferred to larger ones to control volume.
  - Use caution if prior surgical procedure in area (i.e., rhinoplasty, face lift).
  - Consider using a cannula to reduce the chance of entering a blood vessel (i.e., highly vascularized areas such as tear trough).
- Management
  - If ocular pain or vision changes, stop injecting at once.
  - Immediately contact an ophthalmologist or oculoplastic surgeon and transfer the patient directly there.
  - Consider treating the injected area and surrounding tissue with hyaluronidase.
  - Consider retrobulbar injection of 300 to 600 units (2 to 4 mL) of hyaluronidase, regardless of which filler is used.
  - Consider reduction of intraocular pressure (i.e., ocular massage, intravenous mannitol).
  - Monitor the patient's neurologic status and order relevant imaging studies (high prevalence of central nervous system [CNS] complications accompany blindness).

Modified from Beleznay K, Carruthers JD, Humphrey S, Jones D. Avoiding and treating blindness from fillers: a review of the world literature. *Dermatol Surg*. 2015;41:1097–1117.

PEARL 8 The first step in the management of most inflammatory and noninflammatory papules and nodules is to rule out infection or abscess by physical exam and history and to institute antimicrobials if necessary. Noninflammatory nodules are usually immune mediated and thus respond to anti-inflammatories such as oral or intralesional steroids.

Granulomas

A granuloma is a nonallergic inflammatory reaction that is comprised predominantly of macrophages. As this reaction matures, macrophages fuse to become multinucleated giant cells. Local and regional, as well as delayed and recurrent granulomatous, reactions may complicate dermal filler injections. Clinically, these typically manifest as persistent nodules arising between 6 and 24 months following filler placement. While there have been reports of delayed granulomas arising years after filler administration, the precise pathophysiology of these delayed granulomas is not fully understood and may not follow classic mechanisms.

Granuloma formation occurs over five phases, including inflammation, protein adsorption, macrophage adhesion, macrophage fusion, and, finally, cellular crosstalk. The degree and severity of foreign body granulomas can be classified into four grades, as proposed by Duranti et al.,[30] depending on their clinical and histologic characteristics. The development of foreign body granulomas after filler injection is uncommon, and the reported frequency varies considerably and depends on the type of filler used. For example, the incidence of foreign body granulomas occurring after HA filler injection, the most common filler type used, is reported between 0.02% and 0.4%. Factors that may influence the propensity for granuloma formation include the volume of injected material, whether repeat injections were performed, particle size and particle texture of the filler, presence of impurities, and the hydrophilicity and surface charge of the filler.

Virtually all synthetic fillers may act as foreign bodies, and the host response can vary on a spectrum ranging from sparsely distributed macrophages to an exuberant foreign body reaction with fibrosis depending on the filler type and the patient's individual immune response. The filler composition, presence of differential cross-linking, and particle size may all correlate with the risk of developing a granulomatous reaction. Furthermore, as mentioned previously, there may be an increased incidence in delayed-onset nodules for HA-based fillers that incorporate Vycross Technology, a proprietary cross-linking method of manufacturing, according to recent studies by Sadeghpour et al. in 2019 and Humphrey et al. in 2020. Caution should be exercised in patients with a known history of autoimmune connective tissue disorders and is contraindicated in patients with known sarcoidosis. Patients with any autoimmune connective tissue diseases should be properly counseled beforehand that their risks of granuloma formation from soft tissue fillers may be higher than the general population. Thus, filler and patient characteristics should all be considered on an individual basis when determining which product and filler type, if any, may be used safely and appropriately.

For specific fillers, such as PLLA (Sculptra) and CaHA (Radiesse), a fibrotic response by the patient actually drives the resultant and more prolonged volumization. Interestingly, CaHA tends to be associated with a high incidence of nodules when injected into the lips, but these nodules are noninflammatory in nature. Histologically, microspheres of CaHA tend to recruit small numbers of macrophages, which surround the product, but foreign body reactions are not elicited. Nevertheless, due to the unique nongranulomatous lip nodule forming tendency and reports of distant migration with this filler, CaHA should be avoided for augmentation of the lips. In contrast, collagen and its constituents, which are no longer used due to their associated risk of anaphylaxis, are resorbed over a period of approximately 3 to 4 months. As such, the risks of delayed or persistent granuloma formation are quite low. Rare examples of palisading granulomas resembling granuloma annulare and disseminated and recurrent sarcoid-like granulomatous panniculitis have been reported in the past following bovine collagen injections.

Although rare, HA products have been associated with granuloma formation. Clinically, these granulomas manifest as delayed erythema and either painful or nontender swollen nodules. In one case, a patient received an HA product in the vermilion border and subsequently developed discrete nodules, initially associated with eczematous changes of the overlying skin, 6 weeks after injection. Histologic evaluation revealed the presence of a sharply demarcated nodule in the subcutaneous fat, consistent with a granulomatous foreign body reaction to the filler. The underlying mechanisms of these reactions are still poorly understood, although some hypothesize they occur due to an inherent continuous foreign body reaction induced by filler placement, while others favor onset in response to a biofilm. As aforementioned, many reactions that were previously felt to be foreign body granulomas or allergic reactions on the basis of negative bacterial cultures are now thought to be due to biofilms. There is some evidence implicating bacterial contamination at the time of implantation as a potential etiology for these granulomatous responses, although this is not widely accepted.

Regardless of the inciting event, these granulomas have been shown to respond to intralesional and topical steroids as well as topical calcineurin inhibitors. In cases of HA-related granulomatous foreign body reactions that do not respond to initial treatment, the local administration of hyaluronidase may be considered to relieve the problem.

Similar reactions have also been reported and histologically confirmed with non-HA fillers, such as PLLA (Fig. 35.4). The granulomatous reaction to PLLA particles may persist for at least 18 months after injection. Although bacterial etiologies have been implicated as the presumed culprits for these reactions, microorganisms have not been detected by PCR or histological analysis of the granulomatous reaction. There is a particular concern among some experts for a rigorous granulomatous response to PLLA in patients who experience immune reconstitution (IRIS), in which a previously immunodeficient patient becomes immunocompetent while being treated for HIV. In these particular patients, it is hypothesized that these previously immunocompromised patients develop a robust, hyperactive response to implanted infectious or foreign material after their immunity returns. Several authors have reported on significant, visible deformity resulting from foreign body–induced giant cell granulomatous reactions following skin augmentation with PLLA. While some granulomas may resolve spontaneously, management with intralesional steroids, topical imiquimod, and even surgical excision have all been reported to facilitate resolution. Severe systemic adverse effects secondary to PLLA injections are extremely rare; however, one case of anaphylaxis, requiring treatment interruption, and one of angioedema have been reported. As noted previously, with appropriate deposition technique and adequate dilution, late-onset foreign body granulomas are rare (as low as 0.1%). Nevertheless, patients and physicians must be aware of this potential side effect and have strategies in place for management should it arise.

ACUTE, POTENTIALLY CATASTROPHIC DERMAL FILLER COMPLICATIONS

Vascular Complications

Although rare, tissue necrosis, vision loss (both unilateral and bilateral), ophthalmoplegia, and other thrombotic events all represent feared vascular complications that may result from filler injections. It is critical that the injecting clinician be aware of these adverse events, is able to promptly recognize the early signs of these complications and have treatment protocols in place to manage or mitigate these consequences should they arise.

Necrosis

Necrosis of skin and local tissues is a rare but serious complication that may arise from filler injections and has been observed across all filler types. There has been an increase in the incidence of necrosis in recent years, although this may be partially attributable to the rise in the overall number of cosmetic treatments being performed. There is also a growing concern regarding the variable experience level and training backgrounds of individuals offering these treatments, which may further contribute to the increasing incidence of adverse events. Nevertheless, the judicious use of fillers, proper placement and selection of products, as well as the prompt recognition and management of complications are vital to minimizing morbidity. While uncommon, even with proper technique, a vascular incident may be inevitable in any injector's career despite its statistical unlikelihood. As such, the practicing clinician should always be prepared for such a scenario and should possess both the expertise and necessary adjuncts to intervene promptly and attempt to mitigate the ensuing damage.

Necrosis is thought to result from inadvertent placement of filler within the lumen of a vessel or from compression of nearby feeding blood vessels. The resulting vascular occlusion compromises blood flow and results in poor tissue oxygenation, which results in death of the affected skin and local tissue. This may present with a mottled pattern of violaceous or dusky discoloration of the overlying skin in or adjacent to the area in which filler was administered. If not immediately recognized and ameliorated as much as possible, this can further progress to discoloration, pain, ulceration, and eventual scarring of the skin upon healing.

The anatomic area at greatest risk for injection necrosis and complications is the glabellar region. This area corresponds to the supratrochlear artery and accompanying small-caliber branches that supply this "watershed region," which inherently has limited collateral circulation. However, this complication may also arise along the course of the facial artery, angular artery, lateral nasal artery, or any of their branches. A strong understanding of normal facial anatomy, particularly the location and course of major arteries and general differences between regional skin properties and thickness, is of prime importance in minimizing necrosis. To this end, both Beleznay and Carruthers et al. have published practical clinical articles detailing the pertinent facial vascular anatomy in their respective publications.

A number of techniques have been proposed to mitigate the risk of necrosis, including aspirating before injecting, using cannulas, adopting a slow and retrograde manner of injection, and keeping the needle constantly mobile. However, the impact of these injection strategies on decreasing the risk of necrosis is difficult to quantify. The utility of aspiration before injection with HA fillers is controversial because the viscosity of the product may not permit adequate flashback into the syringe when using fine-tipped needles. Furthermore, a 2015 study found that withdrawal of the HA syringe plunger while using slow or fast techniques, even with complete absence of visible blood in the syringe, does not eliminate the possibility of intravascular placement. The proper selection of appropriate agents, for example, using fillers with smaller particle size in superficial injection planes, is also imperative in helping to minimize this complication. It is also generally advised to avoid injection in the immediate vicinity of large named facial vessels. Finally, many experts have adopted and implemented the use of blunt-tipped cannulas, which reduce but do not eliminate the risk of intravascular entry.

Impending necrosis presents in one of three patterns: immediate, early (within 24–48 hours), or delayed (>48 hours). Several protocols exist for managing this complication and the treatment is dependent on the time of onset. First, impending vascular compromise may be evident by blanching, followed by a dusky or purple discoloration of the area. Additionally, a patient may complain of pain out of proportion to normal injection discomfort. Upon prompt recognition of these features, the injection should be immediately discontinued to assess, evaluate, and treat any complications, if necessary. The immediate application of warm compresses and manual massaging of the area will promote vasodilation and improve blood flow. Approximately 0.5 inch (12 mm) of 2% nitroglycerin paste should be massaged onto the affected area, which will often result in revascularization, which is manifested by a pink hue appearing within minutes. Other vasodilatory agents such as sildenafil citrate (Viagra, Pfizer, Inc.), calcium channel blockers, or other similar drugs may also be considered adjunctively to increase blood flow, though their benefits in the acute setting have yet to be determined.

Hyaluronidase, which enzymatically degrades HA, is recommended if the aforementioned treatments prove insufficient or ineffective. It should be noted that anaphylaxis has been reported after retrobulbar injection of hyaluronidase, but not after subcutaneous administration, although anaphylaxis may still theoretically be possible. Because hyaluronidase is one of the active components of bee venom, its administration in patients with a history of allergy to bee stings should be performed cautiously. In the routine use of hyaluronidase, skin testing for hypersensitivity is generally recommended prior to administration of two hyaluronidase formulations: bovine-derived Amphadase (Amphastar Pharmaceuticals, Inc., Rancho Cucamonga, CA) and sheep-derived Vitrase (ISTA Pharmaceutical, Irvine, CA). However, a consensus report on the treatment of filler-induced necrosis did not find it necessary to conduct a skin test prior to administration of hyaluronidase in more urgent situations. In these scenarios, the physician should alternatively be prepared to manage hypersensitivity or anaphylaxis if they should occur.

In addition to enzymatic breakdown of HA, hyaluronidase has been shown to reduce edema, which may minimize external pressure on occluded vessels. As such, hyaluronidase may be of benefit in the management of impending necrosis even if an HA-based filler was not used. In more severe or unresponsive cases of necrosis, Schanz et al. described their success using deep subcutaneous injections of LMW heparin into the affected area. Although a course of oral steroids may decrease inflammation and improve blood flow to the area, corticosteroids also have vasoconstrictive properties, which could exacerbate the vascular occlusion. Thus, the exact role of corticosteroids in this setting is unclear. Fortunately, in many cases, the skin necrosis remodels and the resultant damage are less than expected. Should contour irregularities persist, fillers may be placed to correct depressed areas followed by a series of fractionated laser treatments to improve the contour by stimulating collagen deposition.

> **PEARL 9** Necrosis is a rare but serious complication associated with filler injections and all practicing clinicians should have a treatment protocol in place to effectively manage this. Injections of hyaluronidase may help to minimize impending necrosis across all types of fillers.

Blindness

Although exceedingly rare, blindness is perhaps the most feared and catastrophic complication of filler injection and can be accompanied by ophthalmoplegia, ptosis, skin necrosis, and ischemic stroke. Beleznay's 2015 review of world literature revealed more than 98 cases of vision changes following fillers, ranging from mild impairment to complete vision loss. In the 2019 update, 48 more cases were identified, for a total of 146. Additionally, a systematic review reported a total of 190 cases in the literature. The most common symptoms were immediate vision loss, ocular pain, as well as nausea/vomiting and headache. In both reviews, autologous fat was the most common agent associated with ocular complications (47.9% and 47.4%, respectively), followed by HA fillers (23.5% and 27.9%, respectively). It should be noted that autologous fat had a higher risk of permanent blindness (80.9%) compared with HA (39.1%). This finding could reflect the use of larger volumes, larger syringes, bigger particle sizes, and higher extrusion pressures required for autologous fat injections. Autologous fat may also have a higher propensity to activate the clotting or inflammatory cascade compared to other soft tissue fillers. The injection sites at the highest risk for ocular symptoms in descending order were the glabella (38.8%), nasal region (25.5%), nasolabial fold (13.3%), and forehead (12.2%); however, virtually every anatomic location of the face is at theoretical risk for blindness due to extensive vascular anastomoses and the ability of filler material to travel in retrograde fashion.

Blindness from autologous fat injection has been universally irreversible and has no available injectable antidote, whereas vision loss from HA has been partially reversed in some cases with hyaluronidase. The goal of intervention if impending blindness is suspected is rapid restoration of perfusion to the eye. Carruthers et al. have presented techniques for retrobulbar and peribulbar injection of hyaluronidase in an attempt to restore vision loss. Even if not injected intravascularly, hyaluronidase may be able to cross vessel walls and dissolve intra-arterial HA, which has been demonstrated in facial artery specimens obtained from fresh human cadavers.

It has been shown that damage secondary to retinal ischemia becomes irreversible after 90 minutes; however, many experts feel that this overestimates the time one has to perform sight-saving intervention. It is generally believed that early immediate intervention has the highest likelihood of vision restoration and is preferred. However, there has been an isolated reported case of vision restoration after a 12-hour delay in administration by Sharudin et al. Beleznay et al.[41] have proposed key prevention and management strategies, adapted here in Box 35.3. Ideally, with careful injection technique, iatrogenic blindness from filler may be fully preventable and should never occur, but this complication may become more common with the increasing use of fillers by those less experienced with facial vascular anatomy. Moreover, it is important to note that the use of blunt cannulas may reduce, but does not entirely eliminate, this risk. Therefore, having a blindness protocol (Fig. 35.7) and in-office emergency kit (Fig. 35.8) in place is essential. Several other interventions including systemic steroids, hyperbaric oxygen, systemic antibiotics, and acetazolamide have been described in the literature, but their exact role or benefit is unclear.

Cerebral Infarction and Pulmonary Embolism

Although the exact incidence is unknown, case reports of cerebral infarction and pulmonary embolism attributed to HA-based filler injections have been described. Ischemic stroke is thought to occur when the injected filler material proceeds intra-arterially and travels retrograde into the circle of Willis via the internal carotid artery. In a recently published case series by Sorensen and Council, most reported ischemic strokes occurred in the middle cerebral artery (MCA) distribution, caused permanent hemiparesis, and was independent of filler type. Nevertheless, as both scenarios represent potentially life-threatening situations for the patient, the appropriate emergency and interdisciplinary care should be sought.

Blindness Protocol

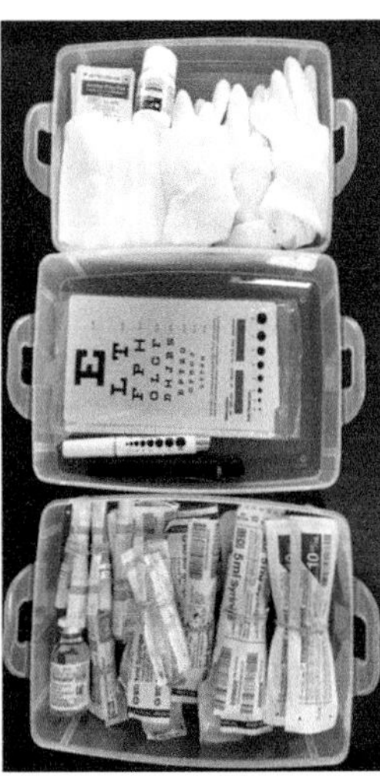

- Vision/Eye examination:
  - Visual acuity chart, swinging flashlight test, extraocular movement, ptosis
- Symptoms:
  - Visual changes, pain, headache, nausea, dizziness, weakness in extremities
- Strength exam of the extremities
- Skin exam, capillary refill
- Document all findings

Courtesy of Dr. Katie Beleznay

Blindness Protocol

- Connect with Ophthalmology ASAP
- 1500 U of HYAL can be injected at site of injection & along path of artery
- Ocular massage, Aspirin, Timolol, Rebreathing in paper bag
- Consider 1000-1500 U HYAL into supraorbital & supratrochlear notch
- Retrobulbar hyaluronidase: Consider retrobulbar injection of 3000 units HYAL (2 cc) (Canadian compounded hyaluronidase 1500 IU/mL)

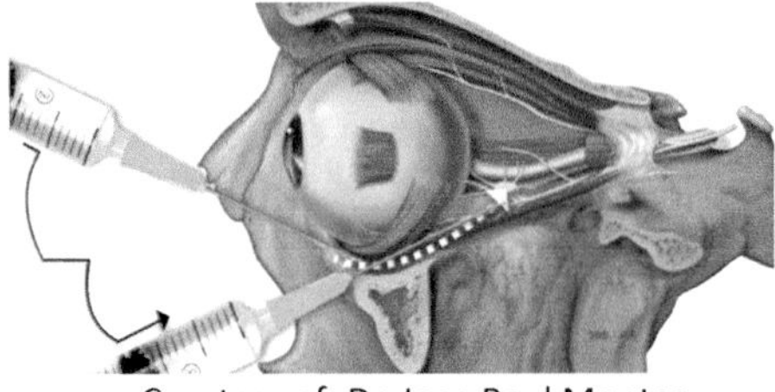

Courtesy of: Dr. Jose Raul Montes

Fig. 35.7 Blindness protocol. (Courtesy of Dr. Katie Beleznay.)

CONCLUSIONS

Soft tissue augmentation with injectable fillers continues to be one of the most commonly performed minimally invasive cosmetic procedures and the number of treatments is expected to continue to rise annually. Under the care of a prudent and judicious clinician, fillers offer an effective, gratifying, reasonably safe, and well-tolerated procedural intervention. Nevertheless, as both the number of patients seeking injections and the repertoire of available fillers and materials expand, it is imperative that injecting physicians have the proper

Blindness Protocol Emergency Kit

- Hyaluronidase vials
- 3 cc syringes, 25 gauge 1.5 inch needles, 30 gauge 1/2 inch needles, 25 gauge cannula, 23 gauge introducer (lots of these)
- Timolol drops
- Aspirin
- Lidocaine (without epinephrine)
- Snellen chart
- Flashlight

Fig. 35.8 Blindness emergency kit. (Courtesy of Dr. Katie Beleznay.)

training and familiarity with their potential complications and resultant management should they arise. Although complication rates are generally low with these agents, they can still occur even in the most experienced of hands, and early recognition and appropriate intervention are critical. The injecting clinician should take every possible measure to ensure the best possible outcomes while minimizing the risk of adverse events with proper technique, proper product selection, and a deep understanding of facial anatomy, but should always be vigilant and prompt in addressing impending complications if additional intervention becomes necessary.

FURTHER READING

Alam, M., & Dover, J. S. (2007). Management of complications and sequelae with temporary injectable fillers. *Plastic and Reconstructive Surgery*, *120*, S98–S105. https://doi.org/10.1097/01.prs.0000248859.14788.60.

Alam, M., & Tung, R. (2018). Injection technique in neurotoxins and fillers: Planning and basic technique. *Journal of the American Academy of Dermatology*, *79*(3), 407–419. https://doi.org/10.1016/j.jaad.2018.01.034.

Alijotas-Reig, J., Fernandez-Figueras, M. T., & Puig, L. (2013). Inflammatory, immune-mediated adverse reactions related to soft tissue dermal fillers. *Seminars in Arthritis and Rheumatism*, *43*, 241–258. https://doi.org/10.1016/j.semarthrit.2013.02.001.

Alsaad, S., Fabi, S. G., & Goldman, M. P. (2012). Granulomatous reaction to hyaluronic acid: A case series and review of the literature. *Dermatologic Surgery*, *38*(2), 271–276. https://doi.org/10.1111/j.1524-4725.2011.02214.x.

Apikian, M., Roberts, S., & Goodman, G. J. (2007). Adverse reactions to polylactic acid injections in the periorbital area. *Journal of Cosmetic Dermatology*, *6*(2), 95–101. https://doi.org/10.1111/j.1473-2165.2007.00303.x.

Artzi, O., Loizides, C., Verner, I., & Landau, M. (2016). Resistant and recurrent late reaction to hyaluronic acid-based gel. *Dermatologic Surgery*, *42*, 31–37. https://doi.org/10.1097/DSS.0000000000000562.

Artzi, O., Cohen, J. L., Dover, J. S., et al. (2020). Delayed inflammatory reactions to hyaluronic acid fillers: A literature review and proposed treatment algorithm. *Clinical, Cosmetic and Investigational Dermatology*, *13*, 371–378. https://doi.org/10.2147/CCID.S247171.

Avram, M., Bertucci, V., Cox, S. E., Jones, D., & Mariwalla, K. (2020). *Guidance regarding SARS-CoV-2 mRNA vaccine side effects in dermal filler patients*. American Society of Dermatologic Surgery.

Baeva, L. F., Lyle, D. B., Rios, M., Langone, J. J., & Lightfoote, M. M. (2014). Different molecular weight hyaluronic acid effects on human macrophage interleukin 1β production. *Journal of Biomedical Materials Research. Part A*, *102*, 305–314. https://doi.org/10.1002/jbm.a.34704.

Beer, K. (2014). Avoiding complications with fillers. *Dermatologist*, *22*(11), 20–21.

Beleznay, K., Carruthers, J. D., Carruthers, A., Mummert, M. E., & Humphrey, S. (2015). Delayed-onset nodules secondary to a smooth cohesive 20 mg/mL hyaluronic acid filler: Cause and management. *Dermatologic Surgery*, *41*, 929–939. https://doi.org/10.1097/DSS.0000000000000418.

Beleznay, K., Carruthers, J. D., Humphrey, S., & Jones, D. (2015). Avoiding and treating blindness from fillers: A review of the world literature. *Dermatologic Surgery, 41*, 1097–1117. https://doi.org/10.1097/DSS.0000000000000486.

Beleznay, K., Carruthers, J. D., Humphrey, S., Carruthers, A., & Jones, D. (2019). Update on avoiding and treating blindness from fillers: a recent review of the world literature. *Aesthetic Surgery Journal, 39*(6), 662–674. https://doi.org/10.1093/asj/sjz053.

Berlin, A. L., & Cohen, J. L. (2016). Improving bruising after facial filler injections. *Dermatologist, 24*(1), 20–21.

Brandt, F., Bassichis, B., Bassichis, M., O'Connell, C., & Lin, X. (2011). Safety and effectiveness of small and large gel-particle hyaluronic acid in the correction of perioral wrinkles. *Journal of Drugs in Dermatology, 10*, 982–987.

Broughton, G., Crosby, M. A., Coleman, J., & Rohrich, R. J. (2007). Use of herbal supplements and vitamins in plastic surgery: A practical review. *Plastic and Reconstructive Surgery, 119*(3), 48e–66e. https://doi.org/10.1097/01.prs.0000252661.72071.8d.

Carey, W., & Weinkle, S. (2015). Retraction of the plunger on a syringe of hyaluronic acid before injection: are we safe? *Dermatologic Surgery, 41*, S340–S346. https://doi.org/10.1097/DSS.0000000000000557.

Carruthers, J., Fagien, S., & Dolman, P. (2015). Retro or peribulbar injection techniques to reverse visual loss after filler injections. *Dermatologic Surgery, 41*, S354–S357. https://doi.org/10.1097/DSS.0000000000000558.

Chatrath, V., Banerjee, P. S., Goodman, G. J., & Rahman, E. (2019). Soft-tissue filler–Associated blindness: A systematic review of case reports and case series. *Plastic and Reconstructive Surgery. Global Open, 7*(4), e2173. https://doi.org/10.1097/GOX.0000000000002173.

Chiang, Y., Pierone, G., & Al-Niaimi, F. (2017). Dermal fillers: Pathophysiology, prevention and treatment of complications. *Journal of the European Academy of Dermatology and Venereology, 31*, 405–413. https://doi.org/10.1111/jdv.13977.

Christensen, L. (2007). Normal and pathologic tissue reactions to soft tissue gel fillers. *Dermatologic Surgery, 33*(suppl 2), S168–S175. https://doi.org/10.1111/j.1524-4725.2007.33357.x.

Christensen, L. (2009). Host tissue interaction, fate, and risks of degradable and nondegradable gel fillers. *Dermatologic Surgery, 35*(suppl 2), S1612–S1619. https://doi.org/10.1111/j.1524-4725.2009.01338.x.

Christensen, L., Breiting, V., Janssen, M., Vuust, J., & Hogdall, E. (2005). Adverse reactions to injectable soft tissue permanent fillers. *Aesthetic Plastic Surgery, 29*(1), 34–48. https://doi.org/10.1007/s00266-004-0113-6.

Cohen, J. L. (2008). Understanding, avoiding, and managing dermal filler complications. *Dermatologic Surgery, 34*(suppl 1), 92–99. https://doi.org/10.1111/j.1524-4725.2008.34249.x.

Cohen, J. L., Biesman, B. S., Dayan, S. H., et al. (2015). Treatment of hyaluronic acid filler-induced impending necrosis with hyaluronidase: Consensus recommendations. *Aesthetic Surgery Journal, 35*(7), 844–849. https://doi.org/10.1093/asj/sjv018.

Coleman, S. R. (2006). Cross-linked hyaluronic acid fillers. *Plastic and Reconstructive Surgery, 117*, 661–665. https://doi.org/10.1097/01.prs.0000200913.34368.79.

Dayan, S. H., Arkins, J. P., & Brindise, R. (2011). Soft tissue fillers and biofilms. *Facial Plastic Surgery, 27*(1), 23–28. https://doi.org/10.1055/s-0030-1270415.

de Felipe, I., & Redondo, P. (2015). The liquid lift: Looking natural without lumps. *Journal of Cutaneous and Aesthetic Surgery, 8*(3), 134–138. https://doi.org/10.4103/0974-2077.167267.

DeLorenzi, C. (2014). Transarterial degradation of hyaluronic acid filler by hyaluronidase. *Dermatologic Surgery, 40*(8), 832–841. https://doi.org/10.1097/DSS.0000000000000062.

Dover, J. S., Rubin, M. G., & Bhatia, A. C. (2009). Review of the efficacy, durability, and safety data of two non-animal stabilized hyaluronic acid fillers from a prospective, randomized, comparative, multicenter study. *Dermatologic Surgery, 35*(suppl 1), S322–S331. https://doi.org/10.1111/j.1524-4725.2008.01060.x.

Duranti, F., Salti, G., Bovani, B., Calandra, M., & Rosati, M. L. (1998). Injectable hyaluronic acid gel for soft tissue augmentation. A clinical and histological study. *Dermatologic Surgery, 24*(12), 1317–1325.

Forbat, E., & Al-Niaimi, F. (2019). Nonvascular uses of pulsed dye laser in clinical dermatology. *Journal of Cosmetic Dermatology, 18*(3), 1186–1201. https://doi.org/10.1111/jocd.12924.

Fulton, J., Caperton, C., Weinkle, S., & Dewandre, L. (2012). Filler injections with the blunt-tip microcannula. *Journal of Drugs in Dermatology, 11*(9), 1098–1103.

Galadari, H., Mariwalla, K., Delobel, P., & Sanchez-Vizcaino, E. M. (2020). Pain and bruising levels after lip augmentation: A comparison of anterograde and retrograde techniques using an automated motorized injection device. A blinded, prospective, randomized, parallel, within-subject trial. *Dermatologic Surgery, 46*(3), 395–401. https://doi.org/10.1097/DSS.0000000000002055.

Gilbert, E., Hui, A., Meehan, S., & Waldorf, H. A. (2012). The basic science of dermal fillers: Past and present part II: Adverse effects. *Journal of Drugs in Dermatology, 11*(9), 1069–1079.

Glashofer, M. G., & Cohen, J. L. (2010). Complications from soft-tissue augmentation of the face: A guide to understanding, avoiding, and managing periprocedural issues. In D. Jones (Ed.), *Injectable fillers, principles and practice* (pp. 121–139). Oxford: Wiley-Blackwell.

Grunebaum, L. D., Allemann, I., Dayan, S., Mandy, S., & Baumann, L. (2009). The risk of alar necrosis associated with dermal filler injection. *Dermatologic Surgery*, *35*(suppl 2), S1635–S1640. https://doi.org/10.1111/j.1524-4725.2009.01342.x.

Guardiani, E., & Davison, S. P. (2012). Angioedema after treatment with injectable poly-l-lactic acid (Sculptra). *Plastic and Reconstructive Surgery*, *129*(1), 187e–189e. https://doi.org/10.1097/PRS.0b013e3182365e58.

Hamilton, R. G., Strobos, J., & Adkinson, N. F. (2007). Immunogenicity studies of cosmetically administered nonanimal-stabilized hyaluronic acid particles. *Dermatologic Surgery*, *33*(suppl 2), S176–S185. https://doi.org/10.1111/j.1524-4725.2007.33358.x.

Hamilton, D. G., Gauthier, N., & Robertson, B. F. (2008). Late-onset, recurrent facial nodules associated with injection of poly-l-lactic acid. *Dermatologic Surgery*, *34*, 123–126. https://doi.org/10.1111/j.1524-4725.2007.34027.x.

Hirsch, R. J., & Cohen, J. L. (2007). Surgical insights: Challenge: Correcting superficially placed hyaluronic acid. *Skin Aging*, *15*, 36–38.

Hirsch, R. J., Cohen, J. L., & Carruthers, J. D. (2007). Successful management of an unusual presentation of impending necrosis following a hyaluronic acid injection embolus and a proposed algorithm for management with hyaluronidase. *Dermatologic Surgery*, *33*, 357–360. https://doi.org/10.1111/j.1524-4725.2007.33073.x.

Ho, D., Jagdeo, J., & Waldorf, H. A. (2016). Is there a role for arnica and bromelain in prevention of post-procedure ecchymosis or edema? A systematic review of the literature. *Dermatologic Surgery*, *42*, 445–463. https://doi.org/10.1097/DSS.0000000000000701.

Humphrey, S., Jones, D. H., Carruthers, J. D., et al. (2020). Retrospective review of delayed adverse events secondary to treatment with a smooth, cohesive 20-mg/mL hyaluronic acid filler in 4500 patients. *Journal of the American Academy of Dermatology*, *83*(1), 86–95. https://doi.org/10.1016/j.jaad.2020.01.066.

Ibrahim, O., Overman, J., Arndt, K., & Dover, J. (2018). Filler nodules: Inflammatory or infectious? A review of biofilms and their implications on clinical practice. *Dermatologic Surgery*, *44*, 53–60. https://doi.org/10.1097/DSS.0000000000001202.

Jang, J. G., Hong, K. S., & Choi, E. Y. (2014). A case of nonthrombotic pulmonary embolism after facial injection of hyaluronic acid in an illegal cosmetic procedure. *Tuberculosis and Respiratory Diseases*, *77*(2), 90–93. https://doi.org/10.4046/trd.2014.77.2.90.

Karen, J. K., Hale, E. K., & Geronemus, R. G. (2010). A simple solution to the common problem of ecchymosis. *Archives of Dermatology*, *146*(1), 94–95. https://doi.org/10.1001/archdermatol.2009.343.

Kassir, M., Gupta, M., Galadari, H., et al. (2020). Complications of botulinum toxin and fillers: A narrative review. *Journal of Cosmetic Dermatology*, *19*, 570–573. https://doi.org/10.1111/jocd.13266.

Kim, E. G., Eom, T. K., & Kang, S. J. (2014). Severe visual loss and cerebral infarction after injection of hyaluronic acid gel. *The Journal of Craniofacial Surgery*, *25*(2), 684–686. https://doi.org/10.1097/SCS.0000000000000537.

Lafaille, P., & Benedetto, A. (2010). Fillers: Contraindications, side effects and precautions. *Journal of Cutaneous and Aesthetic Surgery*, *3*, 16–19. https://doi.org/10.4103/0974-2077.63222.

Lafaurie, M., Dolivo, M., Porcher, R., et al. (2005). Treatment of facial lipoatrophy with intradermal injections of polylactic acid in HIV-infected patients. *Journal of Acquired Immune Deficiency Syndromes*, *38*(4), 393–398. https://doi.org/10.1097/01.qai.0000152834.02912.98.

Lam, S. M. (2016). Periorbital and midfacial volume enhancement with cannula. *JAMA Facial Plastic Surgery*, *18*(1), 71–72. https://doi.org/10.1001/jamafacial.2015.1192.

Landau, M. (2015). Hyaluronidase caveats in treating filler complications. *Dermatologic Surgery*, *41*, S347–S353. https://doi.org/10.1097/DSS.0000000000000555.

Lazzeri, D., Spinelli, G., Zhang, Y. X., Nardi, M., & Lazzeri, S. (2014). Panophthalmoplegia and vision loss after cosmetic nasal dorsum injection. *Journal of Clinical Neuroscience*, *21*(5), 890. https://doi.org/10.1016/j.jocn.2013.12.017.

Lee, J. M., & Kim, Y. J. (2015). Foreign body granulomas after the use of dermal fillers: Pathophysiology, clinical appearance, histologic features, and treatment. *Aesthetic Plastic Surgery*, *42*(2), 232–239. https://doi.org/10.5999/aps.2015.42.2.232.

Lee, A., Grummer, S. E., Kriegel, D., & Marmur, E. (2010). Hyaluronidase. *Dermatologic Surgery*, *36*, 1071–1077. https://doi.org/10.1111/j.1524-4725.2010.01585.x.

Lee, W. R., Kim, S. J., Park, J. H., et al. (2010). Bee venom reduces atherosclerotic lesion formation via anti-inflammatory mechanism. *The American Journal of Chinese Medicine*, *38*, 1077–1092. https://doi.org/10.1142/S0192415X10008482.

Lemperle, G., Rullan, P. P., & Gauthier-Hazan, N. (2006). Avoiding and treating dermal filler complications. *Plastic and Reconstructive Surgery*, *118*(suppl 3), S92–S107. https://doi.org/10.1097/01.prs.0000234672.69287.77.

Leonhardt, J. M., Lawrence, N., & Narins, R. S. (2005). Angioedema acute hypersensitivity reaction to injectable hyaluronic acid. *Dermatologic Surgery*, *31*, 577–579. https://doi.org/10.1111/j.1524-4725.2005.31166.

Lowe, N. J., Maxwell, C. A., & Patnaik, R. (2005). Adverse reactions to dermal fillers: Review. *Dermatologic Surgery*, *31*, 1626–1633.

Mally, P., Czyz, C. N., Chan, N. J., & Wulc, A. E. (2014). Vibration anesthesia for the reduction of pain with facial dermal filler injections. *Aesthetic Plastic Surgery*, *38*(2), 413–418. https://doi.org/10.1007/s00266-013-0264-4.

Monheit, G. D., & Rohrich, R. J. (2009). The nature of long-term fillers and the risk of complications. *Dermatologic Surgery*, *35*(suppl 2), S1598–S1604. https://doi.org/10.1111/j.1524-4725.2009.01336.x.

Mummert, M. E. (2005). Immunologic roles of hyaluronan. *Immunologic Research*, *31*, 189–206. https://doi.org/10.1385/IR:31:3:189.

Munavalli, G. G., Knutsen-Larson, S., Lupo, M., & Geronemus, R. G. (2021). Oral angiotensin converting enzyme inhibitors for the treatment of delayed inflammatory reaction of dermal hyaluronic acid fillers following COVID-19 vaccination – a model for inhibition of angiotensin ii-induced cutaneous inflammation. *JAAD Case Series*, *10*, 63–68. https://doi.org/10.1016/j.jdcr.2021.02.018.

Munavalli, G. G., Guthridge, R., Knutsen-Larson, S., Brodsky, A., Matthew, E., & Landau, M. (2022). COVID-19/SARS-CoV-2 virus spike protein-related delayed inflammatory reaction to hyaluronic acid dermal fillers: A challenging clinical conundrum in diagnosis and treatment. *Archives of Dermatological Research*, *314*(1), 1–15. https://doi.org/10.1007/s00403-021-02190-6.

Narins, R. S. (2008). Minimizing adverse events associated with poly-l-lactic acid injection. *Dermatologic Surgery*, *34*(suppl 1), S100–S104. https://doi.org/10.1111/j.1524-4725.2008.34250.x.

Narins, R. S., Jewell, M., Rubin, M., Cohen, J., & Strobos, J. (2006). Clinical conference: Management of rare events following dermal fillers—Focal necrosis and angry red bumps. *Dermatologic Surgery*, *32*, 426–434. https://doi.org/10.1111/j.1524-4725.2006.32086.x.

Narins, R. S., Coleman, W. P., & Glogau, R. G. (2009). Recommendations and treatment options for nodules and other filler complications. *Dermatologic Surgery*, *35*, 1667–1671. https://doi.org/10.1111/j.1524-4725.2009.01335.x.

Narukar, V. C. (2018). Post filler ecchymosis resolution with intense pulsed light. *Journal of Drugs in Dermatology*, *17*(11), 1184–1185.

Ortiz, A. E., Ahluwalia, J., Song, S. S., & Avram, M. M. (2020). Analysis of U.S. Food and Drug Administration data on soft-tissue filler complications. *Dermatologic Surgery*, *46*, 958–961. https://doi.org/10.1097/DSS.0000000000002208.

Ozturk, C. M., Li, Y., Tung, R., Parker, L., Piliang, M. P., & Zins, J. E. (2013). Complications following injection of soft-tissue fillers. *Aesthetic Surgery Journal*, *33*(6), 862–877. https://doi.org/10.1177/1090820X13493638.

Percival, S. L., Emanuel, C., Cutting, K. F., & Williams, D. W. (2011). Microbiology of the skin and the role of biofilms in infection. *International Wound Journal*, *9*(1), 14–32. https://doi.org/10.1111/j.1742-481X.2011.00836.x.

Requena, L., Requena, C., Christensen, L., Zimmermann, U. S., Kutzner, H., & Cerroni, L. (2011). Adverse reactions to injectable soft tissue fillers. *Journal of the American Academy of Dermatology*, *64*, 1–34. https://doi.org/10.1016/j.jaad.2010.02.064.

Reszko, A. E., Sadick, N. S., Magro, C. M., & Farber, J. (2009). Late-onset subcutaneous nodules after poly-l-lactic acid injection. *Dermatologic Surgery*, *35*, 380–384. https://doi.org/10.1111/j.1524-4725.2008.01042.x.

Robinson, D. M. (2018). In vitro analysis of the degradation of calcium hydroxylapatite dermal filler: A proof-of-concept study. *Dermatologic Surgery*, *44*(suppl 1), S5–S9. https://doi.org/10.1097/DSS.0000000000001683.

Rzany, B., & DeLorenzi, C. (2015). Understanding, avoiding and managing severe filler complications. *Plastic and Reconstructive Surgery*, *136*, S196–S203. https://doi.org/10.1097/PRS.0000000000001760.

Saade, D. S., & Vashi, N. A. (2019). Treatment of purpura with Nd:YAG laser in skin types IV–VI. *Journal of the American Academy of Dermatology*, *80*, e73–e74. https://doi.org/10.1016/j.jaad.2018.09.003.

Sadeghpour, M., & Dover, J. S. (2019). Understanding hyaluronic acid delayed bruising: Why the molecule and not just the injection matters. *Dermatologic Surgery*, *45*(3), 471–473. https://doi.org/10.1097/DSS.0000000000001817.

Sadeghpour, M., Quatrano, N. A., Bonati, L. M., Arndt, K. A., Dover, J. S., & Kaminer, M. S. (2019). Delayed-onset nodules to differentially crosslinked hyaluronic acids: Comparative incidence and risk assessment. *Dermatologic Surgery*, *45*(8), 1085–1094. https://doi.org/10.1097/DSS.0000000000001814.

Schlesinger, T. E., Cohen, J. L., & Ellison, S. (2013). Purpura and fillers: A review of pre-procedural, intra-procedural, and post-procedural considerations. *Journal of Drugs in Dermatology*, *12*(10), 1138–1142.

Sharudin, S. N., Ismail, M. F., Mohamad, N. F., & Vasudevan, S. K. (2018). Complete recovery of filler-induced visual loss following subcutaneous hyaluronidase injection. *Neuroophthalmology*, *43*(2), 102–106. https://doi.org/10.1080/01658107.2018.1482358.

Sito, G., Manzoni, V., & Sommariva, R. (2019). Vascular complications after facial filler injection: A literature review and meta-analysis. *J Clin Aesthet Dermatol*, *12*(6), E65–E72.

Sorensen, E. P., & Council, M. L. (2020). Update in soft-tissue filler-associated blindness. *Dermatologic Surgery*, *46*(5), 671–677. https://doi.org/10.1097/DSS.0000000000002108.

Urdiales-Gálvez, F., Delgado, N. E., Figueiredo, V., et al. (2018). Treatment of soft tissue filler complications: Expert consensus recommendations. *Aesthetic Plastic Surgery*, *42*, 498–510. https://doi.org/10.1007/s00266-017-1063-0.

US Food and Drug Administration. (2020). *Vaccines and related biological products advisory committee meeting; FDA briefing document for Moderna COVID-19 vaccine*. https://www.fda.gov/media/144434/download.

Vanaman, M., Fabi, S. G., & Carruthers, J. (2016). Complications in the cosmetic dermatology patient: A review and our experience (part 1). *Dermatologic Surgery, 42,* 1–11. https://doi.org/10.1097/DSS.0000000000000569.

Vleggaar, D., Fitzgerald, R., Lorenc, P., et al. (2014). Consensus recommendations on the use of injectable poly-L-lactic acid for facial and nonfacial volumization. *Journal of Drugs in Dermatology, 13*(suppl 4), S44–S51.

Wagner, R. D., Fakhro, A., Cox, J. A., & Izaddoost, S. A. (2016). Etiology, prevention, and management of infectious complications of dermal fillers. *Seminars in Plastic Surgery, 30,* 83–86. https://doi.org/10.1055/s-0036-1580734.

Wang, C., Sun, T., Yu, N., & Wang, X. (2020). Herpes reactivation after the injection of hyaluronic acid dermal filler: a case report and review of literature. *Medicine, 99.* https://doi.org/10.1097/MD.0000000000020394. 24(e20394).

Wang, C., Sun, T., Li, H., Li, Z., & Wang, X. (2021). Hypersensitivity caused my cosmetic injection: Systematic review and case report. *Aesthetic Plastic Surgery, 45*(1), 263–272. https://doi.org/10.1007/s00266-020-01684-4.

Woodward, J., Khan, T., & Martin, J. (2015). Facial filler complications. *Facial Plastic Surgery Clinics of North America, 23,* 447–458. https://doi.org/10.1016/j.fsc.2015.07.006.

Zimmermann, U. S., & Clerici, T. J. (2004). The histological aspects of fillers complications. *Seminars in Cutaneous Medicine and Surgery, 23*(4), 241–250. https://doi.org/10.1016/j.sder.2004.09.004.

36

Complications of Permanent Fillers

Paola Barriera, Shilpi Khetarpal, Allison Sutton, and Jeffrey S. Dover

SUMMARY AND KEY FEATURES

- Permanent fillers comprise mostly synthetic materials that cause collagen deposition via fibroplasia as their mechanism of action.
- Permanent fillers are better at facial volumizing and deep structural augmentation than at "line filling."
- Silicones, polyalkylimides, polyacrylamides, polymethylmethacrylate, and acrylic hydrogels are the most common permanent fillers worldwide.
- All cosmetic fillers, whether temporary or permanent, may induce adverse reactions.
- Permanent filler complications may be due to the injection itself, injector-dependent variables, or host tissue and filler interactions.
- Permanent filler complications are difficult to treat since the product will not dissipate, but rather remains in vivo. Permanent fillers have permanent side effects.
- Foreign-body granulomas and late-onset granulomas are the most challenging permanent filler complications to treat.
- Late-onset granulomas are sometimes due to biofilms from bacteria introduced at the time of injection.
- Effective treatments of granulomas must target bacterial etiologies and host immune response mechanisms.
- Invasive and scarring treatments such as surgery should be reserved and used after more conservative treatments have failed.

INTRODUCTION

Injectable facial fillers have become a cornerstone of aesthetic medicine over the past two decades. Although soft tissue augmentation using industrial-grade silicones can be traced to early last century, widespread adoption of injectable fillers began in the 1970s with the advent of bovine collagen. Since the 1990s, with the US Food and Drug Administration (FDA) approval of hyaluronic acid (HA) temporary fillers, soft tissue augmentation for filling lines and volumizing or recontouring the face has surged to become the second most popular nonsurgical aesthetic procedure in the United States, with more than 2.7 million procedures performed in 2019. Based on the axiom that an aged facial appearance is due in some part to dermal, subcutaneous, and osseous atrophy that naturally occurs over time, injectable facial fillers offer the ability to replace lost volume and restore youthful proportions, providing a foundation for facial rejuvenation.

As with certain other nonsurgical aesthetic modalities, facial filling is a product-driven procedure. Beyond an adroit injection technique, judicious use of the appropriate product in the proper location is a prerequisite to success. To know the art of injection, one must know the products, and the products vary significantly. In 2010, more than 200 fillers from over 60 manufacturers worldwide were available for tissue augmentation. Although some share characteristics that may predict a similar clinical response or comparable side effect profile, inappropriate substitution with a dissimilar product, particularly by a novice injector or non-core aesthetic provider, invites complications and ultimately patient dissatisfaction and compromises patient safety.

Although there is no universally accepted classification for soft tissue fillers, they can be classified based on their origin—natural animal, synthetic, or natural synthetic. Fillers may be further divided based on their longevity: temporary, semipermanent, or permanent. Temporary fillers are typically biologically derived products that are eventually broken down in vivo after a period of a few months to a few years. This category includes collagens and HAs, the most predominant fillers worldwide. In contrast, permanent fillers comprise mostly synthetic materials that have an in vivo, biodynamic mechanism of action, causing collagen deposition via fibroplasia. They are composed of nonabsorbable, permanent material. For this reason, permanent fillers are better at facial volumizing and deep structural augmentation than at "line filling," which is better accomplished with temporary fillers. Note that "permanence" refers to a lack of degradation of the in vivo material over time rather than to a "permanent" cosmetic result. Once placed, permanent fillers remain in the skin and subcutaneous tissues indefinitely. Permanent aesthetic results are seldom possible owing to continued tissue volume loss, bone resorption, and other factors associated with the aging face. Nevertheless, duration of correction is more extensive than with temporary fillers. As such, permanent fillers are less "forgiving." Experience and precise technique are required to achieve favorable outcomes.

LIQUID INJECTABLE SILICONE

Silicone is one of the oldest and longest-lasting injectable fillers. Liquid injectable silicone (LIS) received FDA approval in 1959 for intraocular use as a retinal stabilizing agent during vitreous surgery. Its off-label use as a filler is controversial due to potential long-term complications. The FDA-approved medical-grade silicone oils that are recommended for cosmetic use including Silkon-1000 (Alcon, Fort Worth, TX) and Adatosil-5000 (Bausch & Lomb, Rochester, NY). Although injectable silicone has been effectively used for more than 50 years, its use remains controversial owing to the historical widespread reports of complications, most of which are confounded with unknown or impure products labeled as "silicone" and purified silicones injected by improper techniques. When critically evaluating silicone, the distinction must be made between modern products intended for injection (LIS) in contrast to adulterated or impure products lumped under the "silicone" label that is manufactured outside the United States. LIS demonstrates a unique aptness for the correction of specific cutaneous and subcutaneous atrophies owing to its versatility, permanence, excellent cost–benefit profile, and natural texture in vivo. Furthermore, evidence continues to mount demonstrating that modern silicone oils approved by the FDA for injection into the human body may be successfully used off-label when injected according to strict protocol, which includes using the microdroplet serial puncture technique (defined as the injection of ≤ 0.1 mL at 2 to 10 mm intervals subdermally with a small diameter needle) with limited quantities per session and adequately spaced treatment sessions. In contrast, adulterated and impure silicone products, even when labeled "medical grade," are rife with complications.

POLYALKYLIMIDE GEL

Bio-Alcamid (Polymekon, Italy) was first launched in 2000 and has been used in more than 20 countries. It does not require skin allergy testing prior to use (Protopapa, Sito, Caporale, & Cammarota, 2003). Its use was originally as an "endoprosthesis" for the treatment of pectus excavatum and postoperative defects as well as aesthetic use in the lips, cheeks, and nasolabial folds (Fig. 36.1). It contains a nonbiodegradable,

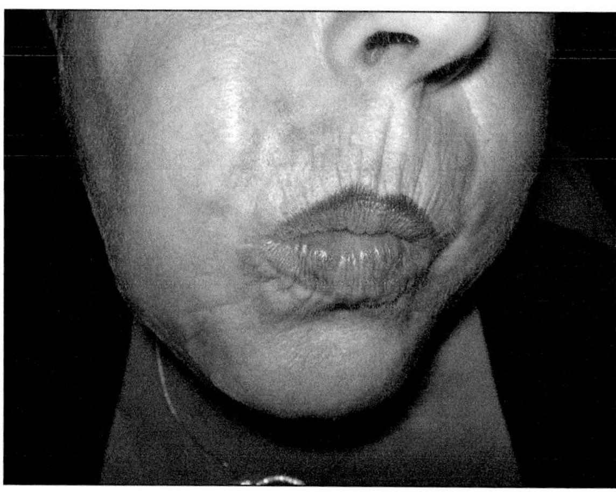

Fig. 36.1 Granuloma of the nasolabial fold 4 years after injection of Bio-Alcamid.

nontoxic, nonimmunogenic synthetic polyalkylimide cross-linked polymer suspended in water. Although it is approved in Europe, it is not approved by the FDA. Bio-Alcamid contains a ratio of 3% alkylamide polymer to 97% sterile water. The product is a gel that is injected as a large bolus subcutaneously. After injection, the polyalkylimide gel is completely covered by a thin collagen capsule (0.02 mm) that isolates it from host tissues, making it a type of endogenous prosthesis (Formigli et al., 2004). It has been successful and safe in treating human immunodeficiency virus (HIV)–associated facial lipoatrophy and showed persistent correction at 18 months. There have been reported cases of product migration and infection that occurred 12 months after injection (Karim, Hage, van Rozelaar, Lange, & Raaijmakers, 2006).

POLYACRYLAMIDE GELS

Polyacrylamide hydrogels contain a nondegradable, nontoxic, nonimmunogenic synthetic polyacrylamide crosslinked polymer suspended in water that belongs to the family of acryl derivatives. Polyacrylamide products are available in Europe and Asia; however, none are currently available for use in the United States. Aquamid (Contura International, Denmark) contains a 2.5% cross-linked polyacrylamide gel in 97.5% sterile water. It has been in use in Europe and worldwide since 2001, primarily for augmentation of nasolabial folds and lips, facial contouring, and correction of HIV facial lipoatrophy. On histology, Aquamid appears as a multivacuolated nonbirefringent material with a surrounding layer of thin fibrous connective tissue, macrophages, multinucleated giant cells, and lymphocytes. Amazingel (NanFeng Medical Science and Technology Development Co. Ltd, Shijiazhuang, People's Republic of China) is a product manufactured in China and available throughout Asia. Although it is readily available for purchase through internet distributors, it has not been extensively studied in the Western medical literature. There have been reports of Amazingel being used for breast augmentation, lip enhancement, and correction of facial scarring. Late-onset complications have been reported, including induration, nodules, hematoma, inflammation, and infection. Surgical removal of the product has led to resolution (Do & Shim, 2012).

POLYMETHYLMETHACRYLATE

Polymethylmethacrylate (PMMA) is a nonresorbable, biocompatible material first synthesized in the early 1900s and used for varied medical purposes, including intraocular implants and bone cements. It was first engineered for soft tissue augmentation in the early 1980s in an attempt to provide a safe implant, with the theory that such a synthetic material might induce long-lasting tissue fibroplasia, in contrast to the temporary volume displacement seen with collagens. Currently available PMMA products are biphasic and suspended in either bovine collagen (Artefill, Suneva Medical, San Diego, CA) or carboxyglutamate (Metacril, private lab, Rio de Janeiro, Brazil). Arteplast was the first-generation commercial PMMA product with less than 20 μm microspheres suspended in a gelatin carrier. It was used in Germany through the early 1990s but was found to have a high incidence of granuloma formation within the first 18 months of implantation. Such complications were likely due to an inconsistent particle size and the presence of surface impurities found with processing methods. Artecoll (Rofil Medical International, Breda, the Netherlands) (Fig. 36.2) was then introduced in 1992 as a second-generation product with an improved processing and washing method that reduced impurities. Significantly, the carrier was also reformulated, and the PMMA was suspended as a 20% product in 80% bovine collagen with 0.3% lidocaine for improved comfort. The PMMA particles were larger at 30 μm, leading to lower rates of foreign body reaction. Because of the bovine collagen component, Artecoll requires allergy testing prior

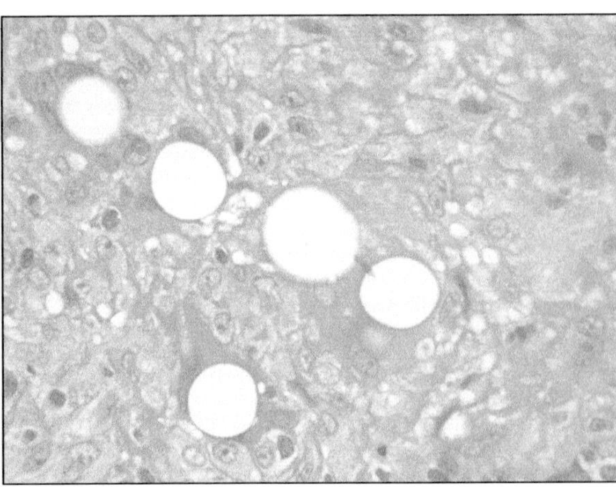

Fig. 36.2 Artecoll.

to injection. As such, Artecoll is considered a biphasic implant, inducing augmentation through displacement with an early collagen component and later through a fibroblastic component caused by PMMA. In 1998, Artecoll was approved in Canada, and processing methods were further improved to reduce particle size variability, resulting in fewer incidences of late-granuloma formation compared with Arteplast. Histology of skin biopsy specimens from areas treated with Artecoll show round, sharply circumscribed, translucent, nonbirefringent particles, epithelioid histiocytes, multinucleated giant cells, lymphocytes, and occasional eosinophils surrounding the microspheres. Artefill, now known as Bellafill, the third-generation iteration of PMMA, was further improved by enhancing the uniformity of the PMMA particle size (30–50 μm) and by eliminating nanoparticles that had plagued earlier formulations. The collagen matrix was also improved, and Artefill was approved by the FDA in 2006 for use in the nasolabial folds based on safety studies performed earlier in the United States with Artecoll. Bellafill was additionally approved for moderate to severe, atrophic, distensible facial acne scars on the cheeks in 2014. Importantly, Bellafill is the only permanent filler currently approved by the FDA for aesthetic use.

ACRYLIC HYDROGEL PLUS HYALURONIC ACID

Dermalive and Dermadeep (Dermatech, Paris, France) are biphasic permanent fillers composed of a mixture of 40% hydroxyethylmethacrylate and ethylmethacrylate particles and 60% biodegradable, fluid cross-linked, bacterially derived HA (Fig. 36.3). The acrylic particles are hydrophobic and irregularly shaped in a polygonal fashion. Dermalive contains acrylic particles 45 to 65 μm in diameter, whereas Dermadeep contains particles 80 to 110 μm in diameter. Both products are intended for injection in the deep dermis and subcutaneous regions, with the Dermadeep product indicated for deep subcutaneous injection only. As with most permanent fillers, injections into the superficial and mid-reticular dermis are not recommended. Both products were CE approved and available in Europe in 1998 but were withdrawn several years ago owing to the high incidence of complications. Neither product has ever been FDA approved for use in the United States. The histology of acrylic hydrogels in tissue reveals pseudocystic structures of different sizes and shapes containing polygonal, pink, translucent, nonbirefringent foreign bodies with a surrounding granulomatous reaction consisting of epithelioid histiocytes, multinucleated giant cells, some lymphocytes, and occasional eosinophils.

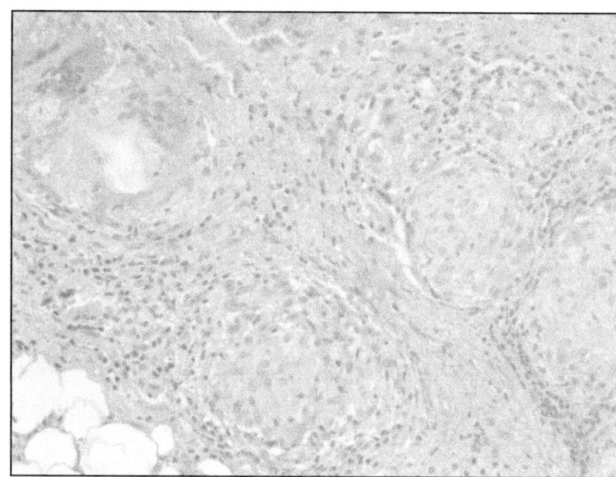

Fig. 36.3 Dermalive.

TREATMENT SITES

Although appropriate indications and uses are beyond the scope of this chapter, it is worthwhile to note that permanent fillers have been extensively used throughout the face and body, and complications in each area have been reported. Documented facial complications have occurred in the eyelids, eyebrows, glabella, temples, cheeks, nose, nasolabial folds, labiomental folds, lips, and pre-jowl sulci. Traumatic surgical scars and atrophic acne scars have also been treated with permanent fillers and have also been noted to have complications. Nonfacial complications have been reported in the chest, breasts, penis, and buttocks, particularly when large amounts are injected in a single session.

COMPLICATIONS

Most permanent fillers are used outside North America, including Europe, Asia, and South America. They are less commonly used in Canada and uncommon in the United States, primarily because of the stringent FDA approval requirements. Those submitted for approval to the FDA must undergo a rigorous clinical trials process prior to approval. The upside of such a process with respect to patient safety is that many complications are identified prior to widespread use. Such is the case for Bellafill, the only permanent filler currently approved in the United States.

Outside the United States, standards are less stringent. Europe requires all products used in the European Union to have a CE certificate. However, such a certificate ensures only the technically correct manufacturing of the preparation and is not a guarantee of biological safety. Because clinical trials are not held before product approval, identification of filler complications must be performed retrospectively and gathered through anecdotal evidence. This system allows the widespread use of most permanent filler products prior to the assurance of safety, and therefore, the largest numbers of reports of permanent filler complications originate in Europe. All cosmetic fillers, regardless of their longevity, can have adverse reactions (Table 36.1). Complications can be divided into early (0–14 days), late (14 days to 1 year), and delayed (> 1 year) reactions. Early reactions include erythema, pain, edema, bruising, and bleeding. Such reactions are inherently due to the invasive nature of the injection itself, are usually mild to moderate, and are typically self-limited to the first 14 days. However, they may be exacerbated by poor technique.

> **PEARL 1** Select patients carefully when considering permanent fillers. The best candidate is a patient who has extensive prior experience with temporary fillers and who desires longstanding correction.

Other early and late complications that may occur with both temporary and permanent fillers are influenced by injector variables. Inexperience and poor technique increase the risk of complications such as discoloration, vascular occlusion, embolism, cutaneous necrosis, undercorrection or overcorrection, asymmetry, contour irregularity, textural irregularity, and migration. Complications, when seen with short-term resorbable and even long-term resorbable fillers, will eventually resolve as the product is resorbed. However, complications from the use of a permanent filler will not dissipate as the product remains in vivo and serves as a continuous source of complication.

> **PEARL 2** Thorough injector training is crucial with permanent fillers.

Extensive injector experience with temporary fillers is required prior to successful injection with a permanent filler.

However, the most vexing complications occur because of poorly understood phenomena that result from host tissue interactions with the injected product in addition to bacterial interference. This may be related either to the product itself or to the biological interaction of the product and host response to a foreign body, or foreign antigen in residence on the foreign body. Inflammation, infection, biofilm formation, foreign body granulomas, and late-onset granulomas may all occur with both temporary and permanent fillers, but they occur more commonly with permanent ones. These complications can occur any time after product placement but are skewed toward the late and delayed periods with permanent products. With permanent fillers increasing dramatically during the past decade, both in number of fillers and in number of patients treated, delayed adverse events are now more commonly seen. Furthermore, they are increasingly recognized as the most challenging aspects of permanent tissue augmentation, owing to their tenacity and resistance to treatment. The characteristic of duration that makes a permanent product seemingly advantageous with respect to good results is also the one that engenders the least desirable group of complications. However, not all complications are created equally, and the following adverse reactions are exacerbated owing to the permanent nature of the product.

> **PEARL 3** Avoid using permanent fillers in patients with active concomitant infectious or inflammatory processes.

Asymmetry may occur with all permanent fillers by a similar mechanism (delayed fibroblastic augmentation), and care should be taken to ensure that equal amounts of product are symmetrically placed. Such a strategy is elementary but may sometimes prove challenging when working with permanent filler products that do not show an immediate volume correction. Cognizance of how much product is being placed as one proceeds through the injection is important, and the amount injected in each site or region should be recorded. Allowing adequate time between injection sessions is also important to avoid placing too much product in a particular area. Contour and textural irregularities may

TABLE 36.1 **Filler Complications and Management**

Complications	Timing of Occurrence	Therapy
Hematoma	Within minutes to hours	• Compression for a few minutes • Heparin or vitamin K ointment for 7 days • Topical arnica • IPL, KTP, and PDL
Neovascularization	Within days to weeks	• Mostly self-limiting in 3–12 months • Laser/IPL
Hyperpigmentation	Within days to weeks	• Sun protection • Topical hydroquinone • Topical tretinoin • IPL (skin type I–IV) • Nd:YAG laser (skin type V–VI)
Postinterventional edema	Within minutes to hours	• Cooling • Keep head elevated at night • Bromelain
Immediate type allergy (type I)	Within minutes to hours	• Cooling • Antihistamine • Prednisone
Erysipelas, cellulitis	Within days	• Amoxicillin clavulanate 625 mg TID for 7–10 days • If penicillin allergy ➔ clindamycin 600 mg TID for 7–10 days
Abscess	Within days	• Culture and treat based on isolate
Herpes Simplex	Within days	• Valacyclovir or famciclovir 500 mg TID for 5 days
Peripheral ischemia with impending necrosis	Variable—depends on the clinical presentation	• Stop injections immediately • Warm compresses • ASA 500 mg orally, then 75–100 mg OD for 7 days • Further options (low level of evidence): • Pentoxifylline 400 mg TID • LMWH • HBOT • Wound care
Retinal ischemia	During injection or immediately after injection	• Stop injections immediately • Place patient in supine position • Call emergency medical service and prepare to transfer the patient to a hospital setting immediately. • Reduce intraocular pressure: • Timolol 0.5% one to two drops to the affected eye • Encourage the patient to "rebreathe" in a paper bag to increase CO_2. • Dislodge embolus to a more peripheral position by massaging the globe with repeated increasing pressure. • Consider administration of hyaluronidase. • MRI of the brain to rule out cerebral ischemia

ASA, Aspirin; *HBOT*, hyperbaric oxygen therapy; *IPL*, intense pulsed light; *KTP*, potassium titanyl phosphate; *LMWH*, low-molecular-weight heparin; *MRI*, magnetic resonance imaging; *Nd:YAG*, neodymium-doped yttrium aluminum garnet; *OD*, once daily; *PDL*, pulsed dye laser; *TID*, three times a day.

also occur with all of the permanent fillers and are due either to placement of the filler product too superficially (textural irregularity) or to placement of too much product too superficially (contour irregularities). As a rule, permanent fillers are best for deep placement and should rarely be placed more superficial than the deep reticular dermis. Most should be placed in the subcutaneous layer or deeper. Moreover, the particulate nature of some permanent fillers, such as PMMA and the acrylic hydrogels, does not allow for the smooth, soft, and pliable texture desirable for superficial placement. However, LIS is soft and pliable but may still lead to textural and contour irregularities when placed superficially. Fibroblastic fillers are essentially best used as deep fillers rather than superficial ones to avoid these complications. Caution should also be taken when injecting permanent fillers into areas with overlying thin skin.

PEARL 4 Fill only the appropriate defects. Some treatment areas, such as lips, have a higher rate of complications with permanent fillers. The lips are a notoriously unforgiving site for textural and contour irregularities, owing to their anatomic characteristics—a thin cutaneous and mucosal layer overlying a region particularly sensitive to volume changes. All but the most experienced of injectors should avoid permanent fillers in the lips.

PEARL 5 When injecting permanent fillers, fill at the appropriate tissue level. Place the product in the subcutaneous tissue and avoid placement of permanent fillers in the superficial and mid-dermis.

Migration refers to the presence of filler at a location remote from the primary injection site. This complication has several potential mechanisms, and although not every mechanism has been reported or is applicable for every filler, it is important to be aware of them.

- *Injection technique–related* explanations refer to poor technique (filler is inadvertently injected into an adjacent area), high volume of filler injection (filler overflows into an adjacent area), and filler injection under high pressure (filler travels along planes of least resistance when excessive pressure is applied to the syringe). With LIS, using the microdroplet serial puncture technique prevents migration from occurring because the total surface area and resulting surface tension of a given volume of LIS are greatly increased when divided into multiple microdroplets. The increased surface tension holds the microdroplet in place.
- Overzealous *massage* of the filler after injection may be responsible for its displacement into adjacent areas.
- Recurrent *muscle activity* may propel the migration of filler into adjacent areas. Injections of fillers in areas of high muscular activity, such as the lips and perioral folds, impair capsule formation around the implant, induce instability of an already existing capsule even years after the infiltration, and facilitate migration from the spot of injection into surrounding tissue layers. On the other hand, the pump function of the orbicularis oris muscle can make the filler material coalesce into nodules. Injections in these highly mobile areas, therefore, should be avoided.
- *Gravitational forces* may explain the downward movement of tissue filler.
- *Pressure-induced displacement* (dislodgement) refers to forced migration of a previously placed filler by additional filler injection at the same site.
- *Lymphatic spread* may explain cryopreserved fat and silicone migration. It has been proposed that microdroplets may undergo phagocytosis and be transported to other sites through lymphatics.
- *Intravascular injection* of filler with spread to distant soft tissue sites (e.g., liver, lung, kidney, or brain) is another consideration.

PEARL 6 Use the appropriate technique. With LIS, a microdroplet serial puncture technique spaced over several sessions is necessary for success.

Many complications are due to the host response to a foreign body or product and host tissue interactions. Inflammation, foreign body granulomas (Figs. 36.4 and 36.5), and late-onset granulomas (Fig. 36.6) may be due to the host immune response independent of infection, in which case the filler serves as the foreign body. However, they may also be due to bacterial biofilm formation, in which case both the filler and biofilm colony serve as a foreign body nidus for pathologic inflammation. Such complications have been seen but are poorly understood. Only in the past decade have theories regarding the etiology of such complications begun

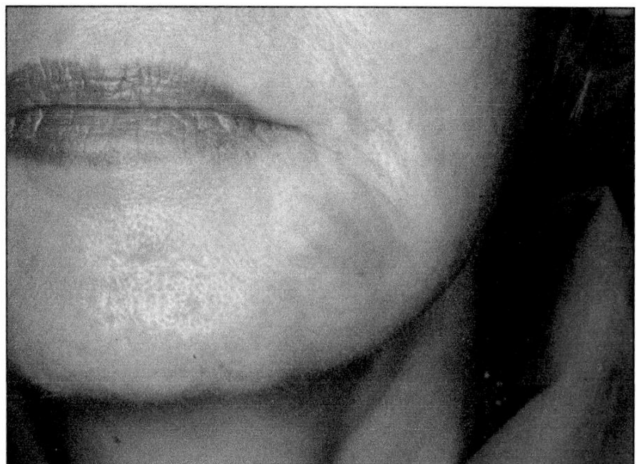

Fig. 36.4 Silicone granuloma (foreign body granuloma).

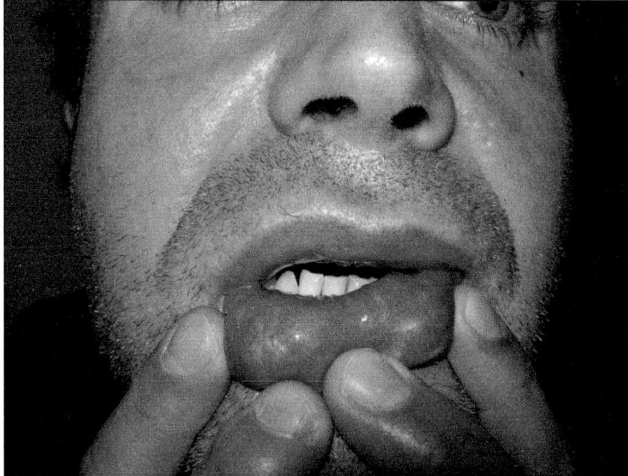

Fig. 36.5 Lower lip granuloma 6 months after injection of Aquamid.

to evolve, and although biofilms are now viewed as the likely culprit, more research is needed to fully understand all mechanisms involved.

Although an exhaustive discussion of bacterial biofilms is beyond this chapter, this phenomenon is increasingly recognized as a possible etiology of permanent filler complications, including inflammation, recurrent infection, and granulomas. Bacterial biofilms are durable subclinical infections on the surface of a foreign body or prosthesis. They are living colonies that adhere to the foreign body surface, in this case a microdroplet or bolus of permanent filler, and are self-encapsulated by a protective matrix to help to avoid a host response. This protective capsule also helps the biofilm to avoid

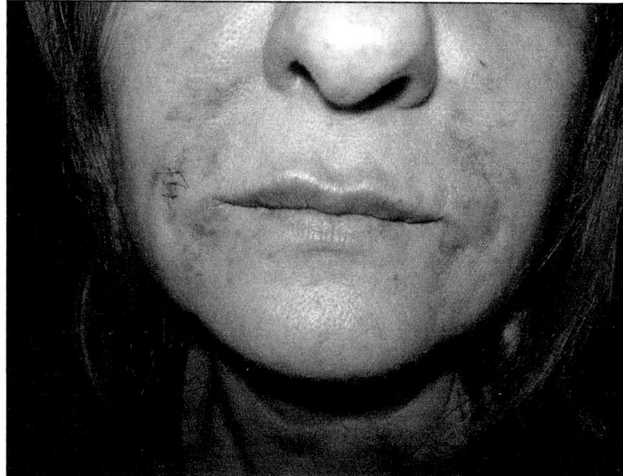

Fig. 36.6 Delayed-onset granuloma 2.5 years after injection with Dermalive.

penetration and destruction by antibiotics. Bacteria in biofilms may remain quiescent for months or years, then reactivate to a free planktonic state to cause inflammatory and infectious sequelae. Importantly, biofilm colonization may remain subclinical because bacteria in the biofilm state are resistant to culture, likely explaining the "sterile" abscesses seen at times with permanent fillers. The irregularities of particulate fillers (PMMA and acrylic hydrogels) may support biofilms, but they may also be found on the smooth surfaces of LIS microdroplets and any other permanent substrate. Biofilms may occur with temporary fillers as well, although they are less significant owing to the lack of substrate permanence. Bacteria that cause biofilms are likely introduced during injection through the skin or mucosa, and although the normal flora encountered during injection can never be completely eliminated, some authors have begun to advocate adopting a sterile approach when injecting permanent fillers, in contrast to the clean approach that is used for temporary fillers, with the idea that the chance for introduction of bacteria and subsequent biofilm formation may be reduced. Biofilms may play a more important causative role in hydrophilic gels in contrast to hydrophobic fillers. Christensen and colleagues found in polymer nonbiodegradable gels that the major cause of foreign body granuloma was likely biofilm formation, which they found in all specimens of patients treated with Aquamid. Such a distinction has strategic implications for treatment, as biofilm causation on hydrophilic products may respond very well to antibiotic treatment. In contrast, hydrophobic fillers with microspheres may not be associated with biofilms and may respond better to steroid treatment. Luitgart Wiest has collected data on 52 patients with foreign body granulomas after Artecoll or Dermalive. Neither biofilms nor bacteria could be detected in any patient with electron microscopy (EM) (Luitgart G. Wiest, personal communication).

Inflammation manifesting as tissue erythema and swelling has been reported as a complication during both the late and delayed periods. It has been reported with both LIS and PMMA products but appears particularly prevalent with the polyalkylimide gels, polyacrylamide gels, and acrylic hydrogels.

Nodules, either inflammatory or noninflammatory, can arise from several causes. Nodule is a clinically descriptive term used in the absence of histologic assessment.

Noninflammatory nodules occur due to overcorrection, incorrect filler selection for the anatomical area, and filler injection into areas with high muscular activity. Overcorrection is an injector-dependent iatrogenic complication that is particularly troublesome with permanent fillers and may occur with any of the permanent fillers (see Table 36.1). Overcorrection may be due to both too much product placed in a particular area and an underestimation of the degree of fibroplasia that will occur over time. With bovine collagens in the 1980s and 1990s, slight overcorrection was intentional at the time of treatment because a significant degree of the immediate correction achieved in the office would dissipate over the next few days. Gross volume displacement was the mechanism for achieving results with collagen alone, and further augmentation by fibroplasia was not expected. However, such a strategy does not translate well into the realm of permanent fillers because these depend heavily on augmentation by fibroplasia over time in addition to immediate volume displacement. To apply the overcorrection strategy of collagens to the permanent fillers is to invite disaster because products that work by inducing collagenous deposition will continue to effect augmentation over several weeks to months afterward. That is, tissue will be augmented beyond the immediate gross displacement due to product volume. For this reason, most permanent fillers should be placed in smaller amounts over multiple sessions spaced several weeks to months apart to allow adequate time for tissue augmentation to occur between sessions.

Inflammatory nodules are often called *granulomas*, that is, a manifestation of the host's natural immunologic response to a foreign body. Indeed, injecting a foreign body into the host, even a biocompatible, nontoxic, inert one as the permanent fillers are, naturally elicits a granulomatous response, characterized by the appearance of macrophages and foreign body giant cells that arrive to both phagocytose the foreign material and deposit a fibroplastic collagenous response in an effort to "wall-off" or neutralize it. This is, after all, the main mechanism of action for fibroblastic tissue augmentation. Ideally, the foreign body granulomatous reaction creates a controlled fibrous area around the surface of the implanted filler, and augmentation proceeds in a controlled, limited, and predictable manner. However, if the fibroplastic response does not cease, either because of an ongoing interaction with the foreign product itself or because of the synergistic presence of bacteria, possibly present in a bacterial biofilm, the fibroblastic response will manifest as a foreign body granulomatous complication. Late-onset granulomas result from the same phenomena but typically occur at least 1 year after injection. These may be explained by continued host–filler interactions because there is evidence that the "permanent" microparticles and gels can be further modified by the host immune response even years after injection. Alterations to the surface of Dermalive particles have been documented by EM at 2 years, suggesting that the product is altered in some fashion over time. This may be due to incomplete polymerization, in which low-molecular-weight oligomers are left in the copolymer after final processing, or ongoing hydrolyzation. However, most late-onset granulomas are likely explained by bacteria being introduced during injection having the opportunity to establish a biofilm around the injected product, and the biofilm being reactivated or triggered to cause a host response, either by distant inflammation or infection or by further mechanical insult (Box 36.1). Other causes of late inflammatory reactions include viral infections, vaccinations, dental procedures, and medications (e.g., interferon (IFN) therapy). These may trigger a granulomatous process at sites of filler implants via immunostimulation, which suggests that reactivity levels of an individual's immune system play a crucial role.

Vascular compromise is the most severe and feared complication associated with the use of dermal fillers. Although reports of ischemic events are exceptionally

BOX 36.1 Reported Possible Triggers of Granulomas

- Injecting different types of fillers in the same location
- Systemic infections
- Sinusitis
- Pharyngitis
- Bronchitis
- Pleurisy
- Enteritis
- Pyelonephritis
- Flulike syndrome
- Autoimmune thyroiditis
- Acupuncture
- Hyperthyroidism
- Ulcerative colitis
- Crohn disease
- Pemphigus
- Sarcoidosis
- Breast cancer
- Psychologic shock
- Facial trauma
- Facelift operation
- Dental focus of infection
- Periodontal disease/inflammation

rare, their incidence appears to be on the rise due to the increasing popularity of these cosmetic treatments. Accidental intravascular injection can lead to tissue necrosis and, more rarely, visual compromise. The latter occurs when the dermal filler inadvertently enters the ocular circulation via retrograde arterial flow into the ophthalmic artery, potentially causing permanent blindness. The clinical presentation of vascular occlusion is characterized by the following:

- Pain. The initial presentation may include pain and discomfort disproportionate to what is typically experienced following filler treatments. However, pain may be absent if anesthetics are given. Absence of pain is therefore unreliable in the early stages of injury.
- Color changes. Temporary blanching or pallor may occur immediately after intra-arterial occlusion. If epinephrine is included in the filler formulation or anesthetic, pallor may be secondary to vascular contraction. Blanching is typically followed, minutes to hours later, by a violaceous, mottled, and net-like discoloration known as livedo reticularis. This pattern may also represent a cold sensitivity or a preexisting medical condition. As local tissue oxygen depletes, a deep blue-black discoloration is seen which progresses to frank necrosis.
- Skin breakdown. In the advanced state of necrosis, the epithelial integrity is lost and skin sloughing begins. When inflammation subsides, repair begins via secondary intent. At this stage, anaerobic bacteria predominate due to the lack of oxygen in tissues; antibiotics may need to be considered.

To minimize the risk of vascular occlusion, detailed knowledge of the vascular anatomy of the face is mandatory. Increased caution should be exerted in the central upper and mid face as these areas have several arteries in close proximity to the ophthalmic circulation (supratrochlear artery, supraorbital artery, dorsal nasal artery and lateral nasal artery). Aspiration prior to injection so as to ascertain that the injection is not intravascular can be helpful. Areas of scarring should be avoided as scars may change vessel anatomy and fix arteries in place, making them easier to penetrate with small sharp needles. Blunt cannulas may reduce the risk of accidental intra-arterial injection. Practitioners should avoid bolus injections since larger amounts of product can cause a proportionally greater degree of arterial obstruction.

EVALUATION METHODS FOR NODULES

Histopathology, scanning EM, high-frequency ultrasound, bacterial culture, polymerase chain reaction (PCR), and fluorescent in situ hybridization (FISH) have all been used to evaluate granulomatous and infectious complications due to permanent fillers. Two questions naturally arise when a granulomatous complication ensues: (1) What product was placed? (2) Is the area infected? The first question is best addressed through histopathology rather than history. Histopathological study of the lesions is the "gold standard" technique to identify the responsible filler. With modern products, the particles of each filler have specific microscopic characteristics that allow identification (Fig. 36.7). EM may be used if histopathological studies prove inconclusive or further research is warranted (Fig. 36.8). High-frequency ultrasound has also been reported to identify and quantify the presence of filler in vivo, as well as to detect inflammation, granulomas, and the presence of different fillers in the same area. Evaluation of the exact offending agent may prove difficult when a patient presents with a history of

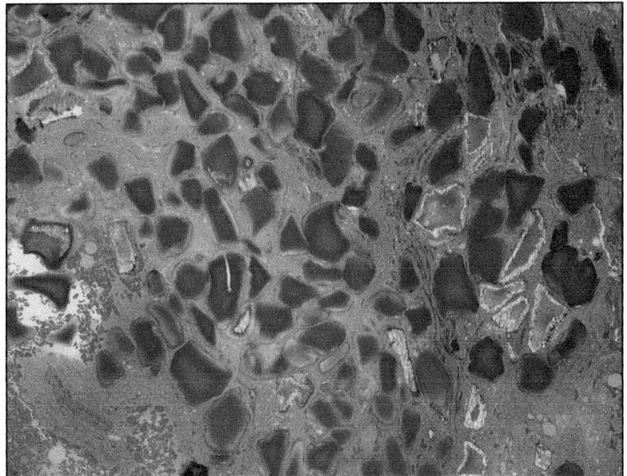

Fig. 36.7 Histology of Dermalive particles 4 years after injection, showing incomplete polymerization.

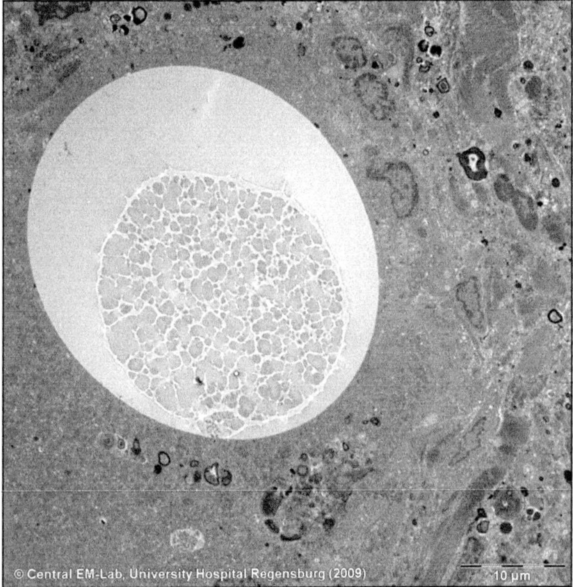

Fig. 36.8 Electron microscopic photograph of an Artecoll microsphere surrounded by a multinucleated giant cell. (Courtesy Dr. Josef Schroeder, Central EM-Unit, Department of Pathology, University Hospital Regensburg, Germany.)

injection with an "unknown" product or an illicitly injected one. Nevertheless, because facial fillers have their own characteristics and density, knowledge of ultrasound patterns can aid in noninvasive diagnosis when interpreted in conjunction with clinical findings. A history of "silicone" injections most often eludes detection. Although silicone may be detected on histopathology, the clinician has no method of testing whether or not adulterants were also present in the injected material. Nonpurified and unknown products are often lumped under "silicone" injections by patient history, and these should be distinguished from modern purified products meant for human soft tissue augmentation and appropriately injected (Fig. 36.9).

> **PEARL 7** In the case of granulomas, identify the agent used and treat according to the properties of the filler.

Detection of infection may be accomplished through routine bacterial cultures of tissue samples or exudate, but granulomas will often be negative on culture. This should not allay the concern for latent bacterial infection because biofilms may be present in the face of negative cultures. In such cases, PCR may be used to detect bacterial presence but has also reportedly been negative in the setting of a suspected infection. FISH analysis may also help to detect bacterial presence in the setting of a negative Gram stain and bacterial culture.

TREATMENT

Treatment of transient, self-limited filler complications due to injection, including erythema, bleeding, bruising, edema, pain, and herpes simplex virus activation, has been well documented in the literature. However, treatment of permanent filler complications in the second and third categories (see Table 36.2) presents a greater challenge. Several treatment methods have been reported in the literature, including topical products, systemic medications, minimally invasive procedures and modalities, and surgical excision. Treatment options are dependent upon the specific product and patient reaction and should be individualized. One tenet is to avoid surgical excisions that will result in scarring until all other treatment options have been exhausted.

Treatment of complications in the second category, those due to procedural technique, becomes more challenging when the product placed is permanent, as there is generally no reversing agent as is seen with hyaluronidase for HA products. *Discoloration* can result from neovascularization, hyperpigmentation, and the Tyndall effect. Neovascularization occurs in response to the tissue trauma caused by filler injection. These new vessels

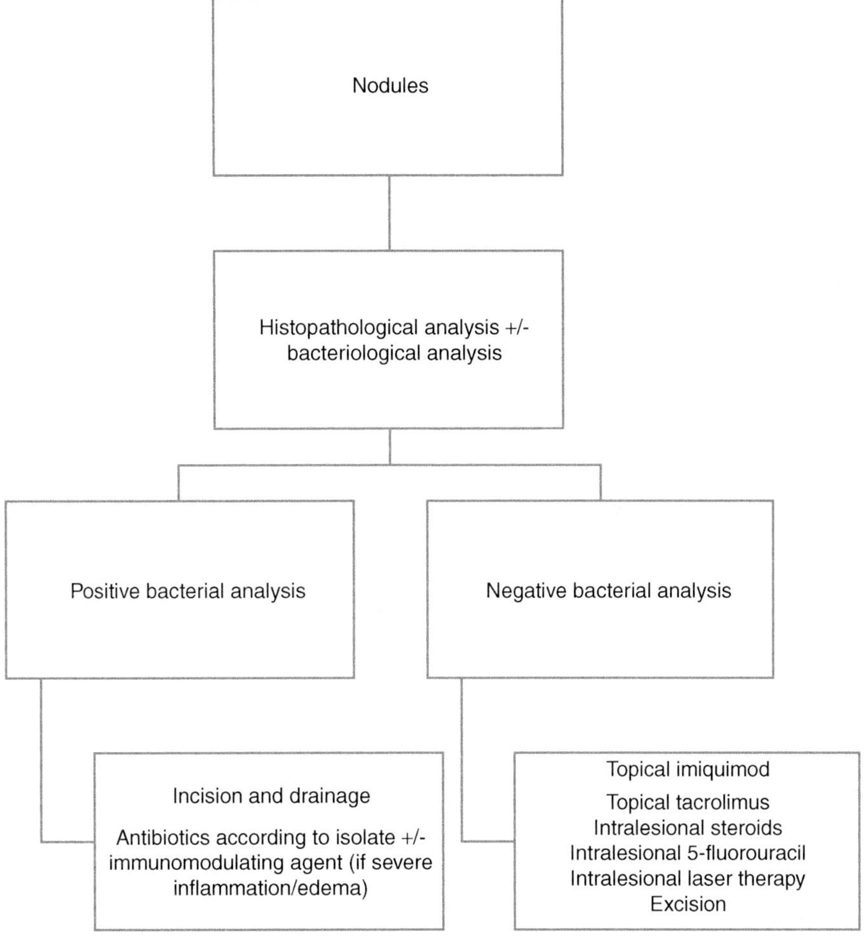

Fig. 36.9 Flowchart summarizing the evaluation and management of nodules.

should fade within 3 to 12 months without further treatment; however, laser treatment has been shown to be effective in recalcitrant cases. Hyperpigmentation is not uncommon especially in patients with Fitzpatrick skin types IV to VI. The therapeutic approach in these cases is with topical bleaching agents such as 4% hydroquinone and tretinoin combined with a daily broad spectrum sunscreen. When discoloration is due to the Tyndall effect, no target chromophore exists. Destruction with a carbon dioxide laser has been reported to be effective.

Vascular occlusion, *embolism*, and *cutaneous necrosis* should be managed aggressively immediately upon recognition. Prompt discontinuation of injections when this is suspected is the first step. Massage with warm compresses and administration of aspirin is reasonable. If the filler contains an HA component (Dermalive, Dermadeep), hyaluronidase may help dissolve a portion of the product. Unfortunately, no other potential reversing agents exist for the permanent fillers. Other therapeutic options to consider include vasodilating agents such as nitroglycerin paste and hyperbaric oxygen. However, recent literature suggests that applying nitroglycerin paste may not improve perfusion and could worsen ischemia via dilation of vessels and further propagation of filler into the smaller arterioles and capillaries. In a rabbit ear model used to create filler- associated skin ischemia, no statistically significant improvement in perfusion was noted after topical application of nitroglycerin paste with indocyanine green imaging. In the case of extensive necrosis, surgical reconstruction may be required.

TABLE 36.2 Selected Permanent Fillers by Category and Composition

Category	Branded Product	Composition
Liquid injectable silicone	Silikon-1000	Purified polydimethylsiloxane polymer
	Adato Sil-ol-5000	Purified polydimethylsiloxane polymer
Other "silicones"	Adulterated and unknown products	Variable and often unknown
Polyalkylimide gels (hydrophilic)	Bio-Alcamid	3% or 4% polyalkylimide gel in 97% or 96% sterile water
Polyacrylamide gels (hydrophilic)	Amazingel	Polyacrylamide gel in sterile water
	Aquamid	2.5% polyacrylamide gel in 97.5% sterile water
Polymethylmethacrylate (hydrophobic)	Arteplast (first generation)	30–42 μm PMMA microspheres in a gelatin carrier
	Artecoll (second generation)	30–50 μm PMMA microspheres in a bovine collagen carrier
	Artefill (third generation)	30–50 μm PMMA microspheres in a bovine collagen carrier
	Bellafill	30–50 μm PMMA microspheres in a bovine collagen carrier
Acrylic hydrogel (hydroxyethylmethacrylate/ ethylmethacrylate) (hydrophobic)	Dermalive	45–65 μm polygonal fragments acrylic hydrogel (40%) in HA (60%)
	Dermadeep	80–110 μm polygonal fragments acrylic hydrogel (40%) in HA (60%)

HA, Hyaluronic acid; *PMMA*, polymethylmetacrylate.
Modified from Prather, C. L., Wiest, L. G. (2013). Soft tissue augmentation, complications of permanent fillers (3rd ed.). USA: Saunders Elsevier.

Undercorrection is simply treated in subsequent sessions. However, overcorrection, asymmetry, contour irregularities, and texture irregularities require the permanent filler to be reduced or removed in some fashion. Needle aspiration, liposuction, extrusion after incision with an angled blade or Nokor needle, and surgical removal have all been reported as effective with permanent fillers. Alternatively, an injected steroid may cause tissue atrophy and help counter slight irregularities, as is done with hypertrophic scarring. However, one must take caution not to create a "doughnut" effect, with residual central prominence and surrounding atrophy. Migration is better avoided than treated, but surgical removal and liposuction are strategies for gross debulking of filler products in this situation.

Treatment of complications in the third category, which includes inflammation, infection, extrusion, and nodule formation, is best geared toward the host immune response and infectious agents, or ultimately by product reduction and removal (Box 36.2). Treatment is difficult, and no one single method has reliably proven effective. Immunomodulators strike at the biological mechanisms underlying the granulomatous response. Topical immunomodulating treatments, such as imiquimod and tacrolimus, have been reported effective for granulomas, likely through dampening of the local host immune response. Injected immunomodulating medications such as corticosteroids and 5-fluorouracil (5-FU) can also be effective for localized inflammation and granulomas (Fig. 36.10A,B). Oral steroids work by systemic, nonspecific immunomodulation and may be required for severe reactions over short to medium durations. Injectable tumor necrosis factor alpha (TNF-α) antagonists such as etanercept and infliximab have also been successful in altering the systemic immune response and decreasing granuloma activation and formation. There have been several reported cases using allopurinol to treat delayed granulomas associated with PMMA. Allopurinol is a xanthine oxidase inhibitor that acts as a catalyst in the formation of superoxide. Allopurinol and its metabolite

BOX 36.2 Anecdotal Treatments of Granulomas

- Triamcinolone intralesional + cryotherapy
- 5-Fluorouracil intralesional
- Bleomycin (1.5 IU/mL) intralesional
- Prednisone (1 mg/kg/day) oral
- Prednisone (60 mg/day) oral + ibuprofen (1800 mg/day)
- Cortivazol (3.75 mg/1.5 mL) intralesional
- Amoxicillin (1.5–3 g twice daily) oral (Christensen)
- Ciprofloxacin (500 mg to 1 g twice daily) oral (Christensen)
- Minocycline (2 Å ~ 100 mg/day) oral
- Minocycline (2Å ~250 mg/day) + prednisolone (4 mg/day) oral
- Cyclosporine (5 mg/kg/day) oral
- Allopurinol (200–600 mg/day) oral
- Imiquimod (Aldara) cream 5% topical
- Tacrolimus cream 0.5% topical
- Laser 532 nm and 1064 nm
- Intense pulsed light

oxypurinol act as free radical scavengers. Free radicals play an important role in the pathogenesis of granulomatous diseases and reduction of their amounts could attribute to the mechanism of action leading to reduced granuloma formation in select patients.

If product reduction or removal is necessary, minimally invasive techniques should be attempted first when practical, including needle aspiration, extrusion after incision, and liposuction. Ultimately, laser destruction or surgical removal may be necessary, but these modalities should be reserved for cases that are particularly problematic or that have not responded to more conservative therapies. Cassuto et al. have described a minimally invasive, minimally scarring technique for laser-assisted evacuation of infectious lesions after hydrogels using a pulsed 532 nm laser as well as a method for intralesional treatment of granulomas caused by gels containing microparticles with an 808 nm diode laser to facilitate product evacuation (Fig. 36.11A,B). Shelke et al. combined an 810 nm diode laser with a 1470 nm diode laser in continuous-wave mode, achieving improvement in 92% of cases. With a special focus on PMMA complications, a study by Goldman et al. brought to action the intralesional neodymium-doped yttrium aluminum garnet (Nd:YAG) laser in analogy to laser lipolysis and laser-assisted liposuction. The laser energy was delivered through an optical fiber fixed in a microcannula with the intent to produce channels (or tunnels) separating the filler material from adjacent tissue and to disrupt the filler's composition facilitating its aspiration via the cannula. The technique is considered safe in the hands of skillful practitioners; complications included seroma (treated with serial aspirations) and transient unilateral temporary paresis of nerve branches. Rivers et al. used long pulsed, 1064 nm Nd:YAG laser treatments at intervals of 2 months to treat seven patients with delayed-onset nodules to PMMA, with improvement in nodule size and skin texture after a median of three treatments.

Particularly with respect to late-onset granulomas, oral and/or intralesional antibiotic therapy should be attempted prior to, or at least alongside, other treatment modalities because biofilms are likely the etiologic agent.

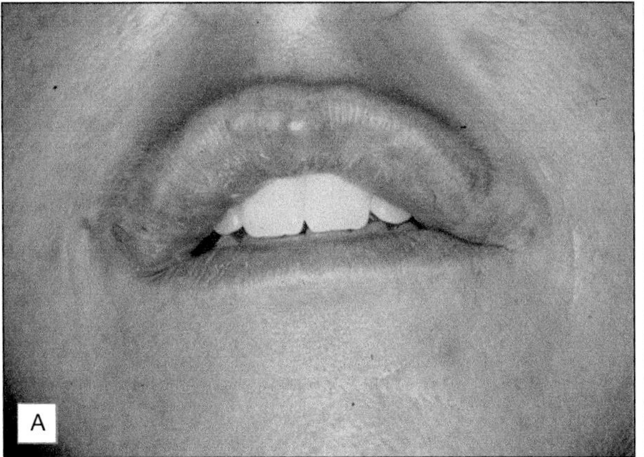

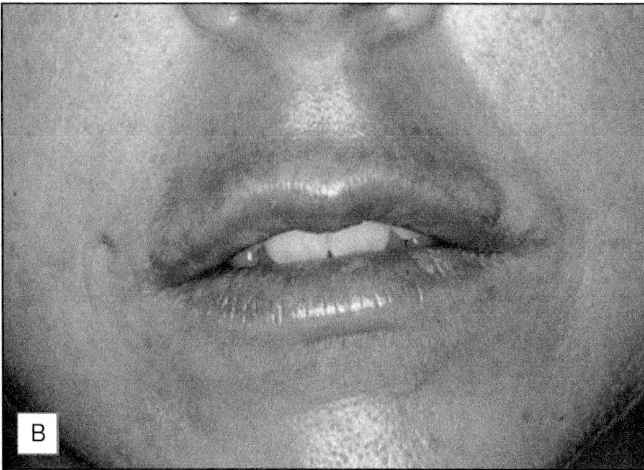

Fig. 36.10 (A) Dermalive granuloma. (B) With improvement after treatment with intralesional 5-fluorouracil and steroids.

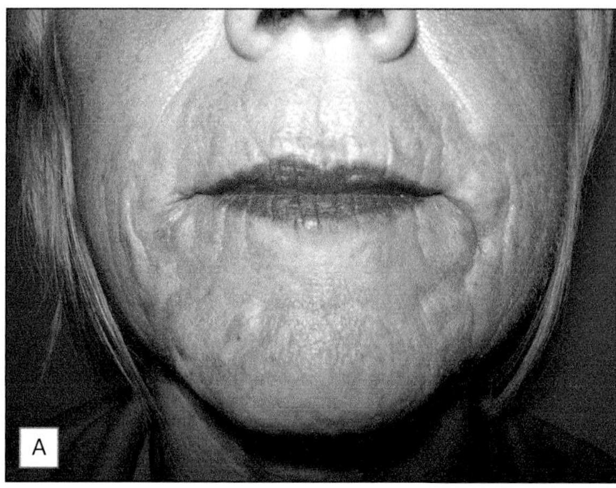

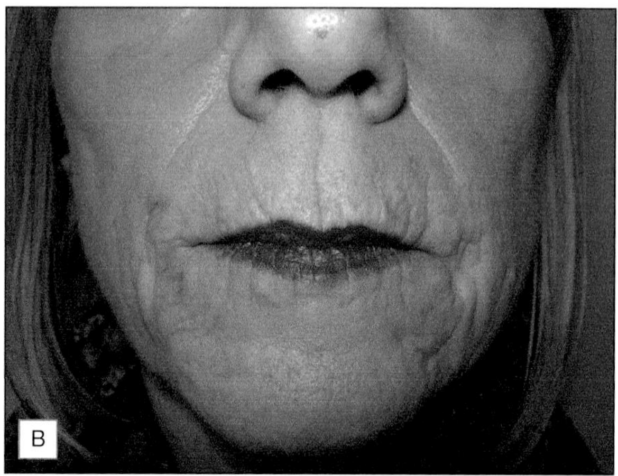

Fig. 36.11 (A) Late-onset granulomas. (B) With improvement after treatment with the method described by Cassuto et al.

Some authors feel that initial treatment with any agent other than antibiotics may allow the biofilm colony to thrive, possibly setting up an opportunity for long-term and recurrent granulomatous sequelae. Ultimately, a multimodal treatment approach may be necessary. A suggested therapeutic ladder for late-onset granulomas includes treatment with antibiotics first and foremost, possibly along with an immunomodulating agent, such as a steroid. Failing that, escalating immunomodulating medications should then be used, followed by minimally invasive and ultimately surgically invasive treatments until a response is achieved.

PEARL 8 Assume that late-onset granulomas are due in some part to bacterial biofilm colonization and direct therapy accordingly.

PEARL 9 Use invasive and surgical options only after all other options have been exhausted.

PEARL 10 Recurrent inflammation and granuloma formation may require chronic suppressive antibacterial therapy.

CONCLUSIONS

All fillers are not created equal, and the aesthetic practitioner who wishes to treat the varied manifestations of facial aging and effectively guide patients to the desired outcome must know which ones will help to accomplish patient goals and which ones will not. Myriad "permanent" products are available, and most fall into particulate and nonparticulate categories. All may cause the full spectrum of filler complications. Permanent fillers share the same complications seen with temporary fillers plus additional ones made more significant by their long-lasting nature. The most difficult complications, foreign body and late-onset granulomas, are increasingly recognized with permanent fillers and may be attributed to product–host interaction, as well as bacterial biofilm formation. A suggested therapeutic ladder includes antibiotic therapy, laser treatment with optic microfiber (as described by Cassuto et al.), immunomodulation, and possibly eventual surgical removal. Permanent fillers abound and will only increase over the next decade, as soft tissue augmentation has become the basis of an ever-expanding worldwide cosmetic industry. Even patients who do not have ready access to permanent fillers (such as in the United States) may easily find them abroad or illicitly for consumption. The modern aesthetic physician must recognize the products, the complications, and the treatment strategies, although there is more work to be done to elucidate underlying causes and best approaches for success.

REFERENCES

Do, E. R., & Shim, J. S. (2012). Long-term complications from breast augmentation by injected polyacrylamide hydrogel. *Archives of Plastic Surgery*, *39*(3), 267–269. https://doi.org/10.5999/aps.2012.39.3.267.

Formigli, L., Zecchi, S., Protopapa, C., Caporale, D., Cammarota, N., & Lotti, T. M. (2004). Bio-Alcamid: An electron microscopic study after skin implantation. *Plastic and Reconstructive Surgery, 113*(3), 1104–1106. https://doi.org/10.1097/01.prs.0000107746.58665.0a.

Karim, R. B., Hage, J. J., van Rozelaar, L., Lange, C. A., & Raaijmakers, J. (2006). Complications of polyalkylimide 4% injections (Bio-Alcamid): A report of 18 cases. *Journal of Plastic, Reconstructive and Aesthetic Surgery, 59*(12), 1409–1414. https://doi.org/10.1016/j.bjps.2006.01.049.

Protopapa, C., Sito, G., Caporale, D., & Cammarota, N. (2003). Bio-Alcamid in drug-induced lipodystrophy. *Journal of Cosmetic and Laser Therapy, 5*(3–4), 226–230. https://doi.org/10.1080/14764170310021922.

FURTHER READING

Al-Qattan, M. M. (2011). Complications related to Artecoll injections for soft tissue augmentation of the hand: 3 case reports. *The Journal of Hand Surgery, 36*(6), 994–997. https://doi.org/10.1016/j.jhsa.2011.03.016.

American Society of Plastic Surgeons. (2020). Plastic Surgery Statistics Report 2019. https://www.plasticsurgery.org/documents/News/Statistics/2019/plastic-surgery-statistics-full-report-2019.pdf.

Cassuto, D., Marangoni, O., De Santis, G., & Christensen, L. (2009). Advanced laser techniques for filler-induced complications. *Dermatologic Surgery, 35*(suppl 2), 1689–1695. https://doi.org/10.1111/j.1524-4725.2009.01348.x.

Cassuto, D., Pignatti, M., Pacchioni, L., Boscaini, G., Spaggiari, A., & De Santis, G. (2016). Management of complications caused by permanent fillers in the face: A treatment algorithm. *Plastic and Reconstructive Surgery, 138*(2), 215e–227e. https://doi.org/10.1097/PRS.0000000000002350.

Chrastil-LaTowsky, B., Wesley, N. O., MacGregor, J. L., Kaminer, M. S., & Arndt, K. A. (2009). Delayed inflammatory reaction to bio-alcamid polyacrylamide gel used for soft-tissue augmentation. *Archives for Dermatological, 145*(11), 1309–1312. https://doi.org/10.1001/archdermatol.2009.266.

Christensen, L. H. (2009). Host tissue interaction, fate, and risks of degradable and nondegradable gel fillers. *Dermatologic Surgery, 35*(suppl 2), 1612–1619. https://doi.org/10.1111/j.1524-4725.2009.01338.x.

Christensen, L., Breiting, V., Janssen, M., Vuust, J., & Hogdall, E. (2005). Adverse reactions to injectable soft tissue permanent fillers. *Aesthetic Plastic Surgery, 29*(1), 34–48. https://doi.org/10.1007/s00266-004-0113-6.

DeLorenzi, C. (2014). Complications of injectable fillers, part 2: Vascular complications. *Aesthetic Surgery Journal, 34*(4), 584–600. https://doi.org/10.1177/1090820X14525035.

Epstein, R. E., & Spencer, J. M. (2010). Correction of atrophic scars with Artefill: An open-label pilot study. *Journal of Drugs in Dermatology, 9*(9), 1062–1064.

Furmanczyk, P. S., Wolgamot, G. M., Argenyi, Z. B., & Gilbert, S. C. (2009). Extensive granulomatous reaction occurring 1.5 years after DermaLive injection. *Dermatologic Surgery, 35*(suppl 1), 385–388. https://doi.org/10.1111/j.1524-4725.2008.01044.x.

Goldman, A., & Wollina, U. (2018). Intralesional neodymium YAG laser to treat complications of polymethylmethacrylate. *Open Access Macedonian Journal of Medical Sciences, 6*(9), 1636–1641. https://doi.org/10.1177/1090820X14525035.

Grippaudo, F. R., & Mattei, M. (2011). The utility of high-frequency ultrasound in dermal filler evaluation. *Annals of Plastic Surgery, 67*(5), 469–473. https://doi.org/10.1097/SAP.0b013e318203ebf6.

Jones, D. H. (2009). Semipermanent and permanent injectable fillers. *Dermatologic Clinics, 27*(4), 433–444, vi. https://doi.org/10.1016/j.det.2009.08.003.

Jordan, D. R., & Stoica, B. (2015). Filler migration: A number of mechanisms to consider. *Ophthalmic Plastic and Reconstructive Surgery, 31*(4), 257–262. https://doi.org/10.1097/IOP.0000000000000368.

Khan, I., Shokrollahi, K., Bisarya, K., & Murison, M. S. (2011). A liposuction technique for extraction of Bio-Alcamid and other permanent fillers. *Aesthetic Surgery Journal, 31*(3), 344–346. https://doi.org/10.1177/1090820X11398476.

Kim, J. H., Ahn, D. K., Jeong, H. S., & Suh, I. S. (2014). Treatment algorithm of complications after filler injection: Based on wound healing process. *Journal of Korean Medical Science, 29*(suppl 3), S176–S182. https://doi.org/10.1097/IOP.0000000000000368.

King, M., Walker, L., Convery, C., & Davies, E. (2020). Management of a vascular occlusion associated with cosmetic injections. *The Journal of Clinical and Aesthetic Dermatology, 13*(1), E53–E58.

Monheit, G. D., & Rohrich, R. J. (2009). The nature of long-term fillers and the risk of complications. *Dermatologic Surgery, 35*(suppl 2), 1598–1604. https://doi.org/10.1111/j.1524-4725.2009.01336.x.

Narins, R. S., Coleman, W. P. 3rd, Rohrich, R., Monheit, G., Glogau, R., Brandt, F., Bruce, S., Colen, L., Dayan, S., Jackson, I., Maas, C., Rivkin, A., Sclafani, A., & Spivak, J. C. (2010). 12-Month controlled study in the United States of the safety and efficacy of a permanent 2.5% polyacrylamide hydrogel soft-tissue filler. *Dermatologic Surgery, 36*(suppl 3), 1819–1829. https://doi.org/10.1111/j.1524-4725.2010.01736.x.

Ono, S., Ogawa, R., & Hyakusoku, H. (2010). Complications after polyacrylamide hydrogel injection for soft-tissue augmentation. *Plastic and Reconstructive Surgery, 126*(4), 1349–1357. https://doi.org/10.1097/PRS.0b013e3181ead122.

Pacini, S., Ruggiero, M., Morucci, G., Cammarota, N., Protopapa, C., & Gulisano, M. (2002). Bio-alcamid: A novelty for reconstructive and cosmetic surgery. *Italian Journal of Anatomy and Embryology, 107*(3), 209–214.

Pallua, N., & Wolter, T. P. (2010). 5-year assessment of safety and aesthetic results after facial soft-tissue augmentation with polyacrylamide hydrogel (Aquamid): A prospective multicenter study of 251 patients. *Plastic and Reconstructive Surgery*, *125*(6), 1797–1804. https://doi.org/10.1097/PRS.0b013e3181d18158.

Park, T. H., Seo, S. W., Kim, J. K., & Chang, C. H. (2012). Clinical experience with polymethylmethacrylate microsphere filler complications. *Aesthetic Plastic Surgery*, *36*(2), 421–426. https://doi.org/10.1007/s00266-011-9803-z.

Prather, C. L., & Jones, D. H. (2006). Liquid injectable silicone for soft tissue augmentation. *Dermatologic Therapy*, *19*(3), 159–168. https://doi.org/10.1111/j.1529-8019.2006.00070.x.

Rauso, R., Freda, N., Parlato, V., Gherardini, G., Amore, R., & Tartaro, G. (2011). Polyacrylamide gel injection for treatment of human immunodeficiency virus-associated facial lipoatrophy: 18 months follow-up. *Dermatologic Surgery*, *37*(11), 1584–1589. https://doi.org/10.1111/j.1524-4725.2011.02131.x.

Requena, L., Requena, C., Christensen, L., Zimmermann, U. S., Kutzner, H., & Cerroni, L. (2011). Adverse reactions to injectable soft tissue fillers. *Journal of the American Academy of Dermatology*, *64*(1), 1–34; quiz 35–36. Erratum (2011) in: *J Am Acad Dermatol*, *64*(6), 1178. doi: 10.1016/j.jaad.2010.02.064.

Rivers, J., Labonté-Truong, N., & Richer, V. (2021). Adjuvant use of a 1,064 nm neodymium-doped yttrium aluminum garnet laser for the management of refractory late-onset nodules related to polymethylmethacrylate fillers. *Dermatologic Surgery*, *47*(3), 432–434. https://doi.org/10.1097/DSS.0000000000002301.

Rossner, M., Rossner, F., Bachmann, F., Wiest, L., & Rzany, B. (2009). Risk of severe adverse reactions to an injectable filler based on a fixed combination of hydroxyethylmethacrylate and ethylmethacrylate with hyaluronic acid. *Dermatologic Surgery*, *35*(suppl 1), 367–374. https://doi.org/10.1111/j.1524-4725.2008.01062.x.

Sachdev, M., Anantheswar, Y., Ashok, B., Hameed, S., & Pai, S. A. (2010). Facial granulomas secondary to injection of semi-permanent cosmetic dermal filler containing acrylic hydrogel particles. *Journal of Cutaneous and Aesthetic Surgery*, *3*(3), 162–166. https://doi.org/10.4103/0974-2077.74493.

Schelke, L., Decates, T., Kadouch, J., & Velthuis, P. (2020). Incidence of vascular obstruction after filler injections. *Aesthetic Surgery Journal*, *40*(8). https://doi.org/10.1093/asj/sjaa086. NP457–NP460.

Schelke, L. W., Van Den Elzen, H. J., Erkamp, P. P., & Neumann, H. A. (2010). Use of ultrasound to provide overall information on facial fillers and surrounding tissue. *Dermatologic Surgery*, *36*(suppl 3), 1843–1851. https://doi.org/10.1111/j.1524-4725.2010.01740.x.

Schuller-Petrović, S., Pavlović, M. D., Schuller, S. S., Schuller-Lukić, B., & Neuhold, N. (2013). Early granulomatous foreign body reactions to a novel alginate dermal filler: The system's failure? *Journal of the European Academy of Dermatology and Venereology*, *27*(1), 121–123. https://doi.org/10.1111/j.1468-3083.2011.04264.x.

Sclafani, A. P., & Fagien, S. (2009). Treatment of injectable soft tissue filler complications. *Dermatologic Surgery*, *35*(suppl 2), 1672–1680. https://doi.org/10.1111/j.1524-4725.2009.01346.x.

Snozzi, P., & van Loghem, J. A. J. (2018). Complication management following rejuvenation procedures with hyaluronic acid fillers—an algorithm-based approach. *Plastic and Reconstructive Surgery Glob Open*, *6*(12), e2061.

Walker, L., & King, M. (2018). This month's guideline: Visual loss secondary to cosmetic filler injection. *The Journal of Clinical and Aesthetic Dermatology*, *11*(5), E53–E55.

Wiest, L. G., Stolz, W., & Schroeder, J. A. (2009). Electron microscopic documentation of late changes in permanent fillers and clinical management of granulomas in affected patients. *Dermatologic Surgery*, *35*(suppl 2), 1681–1688. https://doi.org/10.1111/j.1524-4725.2009.01347.x.

Wolter, T. P., & Pallua, N. (2010). Removal of the permanent filler polyacrylamide hydrogel (aquamid) is possible and easy even after several years. *Plastic and Reconstructive Surgery*, *126*(3), 138e–139e. https://doi.org/10.1097/PRS.0b013e3181e3b506.

Zielke, H., Wölber, L., Wiest, L., & Rzany, B. (2008). Risk profiles of different injectable fillers: Results from the Injectable Filler Safety Study (IFS Study). *Dermatologic Surgery*, *34*(3), 326–335; discussion 335. https://doi.org/10.1111/j.1524-4725.2007.34066.x.

37

Vascular Compromise

Rachel Pritzker and Katie Beleznay

SUMMARY AND KEY FEATURES

- Soft tissue fillers are generally very well tolerated. However, serious vascular complications, including blindness, can occur.
- When filler is injected into blood vessels, ischemic or embolic phenomena may result.
- It is important to understand the depth and location of vessels in all areas of injection, although variation does occur.
- Strategies to prevent vascular compromise are critical and include injecting slowly and with minimal pressure, injecting small volumes at one time, and considering using large-bore, blunt-tipped cannulas.
- A treatment protocol should be instituted urgently at the first sign of vascular compromise. The goal of treatment is rapid restoration of perfusion.

INTRODUCTION

The use of soft tissue fillers continues to grow in popularity, in part, due to their favorable side effect profile. However, serious complications can occur. The most feared and potentially serious complications are vascular in nature. It is critical for injecting physicians to have a firm knowledge of the vascular anatomy and to understand key prevention and management strategies.

Vascular complications occur when filler is injected into blood vessels, resulting in ischemic or embolic phenomena. Skin necrosis occurs when the blood supply to the skin is compromised. Typically, the first indication of vascular compromise of the skin is blanching. This can be subtle and may go unnoticed. It is vital to be looking at all surrounding tissue while injecting dermal filler to possibly catch this subtle sign. Over the following minutes to hours and days, progression to a painful, violaceous, reticulated patch may occur (Fig. 37.1). Necrosis and subsequent scarring may develop.

Blindness results from retrograde embolization of filler into the ocular vessels. Visual complications after filler injection may present with immediate unilateral vision loss, ocular pain, headache, nausea, or vomiting. In addition, central nervous system complications, including infarction and hemiplegia, have been seen in association with blindness. In an updated review article, there were 48 new cases of blindness reported from 2015 to 2018 after filler injection, totaling 146 cases reported since the year 1906. Of the updated cases, most commonly injections were hyaluronic acid (HA) followed by calcium hydroxyapatite (CaHa) injections. These are only the reported cases; likely, a high number more exist. The most high-risk site in descending order was the nose, glabella, forehead, and nasolabial fold, but virtually every anatomic location on the face where filler is injected is at risk for vascular compromise (Fig. 37.2).

ANATOMY

It is important to understand the depth and location of vessels in high-risk sites. In the glabella and forehead, the two major arteries are the supratrochlear artery, which is found along the medial canthal vertical line, and the supraorbital artery, which is more lateral in the region of the medial iris (Fig. 37.3). Both of these arteries start

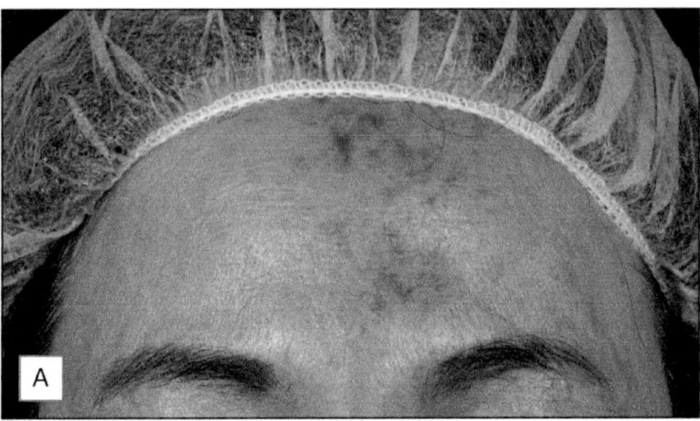

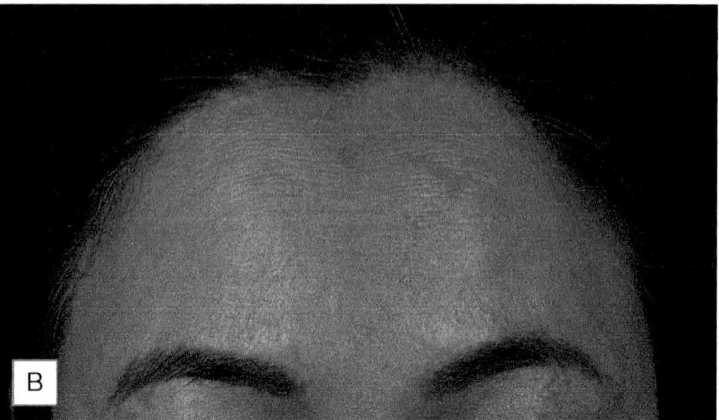

Fig. 37.1 Mottled erythema to forehead, 5 days post injection (A). Resolution of vascular compromise with no sequelae, 2.5 months post injection (B).

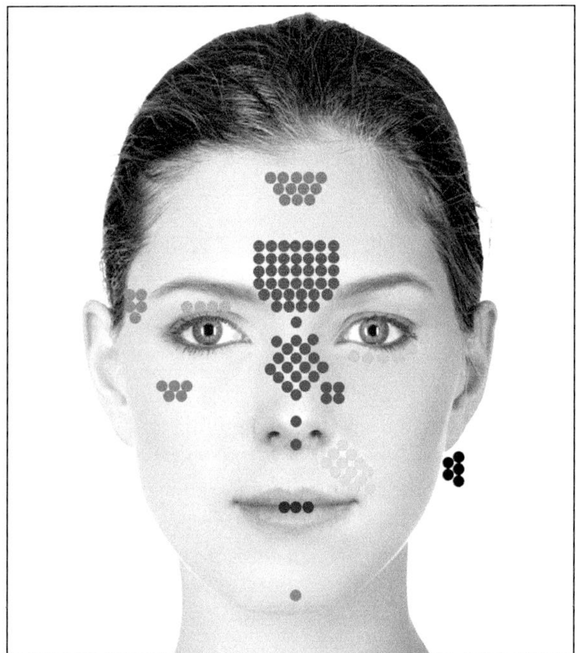

Fig. 37.2 The colored dots are the location of injection for each case of blindness from filler. The five black dots represent cases in which the location was not specified and listed as "face." (With permission from Beleznay K, Carruthers J, Humphrey S, Jones D. Avoiding and treating blindness from fillers: a review of the world literature. *Dermatol Surg*. 2015; 41:1097–1117.)

out deep and become more superficial approximately 15 to 20 mm above the supraorbital rim as they travel superiorly on the forehead. Injections within 2 cm of the supraorbital rim should be superficial. However, injections more superiorly on the forehead should be deep in a supraperiosteal plane. In the nasal region, there are many anastomotic vessels, and as such, filler is most safely placed in the avascular deep supraperiosteal plane. If the patient has had prior surgical procedures to the nose, filler injections should only be performed with extreme caution. One must always ask about prior surgical procedures, traumatic scars, or previous filler injections, as scarring from these can distort the anatomy of the vessels or cause a possible track where the filler may more easily enter a blood vessel. The most high-risk blood vessel for compromise in the medial cheek, nasolabial fold, and medial periorbital area is the angular artery. The angular artery has variable patterns after it branches off the facial artery and can be located more superficially in the subcutaneous layer in the upper third of the nasolabial fold, so it is imperative to be cautious when injecting this region. With multiple anastomoses present, if a needle enters a blood vessel and enough pressure is applied to the plunger when injecting filler, the arterial pressure can be overcome and filler can travel retrograde to the ocular vessels, causing blindness.

PREVENTION

Strategies to prevent vascular compromise are critical because we do not have well-documented standard of care protocols for treating these complications, particularly when it comes to visual compromise from filler. Anatomical knowledge is essential. It is imperative to have a detailed informed consent and have an action plan in your office immediately available for use to manage complications. Methods to help in prevention of occlusion include the use of cannulas, low volumes, low

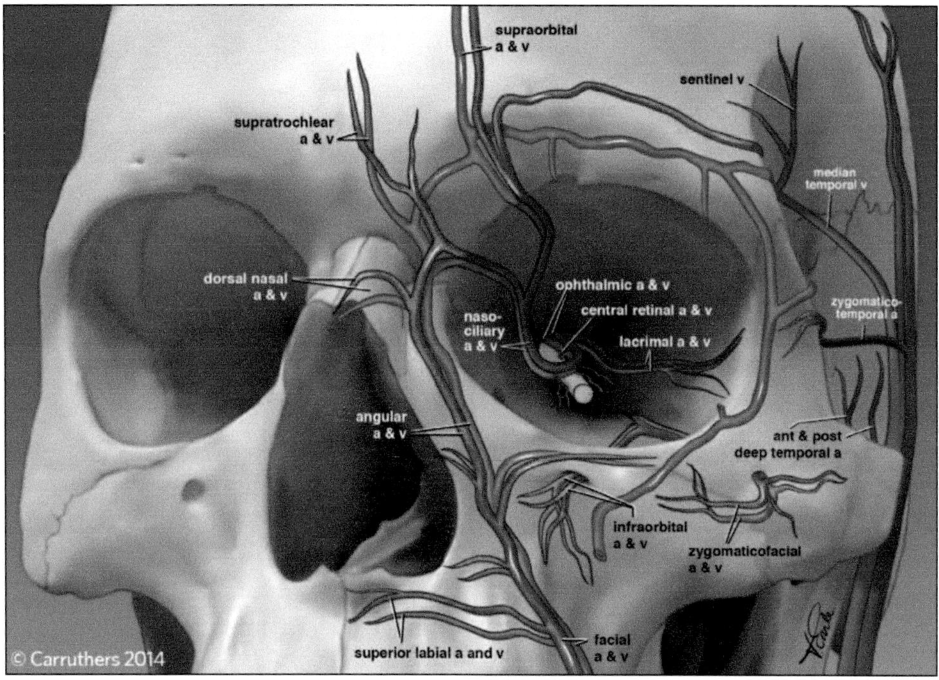

Fig. 37.3 Vascular anatomy of the upper face. *a*, Artery; *v*, vein. (Copyright Jean D. Carruthers, MD, 2014.)

force, and continuous movement as recently reviewed by a prominent consensus panel and are highlighted in Box 37.1.

BOX 37.1 Key Strategies to Prevent Vascular Compromise

- Before injection, obtain a clear informed consent that includes risk of necrosis, blindness, stroke, and the use of hyaluronidase in these situations.
- Before injecting, a detailed history should be obtained. Inquire about previous cosmetic procedures or surgeries, previous fillers, or traumatic scars, as these can distort anatomy.
- Know the location and depth of facial vessels and the common variations. Caution in high-risk areas for blindness, including glabella, nose, forehead, upper nasolabial fold, and medial tear trough.
- Consider using a blunt tip cannula with 25 G or larger lumen.
- Move the needle or cannula tip while injecting, so as not to deliver a large deposit in one location.
- Inject in small increments.
- Inject slowly and with minimal pressure to prevent a large column of filler traveling retrograde.

TREATMENT (Video 37.1)

Increasing popularity of injectable esthetic procedures leads to increasing rates of intravascular occlusion events, yet to date, recommendations on management are based primarily on anecdotal evidence, expert opinion, and a few consensus reports. Advancement in recommendations is progressing quickly, yet there is still a great deal of heterogenicity between protocol recommendations. It is important to read several published articles and combine their opinions to have a plan in place for a possible ischemic event. Treatment should be instituted immediately at the first sign of vascular compromise. The ultimate goal is to restore arterial circulation to the affected tissue.

Hyaluronidase is a soluble protein enzyme that catalyzes the degradation of HA. The use of hyaluronidase is highlighted as the main treatment within the consensus reports to remove the obstruction; even in a consensus recommendation for managing intravascular occlusion while injecting CaHa, hyaluronidase is employed. There are early reports of using sodium thiosulfate (STS) to dissolve CaHa, yet early proof of concept for its intra-arterial use to treat occlusion with CaHa on cadaveric models failed to show efficacy at this time.

Hyaluronidase is injected at the site of injection of the initial HA placement and at all sights of visible tissue ischemia, where one sees blanching or livedoid changes. The dosage of hyaluronidase to use is variable among reports, but a trend toward using higher number of units to flood the area is being seen. In a more recent report based on several anecdotal cases, Dr. DeLorenzi proposes that a minimum of 500 U of hyaluronidase be used per aesthetic unit that is affected with apparent changes of tissue ischemia and that injection be repeated hourly to keep the concentration of hyaluronidase continuously high in the entire area as hyaluronidase can diffuse through the vessel to the obstructed area. A recent consensus recommended the dosage of hyaluronidase be in the order of hundreds of units at each point of time it is injected. The ultimate goal is reperfusion, which can be seen if capillary refill comes back quickly in the affected tissue. With repeated injections of hyaluronidase, and subsequent bruising and swelling in the area, it can be tough to determine if the endpoint has been reached, but one must check for capillary refill and continue hyaluronidase injections until the endpoint of reperfusion is met. If a patient were to leave the office and an ischemic event was not recognized immediately, they may then report hours or days later with pain, atypical patchy skin discoloration, or other complaints of ischemic tissue; therefore, it is imperative that the entire staff be trained to be aware of these changes and bring the patient in for assessment and treatment. Treatment initiated even within 72 hours of onset can lead to successful treatment. Further treatments that should be initiated at the bedside should be oral aspirin, warm compresses, skin massage, and possibly intralesional or systemic corticosteroids. A thorough individual assessment and treatment plan with close follow-up should be initiated for each patient to optimize outcomes. If necrosis does occur, diligent wound care is critical, and long-term scar management should be addressed. Key management strategies for vascular compromise with skin sequelae (Box 37.2) and ocular complications (Box 37.3) are reviewed.

Management of blindness following filler injection is more challenging because there are few reported successful treatments and most commonly vision loss is permanent. In addition, time is of the essence as after approximately 90 minutes, the damage secondary to the retinal ischemia is more likely to be irreversible, and more recent reports have stated that retinal ganglion cells may infarct within 12 to 15 minutes. First and foremost, if the patient complains of ocular pain, vision changes, headache, or nausea, the injection should be stopped at once. The patient should be immediately transferred to an ophthalmologist or oculoplastic colleague. Large volumes of hyaluronidase should be injected at the location of filler injection and surrounding areas, along the path of the vessels leading to the eye, and injecting hyaluronidase at the supraorbital and supratrochlear foramina can also be considered. It has been shown that hyaluronidase can diffuse through the blood vessel walls without needing to be directly injected into the vessel.

BOX 37.2 Recommendation for Treatment of Vascular Compromise

- If blanching occurs, stop the injection immediately.
- Inject hyaluronidase at a high dose, on the order of hundreds of units during each attempt to restore blood flow.
- Apply warm compresses every 10 minutes for the first few hours.
- Massage the affected tissue.
- Consider aspirin 325 mg, under the tongue, immediately and 81 mg daily thereafter.
- Consider oral prednisone.
- Repeat injections of hyaluronidase until goal of reperfusion met.
- Follow the patient daily until improvement. Provide them with clear care instructions and contact information.

BOX 37.3 Treatment of Vascular Compromise With Ocular Complications

- If vision changes, ocular pain, headache, nausea, or vomiting occurs while injecting filler, stop the injection at once. Immediately contact an ophthalmologist colleague and urgently transfer the patient directly there. If there are signs of stroke, immediately send to an emergency room.
- Consider treating the injection site and surrounding area with high-dose hyaluronidase and potentially the area of supraorbital and supratrochlear foramina.
- Document all signs and symptoms related to the event.
- Mechanisms to reduce intraocular pressure should be considered, such as ocular massage, breathing into paper bag, topical timolol, and acetazolamide.

If vision loss occurs after an HA filler, retrobulbar or peribulbar injection of hyaluronidase has been proposed as a potential vision-saving treatment, but more recent recommendations suggest that it remains controversial at this time. Other therapies that have been recommended include treatments that will decrease intraocular pressure, including breathing in to a paper bag, ocular massage, topical timolol, and acetazolamide. Injecting physicians should help to educate their ophthalmology and oculoplastic colleagues about this rare complication and build relationships with them, so if an event occurs, they will be ready to help and understand the rationale and the urgency. Further discussion among experts relating their experiences with this complication and management strategies can help to build consensus that will improve patient safety.

CONCLUSIONS

With the increased use of soft tissue augmentation for revolumization, it is imperative to be aware of the risk of devastating vascular complications. To minimize any adverse events, a thorough understanding of facial anatomy and proper injection technique is critical. Key prevention strategies, such as injecting small amounts under low pressure, using larger-bore cannulas, and injecting slowly with continuous movement of the needle or cannula, should be implemented. Despite proper technique, the possibility of vascular occlusion and embolization of filler into ocular vessels remains. As such, injectors should have a treatment protocol in place, which should include immediate transfer to an ophthalmologist in the case of ocular complications and injection of high doses of hyaluronidase. Immediate and ongoing care ensures optimal outcomes and decreases the risk of permanent complications. Continue to be aware of changing recommendations and be current on the literature as this topic of vascular occlusion from filler injections is continuing to evolve quickly with more literature-based recommendations.

FURTHER READING

Beleznay, K., Carruthers, J. D. A., Humphrey, S., Carruthers, A., & Jones, D. (2019). Update on avoiding and treating blindness from fillers: A recent review of the world literature. *Aesthetic Surgery Journal, 39*(6), 662–674. https://doi.org/10.1093/asj/sjz053.

Cohen, J. L., Biesman, B. S., Dayan, S. H., et al. (2015). Treatment of hyaluronic acid filler-induced impending necrosis with hyaluronidase: Consensus recommendations. *Aesthetic Surgery Journal, 35*(7), 844–849. https://doi.org/10.1093/asj/sjv018.

DeLorenzi, C. (2017). New high dose pulsed hyaluronidase protocol for hyaluronic acid filler vascular adverse events. *Aesthetic Surgery Journal, 37*(7), 814–825. https://doi.org/10.1093/asj/sjw251.

Jones, D. H., Fitzgerald, R., Cox, S. E., et al. (2021). Preventing and treating adverse events of injectable fillers: Evidence-based recommendations from the American Society for Dermatologic Surgery Multidisciplinary Task Force. *Dermatologic Surgery, 47*(2), 214–226. https://doi.org/10.1097/DSS.0000000000002921.

Pavicic, T., Webb, K. L., Frank, K., Gotkin, R. H., Tamura, B., & Cotofana, S. (2019). Arterial wall penetration forces in needles versus cannulas. *Plastic and Reconstructive Surgery, 143*(3), 504e–512e. https://doi.org/10.1097/PRS.0000000000005321.

Scheuer, J. F., 3rd., Sieber, D. A., Pezeshk, R. A., Gassman, A. A., Campbell, C. F., & Rohrich, R. J. (2017). Facial danger zones: Techniques to maximize safety during soft-tissue filler injections. *Plastic and Reconstructive Surgery, 139*(5), 1103–1108.

van Loghem, J., Funt, D., Pavicic, T., et al. (2020). Managing intravascular complications following treatment with calcium hydroxylapatite: An expert consensus. *Journal of Cosmetic Dermatology, 19*(11), 2845–2858. https://doi.org/10.1111/jocd.13353.

Yankova, M., Pavicic, T., Frank, K., et al. (2021). Intraarterial degradation of calcium hydroxylapatite using sodium thiosulfate—An in vitro and cadaveric study. *Aesthetic Surgery Journal, 41*(5). https://doi.org/10.1093/asj/sjab020. NP226–NP236.

38

Reversers

Emily Keller, Rachel Miest, and Kathleen Suozzi

SUMMARY AND KEY FEATURES

- The increasing popularity of soft tissue augmentation requires knowledge of reversal techniques.
- Adverse events due to filler injection can be totally or partially reversed depending on the filler type and timing.
- Nonpermanent fillers are much more forgiving and more easily corrected.
- Hyaluronidase can be considered a treatment "eraser" for many complications arising from the injection of hyaluronic acid, and small doses can be effective.
- Vascular occlusion should be rapidly diagnosed and treated, especially if vision loss is involved, and large doses of hyaluronidase should be considered
- Late-onset inflammatory reactions may require a multifaceted approach, particularly after complications due to permanent filling agents.
- An emerging treatment for calcium hydroxylapatite filler is the use of sodium thiosulfate.

INTRODUCTION

According to the most recent (2019) procedural survey by the American Society for Dermatologic Surgery (ASDS), the use of injectable fillers has increased by 78% since 2012 in the United States. The advent of new, nonpermanent soft tissue fillers, and the resurgence of older, permanent fillers, speaks to the increased demand of the public for soft tissue augmentation. As with all cosmetic procedures, the increase in number of procedures performed increases the chances for complications. Additionally, many of the soft tissue fillers on the market today are injected in locations that are off-label, many of which carry a higher probability of vascular occlusion or other complication. Thus, a profound knowledge of how to reverse filler complications is paramount. Soft tissue fillers can be divided into two categories according to biodegradability: biodegradable (absorbable) or nonbiodegradable (permanent). The innovation of cross-linking techniques with different hyaluronic acid (HA) concentrations determines where fillers may be placed and how long they may provide tissue correction (Table 38.1). Any of the listed products can lead to early or delayed complications, but only HAs can truly be reversed with the use of hyaluronidase. Unlike biodegradable agents, particularly HAs, permanent fillers require a multifaceted approach and can be more difficult to correct in the event of misplacement or serious adverse reactions.

WHY DO WE NEED REVERSERS?

Reversers are necessary secondary to improper placement on depth of filler, overcorrection, vascular occlusion, and late-onset immune-mediated reactions. Looking from the perspective of filler permanence, only HA and collagen can be completely erased by two different enzymes: hyaluronidase and collagenase. An emerging treatment for dissolving calcium hydroxylapatite (CaHA) fillers is the use of sodium thiosulfate (STS), although its use is not as well studied as hyaluronidase and collagenase. If we look at all the adverse events after

TABLE 38.1 **Products According to Biodegradability, Manufacturer, Type of Cross-link or Vehicle, Type of Product and Concentration, and Regulatory Organs approval for United States, Canada, Europe, South America, and Central America**

Product	Manufacturer	Cross-Link Tech/ Vehicle	Type Product and Concentration (mg/mL)	Approval by Country	Biodegradability/ erasability
BIODEGRADABLE PRODUCTS					
Juvéderm Ultra XC	Allergan	Hylacross	HA-24	All	Absorbable/erasable
Juvéderm XC ultra plus	Allergan	Hylacross	HA-24	All	Absorbable/erasable
Juvederm Volux	Allergan	Vycross	HA-25	South, Central America/ Canada/Europe	Absorbable/erasable
Radiesse	Merz	Carboximetilcelullose 70%	Calcium hydroxylapatite 30%	All	Absorbable/ nonerasable
Sculptra	Galderma/Sinclair	Saline and Lidocaine	Poly-l-lactic acid (% depend on dilution)	All	Absorbable/ nonerasable
RHA 2	Teoxane SA	Preserved Network	HA-23	United States/Europe	Absorbable/erasable
RHA 3	Teoxane SA	Preserved Network	HA-23	United States/Europe	Absorbable/erasable
RHA 4	Teoxane SA	Preserved Network	HA-23	United States/Europe	Absorbable/erasable
Juvéderm Voluma XC	Allergan	Vycross	HA-20	All	Absorbable/erasable
Juvéderm Volbella XC	Allergan	Vycross	HA-15	South America/Canada/ Europe	Absorbable/erasable
Juvéderm Volift[a]	Allergan	Vycross	HA-17.5	South, Central America/ Canada/Europe	Absorbable/erasable
Juvederm Vollure XC	Allergan	Vycross	HA-17.5	All (Vilify in other countries)	Absorbable/erasable
Belotero Hydro	Merz	No crosslink, contains glycerol	HA-18	South, Central America/ Canada/Europe	Absorbable/erasable
Belotero Balance	Merz	CPM	HA-22.5	All	Absorbable/erasable

Continued

TABLE 38.1 Products According to Biodegradability, Manufacturer, Type of Cross-link or Vehicle, Type of Product and Concentration, and Regulatory Organs approval for United States, Canada, Europe, South America, and Central America—Cont'd

Product	Manufacturer	Cross-Link Tech/ Vehicle	Type Product and Concentration (mg/mL)	Approval by Country	Biodegradability/ erasability
BIODEGRADABLE PRODUCTS					
Belotero Volume[a]	Merz	CPM	HA-26	South, Central America/ Canada/Europe	Absorbable/erasable
Belotero Intense[a]	Merz	CPM	HA-25.5	South, Central America/ Canada/Europe	Absorbable/erasable
Belotero Soft[a]	Merz	CPM	HA-20	South, Central America/ Canada/Europe	Absorbable/erasable
Emervel Classic[a]	Galderma	OBT	HA-20	South, Central America/ Canada/Europe	Absorbable/erasable
Emervel Lips[a]	Galderma	OBT	HA-20	South, Central America/ Canada/Europe	Absorbable/erasable
Emervel Volume[a]	Galderma	OBT	HA-20	South, Central America/ Canada/Europe	Absorbable/erasable
Emervel Deep	Galderma	OBT	HA-20	South, Central America/ Canada/Europe	Absorbable/erasable
Restylane	Galderma	NASHA	HA-20	All	Absorbable/erasable
Restylane Silk/Vital	Galderma	NASHA	HA-20	All	Absorbable/erasable
Restylane Defyne	Galderma	NASHA	HA-20	All	Absorbable/erasable
Restylane Refyne	Galderma	NASHA	HA-20	All	Absorbable/erasable
Restylane Kysse	Galderma	NASHA	HA-20	All	Absorbable/erasable
Restylane Lyft	Galderma	NASHA	HA-20	All	Absorbable/erasable
Nonbiodegradable products (permanent)					
Silikon 1000	Alcon	—	Polydimethylsiloxane	All (not aesthetic uses)	Nonabsorbable/ nonerasable
Belafill	Suneva Medical	Bovine collagen	PMMA + bovine collagen	North America and Canada	Nonabsorbable/ nonerasable

[a]Products not US Food and Drug Administration approved.

CPM, Cohesive polydensified matrix; *OBT*, optimal balance technology; *NASHA*, nonanimal stabilized hyaluronic acid; *PMMA*, polymethyl methacrylate.

filler application, especially with nonabsorbable fillers, there are complications that can be partially reversed or at least treated with a variety of substances, lasers, or oral medicines (those will be mentioned but not discussed in this chapter). This chapter will focus on the use of substances, procedures, or technology that can alter or change not only the permanence of filler itself, but also change the elements involved in a specific adverse event.

FILLER COMPLICATIONS AND REVERSIBILITY

Adverse effects following soft tissue augmentation are generally classified as early onset (up to 2 weeks after injection), late onset (> 14 days to 1 year), or delayed onset (> 1 year) (Box 38.1). Late- or delayed-onset reactions are more commonly associated with nonabsorbable filling agents but have been more recently described with HA, CaHA, and poly-l-lactic acid (PLLA). Early-onset adverse events are easier to treat and more common than late-onset ones. According to reversibility classification, HA and collagen injection may be a clear advantage over other substances (Figs. 38.1–38.5).

BOX 38.1 Adverse Events Following Soft Tissue Augmentation According to Onset

1. Early onset (immediate to 14 days)
    - Injection site reactions including purpura and edema
    - Noninflammatory nodules (overcorrection or misplacement of injected material)
    - Infection (bacterial, viral)
    - Hypersensitivity reaction/anaphylaxis
    - Vascular occlusion
2. Late onset (from 15 days to 1 year) and delayed (> 1 year)
    - Inflammatory nodules (immune-mediated vs infection/biofilm)
    - Persistent or recurrent edema

Early Adverse Events Treated Without Reversers

Expected early reactions are most commonly injection site reactions, including purpura and edema. Vascular lasers are effective in the treatment of postprocedure purpura. Infections are much less frequent, with herpes virus being the most common. Hypersensitivity and angioedema are

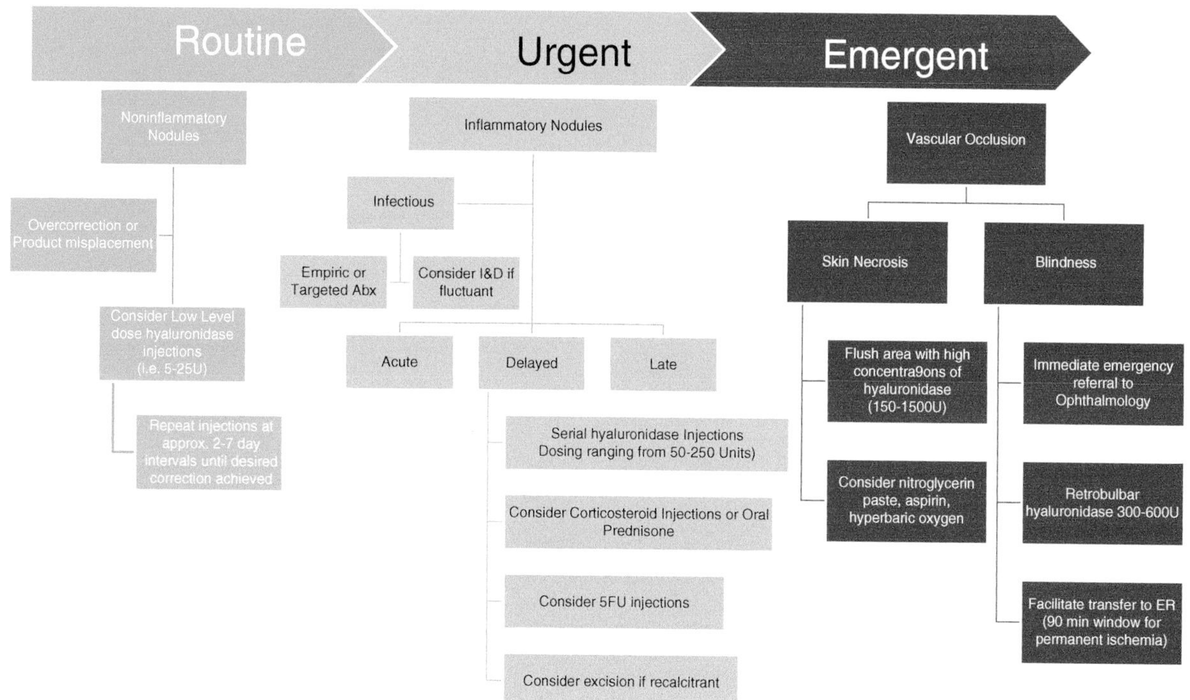

Fig. 38.1 Immediate-onset adverse events totally reversible. *5FU*, 5-Fluorouracil; *I&D*, incision and drainage.

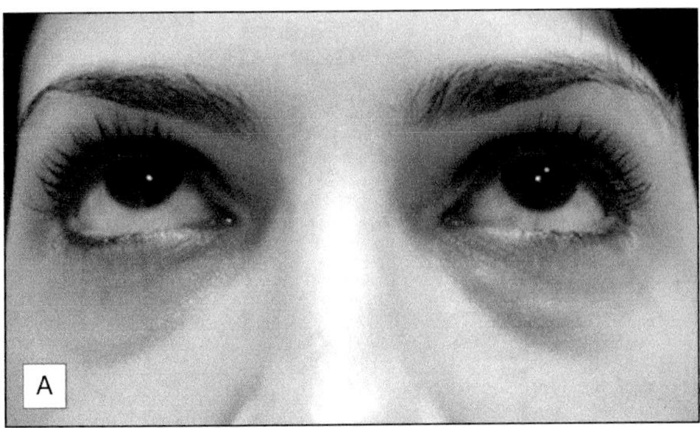

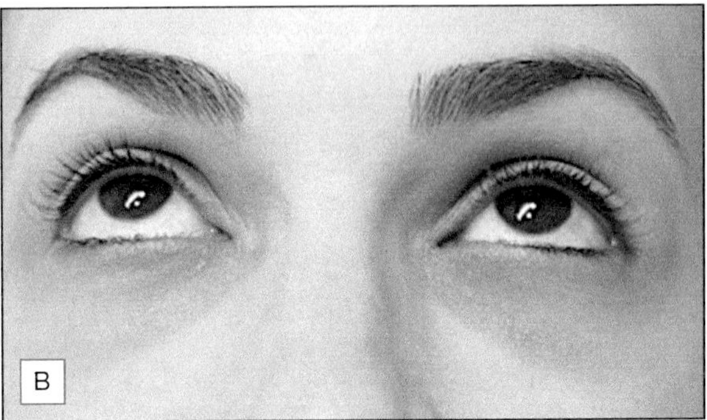

Fig. 38.2 (A) Patient after 6 months of hyaluronic acid filler for tear trough correction and (B) 15 days after 8 U hyaluronidase each side (4 U per lump).

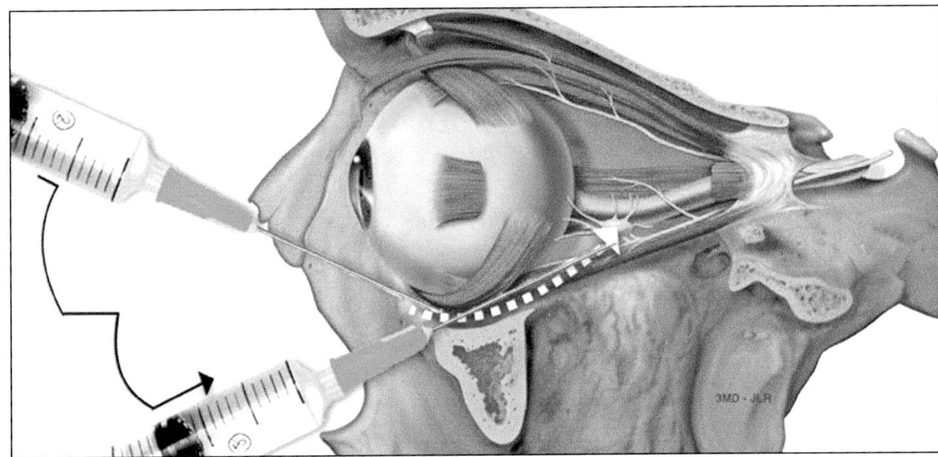

Fig. 38.3 How to perform retrobulbar injection of hyaluronidase if occlusion of ophthalmic artery of retinal artery is suspected.(Original image attribution goes to Patrick J. Lynch, http://commons.wikimedia.org/wiki/Category:Medical_illustrations_by_Patrick_Lynch.)

very rare but can occur with all fillers composed of foreign body material. Anaphylaxis reaction symptoms are pruritus, erythema, urticarial lesions, angioedema, nausea, vomiting, breathlessness, dizziness, syncope, hypotension, or even cardiorespiratory arrest. The physician must be prepared to deal with anaphylaxic reactions. Epinephrine is the most important drug in this clinical emergency, maximally effective when injected promptly. H1-antihistamines are not drugs of choice in initial anaphylaxis treatment because they do not relieve life-threatening respiratory symptoms or shock, although they decrease urticaria and itching. Diphenhydramine can be administered, and glucocorticoids remain in use for anaphylaxis because they potentially prevent biphasic anaphylaxis, reducing the risks of late symptoms. If symptoms are mild, oral prednisone can be prescribed, but more severe cases need intravenous methylprednisolone. It is important to have an oxygen cylinder and β2 agonist medication, such as salbutamol, in the clinic in case of hypoxemia. After clinical stabilization, the physician must decide whether the patient should be taken to the hospital.

Intravascular Occlusion

Among all the adverse events related to filler placement, intravascular injection and its consequences are most concerning and can be devastating. Chapters 35 and 37 discuss the various types of vascular occlusion events and present the relevant anatomical considerations. This section will review the treatment protocols for reversers in more detail. The mechanism of action of hyaluronidase

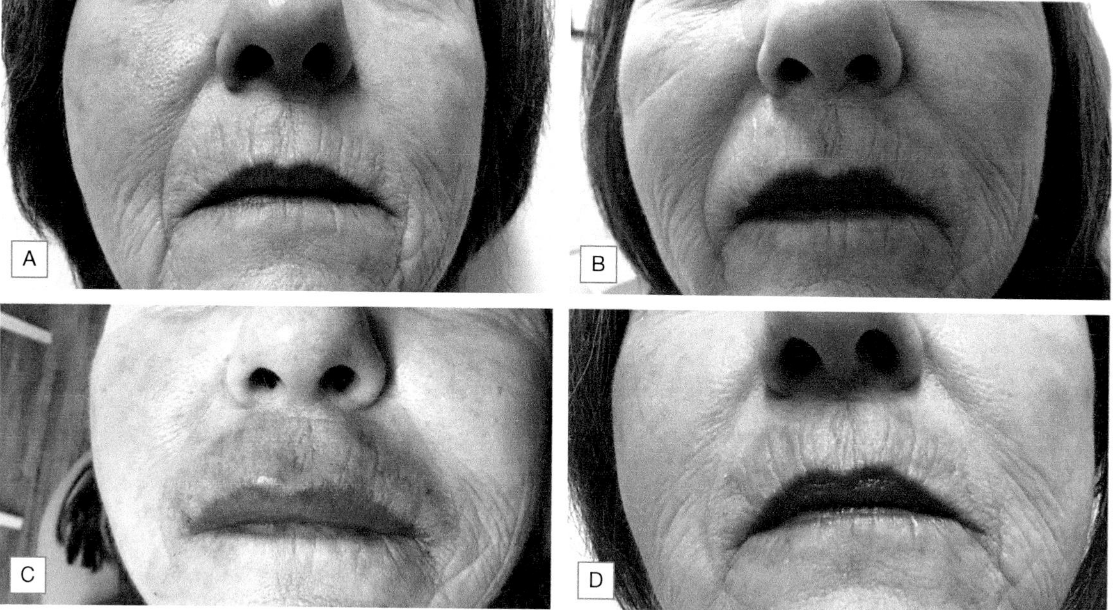

Fig. 38.4 (A) Before and (B) 3 months after 1 cc of hyaluronic acid filler to upper cutaneous vertical lip lines showing granuloma formation. Treated with 1 cc Hylenex, 0.5 cc 1% lidocaine, doxycycline 100 mg BID × 10 days, prednisone 40 mg × 5 days. (C) 4 months, worsening, treated with 2 cc Hylenex, 0.5 cc 1% lidocaine, 0.7 cc ILK 5 mg/cc, prednisone 40 mg × 3 days, 20 mg × 3 days, 10 mg × 3 days. (D) 4.5 months, granuloma resolved.

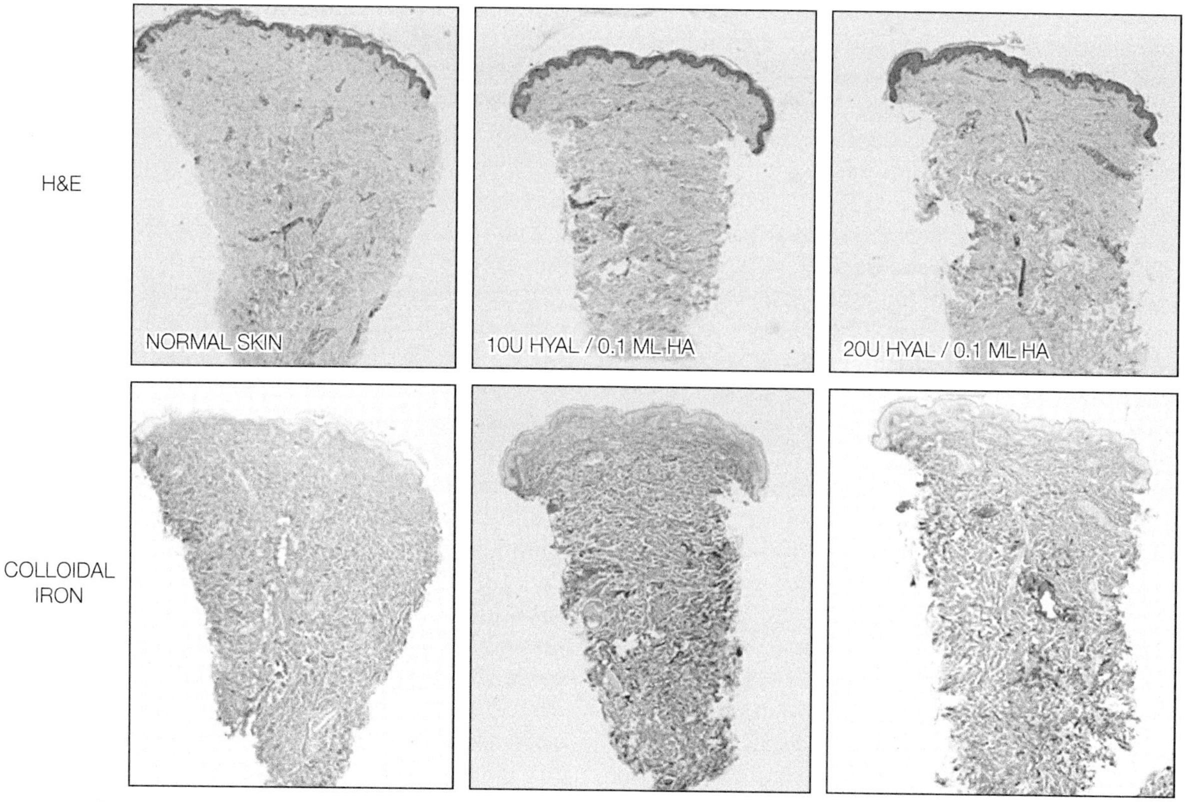

H&E

NORMAL SKIN

10U HYAL / 0.1 ML HA

20U HYAL / 0.1 ML HA

COLLOIDAL IRON

Fig. 38.5 Skin biopsy stained with colloidal iron to compare the amount of hyaluronic acid in normal skin and after 10 and 20 U of hyaluronidase showing no natural hyaluronic acid difference.

in the setting of HA vascular occlusion is bathing the artery in hyaluronidase, which can then readily diffuse across the vessel wall and be carried by arterial flow to the embolism. Selective angiography has also been described, but this technique is highly specialized and requires interdisciplinary care.

Skin Necrosis

Impeding skin necrosis can be predicted by immediate skin reactions after filler injection, including skin blanching, violaceous, or reticular discoloration. According to consensus recommendation, areas of impending necrosis should be treated with hyaluronidase immediately. The recommended injection technique is to space injections approximately 3 to 4 cm apart within the affected area. If no improvement is observed after 60 minutes, the injections should be repeated. Hyaluronidase is able to diffuse readily into a vessel wall to dissolve intraarterial HA, so injections should flood the area of the arterial supply to the necrosed skin. For example, if necrosis is noted, hyaluronidase should be injected within the affected skin region to address peripheral end-vessel embolization, but in addition, injection of hyaluronidase in and around the main feeding vessel allows for hyaluronidase to cross the vessel wall and be carried forward by arterial flow to the area of embolization. According to a systematic review by Nayfeh et al., hyaluronidase amounts injected for treatment of vascular occlusion ranged from 150 to 1500 IU at a median time of 45 hours after the vascular occlusion developed. Over the 100 cases evaluated, 77% of patients recovered from the occlusion event, with 49% of cases experiencing complete resolution. DeLorenzi advocates for high-dose hyaluronidase proportionate to the ischemic surface area, generally 500 IU for smaller regions to 1500 IU for larger regions. Specifically, he describes the dose of hyaluronidase as 500 IU for an area of half an upper lip, 1000 IU if the ischemia involves the nose in addition to the upper lip, and 15,000 IU if it involves a third region, (i.e., cheek or chin). The thickness of the tissue involved is another consideration; the tissue overlying the lateral cheeks in thicker (~ 25 mm) than the upper lip (~ 12 mm) or the glabella (6 mm) and thus hyaluronidase volume should be adjusted accordingly. Combination treatment with topical nitroglycerin 2% paste, aspirin 325 mg, and oral prednisone may also be considered. Fig. 38.1 outlines the treatment protocol for vascular compromise with skin sequalae. The time interval for treatment with a reverser in the setting of vascular compromise is important. Optimal results are achieved when hyaluronidase is injected within 4 hours of the event; however, later treatment can aid in healing of the necrosed tissue.

Blindness

Blindness is the most feared, catastrophic sequalae of soft tissue augmentation. The incidence of visual impairment from fillers is extremely rare, but all practitioners should have a treatment protocol in place. If there is any evidence of a visual problem or sudden ocular pain after dermal filler injection, prompt consultation with an ophthalmologist is recommended. Iatrogenic ophthalmic artery occlusion is characterized by severe ocular pain in the affected eye immediately after injection, but central retinal artery occlusion presents with only decreased vision without ocular pain. Theoretically, there is a 90-minute window to reverse retinal ischemia and prevent tissue necrosis. Nayfeh et al. summarizes the treatment of injection-related visual compromise of 96 patients previously reported in the literature. Various treatment interventions were reported within 1 week of the event. Hyaluronidase injections were performed in 46.9% of patients and ranged in amount from 300 to 9000 IU. Glucocorticoids, antiplatelet and anticoagulation therapy, intraocular pressure lowering drugs, urokinase injections, nitroglycerin, hyperbaric oxygen, and mechanical recanalization were also utilized, but no studies have validated the effectiveness of these interventions.

Carruthers and Fagien have advocated that a large volume of retrobulbar hyaluronidase injection is the single most effective option to prevent retinal infarction after accidental hyaluronic filler embolization. Hyaluronidase 150 to 200 units/mL should be injected along the inferolateral orbit (see Fig. 38.3) and repeated until symptoms improve. The proposed mechanism of action is that flooding the retrobulbar space with hyaluronidase allows for diffusion of the hyaluronidase into a portion of the central retinal artery that is not ensheathed within the optic nerve. Studies have suggested that hyaluronidase is unable to penetrate the nerve sheath of the optic nerve. There is very small, approximately 1 to 10 mm, region of the central retinal artery that is not encased within the ophthalmic nerve, and via entry through this unsheathed portion, the hyaluronidase can be carried via arterial flow to the site of embolus. Alternatively, retrobulbar hyaluronidase may exert its action on the ophthalmic artery, which is not ensheathed within the optic nerve; however, central retinal artery occlusion is thought to be the primary mechanism of vascular occlusion related vision loss. Two studies involving New Zealand rabbits reported differing success with the retrobulbar technique. Hwang et al. injected 1000 IU 30 minutes after simulated occlusion and no improvement was observed. In contrast, Lee et al. used 3000 IU of hyaluronidase 5 to 10 minutes after simulated occlusion and reported retinal reperfusion in three out of four experimental eyes. Chestnut reported the first documented success of using the retrobulbar hyaluronidase technique in a patient. In this case, the patient experienced unilateral eye pain and subjective visual loss (no objective measure of visual loss and no fundus exam performed), which resolved after three retrobulbar injections of hyaluronidase for a total of 450 IU administered within 20 minutes of symptom onset. In 2019, Wibowo et al. reported another case of vision restoration after two injections of 900 IU retrobulbar hyaluronidase given 72 and 96 hours after filler injection. This case is notable in that the injection was performed far outside the 90-minute window thought critical for retinal artery recanalization. The reason for the success in this case is hypothesized to be that the occlusive event did not fully obstruct the central retinal artery or the ophthalmic artery, but likely was a subacute ischemic event with sparing of some of the ophthalmic circulation. Paap et al. reviewed the reports of blindness associated with HA and examined the evidence for use of retrobulbar hyaluronidase injections, identifying 146 reported cases. In addition to the cases previously discussed, there were numerous cases of failed attempts at retrobulbar injections to restore visual loss. Zhu et al. and Thanasarnaksorn et al. reported a total of six patients who were treated with hyaluronidase concentrations of 1200 to 6000 IU with no patient demonstrative improvement in visual acuity or retinal artery recanalization.

Hyaluronidase injection in the region of the supratrochlear and supraorbital arteries has also been described as a technique for treating filler-related blindness. Goodman and Clague describe the technique of injecting hyaluronidase into the region of the supraorbital artery in its location at the supraorbital notch. The proposed mechanism is retrograde flow of hyaluronidase back to the ophthalmic and central retinal arteries.

Selective angiography has also been described for treatment of filler-related blindness. Cannulation of the retinal artery by an interventional radiologist can allow for direct injection of hyaluronidase into the area of embolization. This technique requires multidisciplinary coordination and is challenging to perform within the 90-minute timeframe, particularly outside a tertiary care center. According to Zhang et al., selective angiography was able to establish recanalization of the vessels at least partially, although failing to restore vision in three of the four cases. Combination endovascular treatment of hyaluronidase with urokinase (previously shown to be effective in a rat model) was successfully used by a Chinese group, showing visual improvement in 42% of the patients treated with combination therapy versus 36% of patients experiencing improvement when receiving hyaluronidase alone.

As mentioned previously, to reverse all immediate adverse events, timing is crucial, so we present an algorithm to treat and reverse each one. Every physician who performs filler injections needs to have in mind an algorithm for diagnosis and treatment of those catastrophic complications because timing is crucial to attempt reversal of permanent damage (see Fig. 38.1).

Nodules: Noninflammatory, Inflammatory, and Infectious

Nodules can be classified as noninflammatory, inflammatory, and infectious, as well as by their time to onset (see Fig. 38.1). Early nodules may be related to inappropriate technique or product selection. Late- or delayed-onset nodules are often related to an immune response to the filler with subsequent granuloma formation, although biofilms have also been implicated.

Noninflammatory nodules are usually seen early as an issue of misplaced or excess filler. Delayed noninflammatory fibrotic nodules can also develop, particularly in the setting of CaHA and PLLA. Hyaluronidase can be used to dissolve these typically small, nontender, isolated nodules and has been described as possibly effective for CaHA nodules. However, non-HA fillers generally present a greater challenge. Reassurance of eventual resolution and the addition of HA filler to minimize nodule appearance are options in addition to intralesional treatments (e.g., corticosteroids, lidocaine, 5-fluorouracil, and STS), as well as laser and surgical excision.

Inflammatory nodules are most commonly late or delayed onset. These red, tender nodules may represent a foreign body reaction to the injected material or possible biofilm infection. If fluctuance is present, incision and drainage with subsequent cultures should be the initial step. Empiric antibiotic therapy for at least 2 weeks is recommended with a quinolone and macrolide. Although hyaluronidase can be effective for inflammatory nodules, whether it is advisable to inject directly into an infected area is debatable.

If antimicrobial therapy is ineffective, intralesional corticosteroids are appropriate. Intralesional 5-fluorouracil has also been used successfully, likely due to its antiinflammatory and antimicrobial properties. Laser-assisted treatment has also been described using an 808 nm diode introduced percutaneously. Ultimately, excision may be required but should be pursued only after failure of medical therapy.

REVERSERS

Hyaluronidase

Hyaluronidase is a naturally occurring enzyme (endo-β-N-acetyl-hexosaminidases) that degrades the substrate HA by separating the β-1,4-glucosidic linkages between C1 of the glucosamine moiety and C4 of the glucuronic acid to form tetrasaccharides. After injection, hyaluronidase immediately disperses in tissues to break down the added HA. The duration of hyaluronidase enzyme activity is dependent on the type of tissue. Hyaluronidase acts immediately once in contact with its substrate, and the duration of activity is typically 24 to 48 hours in dermal tissues. However, it has an extended duration in ocular tissues that ranges from 60 to 112 hours. In contrast, the hyaluronidase enzyme is deactivated immediately when injected intravenously. It is hypothesized that the process is antibody mediated; however, the true mechanism of deactivation is unknown. The US Food and Drug Administration (FDA) has approved hyaluronidase to break down and hydrolyze HA for the following three therapeutic indications:

1. Increase the absorption and dispersion of other injected drugs, particularly retrobulbar anesthetic block in ophthalmologic surgery (it reduces the viscosity of extracellular matrix, which facilitates the diffusion of the agent, enlarging the anesthetized area, and shortens diffusion time, increasing the permeability of tissues and enhancing the anesthesia effect).
2. Subcutaneous infusion of fluids (hypodermoclysis), used mostly in the elderly population for mild to moderate dehydration and in young infants or children in whom intravenous administration is not possible.
3. Adjunct for subcutaneous urography, improving the resorption of radiopaque agents.

Therapeutic off-label applications in dermatology have yielded variable success for the treatment of diabetic scleredema, scleroderma, and others. Hyaluronidase can be used after injection of HA fillers to correct asymmetry, overcorrection, the Tyndall effect, granuloma formation, and vascular occlusion.

Available Formulations

North American and Canadian commercial formulations of hyaluronidase include Vitrase, Hylenex, Amphadase, and Hylase Dessau. In most South American countries and Europe, they use US/Canadian versions, or compound their own formulations of hyaluronidase. Those brands found abroad, although not an extensive list, include Hyaluronidase 2000 (Brazil) and Reductonidasa (Spain). The majority of hyaluronidase comes from engineered bovine or ovine testicular cells. Hylenex is the only recombinant human hyaluronidase made by genetically engineered hamster ovary cells (Table 38.2).

Injection Techniques and Dosing

There is no consensus on dose or time comparing all hyaluronidases used in different countries. The dose should depend on the location, the crosslinking used to form the HA filler, and the concentration of HA. Many different HA formulations are available, and each one has a different HA concentration and 1,4-butanediol diglycidyl ether (BDDE)-based cross-linking 1,4 butanedioldiglycidyl ether (Table 38.1). The degree of modification is an important characteristic parameter that can affect the rheologic property, antidegradation ability, and swelling property of modified HA hydrogel in the structural foundation. The modification type (pendent or cross-link modification) also affects the final properties of HA hydrogel. Cross-link modification produces strong covalent bonds to retard the degradation and prolong the duration of the hydrogel. An in vivo study on different hyaluronidase preparations and different HA products was performed by Cassabona et al. to quantify the amount of hyaluronidase and the time needed to dissolve clinical

TABLE 38.2 **Brands, Origin, Manufacturer, Availability by Country, Dilutions, and Dose Recommended for Five Different Hyaluronidase Products**

Product	Manufacturer	Available for Use	Origin of Hyaluronidase	Dose (mL)	Dilution	Amount to Inject 4 U (using 30 U BD syringe) (mL)
Hyaluronidase 2000	Biometil Swiss, Sao Bento do Sul, SC, Brazil	Brazil	Purified bovine testicular	2000 USP/5 mL	5 mL of own diluent	4 UI/0.01
Amphadase	Amphastar Pharmaceuticals, Inc. Rancho Cucamonga, CA	United States, Canada	Purified bovine testicular	150 USP/mL		
Vitrase	Alliance Medical Products, Inc., Irvine, CA	United States, Canada	Purified ovine testicular	200 USP/mL	1.2 mL already diluted	4 UI/0.025
Hylenex	Halozyme Therapeutics, Inc., San Diego, CA	United States, Canada	Recombinant human deoxyribonucleic acid (rDNA), hamster ovary cells	150 USP/mL	1 mL saline 0.9%	4 UI/0.025
Hylase, Dessau	Alliance Medical Products, Inc., Irvine, CA	United States, Canada and Europe	Purified bovine and ovine testicular	150 or 200 USP/mL	1 mL saline 0.9%	4 UI/0.025
Reductonidasa	Mesoestetic Pharma Group, Barcelona, Spain	Europe	Purified bovine testicular	150 UPS/mL	10 mL saline 0.9%	4 UI/0.025

lumps (0.1 and 0.2 mL) of five different HA products immediately and 1 month after injection. According to the study, Vitrase, Reductonidasa, Hylase, Hylenex, and Biometil were all effective at dissolving HA with doses varying from 4 to 28 IU immediately and a month after injected HA. Dosages up to 150 IU showed no compromise to the natural amount of HA of the skin (see Fig. 38.5), as Cavallini et al. reported that ovine hyaluronidase dosages below 14 IU did not affect fibroblast viability

The dilution will depend on the hyaluronidase used (Table 38.2) and a 30- to 32-gauge needle can be used to diminish discomfort. In a prospective, randomized study of intradermal hyaluronidase to reduce dermal augmentation from HA, Vartanian et al. recommended initial injections of 5 to 10 IU to minimize the risk of allergic reaction and to decrease the risk that high concentrations could dissolve native HA in the face, resulting in cosmetic deformity. Current doses in practice vary but range from 0.05 to 0.1 mL (7.5–28 IU) per injection. Slow injections are placed directly into the HA depot. Simple HA nodules generally respond within 24 to 48 hours. Nodules of unknown cause and cases of inflammation may require a greater length of time for complete resolution, although most patients experience some degree of improvement within a few days. For those with significant nodules, hyaluronidase can be combined with intralesional triamcinolone and fluorouracil. As injections tend to be painful, lidocaine can be added to lessen the discomfort. Follow-up at 2 weeks is recommended to assess the result.

Specialized Techniques

Low Unit Hyaluronidase for Filler Correction. Hyaluronidase can also be used in nonemergent scenarios for correction of suboptimal filler results and for adjustments of filler-related asymmetry. Alam et al. investigated the effect of low doses of hyaluronidase on the detectability of filler placed in the arms of patients. Doses of 1.5 to 9 IU were capable of reducing detectability of small depots of filler compared with saline control. This phenomenon can be utilized for correction of small anomalies after filler placement. Minor asymmetries, small nodules, and textural abnormalities can be corrected with small unit injections with serial follow-up and repeat injections as needed. This technique is particularly helpful for periocular filler complications.

Non-Filler-Related Applications. Hyaluronidase has been successfully used for the treatment of microstomia in systemic sclerosis. Melvin et al. reported that serial injections with 20 to 200 IU of hyaluronidase in the perioral area resulted in improvement in perioral wrinkling and improvement in decreased oral aperture. Similarly, Abbas et al. reported success with serial injection of hyaluronidase into sclerotic regions along the jawline of a patient with morphea with marked improvement after 4 injections at 2-week intervals with doses ranging from 15 to 150 IU. Given that patients with scleroderma have overproduction of hyaluronan and collagen types I, III, and VIII, introduction of hyaluronidase into the dermis of these patients can help facilitate extracellular matrix hydrolysis and lead to improvement in microstomia.

Side Effects and Precautions

Adverse effects to hyaluronidase are rare. Local injection site reactions are the most commonly reported reactions and are generally Type 1 immediate hypersensitivity reactions. The incidence of allergic reaction to hyaluronidase is approximately 1/2000, with most cases documented in the ophthalmology literature. Urticaria and edema have been reported to occur after retrobulbar or intravenous injection during ophthalmic surgery, although Andre and Fléchet reported a case of angioedema after ovine hyaluronidase into the upper lip, in which swelling began in the lips and progressed all over the upper face within 15 minutes. According to Balassiano and Bravo's retrospective study of 50 patients after use of hyaluronidase for immediate HA injection, 46% had some kind of reaction, such as erythema, edema, and burning. Vitrase showed the lowest percentage of edema and erythema at the injection site.

Preliminary skin testing is officially recommended prior to using all preparations, particularly those derived from animal sources. An injection of 0.02 mL (3 IU) of a 150 IU/mL solution is placed intradermally; a wheal appearing within 5 minutes and persisting for 20 to 30 minutes with localized itching indicates a positive reaction. However, allergic reaction may not be completely excluded by skin test. Delayed hypersensitivity reactions can occur, and the earlier mentioned skin test will not show positive within the 20- to 30-minute time frame.

Contraindications include hypersensitivity to any of the components, particularly in a patient with a history of allergic response to bovine collagen. Caution should also be used in patients with a history of allergic reaction to bee stings because hyaluronidase is one of the many biologically active components in bee venom. This is not clear cut, as the composition of bee venom has several antigenic compounds and there is no test that can identify this potential cross-reaction. Nevertheless, the incidence of hypersensitivity to hyaluronidase, as mentioned earlier, is rare and the provider should consider risks vs benefits when using hyaluronidase in a patient with bee venom sensitivity. Lastly, the use of hyaluronidase has the potential to spread infection, if present in a nodule or surrounding tissue. Should these be expected, a biopsy for tissue culture is prudent. Treatment should not be delayed while awaiting results, and thus, the use of antibiotics and/or antifungals can be used at onset to decrease the risk of spread.

As mentioned previously, in the presence of infection, hyaluronidase can spread infection and should be used only in conjunction with systemic antibiotics.

Sodium Thiosulfate

An emerging treatment for CaHA is STS. A calcium chelating agent, intravenous and intralesional STS can be used to treat calcinosis cutis and calciphylaxis. A proof-of-concept study by Robinson et al. assessed the efficacy of intralesional STS and topical metabisulfite (SMB) in porcine skin samples and found that intralesional STS was able to dissolve CaHA microspheres. Although monotherapy with topical SMB was also associated with CaHA dissolution, approximately 50% CaHA remained. Subsequent case reports have demonstrated successful STS treatment of CaHA nodules, although it is worth noting that a recent study found limited potential for STS to dissolve intraarterial CaHA. Available data suggest that intralesional STS is safe with low risk for adverse effects.

Collagenase

In February 2010, the FDA approval of collagenase *Clostridium histolyticum* (Xiaflex) for the treatment of patients with Dupuytren's contracture (a genetic disorder of pathologic collagen production) has led to some debate about the enzyme's ability to reverse the effect of collagen-based fillers. However, collagenase is associated with serious potential side effects, including tendon rupture and ligament damage, complex regional pain syndrome, sensory abnormality, injection site hemorrhage, and severe allergic reactions after subsequent treatment sessions, and has not been studied for collagen reversal in the face.

CONCLUSIONS

The use of soft tissue fillers, be they on- or off-label use for augmentation, continues to skyrocket in the world of aesthetics. As their implementation rises, so does the risk of adverse events. Having a solid understanding regarding the filler's composition, cross-linking, and dissolvability is paramount. And while prevention is key, hyaluronidase and collagenase may be used to reverse adverse effects of soft tissue fillers. The nonpermanent fillers tend to more forgiving when using reversing agents than those considered to be permanent and thus are recommended for high-risk areas of augmentation. Regardless of which filler is used, the best results are obtained when adverse events are treated quickly and often with a multifaceted approach. Preparing a plan for treatment of both early- and late-onset events will allow for a scientific, targeted approach to achieve the best outcome.

FURTHER READING

Abbas, L., Coias, J., Jacobe, H., & Nijhawan, R. (2012). Hyaluronidase injections for treatment of symptomatic pansclerotic morphea-induced microstomia. *JAAD Case Rep.*, *5*(10), 871–873. https://doi.org/10.1016/j.jdcr.2019.08.004.

Aguilera, S. B., Aristizabal, M., & Reed, A. (2016). Successful treatment of calcium hydroxylapatite nodules with intralesional 5-fluorouracil, dexamethasone, and triamcinolone. *J Drugs Dermatol.*, *15*(9), 1142–1143.

Alam, M., Hughart, R., & Geisler, A. (2018). Effectiveness of low doses of hyaluronidase to remove hyaluronic acid filler nodules: a randomized clinical trial. *JAMA Dermatol.*, *154*(7), 765–772. https://doi.org/10.1001/jamadermatol.2018.0515.

Andre, P., & Fléchet, M. L. (2008). Angioedema after ovine hyaluronidase injection for treating hyaluronic acid overcorrection. *J Cosmet Dermatol.*, *7*, 136–138. https://doi.org/10.1111/j.1473-2165.2008.00377.x.

Artzi, O., Cohen, J., Dover, J. S., Suwanchinda, A., Pavicic, T., Landau, M., Godman, G. J., Ghannam, S., Al Niaimi, F., van Loghem, J. A., Goldie, K., Sattler, S., Cassuto, D., Lim, T. S., Wanitphakdeedecha, R., Verner, I., Fischer, T. C., Bucay, V., Sprecher, E., & Shalmon, D. (2020). Delayed inflammatory reactions to hyaluronic acid fillers: A literature review and proposed treatment algorithm. *Clinical, Cosmetic and Investigational Dermatology*, *13*, 371–378. https://doi.org/10.2147/CCID.S247171.

Bailey, S. H., Fagien, S., & Rohrich, R. J. (2014). Changing role of hyaluronidase in plastic surgery. *Plast Reconstr Surg.*, *133*(2), 127e–132e. https://doi.org/10.1097/PRS.0b013e3182a4c282.

Balassiano, L., & Bravo, B. (2014). Hyaluronidase: a necessity for any dermatologist applying injectable hyaluronic acid. *Surg Cosmet Dermatol.*, *6*(4), 338–443.

Carruthers, J. D., Fagien, S., Rohrich, R. J., Weinkle, S., & Carruthers, A. (2014). Blindness caused by cosmetic filler injection. *Plast Reconstr Surg.*, *134*(6), 1197–1201. https://doi.org/10.1097/PRS.0000000000000754.

Cassabona, G., Marchese, P. B., Montes, J. R., & Hornfeldt, C. S. (2018). Durability, behavior, and tolerability of 5 hyaluronidase products. *Dermatol Surg.*, *44*(suppl 1), S42–S50. https://doi.org/10.1097/DSS.0000000000001562.

Cassuto, D., Marangoni, O., De Santis, G., & Christensen, L. (2009). Advanced laser techniques for filler-induced complications. *Dermatol Surg.*, *35*(suppl 2), S1689–S1695. https://doi.org/10.1111/j.1524-4725.2009.01348.x.

Cavallini, M., Antonioli, B., Gazzola, R., Tosca, M., Galuzzi, M., Rapisarda, V., Ciancio, F., & Marazzi, M. (2013). Hyaluronidases for treating complications by hyaluronic acid dermal fillers evaluation of the effects on cell cultures and human skin. *Eur J Plast Surg.*, *36*, 477–484. https://doi.org/10.1007/s00238-013-0855-y.

Chatrath, V., Banerjee, P. S., Goodman, G. J., & Raham, E. (2019). Soft-tissue filler-associated blindness: A systematic review of case reports and case series. *Plastic and Reconstructive Surgery. Global Open*, *7*(4), e2173. https://doi.org/10.1097/GOX.0000000000002173.

Chen, J., Ruan, J., Wang, W., Chen, A., Huang, Q., Yang, Y., & Li, J. (2021). Superselective arterial hyaluronidase thrombolysis is not an effective treatment for hyaluronic acid-induced retinal artery occlusion: Study in rabbit model. *Plastic and Reconstructive Surgery*, *147*(1), 69–75. https://doi.org/10.1097/PRS.0000000000007449.

Chestnut, C. (2018). Restoration of visual loss with retrobulbar hyaluronidase injection after hyaluronic acid filler. *Dermatol Surg.*, *44*(3), 435–437. https://doi.org/10.1097/DSS.0000000000001237.

Cohen, J., Biesman, B. S., Dayan, S. H., DeLorenzi, C., Lambros, V. S., Nestor, M. S., Sadick, N., & Sykes, J. (2015). Treatment of hyaluronic acid filler-induced impending necrosis with hyaluronidase: consensus recommendations. *Aesthet Surg J.*, *35*, 1–6. https://doi.org/10.1093/asj/sjv018.

Conejo-Mir, J. S., Sanz Guirado, S., & Angel Muñoz, M. (2006). Adverse granulomatous reaction to Artecoll treated by intralesional 5-fluorouracil and triamcinolone injections. *Dermatologic Surgery*, *32*, 1079–1081. https://doi.org/10.1111/j.1524-4725.2006.32117.x.

Delaere, L., Zeyen, T., Foets, B., Calste, J. V., & Stalmans, I. (2009). Allergic reaction to hyaluronidase after retrobulbar anesthesia: a case series and review. *Int Ophthalmol.*, *29*, 521–528. https://doi.org/10.1007/s10792-008-9258-7.

DeLorenzi, C. (2017). New High dose pulsed hyaluronidase protocol for hyaluronic acid filler vascular adverse events. *Aesthet Surg.*, *37*(7), 814–825. https://doi.org/10.1093/asj/sjw251.

Diwan, Z., Trikha, S., Etemad-Shahidi, S., Virmani, S., Denning, Ca., Al-Mukhtar, Y., Rennie, C., Penny, A., Jamali, Y., & Parrish, N. (2020). Case series and review on managing abscesses secondary to hyaluronic acid soft tissue filler with recommended management guidelines. *The Journal of Clinical and Aesthetic Dermatology*, *13*(11), 37–43. PMID: 33282102.

Fitzgerald, R., Bertucci, V., Sykes, J. M., & Duplechain, J. K. (2016). Adverse reactions to injectable fillers. *Facial Plast Surg.*, *32*(5), 532–555. https://doi.org/10.1055/s-0036-1592340.

Goodman, Gj., & Clague, M. D. (2016). A rethink on hyaluronidase injection, intraarterial injection and blindness: is there another option for treatment of retinal artery embolism caused by intraarterial injection of hyaluronic acid? *Dermatol Surg.*, *42*(4), 547–549. https://doi.org/10.1097/DSS.0000000000000670.

Goldan, O., Georgiou, I., Grabov-Nardini, G., Regev, E., Tessone, A., Liran, A., Haik, J., Mendes, D., Orenstein, A., & Winkler, E., et al. (2007). Early and late complications after a nonabsorbable hydrogel polymer injection: A series of 14 patients and novel management. *Dermatologic Surgery*, *33*(suppl 2), S199–S206. https://doi.org/10.1111/j.1524-4725.2007.33361.x.

Hurst, L. C., Badalamente, M. A., Hentz, V. R., Hotchkiss, R. N., Kaplan, F., Meals, R. A., Smith, T. M., & Rodzvilla, J. (2009). Injectable collagenase clostridium histolyticum for Dupuytren's contracture. *New England Journal of Medicine*, *361*, 968–979. https://doi.org/10.1056/NEJMoa0810866.

Hwang, C. J., Mustak, H., Gupta, A. A., et al. (2019). Role of retrobulbar hyaluronidase in filler-associated blindness: evaluation of fundus perfusion and electroretinogram readings in an animal model. *Ophthal Plast Reconstr Surg.*, *35*, 33–37. https://doi.org/10.1097/IOP.0000000000001132.

Hyunwook, J. (2020). Hyaluronidase: an overview of its properties, applications, and side effects. *Arch Plast Surg.*, *47*(4), 297–300. https://doi.org/10.5999/aps.2020.00752.

Ibrahim, O., Overman, J., Arndt, K., & Dover, J. (2018). Filler nodules: inflammatory or infectious? A review of biofilms and their implications on clinical practice. *Dermatol Surg.*, *44*(1), 53–60. https://doi.org/10.1097/DSS.0000000000001202.

Jones, D. (2018). Update on emergency and nonemergency use of hyaluronidase in aesthetic dermatology. *JAMA Dermatology, 154*(7), 763–764. https://doi.org/10.1001/jamadermatol.2018.0516.

Juhasz, M., Levin, M., & Marmur, E. (2017). The kinetics of reversible hyaluronic acid filler injection treated with hyaluronidase. *Dermatologic Surgery, 43*(6), 841–847. https://doi.org/10.1097/DSS.0000000000001084.

Keller, E. C., Kaminer, M. S., & Dover, J. D. (2014). Use of hyaluronidase in patients with bee allergy. *Dermatol Surg., 40*(10), 1145–1147. https://doi.org/10.1097/DSS.0000000000000123.

Kim, H. J., Kwon, S. B., Whang, K. U., Lee, J. S., Park, Y. L., & Lee, S. Y. (2018). The duration of hyaluronidase and optimal timing of hyaluronic acid (HA) filler reinjection after hyaluronidase injection. *Journal of Cosmetic and Laser Therapy, 20*(1), 52–57. https://doi.org/10.1080/14764172.2017.1293825.

Landau, M. (2015). Hylauronidase caveats in treating filler complications. *Dermatologic Surgery, 41*(suppl 1), S347–S353. https://doi.org/10.1097/DSS.0000000000000555.

Lee, W., Oh, W., Ko, H. S., et al. (2019). Effectiveness of retrobulbar hyaluronidase injection in an iatrogenic blindness rabbit model using hyaluronic acid filler injection. *Plast Reconstr Surg., 144*, 137–143. https://doi.org/10.1097/PRS.0000000000005716.

Lemperle, G., Rullan, P. P., & Gauthier-Hazan, N. (2006). Avoiding and treating dermal filler complications. *Plast Reconstr Surg., 118*(3 suppl), 92S–107S. https://doi.org/10.1097/01.prs.0000234672.69287.77.

Marković-Housley, Z., Miglierini, G., Soldatova, L., Rizkallah, P. J., Müller, U., & Schirmer, T. (2000). Crystal structure of hyaluronidase, a major allergen of bee venom. *Structure, 8*, 1025–1035. https://doi.org/10.1016/s0969-2126(00)00511-6.

Melvin, O. G., Hunt, K. M., & Jacobson, E. S. (2019). Hyaluronidase treatment of scleroderma-induced microstomia. *JAMA Dermatol., 155*(7), 857–859. https://doi.org/10.1001/jamadermatol.2019.0585.

Narins, R. S., Coleman, W. P., 3rd, & Glogau, R. G. (2009). Recommendations and treatment options for nodules and other filler complications. *Dermatologic Surgery, 35*(suppl 2), 1667–1671. https://doi.org/10.1111/j.1524-4725.2009.01335.x.

Nayfeh, T., Shah, S., Malandris, K., Amin, M., Abd-Rabu, R., Oeisa, M., Saadi, S., Rajjoub, R., Firwana, M., Prokop, L., & Murad, M. (2021). A systematic review supporting the American Society of Dermatologic Surgery guidelines on the prevention and treatment of adverse events of injectable fillers. *Dermatol Surg., 47*(2), 227–234. https://doi.org/10.1097/DSS.0000000000002911.

Paap, M. K., Milman, T., Ugradar, S., Goldberg, R., & Silkiss, R. Z. (2020). Examining the role of retrobulbar hyaluronidase in reversive filler induced blindness: a systematic review. *Ophthal Plast Reconstr Surg., 36*(3), 231–238. https://doi.org/10.1097/IOP.0000000000001568.

Reddy, K. K., Brauer, J. A., Anolik, R., Bernstein, L., Brightman, L. A., Hale, E., Karen, J., Weiss, E., & Geronemus, R. G. (2012). Calcium hydroxylapatite nodule resolution after fractional carbon dioxide laser therapy. *Arch Dermatol., 148*(5), 634–636. https://doi.org/10.1001/archdermatol.2011.3374.

Rivers, J., & Mistry, B. (2018). Soft-tissue infection caused by *Streptococcus anginosus* after intramucosal hyaluronidase injection: A rare complication related to dermal filler injection. *Dermatologic Surgery, 44*, S51–S53. https://doi.org/10.1097/DSS.0000000000001625.

Robinson, D. M. (2018). In vitro analysis of the degradation of calcium hydroxylapatite dermal filler: a proof-of-concept study. *Dermatol Surg., 44*, S5–S9. https://doi.org/10.1097/DSS.0000000000001683.

Rullan, P. P., Olson, R., & Lee, K. C. (2020). The use of intralesional sodium thiosulfate to dissolve facial nodules from calcium hydroxylapatite. *Dermatol Surg., 46*(10), 1366–1368. https://doi.org/10.1097/DSS.0000000000002238.

Ryu, C., Lu, J. E., & Zhang-Nunes, S. (2021). Response of twelve different hyaluronic acid gels to varying doses of recombinant human hyaluronidase. *Journal of Plastic, Reconstructive & Aesthetic Surgery, 74*(4), 881–889. https://doi.org/10.1016/j.bjps.2020.10.051.

Rzany, B., & DeLorenzi, C. (2015). Understanding, avoiding, and managing severe filler complications. *Plast Reconstr Surg., 136*(5), 196S–203S. https://doi.org/10.1097/PRS.0000000000001760.

Sadeghpour, M., Quatrano, N., Bonati, L. M., Arndt, K. A., Dover, J. S., & Kaminer, M. S. (2019). Delayed-onset nodules to differentially crosslinked hyaluronic acids: Comparative incidence and risk assessment. *Dermatologic Surgery, 45*(8), 1085–1094. https://doi.org/10.1097/DSS.0000000000001814.

Searle, T., Ali, F., & Al-Niaimi, F. (2020). Hyaluronidase in dermatology: Uses beyond hyaluronic acid fillers. *Journal of Drugs in Dermatology, 19*(10), 993–998. https://doi.org/10.36849/JDD.2020.5416.

Sorensen, E. P., & Council, M. L. (2020). Update in soft-tissue filler-associated blindness. *Dermatologic Surgery, 45*(5), 671–677. https://doi.org/10.1097/DSS.0000000000002108.

Starr, C. R., & Engleberg, N. C. (2006). Role of hyaluronidase in subcutaneous spread and growth of group A streptococcus. *Infection and Immunity, 74*, 40–48. https://doi.org/10.1128/IAI.74.1.40-48.2006.

Sundaram, H., & Fagien, S. (2015). Cohesive polydensified matrix hyaluronic acid for fine lines. *Plastic and Reconstructive Surgery, 136*(suppl 5), 149–163. https://doi.org/10.1097/PRS.0000000000001835.

Thanasarnaksorn, W., Cotofana, S., Rudolph, C., Kraisak, P., Chanasumon, N., & Suwanchinda, A. (2018). Severe vision loss caused by cosmetic filler augmentation: case series with review of cause and therapy. *J Cosmet Dermatol., 17*(5), 712–718. https://doi.org/10.1111/jocd.12705.

Vartanian, A. J., Frankel, A. S., & Rubin, M. G. (2005). Injected hyaluronidase reduces Restylane-mediated cutaneous augmentation. *Arch Facial Plast Surg., 7*, 231–237. https://doi.org/10.1001/archfaci.7.4.231.

Voigts, R., DeVore, D. P., & Grazer, J. M. (2010). Dispersion of calcium hydroxylapatite accumulations in the skin: Animal studies and clinical practices. *Dermatologic Surgery, 36*, 798–803. https://doi.org/10.1111/j.1524-4725.2010.01567.x.

Watt, A. J., Curtin, C. M., & Hentz, V. R. (2010). Collagenase injection as nonsurgical treatment of Dupuytren's disease: 8-year follow-up. *Journal of Hand Surgery, 35*, 534–539. https://doi.org/10.1016/j.jhsa.2010.01.003.

Weber, G., Buhren, B., Schrumpf, H., Wohlrab, J., & Gerber, P. (2019). Clinical applications of hyaluronidase. *Advances in Experimental Medicine and Biology, 1148*, 255–277. https://doi.org/10.1007/978-981-13-7709-9_12.

Wibowo, A., Kapoor, K. M., & Philipp-Dromston, W. G. (2019). Reversal of post-filler vision loss and skin ischaemia with high-dose pulsed hyaluronidase injections. *Aesthetic Plast Surg.*, 1337–1344. https://doi.org/10.1007/s00266-019-01421-6.

Woodward, J., Khan, T., & Martin, J. (2015). Facial filler complications. *Facial Plastic Surgery Clinics of North America, 23*, 447–458. https://doi.org/10.1016/j.fsc.2015.07.006.

Wu, L., Liu, X., Jian, X., Wu, X., Xu, N., Dou, X., & Yu, B. (2018). Delayed allergic hypersensitivity to hyaluronidase during the treatment of granulomatous hyaluronic acid reactions. *Journal of Cosmetic Dermatology, 17*(6), 991–995. https://doi.org/10.1111/jocd.12461.

Yang, B., Guo, X., Zang, H., & Liu, J. (2015). Determination of modification degree in BDDE-modified hyaluronic acid hydrogel by SEC/MS. *Carbohydrate Polymers, 131*, 233–239. https://doi.org/10.1016/j.carbpol.2015.05.050.

Yankova, M., Pavicic, T., Frank, K., Schenck, T., Beleznay, K., Gavril, D. L., Green, J. B., Voropai, D., Robinson, D. M., & Cotofana S. (2021). Intraarterial degradation of calcium hydroxylapatite using sodium thiosulfate—an in vitro and cadaveric study. *Aesthet Surg J. 41*(5):NP226-NP236. https://doi.org/10.1093/asj/sjaa350.

Zhang, L., Lai, L., Zhou, G., Liang, L., Zhou, Y., Bai, X., Dai, Q., Yu, Y., Tang, W., & Chen, M. (2020). Evaluation of intraarterial thrombolysis in treatment of cosmetic facial filler-related ophthalmic artery occlusion. *Plast Reconstr Surg., 145*(1), 42e–50e. https://doi.org/10.1097/PRS.0000000000006313.

Zhang, L., Zuyan, L., Jian, L., Liu, Z., Xu, H., Wu, M., & Wu, S. (2021). Endovascular hyaluronidase application through superselective angiography to rescue blindness caused by hyaluronic acid injection. *Aesthet Surg J., 41*(3), 344–355. https://doi.org/10.1093/asj/sjaa036.

Zhu, G. Z., Sun, Z. S., Liao, W. X., Cai, B., Chen, C., Zheng, L., & Lou, S. (2017). Efficacy of retrobulbar hyaluronidase injection for vision loss resulting from hyaluronic acid filler embolization. *Aesthet Surg J, 38*, 12–22. https://doi.org/10.1093/asj/sjw216.

39

Legal Considerations in Soft Tissue Fillers

Saleh Rachidi and David J. Goldberg

SUMMARY AND KEY POINTS

- The majority of fillers currently used are hyaluronic acid, Poly-L-lactic acid, or calcium hydroxyapatite-based.
- Adverse events range between immediate, early, and late onset events.
- An informed consent discusses the diagnosis, nature and purpose of intervention, risks and benefits, and alternatives.
- The standard of care is outlined based on the expert witness's personal practice, the practice of others observed in their experience, medical literature, statutes and legislative rules, and courses discussing such subjects.
- A cause of action in negligence and a successful claim require four elements: duty, breach of duty, causation, and damage.

INTRODUCTION

Dermal fillers are considered by the US Food and Drug Administration (FDA) as implantable medical devices. Absorbable fillers are approved for nasolabial folds (NLFs), perioral lines, lips, chin, and dorsal hands. Permanent fillers are approved for acne scars and NLFs. Some fillers such as poly-l-lactic acid and calcium hydroxyapatite are approved for human immunodeficiency virus (HIV)–associated lipoatrophy.

Soft tissue fillers are second to only neuromodulators among minimally invasive cosmetic procedures, and their use has increased more than 300% since 2000. Originally, soft tissue fillers were derived from bovine collagen, which were approved by the FDA in the early 1980s. However, hypersensitivity reactions halted their widespread use for a long time. Human collagen then emerged and increased in popularity as a semipermanent filler. Hyaluronic acid (HA) has limited immunogenicity and HA fillers came to address the need for fillers by providing an extracellular matrix polysaccharide instead of a protein to fill wrinkle lines and restore volume. HA also has a more hydrating capacity and longer duration than pure collagen. Two other classes of filler materials are also frequently used. These include poly-l-lactic acid (PLLA) and calcium hydroxyapatite (CaHA).

In this chapter, we discuss the most common types of fillers, complications of fillers, and managing these complications and outline the legal aspects relating to malpractice lawsuits.

COMMONLY USED FILLERS

Hyaluronic acid

HA is a temporary filler that lasts between 6 and 18 months, depending on the filler type and location of placement. HA is a glycosaminoglycan consisting of regular repeating nonsulfated disaccharide units of glucuronic acid and N-acetylglucosamine. HA is a naturally occurring component of the extracellular matrix, with no tissue or species specificity. It is highly hydrophilic, thus can attract water and create turgor, which can withstand compressive forces and provide supportive structure. Given its universal nature and lack of species specificity, HA has low immunogenicity. Different products vary by HA concentration, length and size of each polymer, degree of cross-linking, and presence of anesthetic. The concentration and degree of cross-linking impact the rheology of filler, and thus, its suitability in different anatomic locations.

Poly-l-Lactic Acid

PLLA is an absorbable filler that restores volume and stimulates collagen production. It is FDA approved for antiretroviral therapy–induced lipoatrophy in HIV patients, as well as the correction of NLFs and wrinkles. After the lyophilized powder is reconstituted, it is injected in the deep dermis and subcutaneous tissue and massaged for even distribution. Upon injection, PLLA particles induce an inflammatory response and stimulate collagen synthesis which lasts for 12 to 24 months.

Calcium Hydroxyapatite

CaHA is a biodegradable filler that consists of 30% synthetic CaHA microspheres suspended in a 70% aqueous carboxymethylcellulose gel carrier. In addition to the immediate volume-restoring effect, these microspheres activate fibroblasts and induce collagen production as early as 4 weeks and for 12 to 24 months.

ADVERSE EFFECTS AND COMPLICATIONS ASSOCIATED WITH FILLERS

Early Adverse Events

For the purpose of this discussion, early events are those occurring within the first 2 weeks of injection. Inadvertent superficial placement of filler can lead to lumps immediately postinjection. These resolve with massaging in the majority of times. Infections such as cellulitis or abscesses are uncommon and are typically caused by streptococcus or staphylococcus species. Fungal and viral infections are even less common.

Allergies to anesthesia mixed with the filler include type I hypersensitivity reactions (urticaria, angioedema, anaphylaxis) or type IV (delayed hypersensitivity). Allergy to lidocaine is rare and, in most instances, can be deciphered from history of prior procedures which the patient can recall.

Contact dermatitis to antiseptics manifests between 1 and 7 days after exposure. Chlorhexidine and povidone- iodine rarely cause allergic contact dermatitis, 0.5% for chlorhexidine and 0.4% for povidine-iodine.

Edema and bruising are expected side effects and can be exacerbated by more traumatic techniques. While this side effect resolves inconsequentially in the vast majority of cases, deposition of hemosiderin can lead to undesirable pigmentation. Patients taking over-the-counter supplements predisposing to bruising like vitamin E, fish oils, and garlic should stop them before such procedures. (Figs. 39.1 and 39.2 show swelling after filler injection.)

Inadvertent injection into an artery or external compression of an artery in areas with limited soft tissue expandability can lead to vascular occlusion and overlying skin necrosis (Fig. 39.3). More catastrophically, injection into an artery that communicates with the ophthalmic artery may result in retrograde embolization of the latter and subsequent blindness. Intravascular injections appear to be more frequent than previously assumed. An internet survey of 52 experienced injectors worldwide showed that 62% encountered at least one intravascular injection. Major danger zones for vascular compromise include the glabella, temple, infraorbital region, lips, NLF, and nose. The glabella is the most frequent injection site to result in vision loss due to injection in the supratrochlear and supraorbital arteries, which lie relatively superficial in that area and communicate with the ophthalmic artery.

Ischemic events manifest as skin blanching, dusky discoloration, and possible livedo reticularis, followed days later by skin necrosis, blistering, and sloughing. Particularly in the case of HA fillers, hyaluronidase is first-line treatment. Other treatments include topical nitropaste, aspirin, and warm compresses. Hyaluronidase should always be confirmed to be available, unexpired, and located in a known place in office as early recognition and intervention are key.

Late Adverse Events

Late complications occur beyond 2 weeks of filler placement. They include foreign body reactions (Figs. 39.4 and 39.5), which are a function of the size of filler particles, presence of impurities, and quality of preprocedure preparation to reduce the bacterial biofilm, or could be a result of low-grade infections. It is estimated that 0.01% to 0.1% of filler procedures are complicated by granulomas. Patients often present with subcutaneous nodules several weeks or months after filler injection.

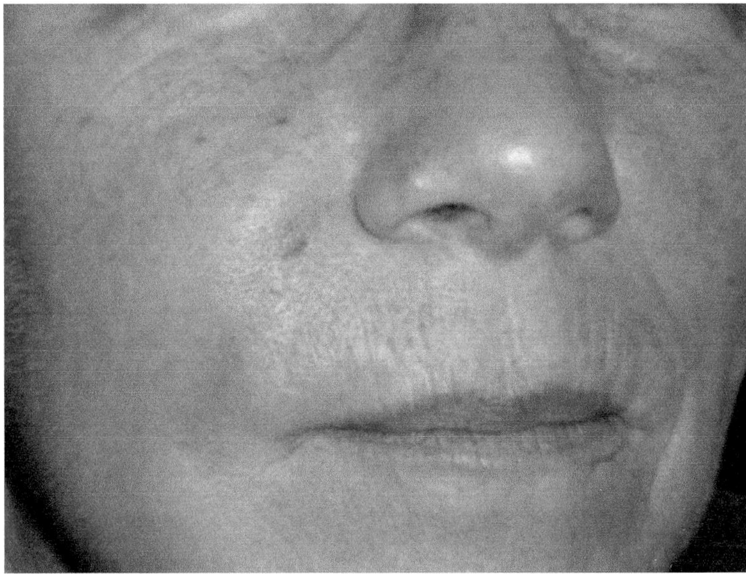

Figure 39.1 Swelling after injection of fillers.

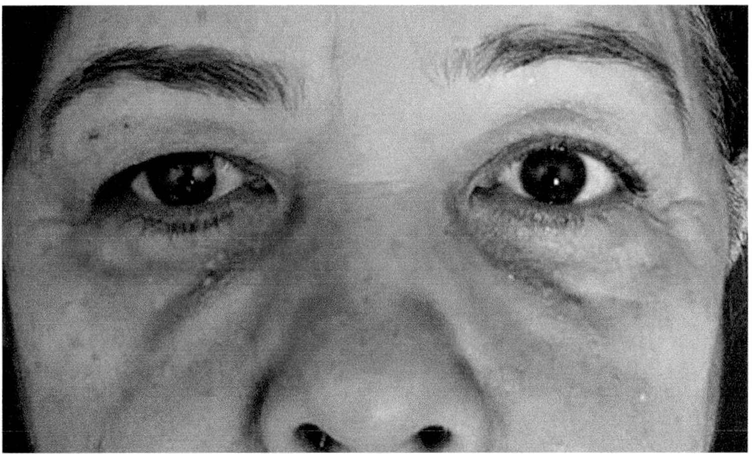

Figure 39.2 Infraorbital swelling after filler injection in the tear troughs.

Thorough disinfection and aseptic technique help avoid such complications.

A retrospective study compared the adverse effects of fillers injected by licensed and unlicensed practitioners between 2009 and 2019. The authors found that illegal fillers were used in 28 of 40 patients who experienced complications (70%), 18 of which were performed by unlicensed practitioners (64%). Adverse effects from illegal fillers lasted longer than legal fillers. Illegal fillers were more likely to cause foreign body reactions and infections.

TREATMENT OF SOFT TISSUE FILLER COMPLICATIONS

Bruising is a common adverse effect, more often seen with injection in the dermis and using fanning or threading techniques. The risk of bruising can be mitigated by slow injection and applying pressure as soon as it appears. Hemoglobin-selective lasers such as pulsed dye laser (PDL) can speed up its resolution. Use of topicals like arnica or vitamin K can help in some cases.

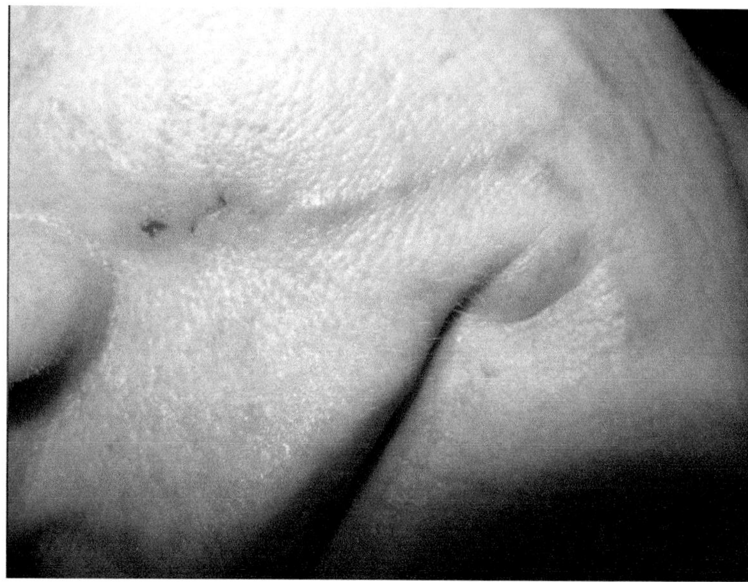

Figure 39.3 Vascular occlusion.

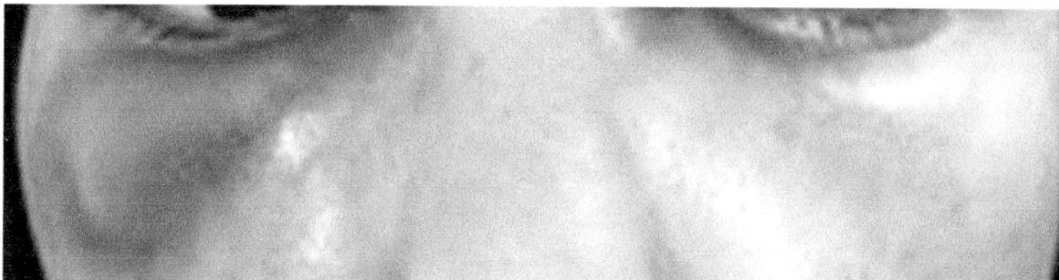

Figure 39.4 Hypersensitivity reaction.

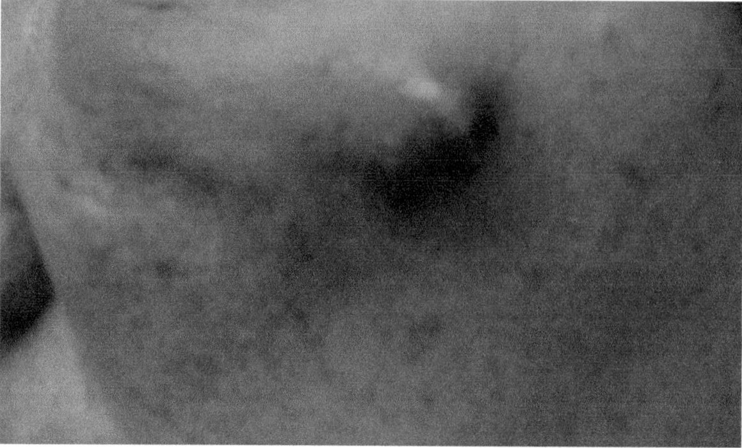

Figure 39.5 Biofilm-induced nodule.

Some swelling is normal after injection, especially in areas like the lips and periorbital regions. Cold compresses and nonsteroidal antiinflammatory drugs could prove effective. Prophylaxis for bacterial infection is not indicated and can be treated as soon as signs or symptoms appear. However, patients with frequent herpes outbreaks should be treated prophylactically with antivirals. Nerve damage during filler injections is exceedingly rare. It can result from direct trauma, injecting filler into the nerve, or nerve compression by the filler. The infraorbital nerve is the most common site. In cases of facial nerve branch injury, transient Bell's palsy or marginal mandibular nerve palsy could last for several weeks. High-dose oral steroids are used for Bell's palsy, as well as protective measures like artificial tears and occlusion. Early lumps or bumps are mostly due to excess or superficial filler placement. If erythema or pain is present, suggesting infection, oral antibiotics should be used. Inflammatory and reactive nodules are treated with antiinflammatories and steroids. Hyaluronidase is used for early HA nodules or even in late reactive nodules.

Early recognition and aggressive treatment of intravascular injections are critical to avoid irreversible complications. When vascular occlusion is suspected (blanching, pain, etc.), injection should be stopped immediately and treatment should be started, including hyaluronidase, massaging, warm compresses, and nitropaste to promote vasodilation. Hyaluronidase should be injected immediately regardless of the filler used, and then injected daily in liberal doses.

RISK MANAGEMENT

Risk management is of paramount importance in aesthetic medicine, particularly in light of the elective nature of procedures and the emphasis of patient satisfaction. Risk management involves appropriate screening of patients and obtaining a complete past medical history including recent infections and procedures. History of prior procedures is of paramount importance because it can provide insight into potential outcomes intrinsic to the procedure, allergies to anesthesia, vasovagal reactions, and postoperative care.

Infection could be due to introduction of bacteria at the time of injection or via systemic spread from another source of infection which can colonize the injected filler. Biofilms that are introduced at time of procedure colonize the product in vivo, are resistant to immune clearance, and incite a foreign body reaction. Filler placement is better avoided in patients with an ongoing urinary or respiratory tract infection, or those who underwent dental procedures or received vaccination in the preceding 2 weeks. Aseptic technique and cleaning with chlorhexidine or diluted bleach decrease the bacterial load of skin flora, thus mitigating the risk of biofilm formation. Cleaning the entire face, avoiding touching the needle, and injecting the lips and perioral regions last is also helpful. Intuitively, immunosuppressed patients are at increased risk of infection and should at least be monitored more carefully. History of autoimmune diseases can also predispose for granuloma formation and patients should be counseled about this risk before injection. Caution should be exercised in patients with prior reconstructive surgeries in the injected areas which can distort normal anatomy. This is particularly important in high-risk areas such as the nose which can lead to skin necrosis and blindness.

A retrospective cohort study of a random sample of 370 board-certified dermatologists showed that the risk of occlusion with any filler was less than 1:5000 syringes. Approximately 29% of dermatologists reported at least one event of vascular occlusion. Cannula injection had 77% lower odds of occlusion. NLFs and lips were most commonly occluded, but occlusions in the glabella were most serious.

Adequate training of the provider is critical in minimizing risks and maximizing benefits. Methodological training in facial dermal filler injection reduces adverse effects. The priority is that for that patient's primary cosmetic concern. Even if it is not the primary problem in the physician's eyes, addressing it is essential for patient's satisfaction. Proper documentation with preprocedure and postprocedure photographs can be very helpful in improving patient satisfaction and, in cases of litigation, in making a case for or against the defense. Providing brochures or other educational material can be helpful for the patient especially if available prior to the day of procedure.

In certain kinds of filler such as collagen, intradermal test spot in the arm is indicated weeks prior to placing the filler. A negative test does not completely exclude the risk of reactivity but indicates lower likelihood of hypersensitivity and provides basis for defense in the event of complications.

INFORMED CONSENT

Informed consent lays the ground for risks and benefits associated with any treatment. Discussing potential complications before a procedure preserves the physician-patient relationship in the event of a complication. The details of the procedure, type of filler, alternatives, and postprocedure course should be explained to the patient.

The informed consent should meet certain minimum standards (Fig. 39.6). A patient must be deemed competent by the provider, and must understand the facts, implications, and future consequences of the intervention. Given that esthetic procedures are not performed

PATIENT CONSENT FOR TREATMENT WITH FILLER AGENTS

The use of and indications for filler agents have been explained to me by my physician. I have had the opportunity to have all questions answered to my satisfaction. I have been specifically informed that the following may occur after the injections: Swelling, redness, pain, itching, discoloration, and tenderness at theimplant site. They typically resolve spontaneously within several days after injection into the skin. There are extremely rare, isolated reports of blindness resulting from filler injection in the forehead.. Other types of reactions are very rare, but rare patients may experience localized reactions thought to be of a hypersensitivity nature. These have usually consisted of swelling at the implant site, sometimes affecting the surrounding tissues. Redness, tenderness, and rarely acne-like formations have also been reported. These reactions have either started a few days after injection or after a delay of 2-4 weeks and have been described as mild to moderate. In most instances, such reactions are self- limiting.

I also understand that the duration of filler agent enhancement may depend on the chosen agent, injection site and my own personal skin. Touch-up and follow-up treatment helps sustain the desired degree of correction. My doctor has explained to me the unique characteristics of each filler agent. I also understand that some products are FDA approved for wrinkles. Others have FDA approval for other uses. For those. thetreatment of wrinkles is considered off-label use.

I agree that **PROVIDER NAME** and/or designated associates may take photographs and/or videotapes of me during and/or immediately after my procedure, as well as subsequent office visits. I understand that these photographs may be published in a variety of sources including all forms of social media. In such an event, I will not be identified by name. I expect no compensation for these photographs and/or videotapes and waive all rights to any claims for payments or royalties. I also release **PRACTICE NAME**, and its associated staff. from any liability in connection with the use of such photographs and/or videos.

The treatment, potential benefits and risks, and alternative treatment options have been explained to my satisfaction. I have read and understand all information presented to me before agreeing and authorizing treatment. I have had all my questions answered. I consent to the proposed treatment today as well as for future treatments if needed.

PATIENT NAME________________________________ DATE______________________

WITNESS____________________________________ DATE______________________

Figure 39.6 Informed consent sample.

on an urgent basis and the patient is voluntarily seeking treatment, the informed consent should also address the likelihood of achieving a certain cosmetic goal that is satisfying to the patient, in addition to discussing the risks. A patient might be seeking a procedure with a certain look or celebrity in mind that they would like to resemble. While the results might be stellar in the physician's expert opinion, it might not meet the expectations of the patient and thus be unsatisfactory. Early discussion of realistic expectations makes sure all parties are in agreement. The patient's motivation for a procedure and, in many cases, careful evaluation of potential psychiatric conditions that could influence their decision-making should be taken into account.

According to the American Medical Association (AMA), an informed consent requires the diagnosis, nature and purpose of an intervention, risks and benefits of intervention, alternatives and their risks and benefits, and risks and benefits of nonintervention. Versions of what constitutes an informed consent vary by state and are spelled out in statutes and laws.

Informed consent can be verbal or written. Written consent may not be required in some states, but careful documentation provides an invaluable defense, and a malpractice case can be lost if a plaintiff proves that informed consent was not obtained. In the period preceding a procedure, taking time to read a written consent form provides an opportunity for the patient to process the information and make a more informed decision. Initial evaluation includes accurately identifying the patient's chief cosmetic concern, which could differ from that perceived by the physician. It is also important to understand the patient's expectations in term of outcomes, timeline, and downtime. The informed consent therefore safeguards the physician and patient from miscommunication and assures that the patient is aware of available techniques, their advantages and disadvantages, and general risks.

MEDICAL PROFESSIONAL LIABILITY AGAINST DERMATOLOGISTS

Soft tissue filler injections have been on the rise, and so is litigation related to them. A study in 2014 that searched public legal documents using the national legal research service WestlawNext for filler-related legal actions between 1995 and 2013 identified 24 legal documents: 19 cases (13 of which physicians were named as defendants) and 5 disciplinary actions. Of the seven cases where a nonphysician was the defendant, six involved a substance injected different from the reported filler. Half of the legal actions were related to a nonphysician performing the procedure. Dermatologists and plastic surgeons had the highest proportion of litigation (17% each). The most common reason for litigation was granuloma formation, and Zyderm was the most encountered filler.

A review of the US FDA's Manufacturer and User Facility Device Experience (MAUDE) database for reported complications from 2013 to 2017 for injectable fillers identified 2813 adverse events. Most common complication sites were the cheeks (n = 915 [32.5%]), lips (n = 503 [17.9%]), and NLFs (n = 412 [14.6%]). Adverse events included swelling (n = 1691 [60.1%]), nodules (n = 948 [33.7%]), and pain (n = 636 [22.6%]). A significant association was observed between the forehead and dorsal nasal injections and intra-arterial complications resulting in necrosis and visual symptoms. Injection with Radiesse was also associated with necrosis and visual symptoms. Upon reviewing the Thomson Reuters Westlaw Edge database, 11 malpractice cases were analyzed. In 10 of the 11 cases, a lack of informed consent had been alleged, and the median award was $600,000.

Another cross-sectional study using the FDA's MAUDE database from 2014 to 2016 to identify complications and the Westlaw Next database to identify jury verdicts analyzed 1748 adverse events. Most cases stemmed from a cheek (n = 751 [43.0%]) or lip (n = 524 [30.0%]) injection. Swelling and infection were the most common events; blindness was associated with dorsal nasal injections, and vascular compromise was associated with Radiesse. Nine malpractice cases were identified, six of which involved allegations on inadequate informed consent, with a median award of $262,000.

A study of the Physician Insurers Association of America registry showed that 2,704 (1.1%) of 239,756 closed claims involved dermatologists, and 28.7% of them resulted in an average indemnity payment of around $137,538. Improper procedure performance, followed by error in diagnosis, was the most common allegation. In a study of 90,743 claims from the same database between 1991 and 2015, 1.2% were against dermatologists. A higher likelihood of legal action was observed against full-time practitioners and those in solo practice, compared to those in institutions and group practices. Of those claims against dermatologists, 67.8% were withdrawn, dismissed, or abandoned. Trial verdicts favoring defendants were 7 times those favoring plaintiffs between 2006 and 2015. The most common reason for claims was procedure-related errors (n = 305), of which 102 were paid. Dyschromia was the most associated adverse outcome.

Another study of 40,916 physicians and 233,738 physician-years of coverage found that dermatology was among the least specialties to be sued (ahead of pediatrics, psychiatry, and family medicine), and the mean indemnity payment ($117,832) was lowest for dermatology.

Dermatologists constitute 1.4% of physicians, and only 0.7% of claims are against dermatologists. Approximately 2% of truly negligent acts lead to malpractice claims, and 17% of all malpractice claims result from true negligence. A survey of Mohs surgeons revealed that lawsuits were due to wrong site (n = 6), functional outcome (n = 6), postprocedure outcome (n = 5), cosmetic outcome (n = 5), recurrent tumor (n = 5), improper consent (n = 3), delayed diagnosis (n = 2), misdiagnosis (n = 1), and other (n = 7).

A 2004 survey of dermatologists in 2004 found substantial variation in medical liability premiums across states. States without $250,000 caps for noneconomic damages had higher premiums. Spending more than 10% of time in cosmetic practice or more than 30% noncosmetic surgery was associated with higher premiums. The rate of premium growth was comparable to other specialties, although premiums were well below those in higher-risk specialties.

LEGAL CONSEQUENCES

A cause of action in negligence and a successful claim require four elements: duty, breach of duty, causation, and damage. A provider has a duty to perform a procedure according to the standard of care. The standard of care is delineated by an expert and what the jury believes. The provider should have the skills ordinarily possessed by a specialist in the field and should have used these skills in the care of a patient under similar circumstances. If the jury is convinced by the testimony of the expert testifying for the defendant, the standard of care is met. The dermatologist is expected to have acted in a reasonable manner by an objective standard, not necessarily in the best possible way. In many jurisdictions, an "error in judgment" leading to an unfavorable outcome by itself is not a violation of the standard of care if the dermatologist acted appropriately prior to exercising this professional judgment.

Evidence for the standard of care is derived from laws, regulations, medical guidelines, peer-reviewed publications, and textbooks. Although variation among states could exist, the standard of care is generally recognized as a national standard. It is the practice followed by the majority of physicians in a similar medical community and the expert should reflect this reality.

The standard of care is typically articulated by an expert witness whose basis is grounded in the following:

1. The witness' personal practice and/or
2. The practice of others observed in their experience; and/or
3. Medical literature; and/or
4. Statutes and/or legislative rules; and/or
5. Courses discussing the subject in a well-defined manner.

The standard of care is thus often an ephemeral concept resulting from differences among the medical profession, the legal system, and the public. While it can be clearly outlined in guidelines or publications, these guidelines are general recommendations, and the physician could (and often should) individualize care based on their best judgment.

Specialty societies such as the American Academy of Dermatology and the American Society for Dermatologic Surgery have invested substantial efforts to place standard guidelines for treating various conditions. These guidelines offer an authoritative statement, and a court has several options when such guidelines are offered as evidence. Practicing in accordance with the guidelines would shield a provider from liability to the same extent as establishing that they followed professional customs. However, if guidelines are not consistent with prevailing medical practice, using them as evidence of professional custom can be problematic. An accepted clinical standard may be presumptive evidence of due care but introducing the standard and establishing its sources and relevance by an expert are still required.

Guidelines often include disclaimers, which undercuts their defensive use in litigation. Per the AMA, guidelines should not be intended to replace physician discretion.

Each of the plaintiff and the physician usually use their own expert to define the standard of care. In addition to referring to clinical practice guidelines, a physician's negligence can be established through (1) admission of negligence by the defendant, (2) examination of the defendant's expert witness, (3) testimony by the plaintiff when they are a medical expert qualified to evaluate the physician's conduct, and (4) common knowledge where understanding the negligence by a lay person does not require the assistance of an expert.

FURTHER READING

Alam, M., Kakar, R., Dover, J. S., et al. (2021). Rates of vascular occlusion associated with using needles vs cannulas for filler injection. *JAMA Dermatology*, *157*, 174–180. https://doi.org/10.1001/jamadermatol.2020.5102.

American Society of Plastic Surgeons. (2017). *2017 Plastic Surgery Statistics Report*. https://www.plasticsurgery.org/documents/News/Statistics/2017/plastic-surgery-statistics-full-report-2017.pdf.

Andre, P., Lowe, N. J., Parc, A., Clerici, T. H., & Zimmermann, U. (2005). Adverse reactions to dermal fillers: A review of European experiences. *Journal of Cosmetic and Laser Therapy*, *7*, 171–176. https://doi.org/10.1080/14764170500344393.

Aremu, S. K., Alabi, B. S., & Segun-Busari, S. (2011). The role of informed consent in risks recall in otorhinolaryngology surgeries: Verbal (nonintervention) vs written (intervention) summaries of risks. *American Journal of Otolaryngology*, *32*(6), 485–4890. https://doi.org/10.1016/j.amjoto.2010.09.012.

Bass, L. S., Smith, S., Busso, M., & McClaren, M. (2010). Calcium hydroxylapatite (Radiesse) for treatment of nasolabial folds: Long-term safety and efficacy results. *Aesthetic Surgery Journal*, *30*, 235–238. https://doi.org/10.1177/1090820X10366549.

Beauvais, D., & Ferneini, E. M. (2020). Complications and litigation associated with injectable facial fillers: A cross-sectional study. *Journal of Oral Maxillofacial Surgery*, *78*, 133–140. https://doi.org/10.1016/j.joms.2019.08.003.

Beer, K., & Avelar, R. (2014). Relationship between delayed reactions to dermal fillers and biofilms: Facts and considerations. *Dermatologic Surgery*, *40*, 1175–1179. https://doi.org/10.1097/01.DSS.0000452646.76270.53.

Chayangsu, O., Wanitphakdeedecha, R., Pattanaprichakul, P., Hidajat, I. J., Evangelista, K. E. R., & Manuskiatti, W. (2020). Legal vs. illegal injectable fillers: The adverse effects comparison study. *Journal of Cosmetic Dermatology*, *19*, 1580–1586. https://doi.org/10.1111/jocd.13492.

Cohen, J. L., Biesman, B. S., Dayan, S. H., DeLorenzi, C., Lambros, V. S., Nestor, M. S., et al. (2015). Treatment of hyaluronic acid filler-induced impending necrosis with hyaluronidase: Consensus recommendations. *Aesthetic Surgery Journal*, *35*, 844–849. https://doi.org/10.1093/asj/sjv018.

De Boulle, K., & Heydenrych, I. (2015). Patient factors influencing dermal filler complications: Prevention, assessment, and treatment. *Clinical, Cosmetic and Investigational Dermatology*, *8*, 205–214. https://doi.org/10.2147/CCID.S80446.

De Oliveira Ruiz, R., Laruccia, M. M., & Gerenutti, M. (2014). Methodology for teaching facial filling with hyaluronic acid. *European Review for Medical and Pharmacological Sciences*, *18*, 3166–3173.

DeLorenzi, C. (2014). Complications of injectable fillers, part 2: Vascular complications. *Aesthetic Surgery Journal*, *34*, 584–600. https://doi.org/10.1177/1090820X14525035.

Engel, E., & Livingston, E. H. (2010). Solving the medical malpractice crisis: Use a clear and convincing evidence standard. *Archives of Surgery*, *145*, 296–300. https://doi.org/10.1001/archsurg.2009.294.

Ericksen, W. L., & Billick, S. B. (2012). Psychiatric issues in cosmetic plastic surgery. *The Psychiatrc Quarterly*, *83*, 343–352. https://doi.org/10.1007/s11126-012-9204-8.

Ezra, N., Peacock, E. A., Keele, B. J., & Kingsley, M. (2015). Litigation arising from the use of soft-tissue fillers in the United States. *Journal of the American Academy of Dermatology*, *73*, 702–704. https://doi.org/10.1016/j.jaad.2015.06.051.

Gladstone, H. B., & Cohen, J. L. (2007). Adverse effects when injecting facial fillers. *Seminars in Cutaneous Medicine and Surgery*, *26*, 34–39. https://doi.org/10.1016/j.sder.2006.12.008.

Glass, G. E., & Tzafetta, K. (2014). Optimising treatment of Bell's palsy in primary care: The need for early appropriate referral. *The British Journal of General Practice*, *64*, e807–e809. https://doi.org/10.3399/bjgp14X683041.

Jena, A. B., Seabury, S., Lakdawalla, D., & Chandra, A. (2011). Malpractice risk according to physician specialty. *The New England Journal of Medicine*, *365*, 629–636. https://doi.org/10.1056/NEJMsa1012370.

Kornmehl, H., Singh, S., Adler, B. L., Wolf, A. E., Bochner, D. A., & Armstrong, A. W. (2018). Characteristics of medical liability claims against dermatologists from 1991 through 2015. *JAMA Dermatology*, *154*, 160–166. https://doi.org/10.1001/jamadermatol.2017.3713.

Lachapelle, J. M. (2005). Allergic contact dermatitis from povidone-iodine: A re-evaluation study. *Contact Dermatitis*, *52*, 9–10. https://doi.org/10.1111/j.0105-1873.2005.00479.x.

Liippo, J., Kousa, P., & Lammintausta, K. (2011). The relevance of chlorhexidine contact allergy. *Contact Dermatitis*, *64*, 229–234. https://doi.org/10.1111/j.1600-0536.2010.01851.x.

Lim, K. S., & Kam, P. C. (2008). Chlorhexidine—pharmacology and clinical applications. *Anaesthesia and Intensive Care*, *36*, 502–512. https://doi.org/10.1177/0310057X0803600404.

Moshell, A. N., Parikh, P. D., & Oetgen, W. J. (2012). Characteristics of medical professional liability claims against dermatologists: Data from 2704 closed claims in a voluntary registry. *Journal of the American Academy of Dermatology*, *66*, 78–85. https://doi.org/10.1016/j.jaad.2010.12.003.

Perlis, C. S., Campbell, R. M., Perlis, R. H., Malik, M., & Dufresne, R. G., Jr. (2006). Incidence of and risk factors for medical malpractice lawsuits among Mohs surgeons. *Dermatologic Surgery*, *32*, 79–83. https://doi.org/10.1111/1524-4725.2006.32009.

Rayess, H. M., Svider, P. F., Hanba, C., Patel, V. S., DeJoseph, L. M., Carron, M., et al. (2018). A cross-sectional analysis of adverse events and litigation for injectable fillers. *JAMA Facial Plastic Surgery*, *20*, 207–214. https://doi.org/10.1001/jamafacial.2017.1888.

Resneck, J. S., Jr. (2006). Trends in malpractice premiums for dermatologists: Results of a national survey. *Archives of Dermatology*, *142*, 337–340. https://doi.org/10.1001/archderm.142.3.337.

Scheuer, J. F., 3rd, Sieber, D. A., Pezeshk, R. A., Gassman, A. A., Campbell, C. F., & Rohrich, R. J. (2017). Facial danger zones: Techniques to maximize safety during soft-tissue filler injections. *Plastic and Reconstructive Surgery*, *139*, 1103–1108. https://doi.org/10.1097/PRS.0000000000003309.

Signorini, M., Liew, S., Sundaram, H., et al. (2016). Global aesthetics consensus: Avoidance and management of complications from hyaluronic acid fillers—Evidence- and opinion-based review and consensus recommendations. *Plastic and Reconstructive Surgery*, *137*, 961e–971e. https://doi.org/10.1097/PRS.0000000000002184.

Wagner, R. D., Fakhro, A., Cox, J. A., & Izaddoost, S. A. (2016). Etiology, prevention, and management of infectious complications of dermal fillers. *Seminars in Plastic Surgery*, *30*, 83–86. https://doi.org/10.1055/s-0036-1580734.

INDEX

Note: Page numbers followed by *f* indicate figures, *t* indicate tables, and *b* indicate boxes.

C

G

M

N

T